The Neuropsychology of Emotion

SERIES IN AFFECTIVE SCIENCE

Series Editors
Richard J. Davidson
Paul Ekman
Klaus R. Scherer

THE NATURE OF EMOTION
Fundamental Questions
edited by Paul Ekman and Richard J. Davidson

BOO!
Culture, Experience, and the Startle Reflex
by Ronald Simons

EMOTIONS IN PSYCHOPATHOLOGY
Theory and Research
edited by William F. Flack, Jr., and James D. Laird

WHAT THE FACE REVEALS
Basic and Applied Studies of Spontaneous Expression
    Using the Facial Action Coding System (FACS)
edited by Paul Ekman and Erika Rosenberg

SHAME
Interpersonal Behavior, Psychopathology, and Culture
edited by Paul Gilbert and Bernice Andrews

AFFECTIVE NEUROSCIENCE
The Foundations of Human and Animal Emotions
by Jaak Panksepp

EXTREME FEAR, SHYNESS, AND SOCIAL PHOBIA
Origins, Biological Mechanisms, and Clinical Outcomes
edited by Louis A. Schmidt and Jay Schulkin

COGNITIVE NEUROSCIENCE OF EMOTION
edited by Richard D. Lane and Lynn Nadel

ANXIETY, DEPRESSION, AND EMOTION
edited by Richard J. Davidson

PERSONS, SITUATIONS, AND EMOTIONS
An Ecological Approach
edited by Hermann Brandstätter and Andrzej Eliasz

THE NEUROPSYCHOLOGY OF EMOTION
edited by Joan C. Borod

THE
NEUROPSYCHOLOGY
OF
EMOTION

Edited by

Joan C. Borod

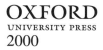
OXFORD
UNIVERSITY PRESS
2000

OXFORD

UNIVERSITY PRESS

Oxford   New York
Athens   Auckland   Bangkok   Bogotá   Buenos Aires   Calcutta
Cape Town   Chennai   Dar es Salaam   Delhi   Florence   Hong Kong   Istanbul
Karachi   Kuala Lumpur   Madrid   Melbourne   Mexico City   Mumbai
Nairobi   Paris   São Paulo   Singapore   Taipei   Tokyo   Toronto   Warsaw

and associated companies in
Berlin   Ibadan

Copyright © 2000 by Oxford University Press, Inc.

Published by Oxford University Press, Inc.,
198 Madison Avenue, New York, New York, 10016
http://www.oup-usa.org
1-800-334-4249

Library of Congress Cataloging-in-Publication Data
The neuropsychology of emotion / edited by Joan C. Borod.
p. ; cm.—(Series in affective science)
Includes bibliographical references.
ISBN 0-19-511464-7
1. Emotions—Physiological aspects.
2. Neuropsychology.
3. Affective disorders—Physiological aspects.
I. Borod, Joan C. II. Series.
[DNLM: 1. Emotions—physiology. 2. Affective Symptoms—psychology.
3. Brain—anatomy & histology. 4. Brain—physiology.
5. Brain—physiopathology. 6. Neuropsychology.
WL 103 N493575 2000]   RC455.4.E46 N48 2000   152.4—dc21   99-045300

9 8 7 6 5 4 3 2 1
Printed in the United States of America
on acid-free paper

To my husband, parents, and sisters

Preface

During the past few decades, the study of the neural mechanisms that underlie emotion has blossomed, even though speculations about such mechanisms date back several centuries. Currently, a wide range of neuroanatomical structures and neurophysiological systems has been implicated in the phenomenon of emotion. Furthermore, many theories have emerged from the neuropsychological literature and from basic emotion research to explain aspects of emotional processing. Evidence for these theories comes from animal and human studies, the latter involving healthy normal, neurological, and psychiatric populations. In addition to elucidating brain mechanisms underlying emotional processing, research pertaining to the neuropsychology of emotion has far-reaching implications for the assessment, diagnosis, treatment, and rehabilitation of individuals with deficits in emotional processing.

For many years, I had wanted to produce a book about the neuropsychology of emotion. The controversy surrounding lateralization for emotion was a motivating factor. Although much was known about laterality for cognitive functions, especially language, hemispheric asymmetries for emotional functioning were less clear-cut. During the 1980s and early 1990s, I organized several symposia on the topic at meetings of the International Neuropsychological Society, some of which led to special journal issues and sections. The first of these issues (Alpert, Borod, & Welkowitz, 1990) presented experimental studies and discussed theoretical implications for a range of neuropsychiatric disorders, focusing on two channels of emotional communication (face and voice). A second endeavor (Borod, 1993) concerned the processing mode component of emotion and included theoretical papers on five different modes: perception, expression, physiology, arousal, and experience. The third contribution (Borod & van Gelder, 1990) had a narrower perspective (i.e., facial asymmetry) and focused on patients with facial paralysis of both central and peripheral origin.

This book takes a more comprehensive approach to the field. It is unique in its organization, choice of topics, and focus on theoretical, experimental, and clinical issues. The book is divided into five sections: (1) Introduction, (2) Background and General Techniques, (3) Theoretical Perspectives, (4) Emotional Disorders, and (5) Clinical Implications. Part I is an introduction that provides a brief summary of each chapter and general information about neuropsychological parameters of emotion, thus embedding the work in a larger theoretical context. This introductory chapter concludes with suggestions for future research and clinical work in the field.

Part II of the book provides historical, evolutionary, and philosophical perspectives on the neuropsychological study of emotion and information about various approaches and techniques to study emotion (i.e., neuroanatomical, neurophysiological, neuroimaging, and neuropsychological assessment). Moving from the pragmatic or technical to the more theoretical, Part III presents contemporary theories about emotion, including overviews of those from the basic psychological and neuropsychological literature. In addition, two specific theories are provided, one from a social-cognitive-neuroscientific perspective and the other from a neurobiological systems perspective. Included in this section are discussions about the relationship between emotion and cognitive functions (e.g., memory).

The next two sections have a more clinical focus. Part IV features a number of discrete emotional response systems and emotional disorders, including elation and mania, sadness and depression, anxiety and stress, anger and impulsivity, and flat affect and apathy. Each chapter reviews the neuropsychological literature pertinent to these discrete systems, drawing on literature from neurological, psychiatric, and life-span disorders. These chapters include theoretical discussions about how knowledge of the anatomical and physiological mechanisms underlying these disorders can inform our understanding of the brain mechanisms underlying emotion.

Part V focuses directly on clinical implications. In contrast to the previous sections, this one addresses specific illnesses (i.e., a range of neurological diseases, depression, and schizophrenia). Here are discussed the emotional deficits accompanying these illnesses and specific treatments for these deficits (e.g., psychotherapy, rehabilitation, psychopharmacology, and psychosurgery). The information in this section should prove useful to a range of health care professionals dealing with patient populations suffering from emotional disorders and affective processing deficits.

This volume contains contributions from some of the most accomplished and innovative researchers in the field. They were all asked to synthesize the major work in their area and to provide an overview of the newer studies. In addition, they were asked to discuss research problems and point out avenues for future research. The central theme of all the chapters is the question of which neural mechanisms underlie emotion.

The main aim of this endeavor is to provide a basic textbook and reference work on emotion for the field of neuropsychology. The volume is designed for emotion researchers, their students and trainees, and clinicians working with neurological, psychiatric, and geriatric populations. Besides neuropsychologists, this volume should be useful to colleagues and students in a wide range of related fields, including clinical and experimental psychology, cognitive neuroscience, speech and hearing sciences, behavioral neurology, biological psychiatry, neuropsychiatry, gerontology, and rehabilitation medicine.

ACKNOWLEDGMENTS

I am most grateful to Jeffrey House, Vice President at Oxford University Press, for his invitation to write this book, for his creative and imaginative inspiration in designing the contents of this book, and for his whole-hearted support and excellent advice along the way. I am also grateful to Fiona Stevens at Oxford for her wise guidance and encouragement at the end of this journey.

Second, I want to thank the contributors for their outstanding chapters, their cheerful enthusiasm (a positive emotion!), and their hard work during the peer review phase. All chapters were anonymously reviewed by two or three contributors, and each chapter was revised in response to the critiques.

Third, I want to thank Scott Sparks for all his support, hard work on this volume, sense of aesthetics, and humor over the years. Nancy Wolitzer's input, assistance, and patience as production editor were invaluable and greatly appreciated.

Fourth, I would like to thank a number of individuals for their support during this project: Elissa Koff, Richie Davidson, and Sarah Raskin in the initial stages of this work; Wendy Heller and Esther Strauss during the middle phase; and Jack Nitschke and Nancy Madigan at the very end. Also, I am grateful to the students in my research laboratory at Queens College and Mount Sinai Medical Center, who have listened to tales about this book over the past few years. A special thanks goes to Matthias Tabert, one of my graduate students, and to Ronald Bloom, my friend and colleague, for all their help, advice, and moral support throughout and for their respective wisdom about emotion research and clinical work in this area.

x

Fifth, I am grateful to my mentors and colleagues who taught me so much about neuropsychological research and assessment at the Aphasia Research Center of the Boston V.A. Hospital: Harold Goodglass, Edith Kaplan, and Nelson Butters. I am especially grateful to Herbert Caron, who kindled my interest in facial expression and brain mechanisms in my earlier years at the Cleveland V.A. Hospital. Justine Sergeant's support of my emotion work over the years has also been greatly appreciated and is now deeply missed.

Finally, I want to thank my family and friends who have waited patiently for me to finish this book so that "life as usual" could resume. In this vein, special acknowledgements go to my dear husband, Paul Kolodner, and my mom, Sylvia Wise, without whose love, support, and encouragement this work would not have been possible.

REFERENCES

Alpert, M., Borod, J., & Welkowitz, J. (Eds.) (1990). Faces, voices, and feelings: Experimental techniques and clinical implications [Special Issue]. *Journal of Communication Disorders, 23(4,5)*.

Borod, J. (Ed.) (1993). Neuropsychological perspectives on components of emotion [Special Section]. *Neuropsychology, 7*, 4.

Borod, J., & van Gelder, R. (Eds.) (1990). Facial asymmetry: Expression and paralysis [Special Issue]. *International Journal of Psychology, 25*, 2.

J.C.B.

September 1999
Flushing, New York

Contents

Contributors, xv

Part I Introduction

1. Neuropsychology of Emotion and Emotional Disorders: An Overview and Research Directions, 3
   Joan C. Borod and Nancy K. Madigan

Part II Background and General Techniques

2. The Epistemology of Reason and Affect, 31
   Ross W. Buck

3. Anatomy and Physiology of Human Emotion: Vertical Integration of Brainstem, Limbic, and Cortical Systems, 56
   Don M. Tucker, Douglas Derryberry, and Phan Luu

4. Neuropsychological Assessment of Emotional Processing in Brain-Damaged Patients, 80
   Joan C. Borod, Matthias H. Tabert, Cornelia Santschi, and Esther H. Strauss

5. Neuroimaging Approaches to the Study of Emotion, 106
   Mark S. George, Terrence A. Ketter, Tim A. Kimbrell, Andrew M. Speer,
   Jeff Lorberbaum, Christopher C. Liberatos, Ziad Nahas, and
   Robert M. Post

Part III Theoretical Perspectives

6. Psychological Models of Emotion, 137
   Klaus R. Scherer

7. A Social Cognitive Neuroscience Approach to Emotion and Memory, 163
   Kevin N. Ochsner and Daniel L. Schacter

8. Neurobiology of Emotion at a Systems Level, 194
   Ralph Adolphs and Antonio R. Damasio

9. Neuropsychological Theories of Emotion, 214
   Guido Gainotti

Part IV Emotional Disorders

10. Elation, Mania, and Mood Disorders: Evidence from
    Neurological Disease, 239
    Robert G. Robinson and Facundo Manes

11. Regional Brain Function in Sadness and Depression, 269
    Richard J. Davidson and Jeffrey Henriques

12. Anxiety, Stress, and Cortical Brain Function, 298
    Jack B. Nitschke, Wendy Heller, and Gregory A. Miller

13. Violence Associated with Anger and Impulsivity, 320
    Angela Scarpa and Adrian Raine

14. Differentiation of States and Causes of Apathy, 340
    Donald T. Stuss, Robert van Reekum, and Kelly J. Murphy

Part V Clinical Implications

15. Neurological Disorders and Emotional Dysfunction, 367
    Kenneth M. Heilman, Lee X. Blonder, Dawn Bowers, and
    Gregory P. Crucian

16. Rehabilitation of Emotional Deficits in Neurological Populations:
A Multidisciplinary Perspective, 413
Sarah A. Raskin, Ronald L. Bloom, and Joan C. Borod

17. Emotional Processing in Schizophrenia: A Focus on Affective States, 432
Christian G. Kohler, Ruben C. Gur, and Raquel E. Gur

18. Therapeutic Brain Interventions in Mood Disorders and
the Nature of Emotion, 456
Sarah H. Lisanby and Harold A. Sackeim

Index, 493

Contributors

RALPH ADOLPHS, PH.D.
Department of Neurology
University of Iowa College of Medicine
Iowa City, Iowa

LEE X. BLONDER, PH.D.
Department of Behavioral Science
University of Kentucky College
  of Medicine
Lexington, Kentucky

RONALD L. BLOOM, PH.D.
Department of Speech-Language-Hearing
  Sciences
Hofstra University
Hempstead, New York

JOAN C. BOROD, PH.D.
Department of Psychology
Queens College and The Graduate Center
The City University of New York
Flushing, New York
and
Department of Neurology
Mount Sinai School of Medicine
New York, New York

DAWN BOWERS, PH.D.
Department of Clinical and Health
  Psychology
University of Florida
Gainesville, Florida

ROSS W. BUCK, PH.D.
Departments of Communication Sciences
  and Psychology
University of Connecticut
Storrs, Connecticut

GREGORY P. CRUCIAN, PH.D.
Department of Neurology
University of Florida
  College of Medicine
Gainesville, Florida

ANTONIO R. DAMASIO, M.D.
Department of Neurology
University of Iowa College of Medicine
Iowa City, Iowa

RICHARD J. DAVIDSON, PH.D.
Department of Psychology
University of Wisconsin
Madison, Wisconsin

DOUGLAS DERRYBERRY, PH.D.
Department of Psychology
Oregon State University
Corvallis, Oregon

GUIDO GAINOTTI, M.D.
Institute of Neurology
Catholic University of Rome
Rome, Italy

MARK S. GEORGE, M.D.
Departments of Psychiatry, Radiology,
  and Neurology
Medical University of South Carolina, and
Psychiatric Neuroimaging
Ralph H. Johnson V.A. Medical Center
Charleston, South Carolina

RAQUEL E. GUR, M.D., PH.D.
Department of Psychiatry
University of Pennsylvania
Philadelphia, Pennsylvania

RUBEN C. GUR, PH.D.
Department of Psychiatry
University of Pennsylvania
Philadelphia, Pennsylvania

KENNETH M. HEILMAN, M.D.
Department of Neurology
University of Florida College of Medicine
Gainesville, Florida

WENDY HELLER, PH.D.
Department of Psychology and Beckman
  Institute for Advanced Science and
  Technology
University of Illinois at Urbana-
  Champaign
Champaign, Illinois

JEFFREY HENRIQUES, PH.D.
Department of Psychology
University of Wisconsin
Madison, Wisconsin

TERRENCE A. KETTER, M.D.
Department of Psychiatry
Stanford University
Palo Alto, California

TIM A. KIMBRELL, M.D.
Biological Psychiatry Branch
National Institute of Mental Health
Bethesda, Maryland

CHRISTIAN G. KOHLER, M.D.
Department of Psychiatry
University of Pennsylvania
Philadelphia, Pennsylvania

CHRISTOPHER C. LIBERATOS, B.S.
Departments of Psychiatry, Radiology,
  and Neurology
Medical University of South Carolina
Charleston, South Carolina

SARAH H. LISANBY, M.D.
Department of Biological Psychiatry
New York State Psychiatric Institute
and
Department of Psychiatry
Columbia University College of
  Physicians and Surgeons
New York, New York

JEFF LORBERBAUM, M.D.
Departments of Psychiatry, Radiology,
  and Neurology
Medical University of South Carolina
Charleston, South Carolina

PHAN LUU, PH.D.
Department of Psychology
University of Oregon
and
Electrical Geodesics, Inc.
Eugene, Oregon

NANCY K. MADIGAN, PH.D.
Department of Psychiatry
Massachusetts Mental Health Center
Boston, Massachusetts

FACUNDO MANES, M.D.
Department of Psychiatry
University of Iowa College of Medicine
Iowa City, Iowa

GREGORY A. MILLER, PH.D.
Departments of Psychology and
Psychiatry and Beckman Institute for
Advanced Science and Technology
University of Illinois at Urbana-Champaign
Champaign, Illinois

KELLY J. MURPHY, PH.D.
Rotman Research Institute
Baycrest Centre for Geriatric Care
University of Toronto
Toronto, Ontario
Canada

ZIAD NAHAS, M.D.
Departments of Psychiatry, Radiology,
and Neurology
Medical University of South Carolina
Charleston, South Carolina

JACK B. NITSCHKE, PH.D.
Department of Psychology
University of Wisconsin
Madison, Wisconsin

KEVIN N. OCHSNER, PH.D.
Department of Psychology
Harvard University
Cambridge, Massachusetts

ROBERT M. POST, M.D.
Biological Psychiatry Branch
National Institute of Mental Health
Bethesda, Maryland

ADRIAN RAINE, D.PHIL.
Department of Psychology
University of Southern California
Los Angeles, California

SARAH A. RASKIN, PH.D.
Departments of Psychology and
Neuroscience
Trinity College
Hartford, Connecticut

ROBERT G. ROBINSON, M.D.
Department of Psychiatry
University of Iowa College of Medicine
Iowa City, Iowa

HAROLD A. SACKEIM, PH.D.
Department of Biological Psychiatry
New York State Psychiatric Institute
and
Department of Psychiatry
Columbia University College of
Physicians and Surgeons
New York, New York

CORNELIA SANTSCHI, PH.D.
Institute of Neurology and
Neurosurgery
Saint Barnabas Medical Center
West Orange, New Jersey
and
Department of Neurology
New York University School of
Medicine
New York, New York

ANGELA SCARPA, PH.D.
Department of Psychology
Virginia Polytechnic Institute and
State University
Blacksburg, Virginia

DANIEL L. SCHACTER, PH.D.
Department of Psychology
Harvard University
Cambridge, Massachusetts

KLAUS R. SCHERER, PH.D.
Department of Psychology
University of Geneva
Geneva, Switzerland

ANDREW M. SPEER, M.D.
Biological Psychiatry Branch
National Institute of Mental Health
Bethesda, Maryland

ESTHER H. STRAUSS, PH.D.
Department of Psychology
University of Victoria
Victoria, British Columbia
Canada

DONALD T. STUSS, PH.D.
Rotman Research Institute
Baycrest Centre for Geriatric Care
and
Departments of Psychology and Medicine
   (Neurology and Rehabilitation
   Science)
University of Toronto
Toronto, Ontario
Canada

MATTHIAS H. TABERT
Department of Psychology
Queens College and The Graduate Center
The City University of New York
Flushing, New York
and
Department of Neurology
Mount Sinai Medical Center
New York, New York

DON M. TUCKER, PH.D.
Department of Psychology
University of Oregon
and
Electrical Geodesics, Inc.
Eugene, Oregon

ROBERT VAN REEKUM, M.D.,
F.R.C.P.C.
Kunin-Lunenfeld Applied Research
   Unit and Department of Psychiatry
Baycrest Centre for Geriatric Care
and
Department of Psychiatry
University of Toronto
Toronto, Ontario
Canada

The Neuropsychology of Emotion

INTRODUCTION

1

Neuropsychology of Emotion and Emotional Disorders: An Overview and Research Directions

JOAN C. BOROD AND NANCY K. MADIGAN

In the past 25 years, the study of neural mechanisms involved in emotional processing has flourished, although findings in this area emanate from the end of the nineteenth century. By *emotion*, we refer to reactions to an appropriately evocative stimulus involving cognitive appraisal (or perception), expressive motoric behavior, subjective experience (or feelings), physiological arousal, and goal-directed behavior (Plutchik, 1984). Researchers have identified numerous neuroanatomical structures and neurophysiological systems that modulate emotion at cortical, subcortical, and limbic levels of the nervous system. From a neuropsychological perspective, a range of theories has been proposed to account for cerebral hemispheric specialization of emotion (e.g., right hemisphere, valence, and motoric-direction hypotheses) and for componential and modular processing. Evidence for these various theories stems from both clinical observation and experimental studies, involving normal, neurological, and psychiatric populations. Experimental studies have employed a variety of methodologies, including behavioral paradigms, the natural lesion method, neurosurgical procedures, electrophysiological techniques, and hemodynamic neuroimaging. In addition to delineating brain mechanisms involved in aspects of emotional processing, this growing body of research has wide-ranging clinical implications for the assessment, diagnosis, treatment, and rehabilitation of neuropsychiatric populations suffering from deficits in emotional processing.

Several critical parameters or factors must be considered in neuropsychological studies of emotional processing (see Borod, 1992, 1996; Heilman & Satz, 1983). Two factors are related to brain organization, one being the interhemispheric or laterality factor (right vs. left cerebral hemisphere) and the other being the intrahemispheric factor, which refers to two different levels of brain organization—caudality (anterior vs. posterior brain structures) and verticality (neocortical vs. limbic/subcortical diencephalic regions). The third factor underscores the importance of the emotional components themselves by distinguishing modes of processing that refer to emotional perception (or comprehension), expression, physiological arousal, experience, and goal-directed activity (Plutchik, 1984). Investigators working with neuropsychiatric and normal populations have studied whether these modes are functionally independent or dependent on one another (Borod, 1993b; Bowers et al., 1993; Gainotti et al., 1993; Semenza et al., 1986). The fourth factor is communication channel or the way in which an emotion is processed. In humans, such modalities typically include the facial, prosodic/intonational, lexical/verbal, gestural, and postural channels. Finally, the fifth factor has been the focus of extensive theoretical debate among emotion theorists (e.g., Ekman & Davidson, 1994; Izard, 1992; Ortony & Turner, 1990; Panksepp, 1992) and refers to the examination of basic, discrete emotions (e.g., happiness, anger, and sadness; Izard, 1977) versus dimensional levels of emotion, such as emotional valence (pleasantness/unpleasantness) and motoric direction (approach/withdrawal).

This volume on the neuropsychology of emotion contains sections on background and general techniques, theoretical perspectives, emotional disorders, and clinical implications. The current chapter provides an introduction (Part I) that summarizes each of the chapters in the volume. In addition, directions for future work in this area are suggested, and research considerations are raised.

BACKGROUND AND GENERAL TECHNIQUES

Part II provides background information about the neuropsychological study of emotion (Chapters 2 and 3) and information about various approaches to the study of emotion—neuroanatomical, neurophysiological, neuroimaging, and neuropsychological assessment (Chapters 3–5).

The background information is provided in two chapters elegantly written by Buck and by Tucker, Derryberry, and Luu. Buck (Chapter 2) provides an epistemological perspective on the evolution of the conceptualization of emotion and cognition, based on both the philosophical tradition developed over several centuries and the more recent contributions from neurobiological research. He thus summarizes the development of relevant philosophical concepts—from mind–body dualism, to rationalism and empiricism, to pragmatism, to positivism. Moreover, Buck reviews the importance and proper use of language in defining such experiential concepts to describe the mind–brain relationship and how an understanding of the neural substrates involved, formalized by LeDoux's research on fear conditioning (1996), can alter such concepts. He provides definitions for motivation, emotion, affect, and cognition derived from a historical perspective and further suggests that these are not distinct but, in fact, interactive phenomena. For cognition, which is equated with knowledge, he delineates the difference between "knowledge-by-acquaintance" and "knowledge-by-description." The former, also termed affective cognition, is self-evident and based on raw perceptual input from physical, social, and internal body environments, whereas the latter, termed rational cognition, is representational in nature and reconstructed from raw perceptual data. A third level of knowledge is one of language competence, termed understanding. Finally, he proposes that these levels of knowledge may be associated with specific neural systems in the brain and that, ultimately, an understanding of emotion may lead to a better understanding of consciousness itself.

Tucker, Derryberry, and Luu (Chapter 3), arguing from a developmental–evolutionary perspective, describe the basic neuroanatomy and neurophysiology of human emotion. The authors describe the subcortical circuits and cortical systems involved in emotion regulation. They maintain that "these combined descending and ascending influences suggest that emotional states facilitate a vertical integration of processing systems across the brain stem, limbic system, and cortex" (p. 64). Throughout the chapter, the classic principles of "hierarchic integration through inhibitory control" (Jackson, 1879) and encephalization are utilized. One of the creative contributions of this chapter is an attempt to delineate the emotional and motivational functions of the dorsal (the spatial or "where" pathway) and ventral (the object or "what" pathway) corticolimbic networks.

The next two chapters in Part II provide some basic information about the techniques used to study emotion: neuropsychological assessment (Chapter 4) and neuroimaging (Chapter 5). Although many experimental paradigms have been used to examine emotional processing, some of the more common are laterality techniques (e.g., dichotic listening, tachistoscopic viewing, and facial asymmetry), the brain lesion method (i.e., studies of individuals with known brain damage), and electrophysiological and functional brain imaging techniques. Studies of patients with unilateral brain lesions and normal adult subjects have provided most of our knowledge base regarding brain–behavior relationships for components of emotional processing in humans. For laterality studies in normal individuals, given the typical contralateral innervation of the central nervous system, superiority of one side of the body (e.g., left ear, left visual field, or left hemiface) implies greater involvement of the contralateral cerebral hemisphere (for reviews, see Borod et al., 1997, 1998a,b; Bruder, 1991; Bryden, 1982; Ley & Strauss, 1986). Studies with brain-damaged patients, in contrast, examine level of performance on tasks involving emotional processing (for reviews, see Borod, 1993b; Heilman et al., Chapter 15, this volume; Ross, 1997; Starkstein & Robinson, 1988). Impaired performance is interpreted as implying that the brain regions damaged are important for the type of processing involved in that particular task. Although these methods have identified functional and anatomical substrates in emotional processing, electrophysiological and functional neuroimaging techniques (for reviews, see Davidson et al., 1999; Heller & Nitschke, 1998) have provided a way to investigate emotional processing "on line" and in real time, thus affording a complementary picture of brain–behavior relationships.

Borod, Tabert, Santschi, and Strauss begin Chapter 4 with a comprehensive review of the literature regarding the neuropsychological assessment of emotional processing in brain-damaged populations. This chapter offers a unique resource, as there is a dearth of information about the assessment of emotion in standard neuropsychological texts and compendia. The chapter is conceptualized via a componential approach (Borod, 1993a), which has as its basic premise that emotion consists of a number of "components" that utilize different brain systems (Cripe, 1997). In their review, the authors selected batteries of emotional measures examining more than one element within a component—a processing mode (i.e., perception, expression, experience, arousal, or behavior) and/or a communication channel (i.e., facial, prosodic, lexical, gestural, postural, or scenic [an environmental/or situational array]). Related studies that include measures of emotion were integrated into this review. Discussion of the 17 sets of batteries and studies includes a brief description of each task; the targeted populations; psychometric properties and normative data, where available; and general research findings. The next part of Chapter 4 contains a summary of information about eliciting and evaluating emotional expression in neurological populations. With respect to evaluation, one approach focuses on external expression and the other on internal states and dispositions. The authors included this summary about expression due to the complexity of such evaluation and to provide a resource for researchers and clinicians working in this area.

In Chapter 5, the final chapter of Part II, George and colleagues concisely and informatively review various neuroimaging approaches and paradigms to the study of emotion and emotional disorders (e.g., depression). A description of such techniques and examples of pertinent emotion research are provided for both structural scanning (i.e., computerized axial tomography [CT] and magnetic resonance imaging [MRI]) and functional imaging (i.e., quantitative electroencephalography [EEG], single photon emission computed tomography [SPECT], positron emission tomography [PET], functional MRI [fMRI], and repetitive transcranial magnetic stimulation [rTMS]). Throughout Chapter 5, George and colleagues highlight important theoretical and methodological issues that must be considered in the design of imaging studies, such as sampling the emotion, determining/selecting the baseline, designing the statistical analysis, and interpreting the results. Interestingly, the authors point out that such studies remind ". . . us of the inextricable links between the mind and the brain . . . [and] offer the potential of forcing us to change our language about emotion into a more exact, neuroscientifically based discourse" (p. 128).

THEORETICAL PERSPECTIVES

Part III, "Theoretical Perspectives," includes four chapters: Chapter 6, an overview of basic psychological theories of emotion (Scherer); Chapter 7, a social-cognitive-neuroscience perspective (Ochsner & Schacter); Chapter 8, a neurobiological approach from a systems perspective (Adolphs & Damasio); and Chapter 9, a review of theories that are specifically neuropsychological (Gainotti).

Borod's own work in this area has focused on hemispheric specialization for emotion. The bulk of the research has suggested that emotion is processed preferentially by the right cerebral hemisphere. In a number of review papers (Borod, 1992, 1993a, 1996; Borod, Bloom, & Haywood, 1998a; Borod & Koff, 1989; see also Tucker, 1981), Borod has speculated on why the right hemisphere may have come to have a special role in emotion. At a psychological level, emotional processing involves strategies (e.g., integrative and holistic) and functions (e.g., nonverbal and visuospatial) for which the right hemisphere is dominant. Cicone et al. (1980, p. 155) have suggested that the critical demand of emotional processing that engages the right hemisphere is an appreciation of "the 'spatial' organization among emotions," that is, a "sensitivity to relations among emotions." At the neurological level, what we know about the right hemisphere is consistent with the strategies and functions associated with emotional processing. In particular, the right hemisphere, as compared with the left hemisphere, has been described as having a greater capacity for multimodal integration (Goldberg & Costa, 1981; Semmes, 1968), greater interlobular organization (Egelko et al., 1988), more neural interconnectivity among regions (Gur et al., 1980; Thatcher et al., 1986; Tucker et al., 1986), more widespread stimulus-evoked physiological activity (Trotman & Hammond, 1989), and overlapping horizontal axonal connectivity (Springer & Deutsch, 1989; Woodward, 1988). In sum, these features of the right hemisphere may be particularly suited to the multimodal, integrative nature of emotional processing.

Other work, however, has pointed to differential hemispheric specialization as a function of emotional dimension or emotion type (e.g., Mandal et al., 1999). A frequently studied dimension of emotion is emotional valence. When laterality findings emerge, most studies indicate that negative emotional states (e.g., disgust) are preferentially processed by the right hemisphere, whereas positive emotions (e.g., happiness) are subserved by the left hemisphere (for reviews, see Heller, 1990; Sackeim et al., 1982; Silberman & Weingartner, 1986). A related dimension, motor direction, suggests that withdrawal-related emotions (e.g., fear) are mediated by the right hemisphere and that approach-related emotions (e.g., happiness) are mediated by the left hemisphere (Davidson, 1984; Kinsbourne & Bemporad, 1984). Hemispheric specialization has been most commonly described in studies of expression and/or experience, although there are also reports that involve perception (e.g., Burton & Levy, 1989; Mandal et al., 1999; Moretti et al., 1996). It has been proposed (Sutton & Davidson, 1997) that dimensions of valence and motoric direction are overlapping concepts, as most approach emotions are pleasant and most withdrawal emotions are unpleasant (Fox, 1991; Gray, 1994; Watson et al., 1999). (Anger, however, is one exception, as it has approach aspects but is negative in tone [Borod et al., 1981; Davidson, 1993].) Most data have implicated frontal and anterior temporal structures in association with these two dimensions (e.g., Davidson, 1993, 1998). A third dimension that is certainly integral to emotional processing is arousal. Level of arousal can affect the characterization of the emotional state experienced or expressed. For instance, fear involves greater arousal than sadness (Mandal, 1986), and joy is more arousing than contentment (Fredrickson, 1998). In terms of its neural substrates, physiological arousal has been associated with the right cerebral hemisphere, in particular the posterior parietal region (Eidelberg & Galaburda, 1984; Heilman et al., 1978; Heller, 1993; Heller et al., 1997; Liotti & Tucker, 1992; Tucker & Williamson, 1984). The chapters to follow not only touch on these models and distinctions, but go beyond them, as well.

In Chapter 6, Scherer provides an overview of current theoretical models in the psychology of emotion, tracing the historical roots and noting current controversies in the research that they have generated. Scherer begins with a "multicomponent" definition of emotion that involves the reaction triad (i.e., physiological arousal, motor expression, and subjective feeling), motivational factors (e.g., action tendencies), and cognitive processes (i.e., evaluation of eliciting events and regulation of ongoing emotional processes). According to Scherer, "Emotions are [relatively brief] episodes of coordinated changes in several components (including at least neurophysiological activation, motor expression, and subjective feeling . . .) in response to external or internal events of major significance to the organism" (pp. 138–139). For clarity, Scherer includes a table that contrasts emotions with other affective phenomena (i.e., mood, interpersonal stances, attitudes, and personality traits). In true definitional fervor, Scherer makes an appeal for clear delineation of the phenomenon being studied as a prerequisite to discovering the underlying mechanisms.

Scherer goes on to describe the historical roots of current psychological models as being built on the thinking of Plato, Descartes, Darwin, and James. The heart of the chapter describes contemporary models, which Scherer organizes into four categories: dimensional, discrete emotion, meaning oriented, and componential. Scherer's own work appears to espouse the componential model, which is based on "the assumptions that emotions are elicited by a cognitive (but not necessarily conscious or controlled) evaluation of antecedent situations and events and that the patterning of the reactions in the different response domains . . . is determined by the outcome of this evaluation process" (p. 149). According to Scherer, one of the major functions of the componential model is the attempt to more explicitly connect elicitation circumstances and response patterning.

In Chapter 7, Ochsner and Schacter draw from theory and research in both social psychology and cognitive neuroscience to provide an informative account of the relationship between emotion and memory. The authors review the literature, which is peppered with delightful anecdotes and examples to illustrate their points. Throughout the chapter, certain cognitive concepts are considered, including attention, perception, appraisal, working memory, effort, and reasoning. The chapter is divided into three main discussions of (1) how emotion guides encoding, (2) elaboration and consolidation of information, and (3) retrieval processes. The chapter also includes important implications for mental health practitioners (e.g., the value of placing a positive spin on stressful life events) and offers useful suggestions for future research vis-à-vis normal aging and neuroimaging.

In Chapter 8, Adolphs and Damasio present a neurobiological systems-level theory of emotion motivated by evolutionary and ecological mechanisms and focused on "knowledge about emotion." Critical to their definition of emotion is the idea that emotions engage neural structures that represent body states and that link perception of external stimuli to body states (Damasio, 1994, 1995). The heart of the chapter is a description of the role of the amygdala in a variety of activities—social judgments, recognition of emotional facial expressions, aversive fear conditioning, and learning and emotional development (see also LeDoux, 1996). Both human and animal experimental data are reviewed, and illustrative case materials are provided. The authors review the neuroanatomical projections of the amygdala, a collection of nuclei located in the anterior mesial temporal lobe, which receives highly processed information about all modalities. A system of numerous reciprocal connections from somatosensory cortices with many other brain structures (e.g., ventromedial frontal cortex, basal ganglia, thalamus, hippocampus, and basal forebrain) and projections to the hypothalamus defines the anatomical amygdala. According to Adolphs and Damasio, "the amygdala is situated so as to link information about external stimuli conveyed by sensory cortices . . . with modulation of decision-making, memory, attention, and somatic, visceral, and endocrine processes" (p. 197). They further point out that all of these processes are influenced by the emotional significance of the external stimulus.

Adolphs and Damasio turn next to the role of right-hemisphere somatosensory cortices in processing emotion, focusing on the parietal cortex. They postulate why emotions should be lateralized and specifically to the right hemisphere, with an emphasis on the processing of somatic information and body states. The chapter is closed with the suggestion that future research focus on the neural systems involved in the sociocultural aspects of emotion and in the social emotions (e.g., jealousy, pride, and embarrassment; Ross et al., 1994). The authors conclude that "ultimately . . . , emotions . . . will be seen to arise from relations between multiple brains and their external environments, embedded in the context of a particular culture" (p. 209), which well portrays their evolutionary and ecological perspective.

Part III ends with Chapter 9, by Gainotti, on neuropsychological theories of emotion, which the author describes as "the set of theoretical models that have accompanied and oriented clinical and experimental studies aiming to clarify the relationships between emotions and the brain" (p. 214). Chapter 9 gives equal consideration to psychological models of emotion and to neurological mechanisms. According to Gainotti, these theories have been influenced by (*1*) the representation and organization of emotions in the human brain (i.e., emotional dimensions vs. discrete emotional categories) and (*2*) the componential nature of emotions, that is, whether there is a "central processor" of emotions or whether emotional components are subserved by different parts of the brain (see also Borod, 1993b). The initial discussion in Chapter 9 reviews studies pertaining to the historical development of neuropsychological theories in terms of subcortical/limbic mechanisms and hemispheric asymmetries.

The second half of Gainotti's chapter describes current neuropsychological theories of emotion with a stronger focus on human than on animal research and with an attempt to take into account the range of neural structures that have been studied. In developing a viable neuropsychology theory, Gainotti contends that the following issues need to be considered: (*1*) the relationship between emotional and cognitive systems, (*2*) the features distinguishing the emotional from the cognitive system (see Table 9.1), (*3*) the componential nature of emotions, and (*4*) the hierarchical organization of the emotional processing system. Gainotti makes a compelling argument for integrated, rather than independent, emotional and cognitive systems. He points out that the general architectures of the two systems are similar, whereas their scopes are quite different. The emotional system is viewed as an emergency one with the ability to rapidly and automatically process stimuli and trigger a response. In contrast, the cognitive system is both a more advanced and a more complex system with the ability to analyze information through the selection of appropriate strategies (see also Oatley & Johnson-Laird, 1987). When discussing the hierarchical nature of emotional processing, Gainotti suggests that the two sides of the brain may play complementary roles in emotional behavior, with the right hemisphere more involved in the automatic, spontaneous, and schematic aspects of emotion and the left hemisphere more instrumental in controlling and modulating emotion (Buck, 1984). He concludes with a discussion of the possible relationships between left/right and cortical/subcortical distinctions. A case is made for both "top-down" (i.e., left-hemisphere cortical dominance for cognitive and control functions) and "bottom-up" (i.e., greater emotional involvement of right-hemisphere subcortical structures [e.g., the amygdala]) processing.

EMOTIONAL DISORDERS

Part IV, "Emotional Disorders," features a spectrum of basic emotional response systems: elation and mania; sadness and depression; anxiety and stress; violence, anger, and impulsivity; and apathy (i.e., the absence of emotion). The authors in this part describe the neurological, psychiatric, and/or life-span disorders associated with each response system and review the neuropsychological literature pertinent to each discrete emotional system. In addition, the authors provide theoretical discussions about how knowledge of the neuroanatomical, physiological, and biochemical substrata underlying these disorders can inform our understanding of brain–behavior relationships for emotion.

Chapter 10 is by Robinson and Manes. It reflects their perspective on elation, mania, and mood disorders after two decades of work focused on the emotional, cognitive, and behavioral changes associated with focal brain injury. They point out that there have been largely two perspectives in investigations of this nature: "One attributes mood disorders to an understandable psychological reaction to the associated impairment; the other, based on a lack of association between severity of impairment and severity of emotional disorder, suggests a direct causal connection between emotional disorders and structural brain damage" (p. 240). The authors begin with an elegant history of a century of work in this area, focusing largely on case descriptions that primarily involve cerebrovascular disease. The authors then review the following emotional changes and associated disorders: mania in stroke, mania in traumatic brain injury, depression in stroke, depression in Parkinson's disease, and depression in traumatic brain injury. In each case, the authors comment on a variety of factors, including lesion location, neural mechanisms, prevalence, risk factors, and longitudinal course. In terms of brain–behavior relationships, the authors suggest that mania is most frequently associated with right-hemisphere cortical lesions, bipolar disorder with right-hemisphere subcortical lesions, and depression with left-hemisphere cortical (frontal) and subcortical (basal ganglia) lesions. Finally, specific treatments are discussed for each disorder and disease. Although the focus of treatment is on psychopharmacology, suggestions for future research into treatment focus on social intervention.

In Chapter 11, Davidson and Henriques provide an excellent review of the brain mechanisms underlying sadness and depression, drawing largely from the normal adult literature, but also from studies of neurological and psychiatric disorders, using electroencephalography, event-related potential, and blood flow procedures. In addition to pointing out various critical methodological issues throughout, the authors provide a theoretical backdrop regarding the approach/withdrawal laterality model (Davidson, 1984) and its relationship to positive/negative affective expression and experience and to anterior brain activation asymmetries (Davidson, 1984, 1998). According to Davidson and Henriques, "absolute anterior asymmetry by itself does not produce a particular pattern of emotional behavior or psychopathology; instead anterior asymmetry is seen as a diathesis (or constitutional predisposition) for the expression of emotional behavior, *given an appropriate affect elicitor*" (p. 270). From the emotion perspective, Davidson maintains that sadness and depression should be associated with reduced left frontal activation, reflecting decreased positive affect. Specifically, individuals who have a characteristic pattern of left frontal hypoactivation should be more susceptible to sad mood induction and should have an increased risk for depression. Importantly, the authors explain that sadness and depression are not the same; sadness is viewed as only one aspect of depression, which also includes loss of pleasure, loss of interest, and social withdrawal. In fact, at the end of Chapter 11, they raise the interesting question of "whether sadness in normal people is a good model system for clinical depression" (p. 287).

In Chapter 12, Nitschke, Heller, and Miller continue the focus on negative emotional states, examining anxiety and stress. In addition, the authors consider the role of stress in anxiety. They review evidence linking different types of anxiety to specific patterns of regional brain function and discuss the implications of these connections in terms of cognition. The major premise on which Chapter 12 is based is that there are two types of anxiety: "anxious apprehension" (AAP), characterized by concern and worry about the future, muscle tension, and verbal rumination about negative expectations and fears; and "anxious arousal" (AAR), associated with panic, feelings of fear, and pounding heart and triggered by threats representing an immediate danger. Conceptually, this distinction differs from the classic distinction between trait and state anxiety. Central to the relationship between these types of anxiety and brain function is the concept of stress, with the authors attending to the important distinction between external stressors and psychological stress.

In terms of brain asymmetry, the authors hypothesize that AAP (in right-handed people) would more likely be associated with increased left-hemisphere activity due to the major verbal component integral to worry and cognitive rumination, whereas AAR would be linked to increased right-hemisphere posterior activity, as there is literature (e.g., Heller, 1993; Heller et al., 1997) linking somatic arousal to posterior regions of the right hemisphere. According to Heller (1993, pp. 480–481), the properties of the right hemisphere, and especially the temporoparietal region, "encompass the cognitive, attentional, and physiological attributes that would be useful for optimal efficiency in responding to environmental events." In support of their hypotheses, the authors provide compelling and consistent evidence from studies cutting across technique domains (i.e., electrophysiological, hemodynamic, behavioral, neurological, psychiatric, and cognitive). An important point made by the authors pertains to the comorbidity between anxiety and depression. The authors point out that, although greater right than left anterior cortical activity has been found in both AAR and depression, increased right posterior activity is unique to AAR, whereas reduced left anterior activity and reduced right posterior activity are unique to depression.

Scarpa and Raine, in Chapter 13, also invoke a dichotomous distinction as the framework for understanding brain–behavior relationships for violence, anger, and impulsivity. Paralleling the categories of defensive and predatory behavior in animals, human aggression has been categorized as "impulsive–emotional" or "controlled–instrumental" (Vitiello & Stoff, 1997). Impulsive aggression occurs suddenly in reaction to threat or provocation within the context of increased anger, emotionality, and impulsivity; it is reactive, affective, and defensive. Controlled aggression, on the other hand, manifests itself as a relatively nonemotional display of aggression directed at obtaining some goal; it is proactive, manipulative, and predatory. From Chapter 13, it appears that the neuropsychology of impulsive-emotional aggression is the better understood of the two. Impulsive aggression is ascribed to greater right-hemisphere activation, especially in frontotemporal regions and connections to limbic and hypothalamic structures, which in turn are important in the expression and regulation of emotion.

The evidence reviewed about these two forms of aggression, with a particular focus on the impulsive type of aggression, are from studies involving neuropsychological testing, neurological disorders (e.g., temporal lobe epilepsy), neuroimaging, neurochemistry, hormonal levels, and psychophysiology (i.e., skin conductance, heart rate, EEG activity, and ERP). Typically, low levels of autonomic activity appear to be related to antisocial behavior and nonviolent crimes, whereas increased autonomic reactivity is related to the impulsive–emotional form of aggression. Scarpa and Raine explain that psychophysiological reactivity is related to aggression in the context of increased negative affect and thought processes. Reminiscent of theorizing by Davidson and Henriques (Chapter 11, this volume). Chapter 13 concludes with the point that biological predispositions and cognitive deficits interact with adverse social and environmental factors to produce impulsive-emotional behavior.

Chapter 14, the final one in this part, examines apathy, whose dictionary definitions are the "absence of emotion" and the "lack of interest or concern," thus representing an endpoint on the spectrum of emotional disorders. The objectives of the authors (Stuss, van Reekum, & Murphy) are to revisit historical concepts and definitions, to review the evidence from the neuropsychiatric literature, and to creatively determine their own neuropsychologically relevant definition of apathy. The definition of apathy arrived at by Stuss, van Reekum, and Murphy is "an absence of responsiveness to stimuli as demonstrated by a lack of self-initiated action" (p. 342). According to the authors, there are many advantages to this definition: (*1*) it provides for objective behavioral measurement, (*2*) it is neither a single state nor a syndrome, and (*3*) it can be divided into different states (or types) that are separable in terms of both the psychological mechanisms and the neural substrates involved. Their definition is intrinsically flexible, because, by using an adjectival descriptor that denotes the major qualities of the kind of apathetic behavior referred to, both increased scope and increased specificity are permitted.

In the course of Chapter 14, the authors provide a unique review of the causes of and disorders associated with apathy disturbances, including localized brain dysfunction (e.g., frontal lobes, basal ganglia, thalamus, and medial forebrain bundles), dementia (e.g., frontal lobe dementia, Huntington's disease, and Alzheimer's disease), and psychiatric disorders (e.g., depression and negative-symptom schizophrenia). From their review of the literature, the authors conclude that neurologically based apathy typically involves frontal/subcortical or frontolimbic system circuitry. The review is followed by a thoughtful discussion of the authors' conceptualization of apathy states in relation to disturbances of arousal and to other theoretical perspectives. The chapter ends with a description of treatment interventions that involve pharmacotherapy (e.g., via increasing dopaminergic activity) and behavioral rehabilitation (e.g., social skills training). The authors conclude that treatment for apathy will be most effective when the underlying psychological and pathophysiological mechanisms are clearly understood (e.g., Stuss, 1987).

CLINICAL IMPLICATIONS

The final section of the book, Part V, focuses on clinical implications. In contrast to Part IV, where a discrete emotional response system or an emotional disorder was emphasized, in Part V a specific illness (i.e., neurological disease, depression, and schizophrenia) is the focus. In addition, information is provided regarding specific treatments for the various disorders, including rehabilitation, psychotherapy, and brain interventions (e.g., pharmacotherapy and psychosurgery). In general, the chapters are filled with theoretical ideas and conceptualizations that provide yet another route to unravel the nature of emotion vis-à-vis neuroanatomical and neurophysiological mechanisms. The information in Part V should be useful to health care professionals dealing with patient populations suffering from emotional disorders and affective processing deficits.

The section begins with Chapter 15, by Heilman, Blonder, Bowers, and Crucian, who discuss how various neurological diseases impact on emotional experience, mood, and the communication of emotion (i.e., comprehension and expression). The brain structures that figure prominently in Chapter 15 are the posterior neocortex, basal ganglia, portions of the limbic system, and frontal lobes. The chapter begins with an excellent review of the literature that describes emotion deficits associated with each disorder and discusses underlying neural mechanisms. The following brain regions and respective diseases are included: cortical dysfunction (e.g., left-hemisphere damage, right-hemisphere damage, and corticobulbar dysfunction), limbic system dysfunction (e.g., amygdalectomy, encephalitis, and complex partial seizures), and basal ganglia diseases (e.g., Parkinson's disease, Huntington's disease, progressive supranuclear palsy, Wilson's disease, striatonigral degeneration, and Sydenham's chorea).

Heilman and colleagues then describe possible mechanisms that link concepts, theories, and neural substrates. In terms of emotional communication disorders, concepts involving iconic representation, motoric representation, and innate cross-cultural mechanisms are discussed. In terms of emotional experience and mood disorders, the discussion of mechanisms focuses on feedback theories (i.e., facial, visceral, and autonomic nervous system) and CNS theories (i.e., subcortical/diencephalic and modular). They also acknowledge the major contribution of neocortical mechanisms, maintaining that "there is overwhelming evidence that in humans the neocortex is critical for interpreting the meaning of many stimuli that induce an emotional experience" (p. 391).

The authors focus mostly on modular theories that postulate, according to the authors, dedicated centers and systems for each emotion or nondevoted systems mediating more than one emotion or specific emotional dimension. According to Heilman (1997), the conscious experience of emotion is mediated by "anatomically distributed modular networks;" these modules determine valence, control arousal, and mediate motor activation (approach vs. avoidance). The chapter provides an excellent critique of the valence dimension. For the arousal dimension, the authors present a discussion about the specific neural mechanisms underlying attention, stimulus novelty and significance, and asymmetric control of physiological arousal. In their discussion of the "motor activation" dimension, the authors maintain that the right hemisphere has a special role in motor activation and intention. In their conclusion, the authors summarize their theory on the neural mechanisms underlying emotional experience, behavior, and communication.

In Chapter 16, Raskin, Bloom, and Borod discuss rehabilitation of a range of emotional deficits, with a focus on neurological disorders. In keeping with the spirit of the volume, a multidisciplinary approach is taken. The authors begin by describing various approaches to rehabilitation, including cognitive remediation, speech–language therapy, multidisciplinary and milieu treatment, and caregiver participation programs. In addition, they describe the assessment and evaluative techniques that accompany rehabilitation and discuss the important principle of treatment generalization.

The chapter's main focus is on the treatment of the emotional deficits that follow neurological disorders and acquired brain injury. Recent work has indicated that affective difficulties in such populations are directly amenable to remediation techniques (e.g., Myers, 1998; Tompkins, 1995), although they have rarely been attempted to date. As a prelude to this part of the chapter, a brief overview is provided regarding some of the emotional deficits associated with common neurological disorders (i.e., traumatic brain injury, stroke, Parkinson's disease, Alzheimer's disease, and multiple sclerosis). Then, specific treatment approaches are described (e.g., cognitive remediation, behavioral therapies, and relaxation training) for depression, anxiety, post-traumatic stress disorder, anger, apathy and indifference, and affective deficits that reflect channel-specific or mode-specific impairments. Chapter 16 concludes with the suggestion that the componential approach to emotional processing described by Borod (1993b), which is similar to the modular theories described by Heilman et al. (Chapter 15, this volume) and the componential perspective provided by Gainotti (Chapter 9, this volume), provides both a potential way to organize and to evaluate the treatment of emotional deficits from a neuropsychological perspective.

This section on clinical implications moves from neurological diseases and brain injury to two chapters on psychiatric disorders. Kohler, Gur, and Gur, in Chapter 17, examine affective processes in schizophrenia, with a focus on mood disorders. They review the schizophrenia literature from a particular conceptual perspective, broadly covering the literature, as well as highlighting their own research pertinent to the topic. The chapter begins with an informative historical review of the development of the concept and symptoms of schizophrenia. The authors then describe affective processes in schizophrenia from the perspective of deficits in emotional expression (e.g., flat affect), emotional experience (e.g., depression), and emotion recognition (e.g., face perception). As a follow-up to this description of deficits, the authors discuss psychopharmacological treatments for aspects of schizophrenia, including psychotic symptoms, depression, schizoaffective disorder, and negative symptoms (i.e., flat affect, alogia, and anhedonia).

Chapter 17 concludes with an explanation of how neurobiological studies (i.e., brain metabolism and blood flow) have advanced the understanding of emotion-related symptoms in schizophrenia. The authors make three interesting points in this regard. First, in their own work (Kohler et al., 1998), schizophrenics with depression had larger temporal lobe volumes. According to the authors, "the association of depression with normal temporal lobe volumes . . . suggests that some integrity of the temporal lobe is necessary for the experience of depression, consistent with evidence for the role of the temporal lobe in emotional experience" (p. 446). Second, depression in schizophrenia is associated with a relative decrease in left compared with right anterior cingulate activity, consistent with lesion studies pointing to greater right hemisphere involvement in negative emotional states (e.g., Gainotti, 1972; Sackeim et al., 1982). Third, because of altered metabolic functioning in frontal regions, the authors conclude that "the neurobiology of depression in schizophrenia has features in common with major depression and depression associated with other brain disorders" (p. 447).

The final chapter, Chapter 18, deals directly with mood disorders (i.e., depression and mania) in psychiatric populations. The authors, Lisanby and Sackeim, present a comprehensive state-of-the-art review of somatic interventions for these disorders, including psychopharmacological agents, electroconvulsive therapy (ECT), functional neurosurgery, and repetitive transcranial magnetic stimulation (rTMS). According to Lisanby and Sackeim, these four different treatments have "mood-altering effects but differ in their mechanisms of action and degree of anatomical specificity" (p. 456). Besides providing a wealth of material about treatment, the authors summarize the knowledge gained during treatment of mood disorders about the neurobiological theories regarding the nature and regulation of emotion.

One of the considerations that emerges from the discussion of psychopharmacology pertains to whether there is a direct relationship between the mechanisms that regulate mood alterations (i.e., sadness and happiness) in healthy normal subjects and those that underlie the psychiatric disorders of major depression and mania. From the evidence reviewed, the authors suggest that the studies in normal individuals may be of limited relevance to the psychiatric studies, and vice versa. Moreover, they suggest that normal people and depressed people may have different neural representations of emotion. One of the promising new speculations emerging from the ECT research is that bilateral frontal ECT may be more effective than the more traditional frontotemporal placement and its associated amnestic effects. In their discussion of psychosurgery, the authors provide an excellent history and review of the procedures utilized to treat psychiatric disorders over the years, including leukotomy, thalamotomy, cingulotomy, subcaudate tractotomy, and limbic leukotomy. In general, the work in this area supports the role of limbic structures in mood regulation.

The authors conclude their chapter with a description of an exciting new technique (i.e., rTMS) that provides a noninvasive method of direct cortical stimulation as we move into the new millenium. The initial studies reviewed here have implications for contemporary theories regarding hemispheric specialization for emotion as a function of valence. Preliminary studies (e.g., George et al., 1996) suggest that rTMS of the dorsolateral prefrontal cortex on the left side leads to transient dysphoria and on the right side leads to mood elevation.[1] Clinically, however, there is some suggestion of therapeutic effects in depression with left-sided stimulation and in mania with right-sided stimulation. Yet again, the findings implicate paradoxical effects in normal versus psychiatric populations.

---

[1]In a similar vein, Borod et al. (2000) found a "reversed valence" effect in a study of verbal pragmatic aspects of discourse production in individuals with unilateral stroke. Right-hemisphere damage was associated with impairment in positive emotion and left-hemisphere damage with impairment in negative emotion.

FUTURE DIRECTIONS AND RESEARCH CONSIDERATIONS

We want here to highlight some of the questions raised in this volume, discuss several related areas of emotion research, and suggest possible directions for further exploration of emotional processing in neuropsychological investigations.

Perhaps the most perplexing question of brain–behavior relationships is why it has been so difficult to delineate the specific neural substrates involved in emotional processing. Intricate brain–behavior models have been proposed in other areas of neural functioning, such as the visual system (Livingstone & Hubel, 1988; Ungerleider & Mishkin, 1982). In part, this is because visual stimuli per se lend themselves to concrete and discernible parameters, such as form, color, movement, and depth perception, variables that are easily tested in animal models. In the current volume, Buck (Chapter 2, this volume) notes the importance of defining the components being examined in emotion research and how such definitions may be altered once the underlying neural organization is understood. Explicit definitions are crucial to furthering our knowledge of how the brain processes emotion (e.g., Scherer, Chapter 6, this volume).

Many of the working definitions for describing components of emotional processing are, however, quite broad, as are the brain regions that have often been implicated. Perhaps this is due to the limitations of the currently available technology for studying human emotional functioning, but, as has been suggested (e.g., Heilman et al., Chapter 15, this volume), it also might reflect very widespread neural substrates underlying these processes. Functional neuroimaging and lesion method studies have clarified the specific brain substrates involved to a degree, but much more work is needed to understand the interplay between such substrates and processing modes.

A recent example of such an attempt is Mayberg's model of depression (1997), which delineates potential neural pathways and altered relationships among various brain regions. Another example, along these lines, is the associative memory, object-based processing subserved by the amygdala (see Adolphs & Damasio, Chapter 8, this volume), investigations of which in humans have been based on models developed from animal studies (e.g., LeDoux, 1992, 1993). Offering theoretical models is an important step (e.g., Davidson & Henriques, Chapter 11; Gainotti, Chapter 9; Nitschke, Heller, & Miller, Chapter 12; and Scherer, Chapter 6, this volume), but the challenge is to develop rigorous tests of these proposals. In other areas, models are awaiting development, such as the interface between emotion and memory (e.g., Hamann et al., 1999; LeDoux, 1996; Oschsner & Schacter, Chapter 7, this volume), as well as the interaction between emotion and other aspects of cognition (e.g., attention; LeDoux, 1996).

Most authors in this volume emphasize the need for clear and concise definitions of emotional parameters in order to design experiments that can further our knowledge regarding the brain substrates implicated by clinical neuropsychological and functional neuroimaging studies. This includes the importance of subtyping clinical disorders based on specific symptoms, not only to enhance our understanding of the neural substrates of emotion but also to refine treatment interventions. Such subtyping, which is essential in emotion research, has emerged and is reviewed in this volume for anxiety (Nitschke, Heller, & Miller, Chapter 12), schizophrenia (Kohler, Gur, & Gur, Chapter 17), aggression (Scarpa & Raine, Chapter 13), and apathy (Stuss, van Reekum, & Murphy, Chapter 14). For example, many functional neuroimaging studies indicate altered frontal brain asymmetry in depression, yet the contributing factors (e.g., affective, motivational, or cognitive) remain enigmatic. Categorizing individuals with symptoms predominantly representing one type, dimension, or factor may provide further clarification. Moreover, subtyping individuals within a particular disorder may eventually lead to a better understanding of the genetic components involved in certain disease states and how genetic vulnerabilities (i.e., risk factors) interact with environmental or neurological (i.e., brain insult) stressors to result in pathological states.

The issue and need for subtyping individuals parallels the issue concerning individual differences (or subject characteristics) in emotional processing. The primary characteristics studied to date are age and gender. In terms of affective changes with age, most studies have focused on psychopathology and emotional experience. For example, most studies have reported an increase in depression with age, whereas most have not found any significant age-related changes in emotional experience per se (for review, see Grunwald et al., 1999). For emotional expression, studies examining posed facial expressions have found older participants to be less accurate than younger participants (Levenson et al., 1991; Malatesta & Izard, 1984; Yecker et al., 2000). In contrast, investigations of spontaneous expression have found either no age-related changes as a function of age (Levenson et al., 1991; Malatesta et al., 1987) or greater expressivity in older adults (Malatesta et al., 1992).

In terms of gender, several investigations indicate that women are better decoders of emotional stimuli than men (e.g., Brody, 1985; Duda & Brown, 1985; Grunwald et al., 1999; Hall, 1978; LaFrance & Banaji, 1992; Otta et al., 1996; Shields, 1991) and that women are more emotionally expressive than men (e.g., Ashmore, 1990; Brody & Hall, 1993). The findings regarding differences in emotional experience between men and women are, however, equivocal, with some studies finding that women report experiencing emotion more intensely than men (Choti et al., 1987; Grunwald et al., 1999; Gross & Levenson, 1993) and other investigations finding no sex differences (Cupchik & Poulos, 1984; Kring & Gordon, 1998; Lanzetta et al., 1976; Wagner et al., 1993; Zuckerman et al., 1981). Finally, gender may be an important moderating variable in lateralization studies of emotion, as there is evidence that there is more bilateral hemispheric representation of function in women than in men (e.g., Crucian & Berenbaum, 1998;

Gur et al., 1982, 1999; McGlone, 1980). Thus, interpretations of findings regarding neural correlates of emotion and emotional regulation must take subject characteristics into account.

Although the emphasis in many neuropsychological studies of emotion has been on pathological and deficit states, a focus on emotional *function* (rather than dysfunction) and the study of positive emotion may also yield important findings. For instance, Tomarken (1998) recently described how pharmacological treatment of depression may differentially influence the appearance of positive versus negative affect in depression. Indeed, most studies of emotion have focused predominantly on negative emotions (see Fredrickson, 1998). Fredrickson (1998) proposed that positive emotions differ from negative ones in that specific effector response systems are not elicited by positive emotional states. Rather, she proposed a "broaden and build" model of positive emotions in which positive emotions elicit thought/action repertoires that serve to alter attentional focus and cognitive flexibility. Thus, exploring positive affect in neuropsychological studies may lead to a richer understanding of emotion in general and may serve to better predict favorable outcomes in individuals with emotional dysfunction.

In the relatively few neuropsychological studies that examine positive emotion, the findings suggest an involvement of temporal regions. For example, when true periods of happiness (indicated by a "felt" or Duchenne smile) were elicited in healthy participants, there was greater activation of left temporal and parietal regions (Ekman et al., 1990). Similarly, in a case study, laughter and feelings of mirth were elicited in two patients with gelastic seizures after stimulation of basal temporal regions, specifically fusiform and parahippocampal gyri (Arroyo et al., 1993). The findings from functional neuroimaging studies in healthy populations are less clear and suggest a great deal of overlap between pleasant and unpleasant emotional states (e.g., appetitive and aversive motivational systems) (George et al., 1995; Lane et al., 1997a,b). Clearly, further work is needed to distinguish specific neural correlates involved in particular kinds of emotion, especially for positive emotional states.

Finally, as several of the authors have proposed, neuropsychologists need to broaden the scope of their research to examine elements of social functioning and its interaction with emotional processing and regulation. Stuss, van Reekum, and Murphy (Chapter 14, this volume) note the injurious effects of apathy, with one subtype leading to "the absence of an abstract model of one's self in society" (p. 356). Their work highlights the importance of multifaceted treatments of such disorders, including both pharmacological and social skill training interventions. Perhaps models and experimental paradigms from neurodevelopmental disorders (namely autism) can be used to explore social–emotional functioning in other psychiatric and neurological disorders (for review, see Brozgold et al., 1998). Oschner and Schacter (Chapter 7, this volume) have attempted to understand how emotion can interact with encoding and retrieval mechanisms of memory to function within the social context of goals and personal motivations. Scherer (Chapter 6, this volume) notes the importance of emotional appraisal in eliciting specific emotions, and much work has been done regarding cultural differences in appraisal processes, as in the social–emotional construct view of emotion (e.g., Mesquita & Frijda, 1992). In contrast, to our knowledge, few neuropsychological studies have examined the role of appraisal and its relationships to other parameters of emotional processing, such as the dimensions of valence and appetitive–aversive components. A final point regarding social–emotional functioning concerns complex social emotions, like shame, embarrassment, jealousy, and pride. As Adolphs and Damasio (Chapter 8, this volume) point out, "the next task will be to elucidate what distinguishes emotion in humans from emotion in other animals" (p. 209). There are almost no studies examining the role of such emotions in clinical populations, with the exception of Ross, Homan, and Buck's study (1994) exploring hemispheric differences between primary and social emotions in epileptic patients. Thus, little is known about the neural correlates of such complex emotions, and this, too, is another area ripe for future study.

SUMMARY

In summary, there are a number of areas that require further investigation to better define brain–behavior relationships in emotion as we enter the new millennium. These principal themes are echoed and expanded in the chapters that follow.

In terms of theory, greater overlap is needed among theoretical models so that a more direct comparison among different perspectives can be completed. Of considerable help would be a "common language" that not only includes careful definition of concepts but also subscribes to using similar terminology. This would make it easier for investigators to compare findings across studies. Although it is unlikely that there will be one theory to describe all aspects of emotional processing, having such a common language will be helpful when integrating such information.

With respect to the study of specific emotional disorders, further classification and subtyping of such disorders is essential to delineate homogenous samples. In addition, individual differences, which contribute further variability, need to be taken into account. In any case, it is our hope that specific interventions will be further refined and developed to treat the gamut of emotional disorders. Furthermore, understanding social emotions, how to promote positive emotions, and the extent to which these emotions have predictive value in outcome may also be addressed.

In terms of evaluating emotional processing deficits and their disorders, psychometric studies are needed to examine protocols assessing emotional perception, expression, and experience. To date, most batteries are either not readily available for clinical use or are not practical to administer within a clinical setting. Such assessment measures will provide valuable information regarding individual functioning that may otherwise be overlooked.

Functional neuroimaging techniques provide other important assessment tools. As such methods are further refined and allow for greater temporal clarity without sacrificing spatial resolution, additional areas in emotion research can be addressed. These include understanding how and when particular neural structures are normally activated in emotional processing and determining interactions among these structures. Imaging technology can be used to address questions that have been debated for decades by emotion theorists, such as the relationship among modes of processing (e.g., experience vs. expression) and channels of communication (e.g., facial vs. prosodic). Such tools may also allow a greater understanding of the exact nature of particular brain regions (e.g., frontal lobes) in emotional processing. The ultimate goal may be to reconcile paradoxical findings from various techniques (e.g., the brain lesion method, neuroimaging data, and behavioral data from healthy adults), leading to a richer understanding of the underlying neural mechanisms involved and the causes of dysfunction.

The following chapters, then, provide new insight into the problems facing investigators of emotion and into interpretations of the neuropsychological mechanisms that underlie emotional processing. The authors' thoughtful presentations, detailed accounts of the research, and provocative ideas will advance the direction of future research so that many different dimensions and components important in emotion processing can be explored in a variety of clinical populations with a wide range of techniques.

ACKNOWLEDGMENTS

We are very grateful to Jack Nitschke, Ronald Bloom, and Sarah Raskin for their insightful comments and input into this chapter.

REFERENCES

Arroyo, S., Lesser, R.P., Gordon, B., Uematsu, S., Hart, J., Schwerdt, P., Andreasson, K., & Fisher, R.S. (1993). Mirth, laughter, and gelastic seizures. *Brain, 116,* 757–780.

Ashmore, R.D. (1990). Sex, gender, and the individual. In L.A. Pervin (Ed.), *Handbook of Personality: Theory and Research* (pp. 486–526). New York: Guilford Press.

Borod, J. (1992). Interhemispheric and intrahemispheric control of emotion: A focus on unilateral brain damage. *Journal of Consulting and Clinical Psychology, 60,* 339–348.

Borod, J. (1993a). Cerebral mechanisms underlying facial, prosodic, and lexical emotional expression: A review of neuropsychological studies and methodological issues. *Neuropsychology,* 1993, *7,* 445–463.

Borod, J. (1993b). Emotion and the brain—Anatomy and theory: An introduction to the Special Section. *Neuropsychology,* 1993, *7,* 427–432.

Borod, J. (1996). Emotional disorders/emotion. In J.G. Beaumont, P. Kenealy, & M. Rogers (Eds.), *The Blackwell Dictionary of Neuropsychology* (pp. 312–320). Oxford, England: Blackwell Publishers.

Borod, J., Bloom, R., & Haywood, C.S. (1998a). Verbal aspects of emotional communication. In M. Beeman & C. Chiarello (Eds.), *Right Hemisphere Language Comprehension: Perspectives from Cognitive Neuroscience* (pp. 285–307). Mahwah, NJ: Lawrence Erlbaum.

Borod, J., Caron, H.S., & Koff, E. (1981). Asymmetry in positive and negative facial expressions: Sex differences. *Neuropsychologia, 19*, 819–824.

Borod, J., Haywood, C.S., & Koff, E. (1997). Neuropsychological aspects of facial asymmetry during emotional expression: A review of the normal adult literature. *Neuropsychology Review, 7*, 41–60.

Borod, J., & Koff, E. (1989). The neuropsychology of emotion: Evidence from normal, neurological, and psychiatric populations. In E. Perecman (Ed.), *Integrating Theory and Practice in Clinical Neuropsychology* (pp. 175–215). New York: Lawrence Erlbaum.

Borod, J., Koff, E., Yecker, S., Santschi, C., & Schmidt, J.M. (1998b). Facial asymmetry during emotional expression: Gender, valence, and methods. *Neuropsychologia, 11*, 1209–1215.

Borod, J., Rorie, K., Pick, L., Bloom, R., Andelman, F., Campbell, A., Obler, L., Tweedy, J., Welkowitz, J., & Sliwinski, M. (2000). Verbal pragmatics following unilateral stroke: Emotional content and valence. *Neuropsychology, 14*, 112–124.

Bowers, D., Bauer, R.M., & Heilman, K.M. (1993). The nonverbal affect lexicon: Theoretical perspectives from neuropsychological studies of affect perception. *Neuropsychology, 7*, 433–444.

Brody, L.R. (1985). Gender differences in emotional development: A review of theories and research. *Journal of Personality, 53*, 102–149.

Brody, L.R., & Hall, J.A. (1993). Gender and emotion. In M. Lewis & J.M. Haviland (Eds.), *Handbook of Emotions* (pp. 447–460). New York: Guilford Press.

Brozgold, A., Borod, J., Martin, C., Pick, L., Alpert, M., & Welkowitz, J. (1998). Social functioning and facial emotional expression in neurological and psychiatric disorders. *Applied Neuropsychology, 5*, 15–23.

Bruder, G. (1991). Dichotic listening: New developments and applications in clinical research. *Annals of the New York Academy of Sciences, 620*, 217–232.

Bryden, M.P. (1982). *Laterality: Functional Asymmetry in the Intact Brain.* New York: Academic Press.

Buck, R. (1984). *The Communication of Emotion.* New York: Guilford Press.

Burton, L.A., & Levy, J. (1989). Sex differences in the lateralized processing of facial emotion. *Brain and Cognition, 11*, 210–228.

Choti, S., Marston, A.R., Holston, S.G., & Hart, J.T. (1987). Gender and personality variables in film-induced sadness and crying. *Journal of Social and Clinical Psychology, 5*, 535–544.

Cicone, M., Wapner, W., & Gardner, H. (1980). Sensitivity to emotional expressions and situations in organic patients. *Cortex, 16*, 145–158.

Cripe, L.I. (1997). Personality assessment of brain-impairment patients. In M.E. Mariush & J.A. Moses, Jr. (Eds.), *Clinical Neuropsychology: Theoretical Foundations for Practitioners* (pp. 119–142). Hillsdale, NJ: Erlbaum.

Crucian, G.P., & Berenbaum, S.A. (1998). Sex differences in right hemisphere tasks. *Brain and Cognition, 36*, 377–389.

Cupchik, G.C., & Poulos, C.X. (1984). Judgments of emotional intensity in self and others: The effects of stimulus, context, sex, and expressivity. *Journal of Personality and Social Psychology, 46,* 431–439.

Damasio, A.R. (1994). *Descartes' Error: Emotion, Reason, and the Human Brain.* New York: Grosset/Putnam.

Damasio, A.R. (1995). Toward a neurobiology of emotion and feeling: Operational concepts and hypotheses. *The Neuroscientist, 1,* 19–25.

Davidson, R.J. (1984). Affect, cognition, and hemispheric specialization. In C.E. Izard, J. Kagan, & R. Zajonc (Eds.), *Emotions, Cognition, and Behavior* (pp. 320–365). Cambridge, England: Cambridge Press.

Davidson, R.J. (1993). Parsing affective space: Perspectives from neuropsychology and psychophysiology. *Neuropsychology, 7,* 464–475.

Davidson, R.J. (1998). Affective style and affective disorders: Perspectives from affective neuroscience. *Cognition and Emotion, 12,* 307–330.

Davidson, R.J., Abercrombie, H., Nitschke, J.B., & Putnam, K. (1999). Regional brain function, emotion, and disorders of emotion. *Current Opinion in Neurobiology, 9,* 228–234.

Duda, P.D., & Brown, J. (1985). Lateral asymmetry of positive and negative emotions. *Cortex, 20,* 253–261.

Egelko, S., Gordon, W., Hibbard, M., Diller, L., Lieberman, A, Holliday, R., Ragnarsson, K., Shaver, M., & Orazen, J. (1988). Relationship among CT scans, neurological exam, and neuropsychological test performance in right-brain–damaged stroke patients. *Journal of Clinical and Experimental Neuropsychology, 10,* 539–564.

Eidelberg, D., & Galaburda, A.M. (1984). Divergent architectonic asymmetries in the human brain. *Archives of Neurology, 41,* 843–852.

Ekman, P., & Davidson, R.J. (1994). Afterward: Are there basic emotions? In P. Ekman & R.J. Davidson (Eds.), *The Nature of Emotion: Fundamental Questions* (pp. 45–47). New York: Oxford University Press.

Ekman, P., Davidson, R.J., & Friesen, W. (1990). The Duchenne smile: Emotional expression and brain physiology II. *Journal of Personality and Social Psychology, 58,* 342–353.

Fox, N.A. (1991). If it's not left, it's right. *American Psychologist, 46,* 863–872.

Fredrickson, B.L. (1998). What good are positive emotions? *Review of General Psychology, 2,* 300–319.

Gainotti, G. (1972). Emotional behavior and hemispheric side of the lesion. *Cortex, 8,* 41–55.

Gainotti, G., Caltagirone, C., & Zoccolotti, P. (1993). Left/right and cortical/subcortical dichotomies in the neuropsychological study of human emotions. *Cognition and Emotion, 7,* 71–93.

George, M.S., Ketter, T.A., Parekh, P.I., Horwitz, B., Herscovitch, P., & Post, R.M. (1995). Brain activity during transient sadness and happiness in healthy women. *American Journal of Psychiatry, 3,* 341–351.

George, M.S., Wasserman, E.M., Williams, W., Steppel, J., Pascual-Leone, A., Basser, P., Hallett,, M., & Post, R.M. (1996). Changes in mood and hormone levels after rapid-rate transcranial magnetic stimulation (rTMS) of the prefrontal cortex. *Journal of Neuropsychiatry and Clinical Neurosciences, 8,* 172–180.

Goldberg, E., & Costa, L. (1981). Hemisphere differences in the acquisition and use of descriptive systems. *Brain and Language, 14,* 144–173.

Gray, J.A. (1994). Three fundamental emotion systems. In P. Ekman & R.J. Davidson

(Eds.), *The Nature of Emotion: Fundamental Questions* (pp. 243–247). New York: Oxford University Press.

Gross, J.J., & Levenson, R.W. (1993). Emotional suppression: Physiology, self-report and expressive behavior. *Journal of Personality and Social Psychology, 64*, 970–986.

Grunwald, I., Borod, J., Obler, L., Erhan, H., Pick, L., Welkowitz, J., Madigan, N., Sliwinski, M., & Whalen, J. (1999). The effects of age and gender on the perception of lexical emotion. *Applied Neuropsychology, 6*, 226–238.

Gur, R.C., Gur, R.E., Obrist, W.D., Hungerbuhler, J.P., Younkin, D., Rosen, A.D., Skolnick, B.E., & Reivich, M. (1982). Sex and handedness differences in cerebral blood flow during rest and cognitive activity. *Science, 217*, 659–661.

Gur, R.C., Packer, I., Hungerbuhler, J., Reivich, M., Obrist, W., Amarnek, W., & Sackeim, H. (1980). Differences in the distribution of gray and white matter in human cerebral hemispheres. *Science, 207*, 1226–1228.

Gur, R.C., Turetsky, B.I., Matsui, M., Van, M., Bilker, W., Hughett, P., & Gur, R.E. (1999). Sex differences in brain gray and white matter in healthy young adults: Correlations with cognitive performance. *Journal of Neuroscience, 19*, 4065–4072.

Hall, J.A. (1978). Gender effects in decoding nonverbal cues. *Psychological Bulletin, 85*, 845–857.

Hamann, S.B., Ely, T.D., Grafton, S.T., & Kilts, C.D. (1999). Amygdala activity related to enhanced memory for pleasant and aversive stimuli. *Nature Neuroscience, 2*, 289–293.

Heilman, K.M. (1997). The neurobiology of emotional experience. *Journal of Neuropsychiatry and Clinical Neuroscience, 9*, 439–448.

Heilman, K.M., & Satz, P. (1983). *Neuropsychology of Human Emotion.* New York: Guilford Press.

Heilman, K.M., Schwartz, H.D., & Watson, R.T. (1978). Hypoarousal in patients with the neglect syndrome and emotional indifference. *Neurology, 28*, 229–232.

Heller, W. (1990). The neuropsychology of emotion: Developmental patterns and implications for psychopathology. In N. Stein, B.L. Leventhal, & T. Trabasso (Eds.), *Psychological and Biological Approaches to Emotion* (pp. 167–211). Hillsdale, NJ: Lawrence Erlbaum.

Heller, W. (1993). Neuropsychological mechanism of individual differences in emotion, personality, and arousal. *Neuropsychology, 7*, 476–489.

Heller, W., & Nitschke, J.B. (1998). The puzzle of regional brain activity in depression and anxiety: The importance of subtypes and comorbidity. *Cognition and Emotion, 12*, 421–447.

Heller, W., Nitschke, J.B., & Lindsay, D.C. (1997). Neuropsychological correlates of arousal in self-reported emotion. *Cognition and Emotion, 11*, 383–402.

Izard, C.E. (1977). *Human Emotions.* New York: Plenum Press.

Izard, C.E. (1992). Basic emotions, relations among emotions and emotion-cognition relations. *Psychological Review, 99*, 561–565.

Jackson, H.J. (1879). On affections of speech from diseases of the brain. *Brain, 2*, 203–222.

Kinsbourne, M., & Bemporad, B. (1984). Lateralization of emotion: A model and the evidence. In N. Fox & R. Davidson (Eds.), *The Psychobiology of Affective Development* (pp. 259–291). Hillsdale, NJ: Lawrence Erlbaum.

Kohler, C.G., Swanson, C.L., Gur, R.C., Mozley, L.H., & Gur, R.E. (1998). Depression in schizophrenia: II. MRI and PET findings. *Biological Psychiatry, 43*, 173–180.

Kring, A.M., & Gordon, A.H. (1998). Sex differences in emotion: Expression, experience, and physiology. *Journal of Personality and Social Psychology, 74*, 686–703.

LaFrance, M., & Banaji, M. (1992). Toward a reconsideration of the gender–emotion relationship. In M.S. Clark (Ed.), *Emotion and Social Behavior: Review of Personality and Social Psychology*, Vol. 14 (pp. 178–201). Newbury Park, CA: Sage.

Lane, R.D., Reiman, E.M., Ahern, G.L., Schwartz, G.E., & Davidson, R.J. (1997a). Neuroanatomical correlates of happiness, sadness, and disgust. *American Journal of Psychiatry, 154*, 926–933.

Lane, R.D., Reiman, E.M., Bradley, M.M., Lang, P.J., Ahern, G.L., Davidson, R.J., & Schwartz, G.E. (1997b). *Neuropsychologia, 35*, 1437–1444.

Lanzetta, J.T., Cartwright-Smith, J., & Kleck, R.E. (1976). Effects of nonverbal dissimulation on emotional experience and arousal. *Journal of Personality and Social Psychology, 33*, 354–370.

LeDoux, J.E. (1992). Emotion and the amygdala. In J.P. Aggleton (Ed.), *The Amygdala: Neurobiological Aspects of Emotion, Memory, and Mental Dysfunction* (pp. 339–352). New York: Wiley-Liss.

LeDoux, J.E. (1993). Emotional memory systems in the brain. *Behavioral Brain Research, 58*, 69–79.

LeDoux, J.E. (1996). *The Emotional Brain*. New York: Simon & Schuster.

Levenson, R.W., Carstenson, L.L., Friesen, W.V., & Ekman, P. (1991). Emotion, physiology, and expression in old age. *Psychology and Aging, 6*, 28–35.

Ley, R.G., & Strauss, E. (1986). Hemispheric asymmetries in the perception of facial expressions in normals. In R. Bruyer (Ed.), *The Neuropsychology of Face Perception and Facial Expression* (pp. 269–289). Hillsdale, NJ: Lawrence Erlbaum.

Liotti, M., & Tucker, D.M. (1992). Right hemisphere sensitivity to arousal and depression. *Brain and Cognition, 18*, 138–151.

Livingstone, M., & Hubel, D. (1988). Segregation of form, color, movement and depth: Anatomy, physiology and perception. *Science, 240*, 740–749.

Malatesta, C.Z., & Izard, C.E. (1984). The facial expression of emotion: Young, middle-aged, and older adult expressions. In C.A. Malatesta & C.E. Izard (Eds.), *Emotion in Adult Development* (pp. 253–273). Beverly Hills, CA: Sage.

Malatesta, C.Z., Izard, C.E., Culver, C., & Nicholich, M. (1987). Emotion communication skills in young, middle-aged, and older women. *Psychology and Aging, 2*, 193–203.

Malatesta, C., Jonas, R., Shepard, B., & Culver, C. (1992). Type A behavior pattern and emotion expression in younger and older adults. *Psychology and Aging, 7*, 551–561.

Mandal, M. (1986). Judgment of facial affect among depressives and schizophrenics. *British Journal of Clinical Psychology, 25*, 87–92.

Mandal, M., Borod, J., Asthana, H.S., Mohanty, A., Mohanty, S., & Koff E. (1999). Effects of lesion variables and emotion type on the perception of facial emotion. *The Journal of Nervous and Mental Disease, 187*, 603–609.

Mayberg, H.S. (1997). Limbic-cortical dysregulation: A proposed model of depression. *Journal of Neuropsychiatry, 9*, 471–481.

McGlone, J. (1980). Sex differences in human brain asymmetry: A critical survey. *The Behavioral and Brain Sciences, 3*, 215–263.

Mesquita, B., & Frijda, N.H. (1992). Cultural variations in emotion: A review. *Psychological Bulletin, 112*, 179–204.

Moretti, M., Charlton, S., & Taylor, S. (1996). The effects of hemispheric asymmetries and depression on the perception of emotion. *Brain and Cognition, 32*, 67–82.

Myers, P. (1998). *Right Hemisphere Damage: Disorders of Communication and Cognition*. San Diego, CA: Singular Publishing Group.

Oatley, K., & Johnson-Laird, P. (1987). Toward a cognitive theory of emotions. *Cognition and Emotion, 1*, 29–50.

Ortony, A., & Turner, T.J. (1990). What's basic about basic emotions? *Psychological Review*, *97*, 315–331.

Otta, E., Abrosio, F.F.E., & Hoshino, R.L. (1996). Reading a smiling face: Messages conveyed by various forms of smiling. *Perceptual and Motor Skills*, *82*, 1111–1121.

Panksepp, J. (1992). A critical role for "affective neuroscience" in resolving what is basic about basic emotions. *Psychological Review*, *99*, 554–560.

Plutchik, R. (1984). Emotions: A general psychoevolutionary theory. In K.R. Scherer & P. Ekman (Eds.), *Approaches to Emotion* (pp. 197–219). Hillsdale, NJ: Lawrence Erlbaum.

Ross, E.D. (1997). Right hemisphere syndromes and the neurology of emotion. In S.C. Schachter & O. Devinsky (Eds.), *Behavioral Neurology and the Legacy of Norman Gerschwind* (pp. 183–191). Philadelphia: Lippincott-Raven.

Ross, E.D., Homan, R.W., & Buck, R. (1994). Differential hemispheric lateralization of primary and social emotions: Implications for developing a comprehensive neurology for emotions, repression, and the subconscious. *Neuropsychiatry, Neuropsychology, and Behavioral Neurology*, *7*, 1–19.

Sackeim, H.A., Greenberg, M.S., Weiman, A.L., Gur, R.C., Hungerbuhler, J.P., & Geschwind, N. (1982). Hemispheric asymmetry in the expression of positive and negative emotions: Neurologic evidence. *Archives of Neurology*, *39*, 210–218.

Semenza, C., Pasini, M., Zettin, M., Tonin, P., & Portolan, P. (1986). Right hemisphere patients' judgments on emotion. *Acta Neurologica Scandinavica*, *74*, 43–50.

Semmes, J. (1968) Hemispheric specialization: A possible clue to mechanism. *Neuropsychologia*, *6*, 11–26.

Shields, S.A. (1991). Gender in the psychology of emotion: A selective research review. In K.T. Strongman (Ed.), *International Review of Studies on Emotion*, Vol. I (pp. 227–245). New York: John Wiley & Sons.

Silberman, E.K., & Weingartner, H. (1986). Hemispheric lateralization of functions related to emotion. *Brain and Cognition*, *5*, 322–353.

Springer, S., & Deutsch, G. (1989). *Left Brain, Right Brain* (3rd ed.). New York: Oxford University Press.

Starkstein, S.S., & Robinson, R.G. (1988). Lateralized emotional response following stroke. In M. Kinsbourne (Ed.), *Cerebral Hemisphere Function in Depression* (pp. 25–47). Washington, DC: American Psychiatric Press.

Stuss, D.T. (1987). Contribution of frontal lobe injury to cognitive impairment after closed head injury—Methods of assessment and recent findings. In H.S. Levin, J. Grafman, & H.M. Eisenberg (Eds.), *Neurobehavioral Recovery after Head Injury* (pp. 166–177). New York: Oxford University Press.

Sutton, S.K., & Davidson, R.J. (1997). Prefrontal brain asymmetry: A biological substrate of the behavioral approach and inhibition systems. *Psychological Science*, *8*, 204–210.

Thatcher, R., Krause, P., & Hrybyk, M. (1986). Cortico-cortical associations and EEG coherence. *Electroencephalography and Clinical Neurophysiology*, *64*, 123–143.

Tomarken, A.J. (1998). Relevance of positive and negative affect constructs of unipolar depression: Evidence from a treatment outcome study. In R.W. Levenson (Chair), *Emotion and Psychopathology*, Symposium conducted at the Tenth American Psychological Society Meeting, Washington, D.C.

Tompkins, C. (1995). *Right Hemisphere Communication Disorders: Theory and Management*. San Diego, CA: Singular Publishing Group.

Trotman, S., & Hammond, G. (1989). Lateral asymmetry of the scalp distribution of somatosensory evoked potential amplitude. *Brain and Cognition*, *10*, 132–147.

Tucker, D.M. (1981). Lateral brain function, emotion, and conceptualization. *Psychological Bulletin*, *89*, 19–46.

Tucker, D.M., Roth, D., & Blair, T. (1986). Functional connections among cortical regions: Topography of EEG coherence. *Electroencephalography and Clinical Neurophysiology, 63*, 242–250.

Tucker, D.M., & Williamson, P. (1984). Asymmetric neural control systems in human self-regulation. *Psychological Review, 91*, 185–215.

Ungerleider, L.G., & Miskin, M. (1982). Two cortical visual systems. In D.J. Ingle, M.A. Goodale, & R.J.W. Mansfield (Eds.), *Analysis of Visual Behavior* (pp. 549–580). Cambridge, MA: MIT.

Vitiello, B., & Stoff, D.M. (1997). Subtypes of aggression and their relevance to child psychiatry. *Journal of the American Academy of Child and Adolescent Psychiatry, 36*, 307–315.

Wagner, H.L., Buck, R., & Winterbotham, M. (1993). Communication of specific emotions: Gender differences in sending accuracy and communication measures. *Journal of Nonverbal Behavior, 17*, 29–52.

Watson, D., Wiese, D., Vaidya, J., & Tellegen, A. (1999). The two general activation systems of affect: Structural findings, evolutionary considerations, and psychobiological evidence. *Journal of Personality and Social Psychology, 76*, 820–838.

Woodward, S.H. (1988). An anatomical model of hemispheric asymmetry [abstract]. *Journal of Clinical and Experimental Neuropsycholology, 10*, 68.

Yecker, S., Borod, J.C., Moreno, C., Welkowitz, J., & Alpert, M. (2000). The accuracy of posed facial emotional expression changes with age [abstract]. *Journal of the International Neuropsychological Society*, in press.

Zuckerman, M., Klorman, R., Larrance, D.T., & Spiegel, N.H. (1981). Facial, autonomic, and subjective components of emotion: The facial feedback hypothesis versus the externalizer-internalizer distinction. *Journal of Personality and Social Psychology, 41*, 929–944.

II

BACKGROUND AND GENERAL TECHNIQUES

2

The Epistemology of Reason and Affect

ROSS W. BUCK

The overwhelming question in neurobiology today is the relation between the mind and the brain.

(Crick & Koch, 1997, p. 19)

Emotions have traditionally been regarded as extras in psychology, not serious mental functions like perception, language, thinking, learning.

(Oatley & Jenkins, 1996, p. 122)

Contemporary investigators interested in the relationship between mind and brain and in the associated questions of knowledge, experience, and consciousness have for the most part centered on higher order cognitive functions—what Oatley and Jenkins (1996) in the above quotation termed *serious mental functions*—and have eschewed the detailed consideration of emotion. Historically, however, emotion more than other psychological phenomena has been intimately connected with the mysterious "mind stuff" of subjective experience. As B.F. Skinner (1953, p. 257) noted, such "private events" are outside the realm of objective observation: They are defined by their "limited accessibility (to the community) but not, so far as we know, by any special structure or nature."

Some advances in the techniques of observing the neurochemical correlates of emotion are relevant to the understanding of subjective experience in general, perhaps making consciousness itself more accessible to objective scrutiny. With this accessibility, comes the opportunity to accommodate our theories to these new observations: to develop a more consensual, formal language with which to describe subjective experience, consciousness, and knowledge. To explore the implications of the new advances in the observation of subjective events, this chapter examines how the public/private distinction has been drawn and the nature of meanings attributed to private events, in modern conceptual philosophy.[1] The chapter outlines the history of philosophical conceptualizations of cognitive and emotional meaning, specifically those of pragmatism, positivism, and ordinary language philosophy, and discusses these with regard to recent advances in understanding the neurobiological bases of emotion.

EPISTEMOLOGY AND NEUROBIOLOGY

Epistemology is the theory of the origin, structure, and validity of knowledge and has generally been considered a branch of philosophy (Runes, 1962). In modern philosophy there is a fundamental distinction between knowledge and discourse that is open to public verification and knowledge and discourse that is not. The epistemological validity of the latter is in dispute: Some consider it to be "meaningless," while others acknowledge that, under some circumstances, what have been termed *emotive* knowledge and discourse have meaning and value. Historically, this debate has been influenced by the degree to which adherents of the different positions recognized the importance of biological processes in thinking and knowing. By and large, those conceptual philosophers who saw value in emotive knowledge were more influenced by biology, particularly Darwin's theory of evolution, and they tended to define the value of emotive knowledge in biological terms.

As conscious experience and thought were increasingly associated with the functioning of the brain, *neurological epistemology* arose from "a need to deal with epistemology on a neurological basis" (Kuhlenbeck, 1965, p. 147). MacLean (1990) coined the term "epistemics" for the study of the subjective brain. Clearly, the facts of neural organization set constraints for epistemology (LeDoux, 1994a, 1996). Moreover, advances in the capacity to observe emotional phenomena—both in the neurology of emotional responding in the brain and in the observation and analysis of the nuances of emotional expression—have opened aspects of private consciousness that were heretofore closed to public verification. Skinner in fact anticipated such advances in his analysis of private events. He wrote, "The line between public and private is not fixed. The boundary shifts with every discovery of a technique for making private events public" (Skinner, 1953, p. 282). These observations are fundamental to understanding the epistemological validity of emotional knowledge. This new understanding offers opportunities both to examine the adequacy of philosophical conceptualizations and to use those conceptualizations to identify important

---

[1]Experiential philosophers, such as the existentialists, also have much to say about consciousness and emotion, but their views are not considered here due to space limitations. See, for example, Sartre (1948, 1957).

questions in the neurobiology of emotion that may have thus far gone unan-swered, or unasked.

PHILOSOPHICAL CONCEPTUALIZATIONS OF COGNITION AND EMOTION

Classical Roots: Monism and Dualism

Since the time of classical Greece in the fifth century B.C., Western thought has distinguished between animalistic energies characteristic of the body and ratio-nal processes associated with "mind" or "soul" unique to human beings. In this *dualistic* position, mind and soul were seen as immaterial and beyond investi-gation except by rational means, that is, by metaphysical speculation. A con-trasting idea of *materialistic monism*, that there is only matter, also appeared in early Greek thought but had less influence at the time. Examples of dualistic thinking are found in the writings of Plato and Aristotle, who presumed that non-human animals have rudimentary "souls" capable of dealing with basic bodily functions but not "rational souls," which were the foundation of human reason and logic. Aristotle distinguished three grades of soul: the *vegetative*, found in all living things; the *sensitive*, characteristic of animals and humans; and the *ra-tional*, possessed only by humans. Following his example, Thomas Aquinas equipped humans with both a "sensitive soul," shared with animals, and a ratio-nal soul (Cofer & Appley, 1964).

In *Meditations* (1641), Rene Descartes contributed the first systematic con-ceptualization of the interaction between mind, or soul, and body. The body is mechanical, public, tangible, visible, and extended in space; the mind/soul is pri-vate, intangible, and invisible. Descartes distinguished between nonhuman ani-mal behavior, which could be accounted for by the reflex-like actions of me-chanical "animal spirits," and human behavior, which was partly mechanical but partly influenced by a rational soul. In his conception, a rational soul makes con-tact with the body at the pineal gland. Conscious sensation occurs when the ra-tional soul becomes aware of the animal spirits: body affecting mind. Conversely, the rational soul can alter the flow of animal spirits: mind affecting body (Woz-niak, 1992). This interaction between spatial body and unextended mind cannot, for Descartes, be comprehended in either spatial or nonspatial terms: It is beyond our capacity to understand. This dilemma has been termed the *Cartesian impasse* (Vesey, 1965) and is reflected perhaps in the "explanatory gap" acknowledged in contemporary theories of consciousness (see Chalmers, 1995; Clark, 1995).

The philosophic tradition from Descartes flowed in two streams: the rational-ism of Spinoza and Leibniz and the empiricism of Locke, Berkeley, and Hume.

Both rationalists and empiricists recognized both *analytic* statements of logic and mathematics and *synthetic* statements of fact and regarded this classification as mutually exclusive. To Hume, it was mutually exhaustive as well: Metaphysical speculation that was neither analytic nor synthetic could be nothing but "sophistry and illusion" (Levi, 1959, p. 333). This argument was to support and sustain a resurgence of materialistic monism in the form of positivism.

Pragmatism

American pragmatism derived its emphasis on science and "hard" facts from the tradition of British empiricism. This was combined, however, with the idea that truth is not absolute and that when we say "this is true" we mean that it is *useful* in some way (Hill, 1961). This doctrine of the functional nature of truth reflected a basic compatibility between pragmatism and evolutionary theory.

Pragmatism has ties to nineteenth century idealism in its doctrine that *the knower conditions the known*: "reality is and can be nothing more than reality-as-known. . . . '[O]bjective' reality is nothing but the most inclusive and coherent system of ideas that the human mind can entertain" (Aiken, 1962a, p. 54). The mind is conceived of as an active agent, not a passive acceptor of sense data. What is "given" in experience is already invested with meaning and significance. A related similarity with idealism is the notion that ideas relate to their cultural and historical context. Furthermore, ideas are purposive: They are always goal-oriented and change with our needs and interests. These themes occur also in recent contextualism and hermeneutic analysis (Taylor, 1992). The pragmatists, however, differ from the idealists and recent theorists in their empirical and behavioral concept of mind and in their emphasis on sense perception and the guidance of the scientific method (when practical) as the best way to reach the objectives of thought. Also, the influence of Darwin's theory on pragmatism placed its spirit worlds apart from that of idealism. Pragmatists regarded thought to be a product of the natural order and conceived of it in essentially biological terms (Aiken, 1962a).

Early nineteenth century philosophy was dominated by what William James was to term "tender-minded" philosophies, such as Emersonian trancendentalism in the United States and neo-Hegelian idealism in England. Darwin's *Origin of Species* (1859) and other scientific advances threatened the adherents of these philosophies: They had to defend their concerns for inner self and spiritual values against the encroachments of positivistic and materialistic scientism, which were supported by Darwin's findings and were actively advanced by Darwinists such as Spencer. The pragmatists did not accept either of the "two extremes of crude naturalism on the one hand and transcendental absolutism on the other" (James, 1907, p. 301). They looked consciously for a position that would reconcile these points of view (White, 1955).

C.S. Peirce

C.S. Peirce is regarded by many as the founder of pragmatism. In his *pragmatic theory of meaning*, Peirce (1877/1962) argued that meaningful propositions must be transformable into hypothetical, operational, experimental statements. Propositions must be translatable into the hypothetical form: "If operation X were to be performed on this, then E would be experienced." The "if" clause must mention an operation performed by the experimenter, and the "then" clause must mention something experienced or observed when the testing conditions are met. This procedure tells what a word denotes by "prescribing what you are to *do* in order to gain a perceptual acquaintance with the object of the word" (Peirce, quoted in White, 1955, p.157). If a proposition resisted translation into the proper form, it was considered scientifically meaningless, although it may evoke images or emotions (White, 1955).

Peirce suggested that the pragmatic theory of meaning rendered meaningless many statements in traditional metaphysics and theology and that, moreover, the theory would show many disputes in philosophy to be pseudoarguments over words or concepts that are pragmatically identical, that is, have the same operational translations. His theory of meaning contributed to the verifiability criterion of meaning of the positivists and to the operationism of P.W. Bridgman (1938), S.S. Stevens (1935) and others.

William James

Peirce's pragmatic theory of meaning was borrowed and modified by William James, who used it in his attempt to reconcile "tender-minded" and "tough-minded" doctrines in philosophy. James offered pragmatism as a "new name for some old ways of thinking" that can satisfy both the demands of the spirit and the demands of fact. He contrasted tender-minded rationalism with tough-minded empiricism, where rationalism "starts from wholes and universals, and makes much of the unity of things" and empiricism "starts from the parts, and makes of the whole a collection" (James, 1907, p. 11).

In *The Principles of Psychology*, James (1890) accepted the idea that good science was positivistic: that everything scientifically knowable is public and that an objective psychology must eliminate subjective factors. In the mid-1890s, he began to revise this idea based on evidence from psychopathological conditions involving emotion and subconscious states. He critiqued scientific materialism with a *metaphysics of radical empiricism*, which was empirical in that it confined itself to the facts of experience but radical in that it demanded that science *not ignore any experience*, including emotional experience (Taylor, 1992). James reinterpreted the foundations of science and religion in his *pragmatic theory of truth*. In the process, he broadened the meanings of Peirce's words "operation" and "experience" so that the operation to be performed was a belief in something and the desired experience was a *feeling of satisfaction*. Thus the statement "S is true" is translated into "if you believe S, you will experience a feeling of satisfaction." The "meaning" lies in those experiences to which the belief, if true, will lead. Verification consists of the occurrence of those experiences (White, 1955).

James' reformulation enabled him to formulate an original theory of meaning, truth, and verification that threw light on many speculative statements bypassed by Peirce. The choice between belief and disbelief in God is meaningful because the adoption of one alternative would lead to different life experiences than the choice of the other (Hill, 1961). Thus, subjective human experience was taken as the ultimate test of truth. This implication led James to be hailed as a savior by some and to be brutally caricatured by others. Peirce dissociated himself from James' formulation by renaming his own view "pragmaticism," a term he described as "ugly enough to be safe from kidnappers" (quoted in White, 1955, p. 158).

White (1955, p. 159) summarized James' position succinctly: "The true is what we ought to believe. That which we ought to believe is what is best for us to believe. Therefore, the true is that which is best for us to believe." This view, however, reflected an ambiguity in utilitarian ethics: What is best for whom? James often answered "the individual," but, as Peirce stated in a letter to James, "What is utility, if it is confined to a single person? Truth is public" (quoted by White, 1955, p. 159). This is the particular theme of pragmatism emphasized by John Dewey.

John Dewey

To Dewey, James' account of truth was too individual and capricious. Dewey used Peirce's pragmatic theory of meaning as the foundation for a theory of social and public morality. Where James used pragmatic theory to explain the "true," Dewey used it to explain the "good" and, with George Santayana, the "beautiful" as well (White, 1955). Dewey offered an ethical theory that, like James', attempted to steer a moderate course between ideas of "transcendent eternal values" and the "empirical" view that value is defined by mere personal liking, desire, enjoyment, or interest.

Peirce's question of "what is best for whom?" can be viewed in terms of Darwin's theory: What is best is that which promotes successful adaptation. The idea of adaptation is consonant with pragmatism, and indeed Dewey approached the idea of public good from a Darwinian point of view. He wrote that Darwinism "led straight to the perception of the importance of distinctive social categories especially communication and participation." He continued, arguing that "a great deal of our philosophizing needs to be done over again from this point of view, and that there will ultimately result an integrated synthesis in philosophy congruous with modern science and related to actual needs in education, morals, and religion" (Dewey, 1931, p. 3). One of his contributions was the idea of a "problematic situation," which was at once biologically rooted and socially enveloped.

Conclusions

In pragmatism, one finds the idea of knowledge as a product of the natural order, suggesting that emotional knowledge may be evaluated according to biological criteria. Also, the essence of scientific methodology is distilled in Peirce's operationism: that to be scientifically meaningful, a proposition must be translatable into an operation that must reliably produce an observation or experience. James extended this so that emotional experiences—for example, of satisfaction—could be used as criteria of meaning and truth. Dewey and others suggested that common values, not individual satisfaction, be used as the criterion not of "truth" but of "good" and "beauty." While James' and Dewey's conceptions tended to moderate and expand the venue of Peirce's operationism into the realm of emotional meaning, the logical positivists applied it much more strictly and rigorously.

Positivism

Positivism is the doctrine that the highest form of knowledge is a simple description of sensory phenomena (Carnap, 1937; Runes, 1962). In contrast with the pragmatists, the positivists of the early twentieth century based their conceptualizations on mathematics and logic: They tended to be uncompromisingly "tough-minded" and were not greatly influenced by biological thinking. In logical positivism was found most directly the faith that human beings come to knowledge through erecting abstract concepts that are based ultimately on publicly verifiable operations. The positivists considered that difficulties arise when concepts are not clearly grounded in observations. They considered the function of philosophy to be analysis and clarification, and a major goal of the early positivists was to construct a perfectly simple, clear, and logical artificial language for science that could clarify scientific statements, free of the entanglements of ordinary language. Judgments of value and beauty and statements expressing feeling were seen to be devoid of cognitive content and were largely ignored.

English neorealism

Bertrand Russell and Alfred North Whitehead formulated the basis for the analysis and construction of ideal, artificial systems of language, logic, and mathematics in three volumes of *Principia Mathematica* (1910–1913). Their objective was to demonstrate that mathematics is derivable from logic, and they introduced technical innovations that both contributed to modern symbolic logic and gave positivism a methodology and the model for an artificial but unambiguous symbolic language (Levi, 1959).

Another major contribution of Russell to positivism was his logical atomism in which he attempted a logical reconstruction of physics. This described the physical universe as if it could be described in terms similar in form to those in *Principia Mathematica*. "Logical atoms" were independent, primitive notions used to describe the rest of the universe. It was reasoned that, if the truths of mathematics, science, and common sense can be dealt with in a logically perfect language, it would allow us to know precisely what we are saying and whether it is logically true. The presupposition is that the world of logical discourse is similar in structure to the world of fact and that the elimination of internal inconsistency in the one will provide a clue to the structure of the other. It is in terms of logical atoms that a perfectly logical scientific language would describe the world (Aiken, 1962b; Levi, 1959).

Between 1911 and 1913, the Austrian Ludwig Wittgenstein was at Cambridge and came under the influence of the new logic. In 1922 he published *Tractatus Logico-Philosophicus*, which was a radical restatement of Russell's logical atomism. Wittgenstein argued that statements that describe or mirror atomic facts are the basis of science. A perfect scientific language would provide a mirror for the structure of reality. Ordinary language cannot provide this mirror because it contains impossible problems of meaning and implication. It is for this reason that philosophical analysis exists. Given a logically perfect language, as approximated in *Principia Mathematica*, statements could be mechanically reduced to their basic atomic facts. This language would resemble a calculus, with clear and simple basic terms (Aiken, 1962b). Wittgenstein distinguished between factual, or synthetic, and logical and mathematical, or analytic, propositions. The latter are always tautologies and tell us nothing about the world. They merely tell us what we can infer from true and false statements (Barrett, 1962).

The Vienna Circle

Wittgenstein's logical atomism and distinction between analytic and synthetic propositions impressed a group of philosophers in Vienna. The "Vienna Circle" was founded in 1923 in a seminar organized by Moritz Schlick. Its most important period began in 1926, when Rudolf Carnap joined the university faculty. The Circle published a manifesto in 1929 and a periodical, *Erkenntnis*, beginning in 1930. In 1938, the group broke up with the fall of Austria to the Nazis (Levi, 1959).

The classic viewpoint of the positivists of the Vienna Circle was summarized by Levi (1959, pp. 344–345). It included the proposition that "all cognitively significant (meaningful) discourse is divisible without remainder into analytic or synthetic propositions." This asserts the crucial distinction between the tautologous statements of logic and mathematics and the factual statements of the sciences, which are considered probably true or probably false. Also, "any proposition that purports to be factual or empirical has meaning only if it is possible in principle to describe a method for its verification." This is the verifiability criterion, closely related to Peirce's criterion of meaning. Furthermore, "all metaphysical assertions, being neither analytic nor synthetic, are meaningless" and "all normative assertions . . . are scientifically unverifiable, and are therefore to be classified as forms of non-cognitive discourse." Noncognitive discourse was termed emotive discourse. Emotive statements are not meaningless, for they express how we feel, but they are not "cognitive" (Levi, 1959).

When the Vienna Circle was formed, the positivists thought that they were absolutely right and were spoiling for a fight with other positions. At this time, their principal weapons were simplicity and clarity (Bochenski, 1961). Beginning in the mid-1930s, however, the positivists came to realize that things were not as clear and simple as they had seemed. Their methods were found to be quite limited, and they were forced to become more flexible, moving in the process toward "a rapprochement with pragmatism" (Barrett, 1962, p. 13). One of the changes in the positivist outlook reflected the fact that their definition of cognitive discourse was so restrictive that large areas of experience remained untouched. The neat analytic–synthetic dualism did not deal with the meaning of "emotive discourse," including value statements like "the painting is beautiful" as opposed to the cognitive statement "the painting is red." Also, statements of feeling, while seen as "noncognitive" were not held to be meaningless.

The Analysis of Ordinary Language

Ludwig Wittgenstein

Wittgenstein eventually abandoned the attempt to develop an ideal artificial language and became skeptical of the very foundation of *Principia Mathematica*. Possibly this was in part a result of Goedel's 1933 theorem proving the incompleteness of mathematics: that any mathematical system must contain true but unprovable statements (Levi, 1959). This discovery revealed mathematics in a light different from what Wittgenstein had seen in *Tractatus*: The tautological character of mathematics was no longer so clear (Barrett, 1962). Instead, Wittgenstein came to agree with G.E. Moore that the common sense statements of ordinary language are the proper objects of analysis (Aiken, 1962b).

Rather than pursue unattainable ideals of simplicity and clarity by analyzing unreduceable "logical atoms" and a fixed syntactic calculus, Wittgenstein came to see language as inevitably complex and organic (1965). The forms of words do not represent the structures of things; instead, they represent forms of life (Aiken, 1962b). Wittgenstein compared language to "an ancient city: a maze of little streets and squares, of old and new houses . . . surrounded by a multitude of new boroughs with straight regular streets and new houses" (Levi, 1959, p. 436). Instead of reforming language, Wittgenstein now sought to understand it.

Central to his new conceptualization was the idea of "language games." Wittgenstein suggested that it is pointless to search for a common element in all that we call "language." The elements of language are related to one another in myriad ways, and one common relationship cannot be found. "Language" is the name of these related elements, just as "games" is not an expression of some common trait that can be found in all of the activities that we call "games." That series of relationships and similarities, overlapping and crisscrossing like the twisted fibers, makes up the thread called "language" or "games." This thread of similarities is termed a "family," exhibiting "family resemblances," rather than a unitary "essence" that characterizes all examples of the phenomenon of "language" or "games" (Wittgenstein, 1953).

This concept of language gave Wittgenstein a new viewpoint on philosophical puzzles and their resolution. He became interested in the things that drive philosophers into bizarre and maddening enigmas, suggesting that the origin of such riddles stems from the improper use of language and that such riddles can be eliminated only by the meticulous analysis of language as it is actually used (White, 1955). "Philosophy," he said, "is a battle against the bewitchment of our intelligence by means of language" (Levi, 1959, p. 441).

Gilbert Ryle: The ghost in the machine

One such enigma is the Cartesian impasse: the incomprehensible idea of a purely spiritual mind joined somehow to a purely material body. Gilbert Ryle (1949, pp. 15–16) ridiculed this as the "dogma of the ghost in the machine." Ryle argued that the "Cartesian myth" is an illusion arising from an improper use of language. Specifically, he argued that speaking of mind as if it were a substance in the same logical category as the body is a *category error* analogous to speaking of "the university" as if it were a substance of the same logical category as classrooms, laboratories, libraries, and the like. Actually, mind is an organizing principle of a different logical type than the body, just as the university is an organizing principle encompassing its constituent elements. He noted that the theoretically interesting category mistakes are those where people are perfectly competent in applying a concept in ordinary life but have difficulty when thinking abstractly about the concept, relating it inappropriately with other abstract concepts.

Ryle (1949, p. 83) singled out the realm of emotion as one where Cartesian thinking is particularly intractable: Most philosophers and psychologists, he noted, view emotions as "internal or private experiences. . . . They are occurrences that take place not in the public, physical world but your or my secret, mental world." Ryle suggested that the word "emotion" is used to designate four different kinds of things, including *inclinations* (or motives), *agitations* (similar to conflicts), *moods*, and *feelings*. He argued that inclinations, agitations, and moods are "not occurrences and do not therefore take place either publicly or privately. They are propensities, not acts or states" (Ryle, 1949, p. 83). Thus brittleness is a propensity of glass to break when struck. Although we may say "the glass broke because it is brittle" or "the glass broke because it was struck," only the latter statement denotes an *occurrence*. Ryle (1949, p. 83) continued: "feelings, on the other hand, are occurrences, but the place that mention of them should take in descriptions of human behaviour is very different from that which the standard theories accord to it." He noted that James defined feelings in terms of bodily sensations, but wrote "for our purposes it is enough to show that we talk of feelings very much as we talk of bodily sensations, though it is possible that there is a tinge of metaphor in our talk of the former which is absent from our talk of the latter" (Ryle, 1949, p. 84).

Ryle suggested that feelings are *signs of agitations* and offered an analogy with a stomach ache as a sign of indigestion. He asserted that there are no necessary or sufficient criteria for either: "[Feelings] are signs of agitations in the same sort of way as stomach-aches are signs of indigestion. Roughly, we do not, as the prevalent theory holds, act purposively because we experience feelings; we experience feelings, as we wince and shudder, because we are inhibited from acting purposively" (Ryle, 1949, p. 106). He goes on, "we can induce in ourselves genuine and acute feelings by merely imagining ourselves in agitating circumstances. Novel-readers and theatergoers feel real pangs and real liftings of the heart, just as they may shed real tears and scowl unfeigned scowls. But their distresses and indignations are feigned. They do not affect their owners' appetites for chocolates, or change the tones of voice of their conversations. Sentimentalists are people who indulge in induced feelings without acknowledging the fictitiousness of their agitations" (Ryle, 1949, p. 107).

Discussion

Ryle hoped that the proper use of language would resolve the Cartesian impasse, but that particular quandary remains: In the words of Crick and Koch (1997, p. 19), "the overwhelming question in neurobiology today is the relation between the mind and the brain." The new ability to observe brain functioning may, however, allow us to reformulate the issues in useful ways. In this regard, Barrett (1962, p. 62) pointed out that there are "large areas of experience where our language is not yet ripe for any significant attempt at formalization." As areas amenable to public observation expand with improved techniques for "making private events public," in Skinner's words (1953, p. 282), formalization of language will naturally follow. Arguably this is occurring today in the realm of emotion theory.

In this regard, Barrett (1962, p. 17) also suggested that the positivistic understanding of "cognitive" is constructed on an overly narrow model. He described and critiqued the positivists' position on feeling and emotion, noting that in their writings feelings are "some kind of subcutaneous twinges, throbs, or tremors that in some odd way lie on the opposite side of mind from intellect and reason, which are the truly cognitive faculties." But, he pointed out, "Ordinary language contains plenty of uses where we speak of knowledge in connection with the presence of feeling and ignorance in connection with its absence." He concluded, "Feeling is not a blind stab or spasm of some psychic substance underlying mind, but a form of consciousness that, like every other mode of consciousness, has its own intentionality and revelation."

Barrett's critique (1962) of the positivist view of cognition and emotion is compatible with recent analyses of emotion as constituting a type of cognition. Arguably emotional knowledge is functional—it has survival value in an evolutionary sense—and is "meaningful" from the pragmatic perspective. The next section considers the nature of emotional and cognitive knowledge from a neurobiological viewpoint.

EMOTIONAL AND COGNITIVE KNOWLEDGE

We have seen that many modern philosophers have considered "emotion" and "cognition" to be mutually exclusive, with cognition being associated with public knowledge and discourse and emotion consigned to a "noncognitive" private knowledge of doubtful epistemological status. Recent research in the neurosciences has afforded a greater objective understanding of how the brain processes underlying what have traditionally been termed *emotional* and *cognitive* knowledge differ, and this understanding offers insights into the functions of this knowledge. More specifically, there is evidence that "emotion" and "cognition" differ in level and speed of brain processing.

Level of Brain Processing

In 1927, Bertrand Russell anticipated a major contemporary theory of emotion in an account of a visit to a dentist. Russell (1927, p. 226) discussed the "radical transformation" in the theory of emotion wrought by Cannon (1915), suggesting that certain endocrine secretions are the "essential physiological conditions of the emotions." The dentist had injected adrenaline in the course of administering a local anesthetic. Russell (1927, pp. 226–227) wrote: "I turned pale and trembled, and my heart beat violently; the bodily symptoms of fear were present, as the books said they should be, but it was quite obvious to me that I was not actually feeling fear. . . . What was different was the cognitive part: I did not feel fear because I knew that there was nothing to be afraid of."

The idea that emotion involves an interaction between "cognitive" and "physiological" factors was the basis of the well-known Schachter and Singer (1962) study and self-attribution theory of emotion. This theory suggested that cognitive elements are responsible for the qualitative aspects, and physiological factors the quantitative aspects, of emotion. Russell recognized, however, that "physiological" factors could be responsible for qualitative aspects of emotion as well. He suggested that some emotions such as melancholia, "presumably, can be caused in their entirety by administering the proper secretions" (Russell, 1927, p. 227).

We now know that the physiological bases of emotion involve far more than the autonomic and endocrine systems: There are basic emotion circuits that reflect primal survival demands, prompting rapid and coherent responses. These interact with higher level brain systems that contribute increased flexibility that can reflect strategic considerations (Panksepp, 1994a).

Speed of Brain Processing

The Zajonc-Lazarus debate

The question of the speed of emotional processing was central to one of the classic debates in recent emotion theory, concerning whether "emotion" precedes or follows "cognition." The Zajonc-Lazarus debate is instructive both because it illustrates how differences in the use of language and the definition of terms can produce apparent theoretical quandaries with devout adherents on both sides and because it was resolved by the results of neurobiological research.

The debate began with evidence that subjects could respond preferentially to stimuli without "knowing" what they were: Familiar nonsense syllables and ideograms were rated more positively even though subjects could not recognize them as familiar. On this and other evidence, Robert Zajonc (1980, 1984) argued that affect occurs before, and independently of, cognition. His argument drew a strong response from Richard Lazarus (1982, 1984), who argued, based on his own research, that emotion could not occur without prior "cognitive appraisal."

Examination of the arguments of Zajonc and Lazarus reveals that their disagreement rests on how each defined "cognition." Both had developed verifiable operational definitions of the construct "cognition," but what was not immediately apparent was that these operations were quite different. Zajonc (1984) defined *cognition* as involving some kind of "mental work": some transformation of sensory input or information processing. For Lazarus, *cognition* could involve a "primitive evaluative perception" (1984, p. 124) that was "global or spherical" (1982, p. 1020). In effect, both Zajonc and Lazarus agreed that *some* sort of sensory information is necessary for emotion, but they disagreed on what would constitute "cognition."

The LeDoux resolution

The Zajonc-Lazarus debate was resolved by the findings of LeDoux and his colleagues that fear involves an interaction between fast processing associated with the amygdala and slower but more elaborate representation associated with the neocortex. Specifically, stimuli reach the amygdala directly via the thalamus: a short and fast route. Because it bypasses the cortex, the amygdala receives directly only a "crude, almost archetypical" representation of the stimulus, which is shortly followed by a more accurate representation involving cortical processing (LeDoux, 1996, p. 166). This neural organization indicates that we "begin to respond to the emotional significance of a stimulus before we fully represent that stimulus" (LeDoux, 1994a, p. 221).

LeDoux (1996, p. 202) also found that the memories of fearful experiences involve at least two sorts of neural organization: an *implicit emotional memory* system associated with the amygdala and a *declarative* or *explicit memory* system associated with the hippocampus that is associated with conscious recollection. These normally operate simultaneously and in parallel, but their functioning can be dissociated in experimental animals and in rare case studies in human beings (LeDoux, 1994b).

LeDoux's data suggest that both Zajonc and Lazarus are correct, but the former limits the definition of "cognition" to the slower, representational process and the latter regards the initial fast response as "cognitive." In any event, the labeling becomes trivial once the neural organization is understood. However we choose to label what goes on (relatively) early and late in the response to events, there is a fast initial response that biases slower representational processing and a more elaborate processing that feeds back and alters the fast response.

MOTIVATION, EMOTION, COGNITION, AND KNOWLEDGE

The LeDoux resolution of the Zajonc-Lazarus debate suggests how language can become trivial once we understand the neural organization underlying what we call *emotion* and *cognition*, and objective neurobiological investigation has the potential to inform other semantic puzzles as well. At that level of understanding, what Barrett (1962) termed the *formalization* of language becomes possible, and we move away from everyday language toward a more specific variety more like the sort championed by the positivists. The formalization of language in a given area of inquiry follows naturally upon public verifiability of fundamental phenomena in that area. If phenomena are not publicly observable, it does not necessarily mean that discourse concerning them is meaningless but rather that *consensual and accurate communication using such discourse is difficult to achieve* because of the slippery nature of language. Verifiability lays the groundwork for formalizing language, but at the same time the language per se in a sense becomes less important. If a theoretical statement is testable it is also trivial, in the sense that it is the testing that is really important. This was demonstrated by the definition of *cognition* being rendered secondary to the operations employed in LeDoux's research.

Before we do fully understand a psychological phenomenon objectively at the level of public verification, however, language is anything but trivial. It is *all we have* to communicate and attempt to come to an understanding about that phenomenon, including how to come eventually to measure it. The criteria for meaning in such discourse remain the classic criteria of rhetoric: the internal consistency of the argument; its cogency, cohesiveness, clarity, simplicity, fruitfulness, eloquence. Some aspects of human experience may forever remain in the realm of the poet or experiential philosopher, whose only tools are language: perhaps the more "emotive" the better.[2]

The remainder of this chapter considers the language used to describe the origin, structure, and validity of knowledge, taking into account recent observations involving emotion in the behavioral and neural sciences. It is suggested that "emotion" and "cognition" are not in fact distinct phenomena: that emotion always involves cognition and, more controversially perhaps, cognition always involves emotion. Furthermore, both emotion and cognition always involve "motivation" and vice versa. In the following, conceptual definitions for, and interactions between, "motivation," "emotion," and "cognition" are laid out.

Defining Motivation, Emotion, and Cognition

Developmental–interactionist theory attempts a unified conceptualization of motivation, emotion, and cognition based on the assumption that one cannot coherently describe or define "motivation," "emotion," or "cognition" without considering both of the other terms. Each is involved in both of the others: Motivation intrinsically involves emotion and cognition, cognition involves motivation and emotion, and emotion involves motivation and cognition (Buck, 1985).

Motivation and emotion

Motivation is defined as the potential for behavior that is built into a system of behavior control and *emotion* as the manifestation or *readout* of motivational potential when activated by a challenging stimulus (Buck, 1985, 1988, 1994a; Buck et al., 1997). The relationship between emotion and motivation is seen to be analogous to that between matter and energy in physics. Energy is a potential that is not seen in itself but rather is manifested in matter: in heat, light, force, and so forth. The energy per se is never shown. Similarly, motivation is conceptualized as a potential that is not seen in itself but rather is manifested in emo-

---

[2]Emotion can be communicated *spontaneously* via biologically based sending and receiving mechanisms. This topic is beyond the scope of this chapter, but see Buck and Ginsburg (1997) for a discussion of the evolutionary epistemology of empathy.

tion. Motivation and emotion are thus seen as two sides of the same coin or as aspects of a common core phenomenon: the *motivational–emotional system*. Phylogenetically structured primary motivational-emotional systems (*primes*) are considered to be "special-purpose processing systems" that over the course of development interact with "general purpose processing systems" that reflect the capacity of the species for learning via classical conditioning, instrumental learning, higher order cognitive processing, and, in human beings, language.

Cognition

Cognition is defined as knowledge that is based on "raw" awareness or *knowledge-by-acquaintance*. This basic knowledge, driven and guided by motivational–emotional systems, is spontaneously restructured into representational *knowledge-by-description* over the course of development (Piaget, 1971). Knowledge-by-acquaintance was described by Bertrand Russell (1912/1959, p. 46) as the presentational immediacy of experience that is completely self-evident. William James (1890/1952, p. 144, italics in the original) noted: "I know the color blue when I see it, and the flavor of a pear when I taste it . . . but *about* the inner nature of these facts or what makes them what they are, I can say nothing at all. I cannot impart acquaintance with them to any one who has not made it himself." Thus knowledge-by-acquaintance is always "true," or veridical, in a sense. In contrast, knowldege-by-description is not self-evident and can be false.

Knowledge-by-acquaintance constitutes the raw data of perception based on perceptual systems evolved to detect information in the form of stimulus energy: in light, vibration, and volatile chemical substances physically present in the environment (Gibson, 1966, 1979). James J. Gibson's theory of *ecological realism* provides a coherent and detailed account of the evolution of knowledge from the earliest organisms to human perception. Gibson (1979, p. 255) termed raw perception *awareness*: "To perceive is to be aware of the surfaces of the environment and of oneself in it." Awareness is direct, self-evident, and nonrepresentational: "percepts *qua* percepts are the ultimate actualities and are not experienced as representing something else. . . . " (Kuhlenbeck, 1965, p. 144. Italics in the original).

According to Gibson, species evolved to be sensitive to those aspects of the environment that afford possibilities or opportunities for behavior: *affordances*. There are three sorts of "raw" awareness. First, there is awareness of affordances in the terrestrial environment, such as those provided by physical objects as support, obstacles to motion, and so forth. Second, there is awareness of *social affordances* provided by other animals: "other animals afford, above all, a rich and complex set of interactions, sexual, predatory, nurturing, fighting, playing, cooperating, and communicating" (Gibson, 1979, p. 128). Emotional displays can be considered to be social affordances (Buck, 1984; Buck & Ginsburg, 1997; McArthur & Baron, 1983). Third, Gibson (1966, p. 31) recognized awareness via *interoceptors* of vague sensations of internal origin—feelings and emotions—

the "pangs and pressures of the internal environment." These may be conceptualized as *bodily affordances*, and in the present view subjectively experienced *affects*—feelings and desires—constitute awareness of bodily affordances.

In contrast to raw awareness or knowledge-by-acquaintance, knowledge-by-description is representational, constructed from the restructuring or processing of raw perceptual data. Thus we have direct perceptual acquaintance with events in the terrestrial environment, social environment, and internal bodily environment and representational knowledge *about* these events based on information processing and inference. *Agnosias*, where elementary perception is intact but "stripped of meaning" (Bauer, 1984, p. 457), might constitute an inability to transfer specific sorts of knowledge by acquaintance into knowledge-by-description (Buck, 1990).

Affect

The subjective experience of emotion involves a direct interoceptive knowledge-by-acquaintance of bodily processes serving functions of self-regulation. "Bodily processes" in this context do not refer to feedback from autonomic responses or expressive behaviors; rather, they are specific neurochemical systems of internal perception that have evolved to inform the organism of functionally important events in the bodily milieu. The experiential aspects or *qualia* associated with these interoceptive perceptual systems are feelings and desires (Buck, 1993). The events of which they inform include needs for food (hunger), for water (thirst), for warmth or cold, for sex, and so forth; these are *drives* involving specific bodily needs. We are also informed of more general need states involving *primary affects*, such as happiness, sadness, fear, and anger.

Affect is defined formally as the direct knowledge-by-acquaintance of feelings and desires based on readouts of specifiable neurochemical systems evolved by natural selection as phylogenetic adaptations functioning to inform the organism of bodily events important in self-regulation (Buck, 1985, 1994a). Affects are special-purpose, gene-based, neurochemical readouts. The subjective phenomenal reality of affect is self-evident and is experienced directly and immediately. Also, *affects are always present*: A constant readout of feelings and desires is available at all times. We can always turn our attention to "pick up" how hungry, or thirsty, or warm we are and also how happy, sad, or angry. We tend spontaneously to *notice* this information only when it is strong or sudden, but, like the feel of our shoes on our feet, it is always with us. Relatively strong affects associated with specific elicitors are typically termed *emotions* as compared with *moods*, which last longer and are not so associated with specific elicitors (Ekman & Davidson, 1994).

Affective and rational cognition

Tucker's distinction (1981) between *syncretic* and *analytic cognition* is related to, but not identical with, the knowledge-by-acquaintance versus knowledge-by-description distinction. Knowledge-by-acquaintance is syncretic cognition: hot, holistic, direct, immediate, and self-evident raw acquaintance. In contrast, much but not all knowledge-by-description is analytic cognition: cold, sequential, and linear information processing (an exception involves spatial knowledge-by-description). Combining Tucker's conceptualization (1981) with the present one, we may say that *affective cognition* is syncretic and based on special-purpose systems, while *rational cognition* is analytic and based on general-purpose systems (Buck, 1985; Buck & Chaudhuri, 1994; Chaudhuri & Buck, 1995).

The Interaction of Affective and Rational Cognition

Biologically based primes are considered to be special-purpose systems arranged in a hierarchy in which the interaction with general-purpose systems becomes more important as one goes up the hierarchy (Buck, 1985). The simplest primes are *reflexes* where the response is wholly "hard wired" and innate, with virtually no flexibility. At the next position on the hierarchy are fixed action patterns, or *instincts*, which are quite inflexible when examined closely: One cannot teach salmon to change their migratory behavior. The next level of the primes does, however, involve flexibility. *Drives* involve specific bodily needs that are signaled to the organism by affects: desires like hunger and thirst that function to activate and direct behavior so that the organism explores its surroundings to search out and learn to find relevant resources. The next level of the hierarchy does not involve specific needs: The *primary affects* signal a bodily state but do not influence behavior directly. The individual knows that he or she is happy or angry and may or may not know why; but no specific behaviors are activated. Instead, the affects function to facilitate flexibility and *choice* among alternative behaviors: The individual has a choice about what to do, and if, for example, anger is felt toward a large person or a small person, the behavior will be different.

As one proceeds up the hierarchy from reflexes to instincts, to drives, to affects, the interaction between special-purpose and general-purpose systems increasingly favors the latter. The dimension presented in the upper section of Figure 2.1 arguably more accurately reflects the relationship between affect and reason than does the more usual categorical distinction between "emotion" and "cognition." Also, other phenomena may be usefully placed on this dimension. For example, the dimension mirrors the phylogenetic scale, with simple creatures' behavior (ants, bees) being mostly a matter of reflexes and creatures with significant analytic–cognitive capacities being at the other extreme. The progressive evolution of learning abilities that confer increased behavioral plasticity has been termed *anagenesis* (Gottlieb, 1984). The developmental scale may also be represented, with the more hard-wired infant at the left and the adult at

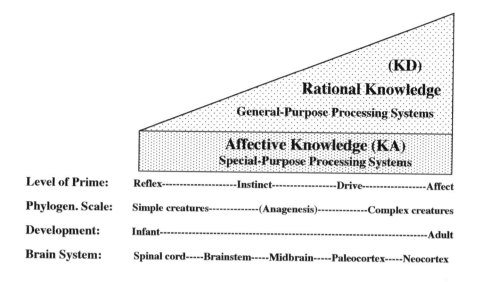

Level of Prime:	Reflex--------------------Instinct-----------------Drive----------------Affect
Phylogen. Scale:	Simple creatures--------------(Anagenesis)--------------Complex creatures
Development:	Infant---Adult
Brain System:	Spinal cord-----Brainstem-----Midbrain-----Paleocortex-----Neocortex

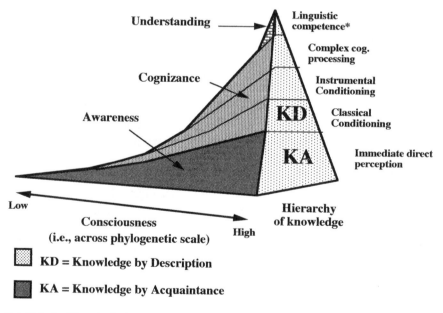

* A.K.A. the Ghost in the Machine (Ryle, 1949).

Figure 2.1. (Upper) The interaction of affective and rational cognition. *Ryle's "ghost in the machine" (1949). (Lower) The hierarchy of knowledge. See text for description.

the right. Finally, the dimension can represent the evolution of the nervous system, with functions served by more "primitive" structures to the left and to the right increasingly complex functions based on brain stem, midbrain, paleocortical, and neocortical processing.

Levels of Knowledge

A hierarchy of knowledge

The relationship between affect and reason can also be presented in terms of three levels of knowledge, which is illustrated in the lower section of Figure 2.1. The most fundamental sort of knowledge is Gibson's *awareness* (1966) constituting knowledge-by-acquaintance: Thus we have an immediate acquaintance with the external physical environment (terrestrial awareness), of other organisms (social awareness), and of oneself (self/bodily awareness). The latter includes the affects. All living creatures, even the simplest, manifest this basic awareness: In this sense it is similar to Aristotle's "vegetative soul." Knowledge-by-description is termed *cognizance*, and Figure 2.1 shows three levels of cognizance: associative classical conditioning, goal-directed instrumental learning, and higher order cognitive processing. These progressively complex sorts of learning came into existence successively over the course of evolution, and they conferred progressively greater behavioral flexibility. Knowledge about the environment is terrestrial cognizance, knowledge about others is social cognizance, and knowledge about the self, including the affects, is self/body cognizance. Such representational knowledge is characteristic both of human beings and other animals and is perhaps analogous to Aristotle's "sensitive soul." The level of knowledge that differentiates human beings and nonhuman animals involves language (Buck, 1994b): Arguably linguistic competence is also what distinguishes Aristotle's "rational soul." Linguistic knowledge might be termed *understanding*, yielding terrestrial understanding, social understanding, and self and body understanding. Self-understanding involves a system of rules that is structured by learning, cognition, and language over the life of the individual, including rules about the experience and expression of affects.

The role of language

These formal rules constitute a system of behavior control that allows human behavior to come under the influence of factors outside the experience of the individual organism. All other creatures are constrained by their own individual experience during development. They can never escape their own experience no matter how powerful their higher order cognitive processes. Human beings, in contrast, can be informed via language by the experiences of those long gone and can imagine events that never have been and indeed never could be experienced, such as counting the number of angels standing on the head of a pin or falling into a black hole. This perhaps is the origin of an essential dualism in the human species apart from the mind–body issue. Language imparts to human behavior a formal, logical structure that does not exist in nonhuman animals. Whereas the forces of natural selection have shaped animal behavior, human behavior is influenced as well by formal, linguistically structured, and socially constructed social rules. This formal linguistic influence is perhaps in fact analogous in some ways to Ryle's "ghost in the machine" (Buck, 1994b). Specifically, language competence involves principles for organizing behavior that are absent in nonhuman animals.

Consciousness

Consciousness is represented in Figure 2.1 as ranging from the raw knowledge-by-acquaintance of simple creatures, through the addition of representational knowledge-by-description, to human linguistic understanding. An assumption here is that consciousness is an emergent function of raw Gibsonian awareness; another is that earlier forms of nonconscious awareness gradually evolved into consciousness but that the earlier forms persist in complex creatures. For example, Panksepp (1994a) has cited evidence that the dream state associated with REM sleep may reflect the functioning of an ancient arousal mechanism associated with emotion.

LeDoux and Panksepp have expressed different but perhaps compatible views regarding emotion and consciousness. LeDoux (1994b) suggested that there is one mechanism of consciousness that is usually filled with the ordinary concerns of daily life, with the capacity to be directed toward objects of interest. When a threatening object is encountered, the emotion network associated with fear takes over, directing consciousness to relevant objects. Panksepp, in comparison, associated different sorts of emotional consciousness with different neural systems. He noted that "there seem to be as many distinct internally experienced affective states as there are basic motivational and emotional systems of the brain" (Panksepp, 1994b, p. 396) and suggested that "all mammals probably experience essentially similar types of basic motivational and emotional feeling states" (p. 399).

It is illuminating to apply these ideas to the example of an emotional situation suggested by Scherer (personal communication, 1996): losing one's luggage at the airport. Typically, at the airport one is filled with ordinary concerns, but if one's baggage is lost attention is directed to coping processes that can involve a variety of affects. One might consider ordinary functioning to be on the right side of the affect–reason model in Figure 2.1 and that losing one's luggage would tend to move functioning to the left, with an increase in the relative ratio of affective to rational functioning. To take the example further, if one loses one's *child* at the airport, the ratio of affective functioning might increase rather more and perhaps particularly involve basic physiological systems associated with panic (Panksepp, 1982). Furthermore, if one loses one's *engines* at the airport, the resulting response might be even more "irrational" and physiologically based. Finally, if the child is found or the emergency landing is made successfully, the relief and joy experienced may similarly overwhelm rational considerations.

SUMMARY

A guiding thesis of the chapter is that a greater scientific understanding of that most "subjective" of phenomena, emotion, can contribute to understanding more general problems of conscious experience: that a well-grounded and valid conceptualization of emotional knowledge is crucial to understanding the relation between the mind and the brain. The chapter has discussed the history of philosophical discussions of the epistemological status of public and private events and suggested that one of the dilemmas with private events is that it is difficult to construct consensual language to define and describe them. As emotional events become more public due to technical advances, conceptual advances in the formalization of language naturally follow. An example is the formalization of the concept of "cognition" from LeDoux's research. In this regard, a conceptualization of how motivation, emotion, and cognition are related is presented. A major proposition is that *emotion in fact involves a kind of cognition, a kind of knowledge*. Analytic "rational" versus syncretic "affective" knowledge are distinguished and related to three levels corresponding roughly with Aristotle's three grades of soul: direct, "raw" acquaintance, or *awareness*; representational knowledge *about* knowledge, or *cognizance*; and formal linguistic knowledge, or *understanding*. These levels can be observed in knowledge of the external world as well as in emotional knowledge and can be associated with levels of neural functioning in the brain, from subcortical systems associated with fast but crude processing to the more accurate, precise, and detailed processing associated with cortical systems.

As for the Cartesian impasse? Perhaps eventually human language and understanding will bridge the gap, but it may involve a reconceptualization of the basic nature of physical reality (see Hameroff & Penrose, 1996).

REFERENCES

Aiken, H.D. (1962a). Introduction. In W. Barrett & H.D. Aiken (Eds.), *Philosophy in the Twentieth Century: An Anthology, Vol. 1: Pragmatism* (pp. 47–81). New York: Random House.
Aiken, H.D. (1962b). Introduction. In W. Barrett & H.D. Aiken (Eds.), *Philosophy in the*

Twentieth Century, Vol. 2: The Rise of Analytical Philosophy in England (pp. 464–496). New York: Random House.

Barrett, W. (1962). Introduction. In W. Barrett & H.D. Aiken (Eds.), *Philosophy in the Twentieth Century: An Anthology, Vol. 3: Positivism* (pp. 5–21). New York: Random House.

Bauer, R.M. (1984). Autonomic recognition of names and faces in prosopagnosia: A neuropsychological application of the guilty knowledge test. *Neuropsychologia, 22*, 456–469.

Bochenski, I.M. (1961). *Contemporary European Philosophy*. Berkeley: University of California Press.

Bridgman, P.W. (1938). *The Intelligent Individual and Society*. New York: Macmillan.

Buck, R. (1984). *The Communication of Emotion*. New York: Guilford Press.

Buck, R. (1985). Prime theory: An integrated view of motivation and emotion. *Psychological Review, 92*, 389–413.

Buck, R. (1988) *Human Motivation and Emotion,* 2nd Ed. New York: Wiley.

Buck, R. (1990) William James and current issues in emotion, cognition, and communication. *Personality and Social Psychology Bulletin. 16(4)*, 612–625.

Buck, R. (1993). What is this thing called subjective experience? Reflections on the neuropsychology of qualia. *Neuropsychology, 7(4)*, 490–499.

Buck, R. (1994a). Social and emotional functions in facial expression and communication: The readout hypothesis. *Biological Psychology, 38*, 95–115.

Buck, R. (1994b). The neuropsychology of communication: Spontaneous and symbolic aspects. *Journal of Pragmatics, 22*, 265–278.

Buck, R., & Chaudhuri, A. (1994). Affect, reason, and involvement in persuasion: The ARI model. In Forschungsgruppe Konsum und Verhalten (Hrsg.), *Konsumentenforschung [Consumer Research]* (pp. 107–117). Munchen: Verlag Franz Vahlen.

Buck, R., & Ginsburg, B. (1997). Communicative genes and the evolution of empathy. In W. Ickes (Ed.), *Empathic Accuracy* (pp. 17–43). New York: Guilford Press.

Buck, R., Goldman, C.K., Easton, C.J., & Norelli Smith, N. (1998). Social learning and emotional education: Emotional expression and communication in behaviorally-disordered children and schizophrenic patients. In W.F. Flack & J.D. Laird (Eds.), *Emotions in Psychopathology* (pp. 298–314). New York: Oxford University Press

Cannon, W.B. (1915). *Bodily Changes in Pain, Hunger, Fear, and Rage*. New York: Appleton.

Carnap, R. (1937). *The Logical Syntax of Language*. New York: Harcourt Brace & Company.

Chalmers, D. (1995). Facing up to the problem of consciousness [keynote paper]. *Journal of Consciousness Studies, 2*, 200–219.

Chaudhuri, A., & Buck, R. (1995). Affect, reason, and persuasion. *Human Comunication Research, 21(3)*, 422–441.

Clark, T.W. (1995). Function and phenomenology: Closing the explanatory gap. *Journal of Consciousness Studies, 2*, 241–255.

Cofer, C.N., & Appley, M.H. (1964). *Motivation: Theory and Research*. New York: Wiley.

Crick, F., & Koch, C. (1997). The problem of consciousness. In J. Rennie (Ed.), *Mysteries of the Mind* (pp. 18–26). New York: Scientific American.

Dewey, J. (1931). *Philosophy and Civilization*. New York: Minton, Balch.

Ekman, P., & Davidson, R. (Eds.) (1994). *The Nature of Emotion: Fundamental Questions*. New York: Oxford University Press.

Gibson, J.J. (1966). *The Senses Considered as Perceptual Systems.* Boston: Houghton Mifflin.

Gibson, J.J. (1979). *The Ecological Approach to Visual Perception.* Boston: Houghton Mifflin.

Gottleib, G. (1984). Evolutionary trends and evolutionary origins: Relevance to theory in comparative psychology. *Psychological Review, 91,* 448–456.

Hameroff, S., & Penrose, R. (1996). Conscious events as orchestrated space–time selections. *Journal of Consciousness Studies, 3,* 36–53.

Hill, T.E. (1961). *Contemporary Theories of Knowledge.* New York: Ronald Press.

James, W. (1890). *The Principles of Psychology.* Chicago: Encyclopedia Britannica, 1953.

James, W. (1907). *Pragmatism: A New Name for Some Old Ways of Thinking.* New York: Longmans, Green, & Company.

Kuhlenbeck, H. (1965). The concept of consciousness in neurological epistemology. In J.R. Smythes (Ed.), *Brain and Mind: Modern Concepts of the Nature of Mind* (pp. 137–161). London: Routledge and Kegan Paul.

Lazarus, R.S. (1982). Thoughts on the relation between emotion and cognition. *American Psychologist, 37,* 1019–1024.

Lazarus, R.S. (1984). On the primacy of cognition. *American Psychologist, 39,* 124–129.

LeDoux, J. (1996). *The Emotional Brain: The Mysterious Underpinnings of Emotional Life.* New York: Simon and Schuster.

LeDoux, J. (1994a). Cognitive–emotional interactions in the brain. In P. Ekman & R.J. Davidson (Eds.), *The Nature of Emotion: Fundamental Questions* (pp. 216–223). New York: Oxford University Press.

LeDoux, J. (1994b). Emotional experience is an output of, not a cause of, emotional processing. In P. Ekman & R.J. Davidson (Eds.), *The Nature of Emotion: Fundamental Questions* (pp. 394–395). New York: Oxford University Press.

Levi, A.W. (1959). *Philosophy in the Modern World.* Bloomington: Indiana University Press.

MacLean, P.D. (1990). *The triune brain in evolution: Role in baleocerebral functions.* New York: Plenum Press.

McArthur, L.Z., & Baron, R.M. (1983). Toward an ecological theory of social perception. *Psychological Review, 90,* 215–238.

Oatley, K., & Jenkins, J.M. (1996). *Understanding Emotions.* Cambridge, MA: Blackwell.

Panksepp, J. (1982). Toward a general psychobiological theory of emotions. *The Behavioral and Brain Sciences, 5,* 407–467.

Panksepp, J. (1994a). Subjectivity may have evolved in the brain as a simple value-coding process that promotes the learning of new behaviors. In P. Ekman & R.J. Davidson (Eds.), *The Nature of Emotion: Fundamental Questions* (pp. 313–315). New York: Oxford University Press.

Panksepp, J. (1994b). Evolution constructed the potential for subjective experience within the neurodynamics of the mammalian brain. In P. Ekman & R.J. Davidson (Eds.), *The Nature of Emotion: Fundamental Questions* (pp. 396–399). New York: Oxford University Press.

Peirce, C.S. (1877/1962). How to make our ideas clear. In W. Barrett & H.D Aiken (Eds.), *Philosophy in the Twentieth Century: An Anthology, Vol. 1: Pragmatism* (pp. 106–122). New York: Random House (first published in 1877).

Piaget, J. (1971). Piaget's theory. In P. Mussen (Ed.), *Handbook of Child Development,* Vol. I. New York: Wiley.

Runes, D.D. (1962). *Dictionary of Philosophy*. Patterson, NJ: Littlefield, Adams & Co.

Russell, B. (1912). *The Problems of Philosophy*. New York: Oxford. 1959

Russell, B. (1927). *An outline of Philosophy*. NewYork: W.W. Norton.

Ryle, G. (1949). *The Concept of Mind*. New York: Barnes & Noble.

Sartre, J.P. (1948). *The Emotions*: *Outline of a Theory*. New York: Philosophical Library.

Sartre, J.P. (1957). *Existentialism and Human Emotions*. New York: Philosophical Library

Schachter, S., & Singer, J.E. (1962). Cognitive, social, and physiological determinants of emotional state. *Psychological Review, 69*, 379–399.

Skinner, B.F. (1953). *Science and Human Behavior*. New York: MacMillan.

Stevens, S.S. (1935). The operational basis of psychology. *Psychological Review, 42*, 512–527.

Taylor, E. (1992). Biological consciousness and the experience of the transcendent: William James and American functional psychology. In R.H. Wozniak (Ed.), *Mind and Body*: *Rene Descartes to William James* (pp. 53–56). Washington, DC: American Psychological Association.

Tucker, D. (1981). Lateral brain function, emotion, and conceptualization. *Psychological Bulletin, 89*, 19–46.

Vesey, G.N.A. (1965). *The Embodied Mind*. London: George Allen and Unwin, Ltd.

White, M. (1955). *The Age of Analysis*. New York: Houghton Mifflin.

Wittgenstein, L. (1953). *Philosophical Investigations*. Oxford: Basil Blackwell (translation by G.E.M. Anscombe).

Wittgenstein, L. (1965). *The Blue and the Brown Books*. New York: Philosophical Library.

Wozniak, R.H. (1992). *Mind and Body*: *Rene Descartes to William James*. Washington, DC: American Psychological Association.

Zajonc, R. (1980). Feeling and thinking: Preferences need no inferences. *American Psychologist, 35*, 151–175.

Zajonc, R. (1984). On the primacy of emotion. *American Psychologist, 39*, 117–123.

3

Anatomy and Physiology of Human Emotion: Vertical Integration of Brain Stem, Limbic, and Cortical Systems

DON M. TUCKER, DOUGLAS DERRYBERRY, AND PHAN LUU

The neural organization of human emotion spans multiple levels of the brain, from the elementary adaptive reflexes of the lower brain stem, to the complex visceral and somatic integration of the hypothalamus and thalamus, to the control of memory and cognition in corticolimbic networks. At each level, there are implications not only for the experience and expression of emotion but also for the effective motivation of behavior.

At the level of the pontine brain stem, for example, there are neural representations of elementary patterns of laughing and crying. These emotional displays become disinhibited when lesions disrupt the fiber tracts that mediate limbic and cortical modulation of the brain stem responses (Rinn, 1984). Anencephalic infants, born with only a brain stem, show well-organized facial displays of pleasure and distress (Buck, 1988). At the pontine level, we also find critical motivational mechanisms in the nuclei of the ascending monoamine projection systems that regulate arousal and alertness according to both internal states and environmental events (Bloom, 1988). The challenge for a neuropsychology of emotion is to explain how the elementary levels of the neuraxis are coordinated with higher cortical systems to control behavior adaptively.

In this chapter, we review the basic outlines of the anatomy and physiology of human emotion, describing the multiple levels of emotional control that have resulted from the progressive elaborations of the mesencephalic, diencephalic,

and telencephalic levels of visceral, reflexive, and behavioral organization in vertebrate evolution. We emphasize the need to understand vertical integration: how
these levels coalesce effectively. Two principles may help with this problem of
understanding vertical integration. The first principle is Jacksonian hierarchic integration through inhibitory control, through which fixed-action lower circuits
are subordinated to the representational flexibility of higher networks. The second, and related, principle is encephalization, through which higher, general-
purpose brain networks take on the functions formerly served by lower, fixed-
action circuits. By sketching the outlines of all of the major emotion control circuits of the mammalian brain, and then considering these in light of the complex
psychological qualities of human emotion, we attempt to formulate more clearly,
even if we cannot answer satisfactorily, the critical question of vertical integration of human brain systems.

OVERVIEW OF EVOLUTIONARY NEUROANATOMY

The hierarchic architecture of the human brain can be understood through a
developmental–evolutionary analysis. From the perspective of engineering or
computer science, the human brain presents a convoluted and confusing circuit
architecture. This architecture makes sense only when it is recognized to be the
end point of the progressive differentiation of the brain in vertebrate evolution.
Given the requirement for continuous functioning of each generation, the foundation circuitry remained in place, and new structures were differentiated to modify, rather than replace, the primordial adaptive mechanisms. The major episodes
of functional transformation were associated with new structures of nerve network anatomy elaborated at the anterior end of the neural tube. These are now
marked by the major divisions of the neuraxis seen in embryogenesis (rhomben-
cephalon, mesencephalon, diencephalon, and telencephalon).

Accounts of human emotion typically emphasize the telencephalic structures
(basal ganglia, limbic circuits, and cortex). It is, however, well-known in clinical neurology that both diencephalic (thalamus, hypothalamus) and mesencephalic (pontine reticular nuclei) structures are critical not only to vegetative
controls and primitive drives but also to the fine regulation of attention and cognition. Many lines of evidence suggest that these subcortical circuits are essential to the cortical representation of emotional experience and behavior as well.
In this chapter, we briefly outline the major control circuits at each level of the
neuraxis, and we provide examples of how mesencephalic and diencephalic influences may be integral to human emotion.

The brain stem circuits have been strongly conserved in vertebrate evolution,
with the core nuclei and connections of the amphibian motor system easily traced
in the human brain stem (Sarnat & Netsky, 1974). In contrast, the architecture

of the telencephalon has become highly unique in each avian and mammalian species. A key insight into mammalian cortical architecture has been achieved in recent years by the study of the connectivity of the primate cortex (Pandya, Seltzer, & Barbas, 1988). This research has suggested that the mammalian neocortex evolved from the limbic structures at two points of origin, with the archicortical base of the cingulate gyrus, parietal lobe, and dorsal frontal lobe (the spatial or "where" pathway) emergent from the hippocampus and the paleocortical base of the inferior temporal and orbital frontal lobe (the object or "what" pathway) emergent from primitive olfactory cortex. A theoretical challenge, thus far unmet, is to determine whether there are unique emotional and motivational properties of these limbic divisions that are integral to their mnemonic and cognitive functions. In this chapter, we outline the anatomical organization of the dorsal and ventral corticolimbic networks, and we raise the question of the differing motivational and emotional functions of these divisions of the cortex.

The human brain has a massive frontal cortex and functionally differentiated cerebral hemispheres. As other chapters in this volume illustrate, these cortical features have been primary targets for theorizing on the uniqueness of human cognition and emotion. In the present chapter, we emphasize that the study of neuroanatomy and neurophysiology not only points out the evolved hierarchy of the human brain; it leads directly to the question of how the flexible operations of the human cortex have come to coexist with the homeostatic drives, arousal mechanisms, and adaptive reflexes of the limbic structures, striatum, and brain stem.

We address this question with two key classic principles of brain function. These emerged from the developmental–evolutionary analysis of the nineteenth century that is again popular in biology (Pennisi & Roush, 1997). The first is Hughlings Jackson's principle of hierarchic integration through inhibitory control (Jackson, 1879). Along with his contemporaries, Jackson was impressed by the evolutionary order in the anatomy of the brain, which is traced by the progressive differentiation in embryogenesis. Observing that brain stem reflexes disappear as the infant matures, but then reappear following cortical lesions, Jackson proposed that the higher (e.g., telencephalic) brain structures evolved to extend, inhibit, and modulate, rather than to replace, the earlier (e.g., mesencephalic) functional systems. Only in rare instances (e.g., the pyramidal motor tract) does a higher brain structure actually replace or bypass lower structures. From this perspective, we may better understand the various forms of disinhibitory psychopathology seen in humans with brain lesions. We may also understand how complex patterns of human emotional experience and behavior are the composite of hierarchic, vertical integration, through which cortical representation networks are regulated by limbic and brain stem control mechanisms.

The second principle is encephalization. It is complementary to Jacksonian hierarchic integration in emphasizing the increasing functional dominance of higher systems with increasing complexity in the phylogenetic order. Encephalization is the evolutionary mechanism through which special-purpose controls in the periphery (e.g., lateral inhibition in the avian retina) are taken over by general-purpose controls in the central nervous system (e.g., lateral inhibition in the mammalian thalamus). A principle such as this is essential to explain how human emotional responses can be so elaborated in time, removed from proximal stimuli. From this perspective, the subcortical circuits that were once complete mechanisms for evaluating the sensory context and motivating fixed-action patterns now must support the more extended adaptive processes of the telencephalon. These are processes of continually integrating past experience, evaluating the significance of events while delaying gratification, and planning the future. Compared with the reflexive fixed-action patterns that comprise the motivational systems of simple vertebrates, the increasing complexity of mammalian emotional systems can be seen as the continued extension of the brain's representation of information in space and time.

In the simplest vertebrates, exemplified in surviving species by *Amphioxus*, the primitive brain responded reflexively to local stimuli, such as tactile contact or pain. With the evolution of sense organs for information from "distant" sources, such as smell or hearing, more complex brain structures, such as the olfactory cortex and thalamus, evolved the specialized synaptic networks to process distant information. Sarnat and Netsky (1974) point out that, by processing distant information in advance of contact, the vertebrates with special senses could afford the increased delay in processing caused by the increased number of synapses in the higher (e.g., diencephalic) nerve networks. We suggest that the human brain represents the continuation of this primordial principle, with progressively greater extension of the reflex arc (stimulus–response complex) in space and time.

The network architecture of the telencephalon shows the limbic structures as pivotal for connecting the sensory representational networks of the posterior brain to the action organization networks of the anterior brain. The limbic circuits and thalamus are also pivotal in funneling the widespread cortical inputs to the key regulatory systems of the brain stem, which then project broadly to tune the arousal and motivational state of the entire neuraxis. The evolutionary trend toward organizing perception and behavior according to "distant" information appears to be extended in the human brain, through memory capacities that allow continual integration of past experience to anticipate the events of the future. These memory capacities cannot be understood by a strictly cognitive analysis. The complex corticolimbic interaction of the massive human cortices is regulated adaptively by motivational and emotional controls of limbic and subcortical systems.

SUBCORTICAL BASES OF EMOTION

Emotions comprise specialized neurophysiological subsystems that control motor, autonomic, and sensory processing. For a coherent theory of emotion, it is necessary to understand how these component subsystems are coordinated by higher level structures to produce adaptive emotional states. A number of advances in integrative capacity appear to have accompanied the evolution of motivational systems within the brain stem and limbic system.

Component Brain Stem Subsystems

The component subsystems arise from cell groups and nuclei located primarily within the spinal cord and lower brain stem. Many of these cell groups serve effector functions through their descending influence on peripheral muscles and organs. Within the caudal medulla, for example, the medial tegmental field controls the axial trunk and head muscles, whereas the more rostral red nucleus controls the distal limb muscles. Other cell groups control specific behaviors such as chewing, vocalization, facial expressions, eye movements, and locomotion. In addition to these somatic functions, medullary cell groups regulate various autonomic reflexes. Some regions appear to control sympathetic activity (e.g., the rostral ventrolateral medulla), whereas others are concerned with parasympathetic functions (e.g., nucleus ambiguus) (Holstege, Bandler, & Saper, 1996; Loewy & Spyer, 1990; Van Bockstaele, Pieribone, & Aston-Jones, 1989).

While these effectors control specific behaviors, additional brain stem systems serve a more general function of adjusting the gain of spinal transmission. These include descending projections employing serotonin (raphe pallidus and raphe obscurus), norepinephrine (locus coeruleus), and dopamine (A 11 cell group). The monoamines' relatively diffuse projections throughout the ventral horn of the spinal cord appear to be modulatory; that is, they do not activate the motorneurons, but enhance responses to inputs converging from other brain stem systems. In addition, they inhibit the transmission of sensory information as it ascends within the dorsal horn, thereby promoting analgesia in stressful situations. These descending modulatory systems appear to adjust the balance between motor and sensory processing within the spinal cord (Holstege, 1991; Holstege, Bandler, & Saper, 1996; White et al., 1996).

A third set of brain stem components includes ascending projections to the forebrain. Traditionally associated with the reticular activating system, these systems include (among others) norepinephrine (locus coeruleus), serotonin (dorsal and median raphe), dopamine (ventral tegmental area), and acetylcholine (nucleus basalis) projections. These cell groups appear responsive to emotional stimuli, and their target effects are primarily modulatory (i.e., facilitating or attenuating converging sensory information). Such effects are consistent with recent studies showing how emotional states regulate attention (Niedenthal & Kitayama, 1993). It has been suggested, for example, that during positive states noradrenergic projections may promote an expansive, present-centered state of cortical processing. In contrast, negative states may recruit dopaminergic projections to promote a more focused, future-oriented attentional state (Tucker & Williamson, 1984).

Integrative Brain Stem Mechanisms

When viewed as a whole, the brain stem consists of discrete subsystems serving somatic, autonomic, and modulatory components. To produce emotional behaviors, however, these components must be coordinated by higher-level structures. Although such coordination is facilitated by limbic and cortical projections, its primitive basis can be found within the brain stem itself. Some of these integrative mechanisms are relatively specific. For example, the nucleus paragigantocellularis provides the main source of sympathetic drive within the organs of the autonomic nervous system while also providing the most potent afferent input to the locus coeruleus. Such projections suggest a mechanism for coordinating the ascending noradrenergic influence on the forebrain with sympathetic tone throughout the body (Aston-Jones, Chiang, & Alexinsky, 1991; Van Bockstaele, Pieribone, & Aston-Jones, 1989).

More rostral brain stem structures appear to provide more elaborate integrative influences. The midbrain periaqueductal gray (PAG) possesses descending projections to somatic, autonomic, and modulatory cell groups, allowing it to coordinate their activities in patterns related to general motivational states. Recent findings indicate that the PAG is organized into columns of cells, with each column related to a motivational pattern. The lateral column organizes active forms of defensive behavior and appears particularly responsive to superficial pain. Stimulation of the intermediate region of the lateral column elicits confrontational defensive behavior (i.e., defensive aggression) and blood flow to the face, whereas stimulation of the caudal region of the lateral column elicits flight behavior and increased blood flow to the limbs. Both of these defensive patterns are accompanied by increased heart rate and a nonopioid analgesia. In contrast, the adjacent ventrolateral column orchestrates a more passive strategy in response to deep pain. This pattern involves a cessation of ongoing motor activity, hyporeactivity, hypotension, decreased heart rate, and opioid-mediated analgesia. In its primitive form, the passive pattern may serve defensive purposes (e.g., playing dead), or it may serve recuperative functions following serious injury (Bandler & Keay, 1996; Bandler & Shipley, 1994). Future studies of the PAG promise a better understanding of some of the brain's most basic emotional functions in terms of both their identity (e.g., defensive, recuperative, and sexual) and their patterned organization.

Integrative Limbic Influences

The more recently evolved limbic structures that surround the brain stem serve a number of functions central to emotion and cognition. In terms of emotion, these circuits provide higher levels of integrative control over the brain stem. At the diencephalic level, the hypothalamic nuclei receive extensive exteroceptive and interoceptive sensory information and innervate multiple brain stem structures. Hypothalamic projections to the motor and autonomic pools of the lower brain stem allow for a fine tuning of homeostatic functions based on a detailed, integrative monitoring of ongoing metabolic conditions (Swanson, 1987). By means of additional projections to the pituitary, the hypothalamus (paraventricular nucleus) can coordinate peripheral endocrine activity in light of ongoing somatic, autonomic, and modulatory activity (Loewy & Spyer, 1990). In addition, hypothalamic projections appear capable of regulating brain stem integrative mechanisms. For example, the ventromedial hypothalamus exerts a descending inhibitory influence on cell groups within the PAG that are responsible for defensive aggression. It has been suggested that such suppression of brain stem aggressive tendencies has been crucial in the evolution of prosocial behaviors involving trust, play, and affection (Panksepp, 1986).

Hypothalamic projections also regulate the fearful forms of defense organized within the brain stem. Gray and McNaughton (1996) suggested that the hypothalamus and PAG function together, along with the amygdala, as part of a distributed fight–flight system. The PAG mobilizes defensive behavior given proximal sources of threat (e.g., pain or a predator) when there is little time for analysis. If the threat is very close and allows no avenue of escape, then fighting is elicited, but, given more distance or more room for escape, undirected flight is elicited. In contrast, the ventromedial hypothalamus mobilizes defense in situations involving more distal threats and more time for sensory analysis. The hypothalamic organization takes the form of directed escape behavior, and it is coordinated by regulating the PAG and recruiting additional brain stem regions involved in orientation (superior colliculus) and locomotion (cuneiform nucleus) functions. It is worth emphasizing that these primitive forms of defensive behavior are based on threats that are physically present and temporally urgent. Several theorists have suggested that they give rise to emotional states of *panic*, which are distinct from the anticipatory states of *anxiety* orchestrated by higher limbic and cortical circuitry (Graeff, 1991; Gray & McNaughton, 1996). The evolutionary progression in motivation can be seen as moving from reflexive responses to systems that engage defensive or other adaptive behavior in the face of proximal stimuli to systems that maintain an emotional state to bias the organization of behavior appropriately (e.g., a threatened posture) over extended intervals of time.

Limbic Anticipatory Functions

in brain stem??

More anticipatory emotional capacities appear to have evolved along with two telencephalic limbic structures, the amygdala and hippocampus. Both of these structures have extensive descending inputs to the hypothalamus, and the amygdala also projects throughout the brain stem. Although the amygdala is a complex structure with multiple nuclei, recent evidence suggests a crucial role in associating exteroceptive information with information concerning rewarding and aversive outcomes. Such learned associations allow the amygdala to organize emotional activity in light of potential rather than actual events. For example, when a rat is exposed to an auditory tone that signals an impending shock, the auditory information is delivered to the amygdala's lateral nucleus. The amygdala can respond based on relatively crude input delivered from the thalamus or on more highly processed information from the cortex. In either case, an immediate conditioned fear response is initiated by projections from the lateral nucleus to the basal nucleus (which projects to the ventromedial hypothalamus) and the central nucleus (which projects to the brain stem) (Davis, 1992; Petrovich, Risold, & Swanson, 1996; Savander et al., 1995).

Although it is supported by activity within the PAG and the hypothalamus, the amygdaloid fear response differs from the more primitive forms of explosive and directed escape. In Gray and McNaughton's terms (1996), the amygdala facilitates anticipatory, active avoidance. Thus, the response integrates a more flexible set of response options in relation to a potential, impending danger. Because these options depend on complex, distal sensory information, the amygdala must be crucially involved in coordinating response and attentional functions. In locomotion, for example, the animal must employ attention to seek out sources of threat (to avoid) and safety (to approach). Such flexibility is based on the amygdala's control over more ballistic brain stem and hypothalamic functions. In addition, projections to response-programming mechanisms within the basal ganglia and frontal cortex allow a finer tuning of selected response options. Furthermore, the amygdala projects (together with the PAG and hypothalamus) to the brain stem's ventral tegmental area, allowing it to adjust the focused attentional state related to the ascending dopaminergic projections. Finally, the amygdala projects extensively on the sensory and association areas within the posterior cortex, allowing a more direct modulation of the sensory information that is converging on the response systems. Thus, the amygdala's integrative capacities are quite extensive, coordinating somatic, autonomic, and sensory processing within the brain stem, limbic system, and cortex.

A final telencephalic structure, the hippocampus, provides a mix of subcortical and cortical functions. In addition to its well-known role in spatial processing (Nadel, 1991), recent findings seem to be converging on a general role of the
hippocampus in memory (Eichenbaum, Otto, & Cohen, 1994). In contrast to the
amygdala, which is involved in associative memory processes involving discrete
objects, the hippocampus appears more concerned with memory for contextual
and relational information. Various researchers have described this capacity in
terms such as *working*, *declarative*, and *configural* memory as opposed to *reference*, *procedural*, and *associative* memory. A simple example involves the conditioning of a fear reaction to background contextual information, apart from the
conditioned stimulus itself (LeDoux, 1995). Consistent with these functions, it
has been suggested that the hippocampus contributes to defensive behavior by
providing contextual information that complements the object information
processed within the amygdala (LeDoux, 1996). This allows another type of anticipatory emotional function based on contextual properties of the environment
rather than on discrete threatening objects.

The hippocampus has also been viewed as central to a behavioral inhibition system (Gray & McNaughton, 1996), which provides a fourth level to the hierarchy
extending from the PAG to the hypothalamus to the amygdala. Gray & McNaughton
(1996) suggest that the hippocampal formation contributes to defensive behavior
when active avoidance is in conflict with an equally strong approach tendency.
Specifically, the behavioral inhibition system performs a conflict resolution function by determining which of the competing tendencies is most appropriate to the
current (often spatial) context and suppressing the inappropriate options (and memories). This capacity relies on hippocampal projections to the fear-related circuits
within the amygdala and hypothalamus, to response programming mechanisms of
the basal ganglia, and to association and motor areas of the cortex. These outputs
orchestrate a complex form of anticipatory anxiety, involving extensive contextual
processing, competing response options, and an emphasis on inhibition.

In summary, subcortical emotional functions are carried out through a hierarchy of projections that integrate multiple motor, autonomic, modulatory, and endocrine subsystems. Although we have emphasized the descending influences,
emotional states also coordinate many ascending subsystems, such as the massive forebrain projections from the locus coeruleus, ventral tegmental area, hypothalamus, amygdala, and hippocampus. These combined descending and ascending influences suggest that emotional states facilitate a vertical integration
of processing systems across the brain stem, limbic system, and cortex. As these
systems evolved, the higher level structures enabled flexible and integrative motivational systems based on increasingly distal and anticipatory sensory processing. This progression continued with the evolution of mammalian cortical
networks.

ANATOMY AND PHYSIOLOGY OF CORTICAL SYSTEMS

In reptiles and amphibians the cortex is only incipient, with a highly undiffer-entiated organization. Based on his comparative anatomical studies, Herrick (1948) proposed that cortical morphogenesis is shaped by adaptation of cortical regions to subcortical inputs. The primitive pallium (hemisphere) can be divided into two fields: the paleocortex (olfactory) and the archicortex (hippocampal). Based on modern anatomical findings and on a consideration of the subcortical and brain stem connections, we can use Herrick's reasoning to see how the two fields of the pallium differentiated under the influence of unique subcortical inputs.

Archicortical and Paleocortical Routes of Corticolimbic Evolution

Evidence for the archicortical and Paleocortical routes of corticolimbic evolution may be traced in Nauta's pivotal study (1964) of the anatomy of the primate frontal lobe. When studying the efferent connections of the prefrontal cortex, Nauta noticed that it was organized into two routes. One route originates from the medial prefrontal areas and travels via the cingulum bundle and terminates in the medial temporal lobe (subiculum and entorhinal areas). The second route (the uncinate faciculus) connects the orbitofrontal cortex with the temporal pole, insula, and amygdaloid complex. Nauta remarked that the observed duality in the organization of prefrontal efferents may reflect something fundamental about the organization of the brain.

The anatomical separations of dorsal and ventral cortical systems led Sanides (1970) to propose that the cerebral cortex evolved along two lines of differenti-ation, one from the primitive paleocortex and the other from the archicortex. The archicortex gave rise to cortices on the mediodorsal surface, and the paleocortex gave rise to cortices on the ventrolateral surface of each hemisphere (Pandya, Seltzer, & Barbas, 1988; Sanides, 1970). For example, the hippocampus gives rise to the cingulate cortex on the medial surface of the cerebral hemisphere. In the frontal lobe, the anterior cingulate gives rise to cortex on the medial (such as the supplementary motor area) and dorsolateral surface. In contrast, the pale-ocortex gave rise to the orbitofrontal cortex and then to the ventrolateral frontal region. In monkeys, the principal sulcus is where the two trends converge on the lateral surface; in humans, it is the inferior frontal sulcus. Sanides (1970) noted that the connectional findings by Nauta (1964) may reflect the differential orga-nization of the cerebral cortex according to these two trends.

More recent evidence has verified the initial work of Sanides and Nauta. Based on extensive studies detailing the architectonic and architecture of cortical con-nections in primates, Pandya, Seltzer, and Barbas (1988) found that cortices and structures within each trend show a preferential pattern of connectivity. Similar to the pattern of connections reported by Nauta, Barbas, and colleagues found that the hippocampus, although projecting to both trends within the prefrontal areas, sends denser projections to the mediodorsal prefrontal cortex (Barbas & Blatt, 1995) and that the amygdala's projections to the prefrontal limbic cortex were densest at the caudal orbitofrontal regions (Barbas & De Olmos, 1990).

The separation of the archicortical (dorsal) and paleocortical (ventral) trends is not limited to connections between limbic structures with the prefrontal cortex. It appears that the dual trends represent a fundamental way in which the brain is organized; this pattern holds for both motor areas (Barbas & Pandya, 1986) and visual areas (Barbas, 1988). For example, the ventrolateral visual cortices (derived from the paleocortex), which are involved in the processing of object information, are preferentially connected with the ventrolateral and basal prefrontal cortex, and the medial and dorsolateral visual cortices, which are involved in visuospatial processing, are preferentially connected with the medial and dorsolateral prefrontal cortex (Barbas, 1988, 1995). This pattern of connections with the visual areas no doubt contributes to the spatial functions of the mediodorsal prefrontal cortex (Fuster, 1989; Goldman-Rakic, Funahashi, & Bruce, 1990) and the object functions of the ventral and lateral prefrontal cortex (Wilson, O'Scalaidhe, & Goldman-Rakic, 1993).

Additionally, Pandya, Seltzer, and Barbas (1988a) and Pandya and Yeterian (1990) noted that corticocortical connections reflect the evolutionary progression of the cortex. That is, the pattern of cortical projections follows the sequence of cortical differentiation such that a given area has dense connections with its precursor and successor and lesser connections with evolutionarily distant regions. More recent areas send projections to older areas via the supragranular layers and receive reciprocal projections to layer I. The older areas receive projections in layer IV and send efferents from their infragranular layers. The functional significance of this architecture is that sensory areas that receive extensively processed information are densely connected with limbic centers involved in the control of motivation and memory. Furthermore, limbic control of information processing occurs most abundantly in the processing layers of sensory areas involved in complex and holistic information.

Corticolimbic Mechanisms of Memory and Cognition

The clarification of cortical anatomy by Pandya and associates has shown the patterns of connectivity that must constrain efforts to frame computational models of memory in neuroanatomical terms (McClelland, McNaughton, & O'Reilly, 1995; Treves & Rolls, 1994). The evolutionary analysis helps to explain why the limbic system forms the base for both sensory integration and motor organization: The cortex evolved by differentiating from limbic structures. This analysis also explains why corticolimbic pathways are essential to memory functions: It is the motivationally significant information that gains consolidation in memory (Kornhuber, 1973). The adaptive significance of sensory information—the extent to which it resonates with core concepts of needs and values—is what determines whether that information will be allocated processing capacity in a limited memory store.

Given the anatomical distinction between archicortical and paleocortical divisions of the cortex, it may be that the dorsal and ventral trends operate under different memory mechanisms, perhaps with different motivational biases. Mishkin and colleagues (see Bachevalier & Mishkin, 1986; Mishkin, 1982; Mishkin & Murray, 1994; Mishkin & Phillips, 1990) have outlined two memory circuits. One circuit consists of the mediodorsal nucleus of the thalamus, the amygdala, and the ventromedial aspects of the prefrontal lobe. We refer to this circuit as the *ventral circuit* to emphasize the paleocortical components within this system. The second circuit involves the anterior nucleus of the thalamus, the hippocampus, and the mediodorsal prefrontal lobe (cingulate). We refer to this circuit as the *dorsal circuit* to emphasize the cingulate cortex and the hippocampus, both belonging to the archicortical trend.

As described above, the hippocampus and the dorsal circuit may be important not only to spatial memory but also to memory for context (Nadel, 1992; Nadel & Moscovitch, 1997). Based on findings that the hippocampus is important to the processing and encoding of nonreinforced stimuli, Pribram (1991) suggested that the hippocampus supports the contextual representation in which behaviors occur. Similarly, Nadel (1992) believes that the hippocampal memory system emphasizes the unique aspects of an event to be remembered. Thus, memory supported by the hippocampal system would resemble a key aspect of episodic memory.

As suggested by the studies of lesions to the inferotemporal pathway (Ungerleider & Mishkin, 1982), the ventral memory circuit is important to memory for objects rather than for spatial locations. Nadel has suggested that the ventral circuit's contribution may be generalized to categorical memory, that is, memory based on identity of objects (Nadel, 1992). Consistent with a context versus category distinction, Gaffan (1994) found that lesions to the fornix and perirhinal regions (dorsal circuit) result in recognition memory for complex scenes, whereas lesions to the amygdala (ventral circuit) result in deficits for food preference learning.

Although the theoretical analysis of corticolimbic function has yet to take advantage of the new insights of connectional anatomy, there have been suggestions that the motivational functions of limbic circuitry may be considered in neuropsychological models of memory. Several lines of evidence show that corticolimbic pathways must be intact for memory consolidation to occur (Squire, 1986). Because patients with hippocampal and medial temporal damage may be impaired in new learning, but not in access to previously learned material, the assumption has been that the neocortex is adequate for storage and retrieval of memory once the limbic structures and paralimbic cortices have participated in the consolidation process (Squire, 1986).

Nadel and Moskovitch (1997) have recently reviewed the literature on human amnesia and have drawn conclusions that may point to the importance of motivational factors in memory access. They point out that the evidence is actually fairly weak for full access to memories laid down before the medial temporal insult, particularly if memory is tested for autobiographical information rather than for general semantic knowledge. Therefore, intact limbic structures may be important to retrieval as well as to consolidation of memory. The fact that the limbic contribution is particularly important to accessing autobiographical memory is consistent with the view that the limbic system is important to evaluating the emotional and motivational significance of information to be retained in memory (Kornhuber, 1973).

Descending Projections for Emotional Control

In addition to showing how subcortical controls are brought to bear on the cognitive functions of the cortex, the evidence on the anatomy of corticolimbic networks provides important insights into the cortical influences on subcortical systems. Nauta's initial delineation (1964) of the dorsal and ventral pathways of the frontal lobe showed the connections through which the frontal lobe can modulate limbic function, and these pathways have been confirmed by recent anatomical studies (Barbas & Pandya, 1986). Two carefully studied examples, the startle response and primate emotional vocalizations, illustrate the role of cortical and limbic networks in regulating brain stem emotional systems.

The startle response shows how emotional states modulate brain stem function in humans as well as rodents and carnivores (Lang, Bradley, & Cuthbert, 1990; Vrana, Spence, & Lang, 1988). The startle response is a simple reflex mediated by a brain stem circuit of five synapses (auditory nerve, ventral cochlear nucleus, nuclei of the lateral lemniscus, nucleus reticularus pontus caudallis, and spinal interneuron) plus the neuromuscular junction. This circuit is modulated by higher control from limbic structures, particularly the amygdala (Davis, Hitchcock, & Rosen, 1987). In humans, complex emotional states, engaging widespread cortical networks (such as when subjects view photographic slides of nudes or mutilated bodies), result in inhibition of the startle response for pleasant states and in facilitation for aversive states (Lang, Bradley, & Cuthbert, 1990; Vrana, Spence, & Lang, 1988). The implication is that the cognitive representations of the cortex are associated with an appropriate adaptive set established across multiple levels of the neural hierarchy. Although startle may not be a significant motivational mechanism in humans, the orderly modulation of this reflex illustrates the role of emotional states in linking a variety of systems, including postural, motor, sensory, and visceral, up and down the neuraxis.

The differential roles of cortical and limbic influences in regulating emotional systems was particularly clear in Ploog's investigations (1981) of the monkey's emotional vocalizations. Ploog showed that the monkey's calls are organized at the most basic level in discrete motor nuclei of the lower brain stem. At the next level, these nuclei are subordinated to the species-specific patterned motor sequences that are organized in the midbrain. For the motor sequences to show modulation by the animal's current emotional state, the contributions of the limbic structures (amygdala and hippocampus) are required. The corticolimbic (cingulate) control of this hierarchy comes into play for what Ploog calls "voluntary call initiation" in which the limbic–brain stem hierarchy is recruited in service of more complex goal-oriented behavior. At the final level, the neocortical control becomes important for "voluntary call formation" in which frontal and motor cortices bypass the midbrain pattern generators to articulate specific vocalizations.

Ploog (1992) suggests that an elaboration of this neocortical control of vocalization may underlie human language capacity. At the same time, he points out that the human brain has undergone expansion of structures such as anterior thalamic nuclei that link frontal cortex to the limbic system. Ploog's analysis is consistent with the observations of disinhibited emotional displays in humans with cortical lesions (Brodal, 1969; Monrad-Krohn, 1947). Human vocalizations can thus be seen to involve not only the direct cortex-to-brain stem pyramidal pathways but also the hierarchy of pathways that integrate limbic with diencephalic and lower brain stem control of emotional vocalization.

VERTICAL INTEGRATION OF MOTIVATIONAL AND EMOTIONAL SYSTEMS

The anatomy and physiology of emotional systems is thus complex, comprising an evolved hierarchy of control processes. For a neuropsychological theory to account for the anatomical and physiological evidence, a critical issue is vertical integration, how the control processes are coordinated across the multiple levels of the neuraxis. Fundamentally, human emotion encompasses the primitive reflexes and homeostatic drives of the vertebrate brain. Vertical integration must explain how these reflexes and drives can act to shape attention and memory while at the same time becoming subordinated to more complex processes of cognitive representation.

In addition to the cortical modulation of subcortical responses, the extensive memory and cognitive capacities of the human cortex depend on adequate regulatory control by limbic and brain stem mechanisms. An important task for a neuropsychological theory of emotion is to explain how subcortical controls have evolved from direct, reflex-like adaptivity to provide generic support functions, such as arousal control, significance evaluation, and action motivation, to support the ongoing, cognitively mediated sensorimotor integration that characterizes human behavior. We suggest that modern neuroanatomy and neurophysiology continue to support Jackson's hierarchic, evolutionary model, specifically as applied to understanding human motivation and emotion.

Hierarchic Anatomy of Emotion and Memory

Connectivity implies function. Although this has always been the assumption of the anatomical method, modern connectionist models provide specific examples of how patterns of connectivity constrain the functional architecture of distributed networks (McClelland, McNaughton, and O'Reilley, 1995; Rumelhart & McClelland, 1986). Papez's initial formulation (1937) of a limbic system came from observations of connectivity, indicated by the propagation of seizures through the dorsal limbic circuitry. The hierarchic organization of emotional behavior was recognized in MacLean's pioneering studies of the limbic system (e.g., MacLean, 1993; Pribram & MacLean, 1953). Maclean emphasized that the development of the cingulate cortex in mammals occurred with the appearance of fundamentally new forms of behavior, including social attachment and play. We now recognize that these new capacities are essential to support the increasingly extended juvenile period that allows the plasticity of the mammalian cortex (Tucker, Luu, & Pribram, 1996).

Several lines of evidence suggest that limbic mechanisms are critical to the integration of motivational controls with the cognitive capacities of human cortical networks. Mesulam (1988) proposes that the ascending cholinergic projections of the nucleus basalis provide modulatory control over the corticolimbic interactions in memory consolidation. Studies of the cholinergic projections to the sensory input pathways of the amygdala show increasingly strong cholinergic modulation as the pathways approach the limbic system. Mesulam suggests that the cholinergic control may be important for gating cortical information exchange into and out of the limbic system.

Most of the cortical areas do not, however, project to the nucleus basalis; rather, it is controlled primarily by the limbic structures and paralimbic cortices. Thus, an important aspect of the memory architecture of the mammalian cortex shows a fan-in of control through which the limbic areas respond to the motivational and emotional content of the corticolimbic traffic and determine the feedback to be applied to the nucleus basalis; the nucleus basalis then projects back in a fan-out pattern to regulate widespread regions of corticolimbic traffic (Mesulam, 1988).

Because connections between cortical regions and limbic structures are required for memory consolidation (Squire, 1992), we can look to corticolimbic physiology for clues to the mechanisms for motivating memory consolidation. The hippocampus shows a particular affinity for the process of long-term potentiation, a model of Hebbian learning in which afferent input to a neuron results in a permanent potentiated response if it is associated with simultaneous activation of that neuron by another source (Gustafsson & Wigstrom, 1988; Teyler, 1986). The reactivity of limbic structures is shown by the electrophysiological phenomenon of kindling. Electrical stimulation anywhere in the cortex tends to elicit responses from the amygdala and hippocampus preferentially. This observation of limbic excitability in animal studies parallels the tendency of epileptic seizures to focalize in the medial temporal lobes in humans. In the animal studies, repeated stimulation may "kindle" increasingly amplified responses from the limbic structures, propagating throughout the cortex. The eventual result may be a pathological facilitation of corticolimbic excitability, evidenced by spontaneous seizures (Dichter & Ayala, 1987).

Long-term potentiation is typically considered to be a model of learning, whereas kindling is typically considered to be a model of epilepsy. The relevance of corticolimbic sensitization to general mechanisms of learning and memory is, however, shown by the finding that kindled seizures can be classically conditioned (Janowsky, Laxer, & Rushmer, 1980). The relevance of motivational control of corticolimbic excitability has been suggested by evidence of limbic sensitization in both normal and pathological forms of emotional responses (Harkness & Tucker, in preparation; Sapolsky, 1992; Tucker & Luu, 1999). Harkness and Tucker propose that a traumatic emotional response induces a pattern of limbic reactivity involving the same electrophysiological and endocrine mechanisms as kindling. Thus, subsequent exposure to a traumatic stimulus may elicit a response that is disproportional to the stimulus unless the sensitization caused by the traumatic history is appreciated (Harkness & Tucker, in preparation).

Mechanisms of Limbic Drive

A different perspective on the contributions of limbic networks to cortical function has been provided by studies of emotional disorders in patients with temporal lobe epilepsy. Flor-Henry (1969) observed that, of those epileptics who develop major psychiatric symptoms, patients with a left temporal focus were more likely to show a schizophreniform disorder, whereas those with a right temporal focus were more likely to show an affective disorder. A consistent set of observations, with a more direct parallel with hemispheric psychological functions, has been gathered in psychometric studies of temporal lobe epileptics by Bear and Fedio (1977).

Bear and Fedio (1977) used both self-ratings and observer ratings of the patients and found what appeared to be an exaggeration of the pathological hemisphere's psychological processes. Consistent with Flor-Henry's observations

(1969), the epileptics with right temporal focus showed affective instability and emotional expressiveness in their behavior, possibly suggesting an exaggeration of the right hemisphere's role in affective prosody and emotional communication. As if reflecting an exaggeration of the left hemisphere's verbal cognitive capacities, the epileptics with left temporal focus were found to show an "ideative" pattern of traits, with a preoccupation with intellectual, philosophical, and religious concerns.

The Bear and Fedio (1977) findings were predictably controversial, but they have been replicated in independent samples (Fedio, 1986; Fedio & Martin, 1983). Although the subsequent findings may seem at first to confirm characterizations of the right hemisphere as emotional and the left hemisphere as nonemotional, closer inspection shows that the psychological operations of the epileptic hemisphere were charged with emotional significance for the left as well as the right sides. The left temporal lobe–affected patients were obsessed with the personal importance of their intellectual concerns, often writing long treatises on the topics. To explain the exaggerated personal significance associated with the intellectual as well as the affective behavior, Bear and Fedio proposed that the epileptic disorder resulted in a "functional hyperconnection" of limbic areas with the cortex.

These several observations on limbic reactivity may provide a way of understanding, in both psychological and neurophysiological terms, how limbic areas use their privileged connectivity with subcortical control systems to motivate memory consolidation and therefore cognitive processing. These observations may also help to integrate the emphasis on vertical integration in the present chapter with the evidence on hemispheric specialization reviewed in other chapters of this volume (Gainotti, Chapter 9, this volume; Davidson & Henriquez, Chapter 11 this volume). The massive human cortices provide extensive, but limited, representational capacity. The selection for a representation to be consolidated within cortical networks is based on the adaptive resonance it recruits within limbic structures and paralimbic (archi and paleo) cortices. The adaptive resonance may be extended in time, as in ruminations, obsessions, and fantasies. The linked networks from sensory areas to limbic cortex (Pandya & Yeterian, 1985) are engaged by this resonance, stabilizing memory representations in a distributed fashion across the paralimbic and neocortical levels.

As Pandya and associates have pointed out, the "back projections" from limbic toward cortical areas are as extensive as the "forward projections" carrying sensory data from primary sensory cortex to the intermediate association areas to paralimbic cortex. In modern psychological theories of perception, the perceptual process is seen as one in which memory and expectations resonate with and shape the organization of sensory input (Shepard, 1984). Shepard (1984) emphasizes the active, constructive role of memory by suggesting that perception is "hallucination constrained by the sensory data." In the context of the corticolimbic architecture for perception, we would add that the resonance is shaped by inherent motivational constraints incorporated with the representation at the paralimbic level. Because they are the most densely interconnected of cortical networks, the paralimbic cortices provide a global, integrative, and yet undifferentiated, mnemonic context for cognition. Given their connectivity to subcortical controls and their intrinsic excitability, the paralimbic cortices may provide the motivational drive for evaluating and consolidating significant contents in memory.

The physiology of motivated perception may thus be seen as a kind of arbitration across layered networks, anchored at the superficial layers by sensory analyzers and energized in the deep layers by a resonance of the information with a global representation of adaptive need states (Derryberry & Tucker, 1991). Because the paralimbic representations are the composite of the person's developmental experience, the "limbic drive" structuring perception is formed not just by immediate homeostatic needs, but by more extended processes of self-representation. In this manner, the self may be understood as the implicit context of autobiographical memory. In normal personalities, there is an effective arbitration of perception between limbic drive, with its inherent motivational, self-referential constraints, and the requirements for maintaining veridical and complex representations in the neocortex. Judging from the personality disorders of temporal lobe epileptics, limbic drive occurs not only in the emotionally expressive right hemisphere but also in the verbal and analytic left hemisphere as well. We may speculate that the charged intellectualizations of epileptics with left temporal lobe focus may have their counterparts in disorders in which limbic kindling may be psychopathological rather than neuropathological, such as in the forced ruminations of the obsessive or the rigid delusions of the paranoid (Shapiro, 1965). In contrast, excessive limbic drive may take a more affectively labile form within the right hemisphere, supporting the loose modes of self-regulation of the histrionic, psychopathic, and impulsive personalities (Tucker, 1981).

Motive Persistence

Although the distorted cognition in emotional disorders may be most easily understood in terms of temporal–limbic dysfunction, there are more subtle deficits of motivation that occur with damage to the frontal lobe that result in profound deficits in life adjustment. Patients with mild frontal lesions may appear entirely normal during clinical examination and cursory neuropsychological testing. Despite the popular "working memory" idea of frontal lobe function, the memory deficits of these patients are typically not a significant feature of their clinical presentation (Squire, 1987). Yet within a short time of returning to work and family life, patients with frontal lesions often experience complete failures of adjustment. The problem seems to be not just a memory defect but also an inability to motivate ongoing behavior in relation to long-term goals (Lezak, 1983; Luria, 1973).

The frontal lobe's expansion in human evolution may support a vertical integration of multiple adaptive systems to allow complex behavior to be organized over time. The massive cortical networks provide cognitive representational capacity, yet this capacity is not effective unless it is controlled in relation to the adaptive challenges that humans must organize over increasingly extended intervals of time. Extended challenges, such as keeping a job or maintaining a relationship, are the tasks at which frontal-lesioned patients fail. As recognized in classic formulations, the frontal cortex mediates between the motivational and emotional representations in limbic areas and the organization of action in premotor areas (Nauta, 1971; Pribram, 1950). In doing so, the frontal networks are able to integrate functions such as arousal control that require contributions from lower as well as higher levels of the neuraxis (Luria & Homskaya, 1970; Yakovlev & Lecours, 1967).

In the extended plasticity of frontal networks through the long human juvenile period, cortical representations appear to form that mirror not only the perceptual operations of the posterior brain but also the regulatory controls of limbic and subcortical structures. The effect seems to be a kind of encephalization of vertical integration such that, toward the end of the juvenile period, human frontal cortical networks may be prepared to take on increasing control of the multiple levels of the neural hierarchy required for effective self-regulation.

Intrinsic Motivation: The Cognitive Means Become the End

The study of neuroanatomy and neurophysiology thus uncovers many mechanisms of emotion and motivation that humans share with primitive vertebrates. It also points to structures and mechanisms that are unique to the human brain. The increasing emphasis on "distant" events, evident in the progression from mesencephalic to diencephalic controls in primitive vertebrates, can be seen as a simple principle that continues to describe evolution of motivation in the executive functions of the human frontal lobes.

Although a thorough knowledge of the vertebrate control systems is essential for understanding human neuropsychology, the human cortex appears to represent and subsume motivational and emotional processes to an extent unknown among other mammals. Instead of stereotyped, species-specific motivations, humans acquire flexible, and highly idiosyncratic, patterns of motivation as neural plasticity shapes and reshapes the cortical mantle over a 20-year juvenile period.

To allow the extended neural plasticity of massive cortical networks, subcortical control systems appear to have become redirected from reflexive, immediate influences on behavior to take on the increasingly complex support operations for the corticolimbic matrix. Thus, the task of arousal control is important not just to facilitate a reflex but also to facilitate memory consolidation across distributed cortical networks. The task of detecting the adaptive significance of a perception is important both to release an endocrine secretion and to code a sensory pattern for the limbic resonance that excites corticolimbic consolidation.

In many ways, the neurophysiology of human motivation has become encephalized in a way that inverts the relation between cortical and subcortical systems. Whereas the cortex was initially a device for elementary representation and memory, supporting the integration between the stimulus and response circuits in the reflexes of the subcortical control systems, in human evolution the tables are turned. The support of cortical operations has now become the primary task of the subcortical systems. Although humans continue to struggle with biological needs, there are now many people who are motivated, at least briefly, by intellectual interests. Activities such as curiosity, reasoning, and the search for understanding are a kind of inversion of the vertebrate control hierarchy. The corticolimbic networks that once served a subordinate support function for brain stem adaptive mechanisms have now commandeered the motivational systems to support cognition as an end in itself.

REFERENCES

Aston-Jones, G., Chiang, C., & Alexinsky, T. (1991). Discharge of noradrenergic locus coeruleus neurons in behaving rats and monkeys suggests a role in vigilance. In C.D. Barnes & O. Pompeiano (Ed.), *Progress in Brain Research, Vol 88: Neurobiology of the Locus Coeruleus* (pp. 501–520). Amsterdam: Elsevier Science Publishers.

Bachevalier, J., & Mishkin, M. (1986). Visual recognition impairment follows ventromedial but not dorsolateral prefrontal lesions in monkeys. *Behavioural Brain Research, 20*, 249–261.

Bandler, R., & Keay, K.A. (1996). Columnar organization in the midbrain periaqueductal gray and the integration of emotional expression. In G. Holstege, R. Bandler, & C.B. Saper (Eds.), *Progress in Brain Research, Vol. 107: The Emotional Motor System* (pp. 285–300). Amsterdam: Elsevier.

Bandler, R., & Shipley, M.T. (1994). Columnar organization in the midbrain periaqueductal gray: Modules for emotional expression? *Trends in Neurosciences, 17*, 379–389.

Barbas, H. (1988). Anatomic organization of basoventral and mediodorsal visual recipient prefrontal regions in the rhesus monkey. *Journal of Comparative Neurology, 276*, 313–342.

Barbas, H. (1995). Anatomic basis of cognitive–emotional interactions in the primate prefrontal cortex. *Neuroscience and Biobehavioral Reviews, 19*, 499–510.

Barbas, H., & Blatt, G.J. (1995). Topographically specific hippocampal projections target functionally distinct prefrontal areas in the rhesus monkey. *Hippocamp* 5, 511–533.

Barbas, H., & De Olmos, J. (1990). Projections from the amygdala to basover mediodorsal prefrontal regions in the rhesus monkey. *Journal of Compara rology, 300*, 549–571.

Barbas, H., & Pandya, D.N. (1986). Architecture and frontal cortical connections of the premotor cortex (area 6) in the rhesus monkey. *Journal of Comparative Neurology*, *256*, 211–228.

Bear, D.M., & Fedio, P. (1977). Quantitative analysis of interictal behavior in temporal lobe epilepsy. *Archives of Neurology*, *34*, 454–467.

Bloom, F.E. (1988). What is the role of general activating systems in cortical function? In P. Rakic & W. Singer (Eds.), *Neurobiology of Neocortex* (pp. 407–421). New York: John Wiley.

Brodal, A. (1969). *Neurological Anatomy in Relation to Clinical Medicine*. New York: Oxford University Press.

Buck, R. (1988). *Human Motivation and Emotion*, 2nd Ed. New York: John Wiley & Sons.

Davis, M. (1992). The role of the amygdala in fear and anxiety. *Annual Review of Neuroscience*, *15*, 353–375.

Davis, M., Hitchcock, J.M., & Rosen, J.B. (1987). Anxiety and the amygdala: Pharmacological and anatomical analysis of the fear-potentiated startle paradigm. In G. Bower (Ed.), *The Psychology of Learning and Motivation* (pp. 263–305). New York: Academic Press.

Derryberry, D., & Tucker, D.M. (1991). The adaptive base of the neural hierarchy: Elementary motivational controls on network function. In R. Dienstbier (Ed.), *Nebraska Symposium on Motivation* (pp. 289–342). Lincoln: University of Nebraska Press.

Dichter, M.A., & Ayala, G.F. (1987). Cellular mechanisms of epilepsy: A status report. *Science*, *237*, 157–164.

Eichenbaum, H., Otto, T., & Cohen, N.J. (1994). The functional components of the hippocampal memory system. *Behavioral and Brain Sciences*, *17*, 449–518.

Fedio, P. (1986). Behavioral characteristics of patients with temporal lobe epilepsy. *Psychiatric Clinics of North America*, *9*, 267–281.

Fedio, P., & Martin, A. (1983). Ideative–emotive behavioral characteristics of patients following left or right temporal lobectomy. *Epilepsia*, *24*, 117–130.

Flor-Henry, P. (1969). Psychosis and temporal lobe epilepsy: A controlled investigation. *Epilepsia*, *10*, 363–395.

Fuster, J. (1989). *The Prefrontal Cortex*. New York: Raven Press.

Gaffan, D. (1994). Dissociated effects of perirhinal cortex ablation, fornix transection, and amygdalectomy: Evidence for multiple memory systems in the primate temporal lobe. *Experimental Brain Research*, *99*, 411–422.

Goldman-Rakic, P.S., Funahashi, S., & Bruce, C.J. (1990). Neocortical memory circuits. *Cold Spring Harbor Symposia on Quantitative Biology*, *55*, 1025–1038.

Graeff, F.G. (1991). Neurotransmitters in the dorsal periaqueductal gray and animal models of panic anxiety. In M. Briley & S.E. File (Eds.), *New Concepts in Anxiety* (pp. 288–312). London: Macmillan.

Gray, J.A., & McNaughton, N. (1996). The neuropsychology of anxiety: Reprise. In D.A. Hope (Ed.), *Nebraska Symposium on Motivation: Perspectives on Anxiety, Panic, and Fear*, Vol. 43 (pp. 61–134). Lincoln: University of Nebraska Press.

Gustafsson, B., & Wigstrom, H. (1988). Physiological mechanisms underlying long-term potentiation. *Trends in Neuroscience*, *11*, 156–162.

Harkness, K., & Tucker D.M. *Kindling as a model of stress-induced psychopathology*. Manuscript in preparation.

Herrick, C.J. (1948). *The Brain of the Tiger Salamander*. Chicago: University of Chicago Press.

Holstege, G. (1991). Descending motor pathways and the spinal motor system: Limbic and nonlimbic components. In G. Holstege (Ed.), *Progress in Brain Research, Vol. 57: Role of the Forebrain in Sensation and Behavior* (pp. 307–421). New York: Elsevier.

Holstege, G., Bandler, R., & Saper, C.B. (1996). *Progress in Brain Research, Vol. 107: The Emotional Motor System.* Amsterdam: Elsevier.

Jackson, J.H. (1879). On affections of speech from diseases of the brain. *Brain, 2*, 203–222.

Janowsky, J.S., Laxer, K.D., & Rushmer, D.S. (1980). Classical conditioning of kindled seizures. *Epilepsia, 21*, 393–398.

Kornhuber, H.H. (1973). Neural control of input into long term memory: Limbic system and amnestic syndrome in man. In H.P. Zippel (ed.), *Memory and Transfer of Information* (pp. 1–22). New York: Plenum.

Lang, P.J., Bradley, M.M., & Cuthbert, B.N. (1990). Emotion, attention, and the startle reflex. *Psychological Review, 97*, 377–398.

LeDoux, J. (1995). In search of an emotional system in the brain: Leaping from fear to emotion and consciousness. In M.S. Gazzaniga (Ed.), *The Cognitive Neurosciences* (pp. 1049–1062). Cambridge, MA: MIT Press.

LeDoux, J. (1996). *The Emotional Brain.* New York: Simon & Schuster.

Lezak, M.D. (1983). *Neuropsychological Assessment.* New York: Oxford University Press.

Loewy, A.D., & Spyer, K.M. (1990). *Central Regulation of Autonomic Functions.* New York: Oxford University Press.

Luria, A.R. (1973). *The Working Brain: An Introduction to Neuropsychology.* New York: Basic Books.

Luria, A.R., & Homskaya, E.D. (1970). Frontal lobe and the regulation of arousal processes. In D. Mostofsky (Ed.), *Attention: Contemporary Theory and Research.* New York: Appleton-Century-Croft.

MacLean, P.D. (1993). Introduction: Perspectives on cingulate cortex in the limbic system. In B.A. Vogt, & M. Gabriel (Eds.), *Neurobiology of the Cingulate Cortex and Limbic Thalamus* (pp. 1–15). Boston: Birkhauser.

McClelland, J.L., McNaughton, B.L., & O'Reilly, R.C. (1995). Why there are complementary learning systems in the hippocampus and neocortex: Insights from the successes and failures of connectionist models of learning and memory. *Psychological Review, 102*, 419–457.

Mesulam, M. (1988). Central cholinergic pathways: Neuroanatomy and some behavioral implications. In M. Avoli, T.A. Reader, R.W. Dykes, & P. Gloor (Eds.), *Neurotransmitters and Cortical Function: From Molecules to Mind* (pp. 237–260). New York: Plenum Press.

Mishkin, M. (1982). A memory system in the monkey. *Philosophical Transactions of the Royal Society of London Series B, 298*, 85–95.

Mishkin, M., & Murray, E.A. (1994). Stimulus recognition. *Current Opinion in Neurobiology, 4*, 200–206.

Mishkin, M., & Phillips, R.R. (1990). A corticolimbic memory path revealed through its disconnection. In C. Trevarthen (Ed.), *Brain Circuits and Functions of the Mind: Essays in Honor of Roger W. Sperry* (pp. 196–210). New York: Cambridge University Press.

Monrad-Krohn, G.H. (1947). Dysprosody or altered melody of language. *Brain, 70*, 405–415.

Nadel, L. (1991). The hippocampus and space revisited. *Hippocampus, 1*, 221–229.

Nadel, L. (1992). Multiple memory systems: What and why. *Journal of Cognitive Neuroscience, 4*, 179–188.

Nadel, L., & Moscovitch, M. (1997). Memory consolidation, retrograde amnesia and the hippocampal complex. *Current Opinion in Neurobiology*, *7*, 217–227.

Nauta, W.J.H. (1971). The problem of the frontal lobe: A reinterpretation. *Journal of Psychiatric Research*, *8*, 167–187.

Nauta, W.J.H. (1964). Some efferent connections of the prefrontal cortex in the monkey. In J.M. Warren & K. Akert (Eds.), *The Frontal Granular Cortex and Behavior* (pp. 397–409). New York: McGraw Hill.

Niedenthal, P., & Kitayama, S. (1994). *The Heart's Eye: Emotional Influences in Perception and Attention*. San Diego, CA: Academic Press.

Pandya, D.N., Seltzer, B., & Barbas, H. (1988). Input–output organization of the primate cerebral cortex. In *Comparative Primate Biology, Vol. IV: Neurosciences* (pp. 39–80). New York: Allen Ardlis, Inc.

Pandya, D.N., & Yeterian, E.H. (1985). Architecture and connections of cortical association areas. In A. Peters & E.G. Jones (Eds.), *Cerebral Cortex, Vol. 4: Association and Auditory Cortices* (pp. 3–61). New York: Plenum Press.

Pandya, D.N., & Yeterian, E. H. (1990). Prefrontal cortex in relation to other cortical areas in rhesus monkey: Architecture and connections. *Progress in Brain Research*, *85*, 63–94.

Panksepp, J. (1986). The psychobiology of prosocial behaviors: Separation distress, play, and altruism. In C. Zahn-Waxler, E.M. Cummings, & R. Iannotti (Eds.), *Altruism and Aggression: Biological and Social Origins* (pp. 19–57). Cambridge, England: Cambridge University Press.

Papez, J. (1937). A proposed mechanism of emotion. *Archives of Neurology and Psychiatry*, *38*, 725–744.

Pennisi, E., & Roush, W. (1997). Developing a new view of evolution. *Science*, *277*, 34–37.

Petrovich, G.D., Risold, P.Y., & Swanson, L.W. (1996). Organization of projections from the basomedial nucleus of the amygdala: A PHAL study in the rat. *Journal of Comparative Neurology*, *374*, 387–420.

Ploog, D. (1981). Neurobiology of primate audio-vocal behavior. *Brain Research Reviews*, *3*, 35–61.

Ploog, D. (1992). Neuroethological perspectives on the human brain: From the expression of emotions to intentional signing and speech. In A. Harrington (Ed.), *So Human a Brain: Knowledge and Values in the Neurosciences* (pp. 3–13). Boston: Birkhauser.

Pribram, K.H. (1950). Psychosurgery in midcentury. *Surgery, Gynecology, and Obstetrics*, *91*, 364–367.

Pribram, K.H. (1991). *Brain and Perception: Holonomy and Structure in Figural Processing*. Hillsdale, NJ: Erlbaum.

Pribram, K.H., & MacLean, P.D. (1953). Neuronographic analysis of medial and basal cerebral cortex: II. Monkey. *Journal of Neurophysiology*, *16*, 324–340.

Rinn, W.E. (1984). The neuropsychology of facial expression: A review of the neurological and psychological mechanisms for producing facial expressions. *Psychological Bulletin*, *95*, 52–77.

Rumelhart, D.E., & McClelland, J.L. (1986). *Parallel Distributed Processing: Explorations in the Microstructure of Cognition, Vol. I: Foundations*. Cambridge, MA: MIT Press.,

Sanides, F. (1970). Functional architecture of motor and sensory cortices in primates in the light of a new concept of neocortex evolution. In C.R. Noback & W. Montagna (Eds.), *The Primate Brain: Advances in Primatology* (pp. 137–208). New York: Appleton-Century-Crofts.

Sapolsky, R.M. (1992). Neuroendocrinology of the stress-response. In J.B. Becker, S.M. Breedlove, & D. Crews (Eds.), *Behavioral Endocrinology* (pp. 287–324). Cambridge, MA: MIT Press.

Savander, V., Go, C.G., LeDoux, J.E., & Pitkanen, A. (1995). Intrinsic connections of the rat amygdaloid complex: Projections originating in the basal nucleus. *Journal of Comparative Neurology, 361*, 345–368.

Shapiro, D. (1965). *Neurotic Styles.* New York: Basic Books.

Shepard, R.N. (1984). Ecological constraints on internal representation: Resonant kinematics of perceiving, imagining, thinking, and dreaming. *Psychological Review, 91*, 417–447.

Squire, L.R. (1986). Mechanisms of memory. *Science, 232*, 1612–1619.

Squire, L.R. (1987). *Memory and Brain.* New York: Oxford University Press.

Squire, L.R. (1992). Memory and the hippocampus: A synthesis of findings with rats, monkeys, and humans. *Psychological Review, 99*, 195–231.

Swanson, L.W. (1987). The hypothalamus. In A. Bjorklund, T. Hokfelt, & L.W. Swanson (Eds.), *Handbook of Chemical Neuroanatomy, Vol. 5: Integrated Systems of the CNS (Part I)* (pp. 1–124). New York: Elsevier.

Teyler, T.J. (1986). Memory: Electrophysiological analogs. In J.L. Martinez, Jr., & R.P. Kesner (Eds.), *Learning and Memory: A Biological View.* Orlando: Academic Press.

Treves, A., & Rolls, E.T. (1994). Computational analysis of the role of the hippocampus in memory. *Hippocampus, 4*, 374–391.

Tucker, D.M. (1981). Lateral brain function, emotion, and conceptualization. *Psychological Bulletin, 89*, 19–46.

Tucker, D.M., & Luu, P. (1998). Cathexis revisited: Corticolimbic resonance and the adaptive control of memory. In R. Bilder (Ed.), *Centennial of Freud's Project for a Scientific Psychology* (pp. 134–152). New York: New York Academy of Sciences.

Tucker, D.M., Luu, P., & Pribram, K.H. (1996). Social and emotional self-regulation. In J. Grafman & F. Boller (Eds.), *Structure and Functions of the Human Prefrontal Cortex* (pp. 213–239). New York: New York Academy of Sciences.

Tucker, D.M., & Williamson, P.A. (1984). Asymmetric neural control systems in human self-regulation. *Psychological Review, 91*, 185–215.

Ungerleider, L.G., & Mishkin, M. (1982). Two cortical visual systems. In D.J. Ingle, R.J.W. Mansfield, & M.A. Goodale (Eds.), *The Analysis of Visual Behavior* (pp. 549–586). Cambridge, MA: MIT Press.

Van Bockstaele, E.J., Pieribone, V.A., & Aston-Jones, G. (1989). Diverse afferents converge on the nucleus paragigantocellularis in the rat ventrolateral medulla: Retrograde and anterograde tracing studies. *Journal of Comparative Neurology, 290*, 561–584.

Vrana, S.R., Spence, E.L., & Lang, P.J. (1988). The startle probe response: A new measure of emotion? *Journal of Abnormal Psychology, 97*, 487–491.

White, S.R., Fung, S.J., Jackson, D.A., & Imel, K.M. (1996). Serotonin, norepinephrine and associated neuropeptides: Effects on somatic motoneuron excitability. In G. Holstege, R. Bandler, & C.B. Saper (Eds.), *Progress in Brain Research, Vol. 107: The Emotional Motor System* (pp. 183–200). Amsterdam: Elsevier.

Wilson, F.A.W., O'Scalaidhe, S.P., & Goldman-Rakic, P.S. (1993). Dissociation of object and spatial processing domains in primate prefrontal cortex. *Science, 260*, 1955–1958.

Yakovlev, P.I., & Lecours, A.-R. (1967). The myelogenetic cycles of regional maturation of the brain. In A. Minkowski (Ed.), *Regional Development of the Brain in Early Life* (pp. 3–70). Oxford: Blackwell.

4

Neuropsychological Assessment of Emotional Processing in Brain-Damaged Patients

JOAN C. BOROD, MATTHIAS H. TABERT,
CORNELIA SANTSCHI, AND ESTHER H. STRAUSS

This chapter reviews literature on the assessment of emotional processing in brain-damaged populations. By *emotion*, we refer to affective behaviors that are relatively brief in duration. We begin with a brief discussion of the current neuropsychological literature pertaining to the assessment of emotion. Next, we turn to the main focus of the chapter, which is a description of batteries of tests that were developed specifically to assess emotional processing in neurological populations. Then, because of the complexity of assessment in this area, we describe procedures commonly used for eliciting and evaluating emotional expression. We conclude with recommendations for future research on the neuropsychological assessment of emotion.

Our focus is on adult brain-damaged and healthy aging populations and not on psychiatric and developmental issues, which are beyond the scope of this chapter. The chapter provides a compendium of emotional processing tests that can be used as a foundation for research, assessment, and rehabilitation purposes. The reader should note, however, that many of these tests are in the developmental stages and may not be commercially available.

BACKGROUND

Within the neuropsychological literature, there is a dearth of information about assessment of emotion (Cripe, 1996; Tarter & Edwards, 1986). This observation was confirmed by our review of recent textbooks focusing on neuropsychological assessment (Filskov & Boll, 1991; Incagnoli, Goldstein, & Golden, 1986; Lezak, 1995; Spreen & Strauss, 1998). In general, these textbooks present a variety of self-report inventories that examine mood, personality, well-being, and social adjustment. For the most part, these inventories (e.g., Beck Depression Inventory, Minnesota Multiphasic Personality Inventory [MMPI], and Symptom Check List-90) were developed for use with psychiatric populations (Reitan & Wolfson, 1997). When clinicians have examined affective behaviors, they have taken a descriptive approach and conducted bedside evaluations, analogous to what is used in a neurological/psychiatric mental status examination (e.g., Ruckdeschel-Hibbard, Gordon, & Diller, 1986). The social functioning inventories tend to focus on evaluating the extent of physical and social dysfunction within the context of activities of daily living (e.g., Tarter & Edwards, 1986). Those authors who do point to the need for assessment procedures for emotional processing indicate methodological and psychometric issues as problematic in standardizing potential measures in this area (e.g., Nelson & Cicchetti, 1995). Furthermore, they often cite the need for theoretical grounding in this area and the need for the development of tools that assess various discrete aspects of emotional functioning (Cripe, 1996).

REVIEW OF THE EMOTIONAL ASSESSMENT LITERATURE: TEST BATTERIES AND RELATED STUDIES OF EMOTIONAL PROCESSING

Our goal has been to simplify and organize the literature on the neuropsychological assessment of emotional processing. We assumed a componential approach (Borod, 1993b), which conceptualizes emotion as consisting of a number of aspects or components that are presumed to be mediated by different neural substrates (Borod et al., in press; Cripe, 1997; Gainotti, Chapter 9, this volume). For our purposes, the components and their respective elements include processing modes (i.e., perception, arousal, experience, expression, and goal-directed behavior) (Plutchik, 1984) and communication channels (i.e., facial, prosodic, lexical, gestural, postural, and scenic). By a *scene*, we refer to the total arrangement and interactions of stimuli that form the environment in which a situation occurs, for example, a line drawing of a man being held at gunpoint for the emotion of fear (Cicone, Wapner, & Gardner, 1980). Given the complexity of the brain–behavior relationships for emotion, the componential approach provides a useful model for organizing this literature. This approach is predicated on a long-standing issue in the overall emotion literature (Buck, Miller, & Caul, 1974; Levitt, 1964; Mebrabian & Reed, 1968), including more recent work in the neuropsychology of emotion literature (e.g., Borod et al., 1986; Bowers, Bauer, &

Heilman, 1993; Gainotti, Caltagirone, & Zoccolotti, 1993; Semenza et al., 1986), namely, whether there are separate or overlapping systems in the brain underlying emotional processing.

Based on this theoretical perspective, we selected batteries of emotion tests with more than one element within a component (i.e., processing mode and/or communication channel). In this review, the primary modes included are perception, expression, and experience, and the channels included are facial, prosodic, lexical, gestural, postural, and scenic. Batteries reviewed were designed or specifically adapted for brain-damaged populations. For each battery, we provide a brief description of each task included; targeted populations; psychometric properties, where available; and general research findings. In addition, related studies including measures of emotion, although not necessarily called "batteries" by the authors of the studies, were reviewed and integrated into this section. Table 4.1 lists the batteries and related studies, specified by mode and channel. Psychometric information regarding reliability, validity, standardization, and norms is not systematically included because it was not provided for many of the published reports reviewed in this chapter. Accordingly, we refer the reader to individual authors. Due to space limitations, our focus here is descriptive. Future reviews of this literature would benefit from a more systematic conceptual and methodological critique of emotion assessment techniques.

A Single Processing Mode via Multiple Channels

Perception

Profile of Nonverbal Sensitivity. Benowitz and colleagues (1983) used the Profile of Nonverbal Sensitivity (PONS) (Rosenthal et al., 1979) to assess emotional perception ability across three channels (facial, prosodic, and body movement). The body movement channel examines the neck to the knee, focusing on gestural and postural expression. Stimuli involved 220 2-second film segments extracted from 20 different emotional scenes portrayed by a woman poser in four emotional categories (positive–dominant, positive–submissive, negative–dominant, and negative–submissive). Each of the 20 scenes is presented in 11 different formats: face (F) alone, body (B) alone, prosody via content-filtered speech (PCF), prosody via randomly spliced speech (PRS), F/B, F/PCF, F/PRS, B/PCF, B/PRS, F/B/PCF, and F/B/PRS. For each item, the subject is required to select one of two alternative descriptions (e.g., positive–dominant). In the Benowitz et al. study (see Benowitz, 1980; Benowitz et al., 1983), the full PONS was administered to seven right brain–damaged (RBD) (*M* age = 48.9 years) and four left brain–damaged (LBD) (*M* = 46.3 years) patients, and an abbreviated version of the PONS (containing 80 items in which only single-channel items

Table 4.1. Literature Included in the Emotional Assessment Review as a Function of Processing Mode and Communication Channel

| CATEGORY | STUDY | BATTERY (IF AVAILABLE) | PROCESSING MODE | | | | | COMMUNICATION CHANNEL | | | | | | |
			PERCEPTION	EXPRESSION	EXPERIENCE	AROUSAL	BEHAVIOR	FACIAL	PROSODIC	LEXICAL	GESTURAL	BODY MOVEMENT	SCENES	MISCELLANEOUS
Single mode/ multiple channels														
	Benowitz et al. (1983)	Profile of Nonverbal Sensitivity (PONS)	X					X	X			X	X	
	Egan et al. (1990)	Perception of Emotion Test (POET)	X					X	X	X				
	Mountain (1993)	Victoria Emotion Perception Test (VERT)	X					X	X					
	Bowers et al. (1991); Blonder et al. (1991)	Florida Affect Battery (FAB); selected study	X					X	X		X			

(Continued)

Table 4.1. Literature Included in the Emotional Assessment Review as a Function of Processing Mode and Communication Channel (*Continued*)

| | | | PROCESSING MODE | | | | COMMUNICATION CHANNEL | | | | | BODY | | |
CATEGORY	STUDY	BATTERY (IF AVAILABLE)	PERCEP-TION	EXPRES-SION	EXPERI-ENCE	AROUSAL	BE-HAVIOR	FACIAL	PROSODIC	LEXI-CAL	GES-TURAL	MOVE-MENT	SCENES	MISCELLA-NEOUS
	Lalande et al. (1992)	Selected study	X						X	X	X			
	Cicone et al. (1980)	Selected study	X					X		X	X		X	
	Heath et al. (1997)	Selected study		X				X	X			X		X*
Single channel/ multiple modes	Ross et al. (1997)	Aprosodia Battery (AB)	X	X					X					
	Meadows & Kaplan (1994)	Selected study			X	X							X	
Multiple modes/ multiple channels	Cancelliere & Kertesz (1990)	Battery of Emotional Expression & Comprehension (BEEC)		X				X	X				X	

Study										
Borod et al. (1992)	New York Emotion Battery (NYEB)	X	X	X		X	X	X		
Hornak et al. (1996)	Selected study	X		X	X	X	X			
Weddell (1994)	Selected study	X	X			X	X	X	X	
					X	X				
Cohen et al. (1994)	Selected study	X	X				X			X
Blonder et al. (1989)	Selected study	X	X			X	X	X		
						X				
Scott et al. (1984)	Selected study	X	X			X	X			
						X				
Borod et al. (1990)	Experimental affect battery	X	X			X	X			

*Affective state.

were presented) was given to one right-hemispherectomized patient (age = 24 years) and four commissurotomized patients (M = 40.3 years). As might be expected, the data revealed right-hemisphere superiority for the ability to evaluate emotional information.

Perception of Emotions Test. The Perception of Emotions Test (POET) (Egan et al., 1990) is a test of emotional perception across three channels (facial, prosodic, and verbal), separately and combined. Stimuli involve 128 6-second video/audio segments with emotional components portrayed by two men and two women. Four emotions are portrayed (anger, happiness, sadness, and neutrality) in each of four conditions: facial expressions without sound; prosodically intoned scripts with neutral content (no video); verbal emotional scripts presented in a neutral tone of voice (no video); and combined scenes with emotional content in all three channels simultaneously. After stimulus presentation, the subject has 8 seconds to respond by pointing to one of four drawings, each with a verbal label depicting each of the emotions. The real-time presentation of emotional stimuli across channels provides a degree of ecological validity. The POET was originally administered to 100 normal adults (M = 22.2 years), 11 LBD patients (M = 65.9 years), and 10 RBD patients (M = 63.6 years) (Egan et al., 1990). In addition, the facial stimuli were adapted for use with positron emission tomography (Egan et al., 1996), showing more frequent right-hemisphere activation.

Victoria Emotion Perception Test. The Victoria Emotion Perception Test (VERT) (Mountain, 1993) evaluates emotional perception across two channels (facial and prosodic), both separately and combined. The VERT is comprised of three subtests (facial, prosodic, and combined), each consisting of 24 paired-items involving photographs of facial emotional expressions and prosodic emotionally intoned strings of nonsense words. There are four emotions (anger, sadness, happiness, and fear) presented at three intensity levels (mild, moderate, and extreme). For each item-pair, the subject is required to make four separate forced-choice judgements: a same–different discrimination with respect to emotional category and intensity level, and an identification of the discrete emotion and the intensity level.

The battery (VERT Research) was designed for use with clinical populations suffering from emotional disorders and was originally normed and standardized on young and elderly normal adults. The VERT Clinical consists of half of the items selected for item stability. The VERT provides age-related norms (based on two samples of young adults [N_1 = 13, M = 27.2 years; N_2 = 18, M = 24.5 years] and one sample of older adults [N = 9, M = 72 years]) *and* reliability data (internal consistency and test–retest). For construct validity, a significant positive correlation was found between the PONS and both versions of the VERT (Mountain & Spreen, 1993).

Florida Affect Battery and related study. The Florida Affect Battery (FAB) (Bowers, Blonder, & Heilman, 1991) is a comprehensive battery, consisting of ten subtests, for the assessment of emotional perception across facial and prosodic channels. For both channels, five emotions are studied (i.e., happiness, sadness, anger, fear, and neutrality), and there are an emotional identification and discrimination task, as well as a nonemotional discrimination task. For face, there are two additional emotional subtests, one involving comprehension and one involving matching. Finally, there are two reciprocal cross-modal subtests involving facial and prosodic emotional stimuli. All subtests for these two channels have 20 items (5 emotions × 4 items) except for the prosodic nonemotional subtest, which has 16 items.

Blonder, Bowers, and Heilman (1991) included two lexical tasks in a study incorporating the FAB. The tasks were comprised of 56 verbal sentence descriptors of nonverbal expressions (face, voice, and gesture; e.g., "tears fell from her eyes" and "she laughed") and comprehension of 75 emotional sentences (e.g., "you were delighted by the bonus"). The latter task contains no words describing facial, prosodic, or gestural signals *and* contains three levels of inferential complexity (denotations, words and phrases associated with particular emotions, and contextual cues requiring inferences).

The FAB and the two lexical tasks were administered (Blonder, Bower, & Heilman 1991) to ten RBD (*M* = 64.1 years), ten LBD (*M* = 59.6 years), and ten normal control (NC) (*M* = 63.2 years) right-handed adults. Right brain–damaged subjects showed deficits in discriminating and matching facial emotion, identifying and discriminating emotional prosody, and identifying sentences depicting nonverbal expressions. The FAB has also been administered to Alzheimer's disease patients (Cadieux & Greve, 1996), who showed some deficits, and to a global aphasic patient with a large left hemisphere lesion (Barrett et al., 1999), who showed preserved performance on nonverbal affect recognition tasks.

Related studies. Lalande et al. (1992) examined verbal and prosodic emotional perception in unilateral right (*N* = 12, *M* = 61.8 years) and nonaphasic left (*N* = 10, *M* = 58 years) stroke patients and in 16 NCs (*M* = 61 years). Six emotions were studied (joy, anger, fear, disgust, surprise, and sadness), and 36 taped phrases were used for all tasks. For the verbal contextual task, neutrally intoned phrases were presented auditorily. For the pure prosody task, hummed phrases with emotional intonation were presented auditorily (e.g., "propulsive growling," "whining," and "screaming"). For single-channel tasks, an identification paradigm was used. For the cross-modal task, a discrimination paradigm was used; 18 phrases were presented in a content-concordant tone, and 18 were discordant. Hemisphere-specific deficits were reported, with RBDs impaired on the pure prosody and cross-modal tasks and LBDs on the verbal contextual task.

Cicone, Wapner, and Gardner (*1980*) studied the perception of positive emotions (happiness, surprise–glee, excitement, and/or love) and negative emotions (i.e., sadness, disgust, fear, and anger) in facial expressions, verbal/phrasal descriptors, and pictorial scenes. Six emotions were used per task, and a multiple-choice recognition paradigm was employed with both verbal and pictorial formats. Subjects were 18 LBD patients (*M* = 49 years) and 21 RBD patients (*M* = 58 years) of various etiologies. Demographically matched and age-matched control subjects were ten hospital patients being treated for non-neurological illness. A second group of control subjects included 13 bifrontal leukotomy patients (*M* = 55 years). Although LBDs showed a selective deficit for linguistic stimuli, RBDs demonstrated a reduction in emotional sensitivity across channels.

Expression

Related study. In a recent innovative study by *Heath et al.* (*1997*) utilizing a naturalistic observational approach, spontaneous expression during a neuropsychological evaluation was observed and rated for the occurrence of facial expression, intonation, eye contact, and affective state. Two ethnographers determined the frequencies of occurrences for each channel, and most subjects were observed more than once. Subjects were unilateral stroke patients with RBD (*N* = 4, *M* = 65.5 years) and LBD (*N* = 7, *M* = 60.7 years) *and* normal hospital controls (*N* = 7, *M* = 69.4 years). Although both stroke groups showed difficulty in facial expressiveness and in conveying affective state, the patients with right-hemisphere pathology also showed selective impairments in intonation and in establishing eye contact.

A Single Channel via Multiple Processing Modes

Prosody

Aprosodia Battery. The Aprosodia Battery (AB), recently described by Ross, Thompson, and Yenkosky (1997), originated in earlier work by Ross in the 1970s and 1980s (see Ross, 1985; Ross & Mesulam, 1979). This battery arose from clinical neurological observations of altered prosodic components of speech in RBDs and was originally developed for bedside evaluation. Furthermore, the basis of the battery and Ross's conceptualization of the aprosodias vis-à-vis the right hemisphere are grounded in neuroanatomical models of language organization for the left hemisphere (e.g., Goodglass & Kaplan, 1983).

The AB examines prosody across expressive (posed repetition and spontaneous) and comprehension (identification and discrimination) processing modes. Six emotional categories (neutral, happiness, surprise, sadness, anger, and disinterested) are examined for all aspects of the battery except for spontaneous expression for which one positive and three negative scenarios are used to elicit responses. The posed repetition tasks include 12 stimuli in each of three conditions (words, monosyllables [e.g., "ba"], and asyllables [e.g., "aaahhhhhhhh"]). The comprehension tasks include 24 stimuli for identification across three conditions (words, monosyllables, and asyllables) and for discrimination across one condition (filtered words). For the identification tasks, subjects are required to select one of six choices presented as line drawings of faces with verbal labels. For the expression tasks, Ross has developed extensive procedures for computer-assisted acoustical analysis (e.g., Ross, 1997; Ross, Edmondson, & Seibert, 1986; Ross et al., 1987). Trained judges also rate the posed voice recordings for affective category and for intensity. Ross's battery has been used to determine the relationship between aprosodic syndromes (e.g., sensory aprosodia and motor aprosodia) and neuroanatomical sites via template mapping of brain lesions for functional-anatomical correlations (Gorelick & Ross, 1987; Ross, 1981). Findings from the work of Ross and colleagues have suggested that anterior portions of the right hemisphere are important for the production of emotional prosody, whereas posterior regions of the right hemisphere are important for the comprehension of emotional prosody.

Emotional situations/scenes

Related study. In a study by *Meadows and Kaplan* (*1994*), autonomic and subjective responses to emotional and neutral slides (Buck, 1978) were evaluated in 12 RBD subjects ($M = 63.2$ years) and nine LBD subjects ($M = 64.6$ years) with cerebrovascular accidents and in 25 NC subjects ($M = 55.8$ years). The communication channel utilized in this study (i.e., "scenes") employed emotionally charged scenarios or scenes. The psychophysiological measures were skin conductance and heart rate, and subjects were required to identify the content of each slide and rate their subjective experience on a 9-point Likert pleasantness scale. Although the groups did not differ in subjective ratings, the RBDs showed a significant reduction in autonomic arousal as measured by skin conductance.

Multiple Processing Modes Via Multiple Channels

Battery of Emotional Expression and Comprehension

The Battery of Emotional Expression and Comprehension (BEEC) (Cancelliere & Kertesz, 1990) assesses posed emotional expression for the prosodic channel and emotional perception for faces, prosody, and scenes. For expression, there are two prosodic subtests, one involving posing to verbal command and the other posing to imitation ("repetition"). Each subtest contains 16 neutral-content sentences, and four expressions are elicited (happiness, sadness, anger, and neutrality). Procedures are described for the evaluation of prosodic expressions, via trained raters, for both valence and pitch (on a 7-point Likert scale). For perception, each identification subtest contains the four expressions mentioned above. There are 20 items for facial and prosodic emotion and 16 items for line drawings of emotional scenes (e.g., a child opening a Christmas gift). The BEEC was administered to unilateral stroke patients (who were relatively acute) (28 RBDs and 18 LBDs [$M = 62.5$ years]) and to 20 NCs ($M = 62.4$ years) and was studied with respect to computed tomography scan lesion localization and aprosodic syndromes (Cancelliere & Kertesz, 1990). Results did not reveal differences as a function of lesion side, but lesion site differences were observed, with deficits most prominent for basal ganglia, anterior temporal, insula, and perisylvian regions.

New York Emotion Battery

The New York Emotion Battery (NYEB) (Borod, Welkowitz, & Obler, 1992) originates in a componential approach to emotional processing (Borod, 1993b) and examines emotional expression (posed and spontaneous), perception (identification and discrimination), and experience across facial, prosodic, and lexical channels. There are three positive emotions (happiness, interest, and pleasant surprise) and five negative emotions (anger, disgust, fear, sadness, and unpleasant surprise). In addition, the battery includes screening measures and nonemotional control tasks for each channel and processing mode. The categories for the nonemotional tasks are characteristics of people (e.g., vision) for perception, everyday activities (e.g., bought something for the house) for spontaneous expression, and relatively abstract imageable words (e.g., space) for posed expression. Subtests of the battery have analogous psychometric properties (e.g., structure and administration procedures) across the three channels. In addition, in developing the perception tasks (Borod et al., 1998), normal adults rated each stimulus item as belonging to a particular emotional category (e.g., happiness) at 80%, on the average, across channels, paradigms, valences, and discrete emotions.

Identification tasks for prosodic and lexical channels consist of 24 items each, and 32 items are included for the facial channel; discrimination tasks include 28 stimulus pairs. For facial stimuli, slides developed by Borod, Welkowitz, and Obler (1992) and by Ekman and Friesen (1976) are used. There are two lexical identification tasks, one with single words and one with complete sentences. For posed expression, the eight emotional expressions are produced to verbal command and imitation. For spontaneous expression, subjects recollect recent experiences ("monologues") for each emotion. For analysis of expression data, raters evaluate facial expressions via video without sound, prosodic expressions via audio, and lexical expressions via transcripts. Trained raters analyze expressions for category accuracy and emotional intensity using procedures developed by Canino et al. (1999) for posed expressions in all three channels, by Montreys and Borod (1998) for spontaneous facial expressions, and by Borod et al. (1996) for spontaneous lexical expression. (See also Tabert et al. [1997] for a word error–type analysis of the posed lexical expression data). Emotional experience is evaluated via Likert-scale self-report measures of intensity and accuracy after each monologue.

The perception measures of the NYEB were administered to 11 RBD stroke patients ($M = 67.1$ years), 10 LBD stroke patients ($M = 63.2$ years), and 15 NC adults ($M = 64.8$ years) (Borod et al., 1998). On identification measures, RBDs were significantly impaired relative to LBDs and NCs across all three channels; for discrimination measures, no group differences emerged. In a follow-up study focusing on language deficits, Cicero et al. (1999) found that the performance of LBDs with language deficits was facilitated, whereas the performance of RBDs was suppressed on the emotional sentence identification task. In addition, parts of or adaptations of aspects of the NYEB have been used in Borod's laboratory to study emotional communication in temporal lobe epileptics (Santschi-Haywood et al., 1996, 1997), hemiparkinson's disease patients (St. Clair et al., 1998), and healthy normal adults across the lifespan (Grunwald et al., 1999), and to examine the recovery of emotional functioning after stroke.

Related studies

Hornak, Rolls, and Wade (1996) examined emotional facial and prosodic perception, subjective experience, and behavior in brain-injured patients with postinjury histories of socially inappropriate behavior. Patients had either head injury or stroke; there were 12 patients with ventral frontal lobe damage ($M = 41.4$ years) and 11 with nonventral (e.g., parietal or basal ganglia) damage ($M = 47.4$ years). For facial perception, the emotions used were happiness, surprise, anger, disgust, fright, sadness, and neutrality; for prosodic perception, the emotions used were contentment, puzzlement, anger, disgust, fright, sadness, and neutrality. The prosodic paradigm involved nonverbal expressions (e.g., "ugh" and "yuck" for disgust) rather than emotionally modulated speech to make it easier for brain-injured patients to process. To evaluate experience, a subjective emotional change questionnaire was used. To evaluate "behavior," a questionnaire was used involving a range of behavioral problems (e.g., disinhibition) occurring in social milieus. A member of the patient's rehabilitation team completed the questionnaire. There was a positive correlation between the degree of altered emotional experience and the severity of behavioral problems. The use of both subjective and objective measures of emotion enables a more refined examination of processing mode relationships and has implications for clinical rehabilitation. The focus of this work (Hornak, Rolls, & Wade, 1996) was on caudality rather than laterality. Results demonstrated that the ventral patients were more impaired than the nonventral patients on the perceptual and experiential measures.

Weddell (1994) examined the effects of subcortical lesion site on emotional expression and perception. Subjects were 10 patients with damage to structures of the third ventricle (M = 43.5 years), 61 patients with focal cerebral lesions (M = 50.7 years; 27 RBDs and 24 LBDs), and 15 non-brain–damaged patients with spinal cord lesions. For expression, both spontaneous and posed facial expressions were elicited and evaluated via the Facial Action Coding System (Ekman & Friesen, 1978). Spontaneous expression included both positive and negative responses (Weddell, Trevarthen, & Miller, 1988); posed expressions included happiness, anger, disgust, and surprise (Weddell, Miller, & Trevarthen, 1990). For perception, facial, prosodic, and lexical channels were evaluated via emotional and neutral-content sentences and utterances; emotions included happiness, sadness, anger, surprise, and neutrality. In addition, a recognition memory paradigm (Weddell, 1989) was used for the facial channel. Finally, behavior was assessed with a semistructured interview that focused on social–emotional behaviors, appetitive disturbances, and psychiatric symptoms. In general, patients with hypothalamic damage exhibited appetitive disorders; patients with cerebral lesions, especially right medial temporal involvement, demonstrated impaired emotional recognition; and patients with frontal and basal ganglia damage displayed impoverished facial emotional expression.

Cohen, Riccio, and Flannery (1994) reported a case study of a 16-year-old girl with a unilateral right-hemisphere basal ganglia embolic stroke that used multiple channels and modes. For perception, the patient was administered a test involving the identification of emotional gesturing via videotape, emotional prosody in audiotaped sentences, and a combination of gesturing and prosody. The emotions used were happiness, sadness, and anger. For expression, the patient was required to intone sentences and to imitate prosodically intoned sentences; expressions were evaluated for appropriateness by two independent raters. The measures were administered immediately after the stroke and again 4 months later. During both assessments, the patient was able to comprehend emotional gestures and prosody but showed a deficit in expressing emotional prosody. Procedures for the evaluation of gestural communication have been previously described by Ross (1985, 1997) for clinical examination and by Blonder et al. (1995) in an experimental paradigm.

In another study examining unilateral hemispheric pathology (in hemiparkinson's disease [HPD]), *Blonder, Gur, and Gur (1989)* evaluated the expression of emotional prosody and the perception of emotion across three channels. There were 14 right HPDs (M = 61 years), 7 left HPDs (M = 62 years), and 17 NCs (M = 62.4 years). For the expressive task, subjects were required to make and imitate semantically neutral sentences in five different emotional tones (happiness, puzzlement, anger, sadness, and neutrality). These expressions were subsequently rated for intensity and/or accuracy. For perception, subjects were required to identify emotions conveyed by facial expressions (Ekman & Friesen, 1975), intoned neutral sentences, and semantically emotional sentences.

Nonemotional control tasks for the prosodic (e.g., receptive linguistic prosody [Weintraub, Mesulam, & Kramer, 1981]) and facial (e.g., identification of famous faces) channels were included to control for cognitive and perceptual deficits (e.g., visuospatial deficits for the facial channel) commonly seen in Parkinson's disease. Although there were expressive and receptive emotional deficits for HPDs relative to NCs, there were no differences as a function of laterality, suggesting bilateral involvement in emotional processing at the subcortical level. To our knowledge, this was the first study to examine emotional processing in HPD.

An evaluation of Parkinson's disease conducted by *Scott, Caird, and Williams* (*1984*) involved 28 patients with Parkinson's disease (*M* = 63 years) and 28 elderly NCs (*M* = 70 years). Perception was evaluated in two channels, and expression was evaluated in one. For expression, prosodic production of a single emotion (i.e., anger) via a brief sentence was examined and scored for accuracy. For perception, matching tasks containing several facial and prosodic emotional stimuli were administered. Overall, the Parkinson's disease patients were impaired relative to NCs in expressing and perceiving emotion.

Finally, we conclude with a study by *Borod et al.* (*1990*) that examined emotional expression and perception in 20 Parkinson's disease patients (*M* = 65.7 years), 19 unilateral right-sided stroke patients (*M* = 63.5 years), psychiatric patients (i.e., 20 schizophrenic [*M* = 39.1 years] and 12 unipolar depressive [*M* = 56.4 years]), and 21 NCs [*M* = 56.9 years]). An experimental affect battery was used to examine the perception and expression of facial and prosodic emotion. As emotional valence was a focus of this study, three positive emotions (happiness, pleasant surprise, and interest) and four negative emotions (anger, sadness, fear, and disgust) were assessed across all tasks. For expression, subjects were required to pose, facially and prosodically, these emotions to oral command. Video and audio recordings of the expressions were later evaluated by naïve judges for emotional intensity, category accuracy, and valence accuracy. For perception, both identification and discrimination paradigms were used, involving photographs of facial emotion (Ekman & Friesen, 1976) and intoned neutral-content sentences (e.g., "fish can jump out of the water"; Tucker, Watson, & Heilman, 1977). Reliability data were provided for the tasks—interrater agreement for expression and internal consistency for perception. Schizophrenics showed the most impairment in expressing and perceiving emotions, followed by RBDs and Parkinson's disease patients, then by unipolar depressive patients, with NCs showing the least impairment. Borod et al. (1990) examined relationships between facial and prosodic channels *and* between expressive and perceptual processing modes. Although there were positive associations between facial and prosodic channels, measures of perception and expression were less strongly correlated.

EMOTIONAL EXPRESSION

This section provides information about examining emotional expression in neurological populations. Note that the procedures described come from basic emotion research with normal people and from the psychiatric literature. Both expression elicitation and evaluation procedures are provided. With respect to evaluation, essentially there are two approaches, one focuses on external expression and the other on internal states and dispositions.

Elicitation Procedures

Typically, for external expression, emotion is induced via elicitation procedures involving the presentation of emotionally evocative stimuli. In work with brain-damaged individuals, both auditory (e.g., mood-induction) and visual (e.g., slide-presentation) stimuli are employed. For example, mood-induction procedures reported in the literature primarily involve verbal statements (e.g., Velten, 1968) and sometimes nonverbal stimuli (e.g., facial expressions [Dimberg, 1982; Schneider et al., 1995] and video clips from movies [Davidson, 1995; Tomarken, Davidson, & Henriques, 1990]). In terms of slide-presentation procedures, for example, one set of stimuli frequently used in neuropsychological research is the set developed by Buck (1978). It consists of 32 photographs (in slide format) representing five separate categories: scenic (e.g., sunset over a lake), pleasant (e.g., young child touching flowers), sexual (e.g., embracing couple), unusual (e.g., multiple exposures of an airport), and unpleasant (e.g., starving child). Another set of slides used extensively in emotion research with normal individuals that can be adapted for use with clinical populations is the International Affective Picture System (IAPS) (Lang, Ohman, & Vaitl, 1988). As described by Lang et al. (1993), the IAPS consists of 240 slides that have been conceptualized across several dimensions, that is, valence (pleasantness/unpleasantness), arousal (calm/arousing), and dominance (or control). Employing another approach that focuses on expression rather than perception to induce a mood, Schiff and Lamon (1989) have used unilateral facial manipulation to induce pleasant and unpleasant mood states.

Evaluation Procedures

Observations of external expression

Once expressions are elicited and recorded, they are typically subjected to ratings by trained judges or to analytical techniques for a specific channel. In the case of ratings, the most commonly used measures with brain-damaged individuals are accuracy (or appropriateness), expressivity (or frequency), and intensity (for review, see Borod, 1993a). Subjects' expressions are recorded (via audio, video, and/or transcription procedures) and then evaluated by judges who are naïve to the characteristics of the patients. It is essential to train the judges and to establish a high degree of interrater reliability. The following references provide examples of rating procedures frequently used, by channel: facial channel— Blonder et al., 1993; Borod et al., 1988; Kolb & Taylor, 1990; Malatesta & Izard, 1984; Oster, Hegley, & Nagel, 1992; Weddell, Miller, & Trevarthen, 1990; prosodic channel—Banse & Scherer, 1996; Borod et al., 1990; Ross, 1997; Sobin & Alpert, 1999; lexical channel—Bloom et al., 1990, 1992; Borod et al., 1996; Cimino et al., 1991; and gestural channel—Blonder et al., 1995; Ross, 1997. Some investigators have developed rating procedures that are standardized across multiple channels (Borod et al., 1990; Canino et al., 1999).

There are also a number of techniques for quantification of features related to each of the communication channels: muscle action units for the facial channel (Facial Action Coding System [Ekman & Friesen, 1978] and the Maximally Discriminative Facial Movement Coding System [Izard, 1983]); acoustical parameters (e.g., frequency, duration, pitch, and amplitude) for the prosodic channel (Alpert et al., 1989; Martz & Welkowitz, 1977; Ross et al., 1987; Shapiro & Danly, 1985; Welkowitz, Bond, & Zelano, 1990); and discourse and word analysis (e.g., length, frequency, structure, and grammatical type) for the lexical channel (Bloom et al., 1994; Davitz, 1964; Tabert et al., 1997). For a review of computerized voice analysis software (i.e., Computerized Speech Laboratory, CSpeech, and Sound Scope), see Bielamowicz et al. (1996).

Observations of internal states and dispositions

To obtain a patient's evaluation of his or her own experience while producing emotional expressions, typically, individuals are asked to produce self-reports about internal subjective experience. Although clinicians often rely on such standard measures as the MMPI-2 (Gasparrani et al., 1978; Greene, 1992), Personality Assessment Inventory (Morley, 1991), Rorschach (Rorschach, 1942), and Thematic Aperception Test (Murray, 1938), our focus here is on novel and often experimental measures developed specifically for neurological populations. Within a neuropsychological context, use of more routine tests, such as the MMPI-2 and Rorschach, may be contraindicated because of their heavy demands on attention, concentration, comprehension, and/or perceptual skills. Neurological insult often results in deficits in these domains, rendering administration and interpretation of test results problematic. In a related vein, some concerns endorsed by patients (e.g., fatigue and hallucinations) may be caused by valid neurological dysfunction and therefore should not be considered a reflection of the patient's emotional state. For a more detailed description of standardized assessment techniques, see Exner (1986), Graham (1993), and Spreen and Strauss (1998).

To assess internal experience, Likert-type scales are generally employed (ranging from minimal to maximal), and the amount of emotional intensity or accuracy is assessed (e.g., via the Differential Emotions Scale [Izard, 1972]). These scales typically apply to one's experience at the moment with respect to the "affect" elicited by a particular stimulus. To evaluate "mood," which is longer lasting and more stable in duration than affect, a number of scales have been developed for use with brain-damaged populations (for review, see Sweet et al., 1992). For depression, examples of scales are the Geriatric Depression Screening Scale (Yesavage et al., 1983), the Post-Stroke Depression Rating Scale (Gainotti et al., 1997), and the Structured Assessment of Depression in Brain-Damaged Individuals (Gordon et al., 1991). Taking a broader approach, Nelson et al. (1989) developed the Neuropsychology Behavior and Affect Profile to use with neurological populations and to assess five areas: inappropriateness, indifference, depression, pragnosia ("defects in the pragmatics of conversational style"), and mania. In a similar vein, Levin et al. (1987) developed the Neurobehavioral Rating Scale, adapted from the Brief Psychiatric Rating Scale (Overall & Gorham, 1962), to document behavioral sequelae of brain damage (e.g., anxiety, depressive mood, lability, and suspiciousness). The scale is designed for patients who are unable to fill in self-report inventories; it is completed by a clinician or interviewer familiar with the patient. Finally, the Portland Adaptability Inventory (O'Brien & Lezak, 1988) was developed to evaluate a patient's emotionality (e.g., irritability, depression, and delusions) and social adaptation (e.g., appropriateness and employment) via a trained observer and a rating scale.

To obtain a sense of a person's inner experience, personality inventories have been used. They typically capture traits and characteristics of personality over an extended period of time. One such questionnaire is the Temporal Lobe Epilepsy Questionnaire developed by Bear and Fedio (1977) to assess characteristics of temporal lobe epilepsy (e.g., circumstantiality, religiosity, emotionality, humorlessness, and euphoria). Another inventory, the Friedes Neuropsychological Personality Survey (Friedes, 1991), attempts to integrate aspects of personality (e.g., endurance, aggression, disorganization, and anxiety) with cortical levels of arousal.

CONCLUSION

In summary, several tests have been developed recently to assess emotional processing in brain-damaged individuals. In their current state, these measures are best regarded as research tools. Although these tests and batteries hold considerable promise, much more work needs to be done if they are to be used in the clinical setting.

Currently, these batteries and procedures have both conceptual and methodological limitations. From a conceptual perspective, there is the issue of construct validity. Many tasks/inventories have been developed, yet few provide both convergent and divergent evidence for construct validity. Furthermore, most studies have been performed by the authors of the particular tests. Data from diverse laboratories are important to provide validating evidence. In addition, large-scale studies of normal persons and a range of patient populations are needed to allow meaningful evaluation of the performance of an individual patient. Another type of validity that needs to be addressed is ecological validity because "the scores derived from such tests may have little bearing on the patient's ability to function in his or her environment or society" (Sbordone, 1996, p. 16). With regard to future work in this area, investigators might want to borrow from the literature on functional communication (e.g., Borod et al., 1989; Holland, 1980; Sarno, 1969) and social skills training (e.g., Brozgold et al., 1998; Mueser et al., 1996); they have dealt with ecological validity in perhaps a more direct fashion and have developed measures that can be used in more naturalistic settings. In general, test validity depends on three elements: content, criterion-related, and construct validity. Although these principles have typically been central to the development of tests within the cognitive domain, attention to such procedures should also help to clarify and refine the meaning of various aspects of emotional processing.

From a methodological perspective, the measures reviewed here need considerable work with respect to psychometric features (e.g., standardization, norms, and reliability). Several emotion tests do provide substantive information about the psychometric properties of the procedures used. These tests focus on a single channel and on a single processing mode and thus were not reviewed above. One is a test of facial emotion identification, using standard slides (Ekman & Friesen, 1976), developed by LeFever (1988) for use with normal adults. A second is a facial emotion discrimination task developed by the Gurs and colleagues for use with normal (Erwin et al., 1992), depressed (Gur et al., 1992), and schizophrenic (Heimberg et al., 1992) individuals. The third is a prosodic emotion identification task (Emotional Perception Test) that has been normed for children (Allen, personal communication, 1998) and for adults across the lifespan (Green, 1996). To move beyond a single channel and mode, in our own work on the NYEB, we are currently establishing reliability for both perception measures (Borod et al., in press) and expression measures (Canino et al., 1999) across multiple channels, and we are developing norms across the lifespan.

An interesting area for future research entails the use of emotional stimuli in neuropsychological evaluations of cognitive functions (e.g., attention via the Emotional Stroop Task [Williams, Matthews, & McLeod, 1996] and memory via the Affective Auditory Verbal Learning Test [Snyder & Harrison, 1997]). In addition, such procedures may allow researchers to unravel the interplay and interdependence between cognitive and emotional processes. Bartolic et al. (1999)

recently demonstrated that cognitive processing (i.e., fluency) associated with the frontal lobes can vary as a function of dysphoric mood induction (figural fluency, right hemisphere) versus euphoric mood induction (verbal fluency, left hemisphere). For discussions that explore the relationship between cognition and emotion, see Oschner and Schacter (Chapter 7, this volume) and Adolphs and Damasio (Chapter 8, this volume).

ACKNOWLEDGMENTS

This project was supported, in part, by NIMH grant MH42172 to Queens College, by PSC-CUNY Research Award 668268 to Queens College, and by the Natural Sciences and Research Council of Canada. We are grateful to Jack Nitschke for his helpful comments on this manuscript.

REFERENCES

Alpert, M., Rosen, A., Welkowitz, J., Sobin, C., & Borod, J.C. (1989). Vocal acoustic correlates of flat affect in schizophrenia: Similarity to Parkinson's disease and right hemisphere disease and contrast with depression. *British Journal of Psychiatry, 154,* 51–56.

Banse, R., & Scherer, K.R. (1996). Acoustic profiles in vocal emotion expression. *Journal of Personality and Social Psychology, 70,* 614–636.

Barrett, A.M., Crucian, G.P., Raymer, A.M., & Heilman, K.M. (1999). Spared comprehension of emotional prosody in a patient with global aphasia. *Neuropsychiatry, Neuropsychology, and Behavioral Neurology, 12,* 117–120.

Bartolic, E., Basso, M., Schefft, B., Glauser, T., & Titanic-Schefft, M. (1999). Effects of experimentally-induced emotional states on frontal lobe cognitive task performance. *Neuropsychologia, 37,* 677–683.

Bear, D.M., & Fedio, P. (1977). Quantitative analysis of interictal behavior in temporal lobe epilepsy. *Archives of Neurology, 34,* 454–467.

Benowitz, L.I. (1980). Cerebral lateralization in the perception of nonverbal emotional cues. *McLean Hospital Journal, 3–4,* 147.

Benowitz, L.I., Bear, D.M., Rosenthal, R., Mesulam, M.-M., Zaidel, E., & Sperry, R.W. (1983). Hemispheric specialization in nonverbal communication. *Cortex, 19,* 5–11.

Bielamowicz, S., Kreiman, J., Gerratt, B., Dauer, M., & Berke, G. (1996). Comparison of voice analysis systems for perturbation measurement. *Journal of Speech and Hearing Research, 39,* 126–134.

Blonder, L.X., Bowers, D., & Heilman, K.M. (1991). The role of the right hemisphere in emotional communication. *Brain, 114,* 1115–1127.

Blonder, L.X., Burns, A.F., Bowers, D., Moore, R.W., & Heilman, K.M. (1993). Right hemisphere facial expressivity during natural conversation. *Brain and Cognition, 21,* 44–56.

Blonder, L.X., Burns, A.F., Bowers, D., Moore, R.W., & Heilman, K.M. (1995). Spontaneous gestures following right hemisphere infarct. *Neuropsychologia, 35,* 203–213.

Blonder, L.X., Gur, R.E., & Gur, R.C. (1989). The effects of right and left hemiparkinsonism on prosody. *Brain and Language, 36,* 193–207.

Bloom, R.L., Borod, J.C., Obler, L.K., & Gerstman, L. (1992). Impact of emotional content on discourse production in patients with unilateral brain damage. *Brain and Language*, *42*, 153–164.

Bloom, R.L., Borod, J.C., Obler, L.K., & Koff, E. (1990). A preliminary characterization of lexical emotional expression in right and left brain-damaged patients. *International Journal of Neuroscience*, *55*, 71–80.

Bloom, R.L., Obler, L.K., DeSanti, S., & Ehrlich, J.S. (1994). *Discourse Analysis and Applications: Studies in Adult Clinical Populations*. Hillsdale, NJ: Lawrence Erlbaum.

Borod, J.C. (1993a). Cerebral mechanisms underlying facial, prosodic, and lexical emotional expression: A review of neuropsychological studies and methodological issues. *Neuropsychology*, *7*, 445–463.

Borod, J.C. (1993b). Emotion and the brain—Anatomy and theory: An introduction to the Special Section. *Neuropsychology*, *7*, 427–432.

Borod, J.C., Cicero, J.C., Obler, L.K., Welkowitz, J., Erhan, H.M., Santschi, C., Grunwald, I.S., Agosti, R.M., & Whalen, J. (1998). Right hemisphere emotional perception: Evidence across multiple channels. *Neuropsychology*, *12*, 446–458.

Borod, J.C., Fitzpatrick, P.M., Helm-Estabrooks, N., & Goodglass, H. (1989). The relationship between limb apraxia and the spontaneous use of communicative gesture in aphasia. *Brain and Cognition*, *10*, 121–131.

Borod, J.C., Koff, E., Lorch, M.P., & Nicholas, M. (1986). The expression and perception of facial emotions in brain-damaged patients. *Neuropsychologia*, *24*, 169–180.

Borod, J.C., Koff, E., Lorch, M.P., Nicholas, M., & Welkowitz, J. (1988). Emotional and non-emotional facial behaviors in patients with unilateral brain damage. *Journal of Neurology, Neurosurgery, and Psychiatry*, *51*, 826–832.

Borod, J.C., Pick, L., Hall, S., Sliwinski, M., Madigan, N., Obler, L.K., Welkowitz, J., Canino, E., Erhan, H., Goral, M., Morrison, C., & Tabert, M. (in press). The relationships among facial, prosodic, and lexical channels of emotional perceptual processing. *Cognition and Emotion*.

Borod, J.C., Rorie, K.D., Haywood, C.S., Andelman, F., Obler, L.K., Welkowitz, J., Bloom, R., & Tweedy, J. (1996). Hemispheric specialization for discourse reports of emotional experiences: Relationships to demographic, neurological, and perceptual variables. *Neuropsychologia*, *34*, 351–359.

Borod, J.C., Welkowitz, J. Alpert, M., Brozgold, A., Martin, C., Peselow, E., & Diller, L. (1990). Parameters of emotional processing in neuropsychiatric disorders: Conceptual issues and a battery of tests. *Journal of Communication Disorders*, *23*, 247–271.

Borod, J.C., Welkowitz, J., & Obler, L.K. (1992). *The New York Emotion Battery*. Unpublished materials, Department of Neurology, Mount Sinai Medical Center, New York, N.Y.

Bowers, D., Bauer, R.M., & Heilman, K.M. (1993). The nonverbal affect lexicon: Theoretical perspectives from neuropsychological studies of affect perception. *Neuropsychology*, *7*, 433–444.

Bowers, D., Blonder, L.X., & Heilman, K.M. (1991). *The Florida Affect Battery, Experimental Edition*. Gainesville, FL: University of Florida.

Brozgold, A. Borod, J.C., Martin, C., Pick, L., Alpert, M., & Welkowitz, J. (1998). Social functioning and facial emotional expression in neurological and psychiatric disorders. *Applied Neuropsychology*, *5*, 15–23.

Buck, R. (1978). The slide-viewing technique for measuring nonverbal sending accuracy: A guide for replication. *Catalog of Selected Documents in Psychology*, *8*, 63.

Buck, R., Miller, R.E., & Caul, W.F. (1974). Sex, personality, and physiological variables in the communication of affect via facial expression. *Journal of Personality and Social Psychology*, *30*, 587–596.

Cadieux, N.I., & Greve, K.W. (1996). Emotion processing in Alzheimer's disease [abstract]. *Journal of the International Neuropsychological Society*, *2*, 59.

Cancelliere, A.E., & Kertesz, A. (1990). Lesion localization in acquired deficits of emotional expression and comprehension. *Brain and Cognition*, *13*, 133–147.

Canino, E., Borod, J.C., Madigan, N., Tabert, M., & Schmidt, J.M. (1999). The development of procedures for rating posed emotional expressions across facial, prosodic, and lexical channels. *Perceptual and Motor Skills*, *89*, 57–71.

Cicero, B., Borod, J.C., Santschi, C., Erhan, H., Obler, L.K, Welkowitz, J., Agosti, R., & Grunwald, I. (1999). Emotional versus nonemotional lexical perception in patients with right and left brain damage. *Neuropsychiatry, Neuropsychology, and Behavioral Neurology*, *12*, 255–264.

Cicone, M., Wapner, W., & Gardner, H. (1980). Sensitivity to emotional expressions and situations in organic patients. *Cortex*, *16*, 145–158.

Cimino, C.R., Verfaellie, M., Bowers, D. & Heilman, K.M. (1991). Autobiographical memory: Influence of right hemisphere damage on emotionality and specificity. *Brain and Cognition*, *15*, 106–118.

Cohen, M.J., Riccio, C.A., & Flannery, A.M. (1994). Expressive aprosodia following stroke to the right basal ganglia: A case report. *Neuropsychology*, *8*, 242–245.

Cripe, L.I. (1996). The MMPI in neuropsychological assessment: A murky measure. *Applied Neuropsychology*, *3–4*, 97–103.

Cripe, L.I. (1997). Personality assessment of brain-impairment patients. In M.E. Maruish & J.A. Moses, Jr. (Eds.), *Clinical Neuropsychology: Theoretical Foundations for Practitioners* (pp. 119–142). Hillsdale, NJ: Erlbaum.

Davidson, R.J. (1995). Cerebral asymmetry, emotion, and affective style. In R.J. Davidson & K. Hugdahl, K. (Eds.), *Brain Asymmetry* (pp. 361–387). Cambridge, MA: MIT Press.

Davitz, J.R. (1964). *The Communication of Emotional Meaning*. New York: McGraw-Hill.

Dimberg, U. (1982). Facial reactions to facial expressions. *Psychophysiology*, *19*, 643–647.

Egan, G., Kilts, C.D., Gideon, D.A., Hoffman, J.M., & Faber, T. (1996). PET analysis of hemispheric involvement in human face emotion perception [abstract]. *The Clinical Neuropsychologist*, *10*, 335.

Egan, G., Morris, R., Stringer, A., Ewert, J., & Collins, L. (1990). Assessment of emotional perception in right and left hemisphere stroke patients: A validation study [abstract]. *Journal of Clinical and Experimental Neuropsychology*, *12*, 51.

Ekman, P., & Friesen, W.V. (1975). *Unmasking the Face*. Englewood Cliffs, N.J.: Prentice-Hall.

Ekman, P., & Friesen, W.V. (1976). *Pictures of Facial Affect*. Palo Alto, CA: Consulting Psychologists Press.

Ekman, P., & Friesen, W.V. (1978). *Facial Action Coding System*. Palo Alto, CA: Consulting Psychologists Press.

Erwin, R.J., Gur, R.C., Gur, R.E., Skolnick, B., Mawhinney-Hee, M., & Smailis, J. (1992). Facial emotion discrimination: I. Task construction and behavioral findings in normal subjects. *Psychiatry Research*, *42*, 231–240.

Exner, J.E. (1986). *The Rorschach: A Comprehensive System*. New York: Wiley-InterScience.

Filskov, S.B., & Boll, T.J. (1991). *Handbook of Clinical Neuropsychology*, Vol. 2. New York: John Wiley & Sons.

Friedes, D. (1991). *Introduction of a Neuropsychological Personality Inventory*. Paper presented at the Pacific Rim Conference, Gold Coast, Queensland, Australia.

Gainotti, G., Azzoni, A., Razzano, C., Lanzillotta, M., Camillo, M., & Gasparini, F. (1997). The post-stroke depression rating scale: A test specifically devised to investigate affective disorders of stroke patients. *Journal of Clinical and Experimental Neuropsychology, 19*, 340–356.

Gainotti, G., Caltagirone, C., & Zoccolotti, P. (1993). Left/right and cortical/subcortical dichotomies in the neuropsychological study of human emotions. *Cognition and Emotion, 7*, 71–93.

Gasparrani, W.G., Satz, P., Heilman, K.M., & Coolidge, F.L. (1978). Hemispheric asymmetries of affective processing as determined by the Minnesota Multiphasic Personality Inventory. *Journal of Neurology, Neurosurgery, and Psychiatry, 41*, 470–473.

Goodglass, H., & Kaplan, E. (1983). *The Assessment of Aphasia and Related Disorders*. Philadelphia: Lea & Febiger.

Gordon, W.A., Hibbard, M.R., Egelko, S., Riley, E., Simon, D., Diller, L., Ross, E.D., & Lieberman, A. (1991). Issues in the diagnosis of post-stroke depression. *Rehabilitation Psychology, 36*, 71–87.

Gorelick, P.B., & Ross, E.D. (1987). The aprosodias: Further functional–anatomic evidence for the organization of affective language in the right hemisphere. *Journal of Neurology, Neurosurgery, and Psychiatry, 50*, 553–560.

Graham, J.R. (1993). *MMPI-2: Assessing Personality and Psychopathology*. New York: Oxford University Press.

Green, W.P. (1996). *Emotional Perception Test*. Durham, N.C.: CogniSyst, Inc.

Greene, R.L. (1992). *The MMPI-2/MMPI: An Interpretive Manual*. Odessa, FL: Psychological Assessment Resources.

Grunwald, I.S., Borod, J.C., Obler, L.K., Erhan, H., Pick, L., Welkowitz, J., Madigan, N., Sliwinski, M., & Whalen, J. (1999). The effects of age and gender on the perception of lexical emotion. *Applied Neuropsychology, 6*, 226–238.

Gur, R.C., Erwin, R.J., Gur, R.E., Zwil, C.H., & Kraemer, H.C. (1992). Facial emotion discrimination: II. Behavioral findings in depression. *Psychiatry Research, 42*, 241–251.

Heath, R., Kryst, S., Rosenbaum, M., & Blonder, L. (1997). Ethonographic observations of unilateral stroke patients [abstract]. *Journal of the International Neuropsychological Society, 3*, 57.

Heimberg, C., Gur, R.E., Erwin, R.J., Shtasel, D.L., & Gur, R.C. (1992). Facial emotion discrimination: III. Behavioral findings in schizophrenia. *Psychiatry Research, 42*, 253–265.

Holland, A.L. (1980). *Communicative Abilities in Daily Living: A Test of Functional Communication for Aphasic Adults*. Baltimore: University Park Press.

Hornak, J., Rolls, E.T., & Wade, D. (1996). Face and voice expression identification in patients with emotional and behavioral changes following ventral lobe damage. *Neuropsychologia, 34*, 247–261.

Incagnoli, T., Goldstein, G., & Golden, C.J. (1986). *Clinical Application of Neuropsychological Test Batteries*. New York: Plenum Press.

Izard, C.E. (1972). *Patterns of Emotions*. New York: Academic Press.

Izard, C.E. (1983). *The Maximally Discriminative Facial Movement Coding System (Max)* (Revised). Newark: University of Delaware, Instructional Resources Center.

Kolb, B., & Taylor, L. (1990). Neocortical substrates of emotional behavior. In N.L. Stein, B. Leventhal, & T. Trabasso (Eds.), *Psychosocial and Biological Approaches to Emotion* (pp. 115–144). Hillsdale, NJ: Erlbaum.

Lalande, S., Braun, C.M.J., Charlebois, N., & Whitaker, H.A. (1992). Effects of right and left hemisphere cerebrovascular lesion on discrimination of prosodic and semantic aspects of affect in sentences. *Brain and Language, 42*, 165–186.

Lang, P.J., Greenwald, M.K., Bradley, M.M., & Hamm, A.O. (1993). Looking at pictures: Evaluative, facial, visceral, and behavioral responses. *Psychophysiology, 30*, 261–273.

Lang, P.J., Ohman, A., & Vaitl, D. (1988). *The International Affective Picture System* [*photographic slides*]. Gainesville: The Center for Research in Psychophysiology, University of Florida.

LeFever, F.F. (1988). A test of facial emotion identification: Norms for accuracy and response bias [abstract]. *Journal of Clinical and Experimental Neuropsychology, 10*, 327.

Levin, H.S., High, W.M., Goethe, K.E., Sisson, R.A., Overall, J.E., Rhoades, H.M., Eisenberg, H.M., Kalisky, Z., & Gary, H.E. (1987). The Neurobehavioral Rating Scale: Assessment of the behavioral sequelae of head injury by the clinician. *Journal of Neurology, Neurosurgery, and Psychiatry, 50*, 183–193.

Levitt, E. (1964). The relationship between abilities to express emotional meaning vocally and facially. In J.R. Davitz (Ed.), *The Communication of Emotional Meaning* (pp. 87–100). New York: McGraw-Hill.

Lezak, M.D. (1995). *Neuropsychological Assessment*. New York: Oxford University Press.

Malatesta, C., & Izard, C.E. (1984). The facial expression of emotion: Young, middle-aged, and older adult expressions. In C. Malatesta & C.E. Izard (Eds.), *Emotion in Adult Development* (pp. 253–273). Beverly Hills, CA: Sage.

Martz, M.J., & Welkowitz, J. (1977). Welmar–computer programs to analyze dialogic time patterns. *Perceptual and Motor Skills, 45*, 531–537.

Meadows, M., & Kaplan, R.F. (1994). Dissociation of autonomic and subjective responses to emotional slides in right hemisphere damaged patients. *Neuropsychologia, 32*, 847–856.

Mebrabian, A., & Reed, H. (1968). Some determinants of communication accuracy. *Psychological Bulletin, 70*, 365–381.

Montreys, C.R., & Borod, J.C. (1998). A preliminary evaluation of emotional experience and expression following unilateral brain damage. *International Journal of Neuroscience, 96*, 269–283.

Morley, L.C. (1991). *Personality Assessment Inventory*. Odessa, FL: Psychological Assessment Resources.

Mountain, M.A. (1993). *The Victoria Emotion Recognition Test*. Unpublished doctoral dissertation, University of Victoria, British Columbia, Canada.

Mountain, M.A., & Spreen, O. (1993). Reliability and validity of the Victoria Emotion Recognition Test [abstract]. *The Clinical Neuropsychologist, 7*, 347.

Mueser, K.T., Doonan, R., Penn, D.L., Blanchard, J.L., Bellack, A.S., Nishith, P., & DeLeon, J. (1996). Emotion recognition and social competence in chronic schizophrenia. *Journal of Abnormal Psychology, 105*, 271–275.

Murray, H.A. (1938). *Explorations in Personality*. New York: Oxford University Press.

Nelson, L.D., & Cicchetti, D.V. (1995). Assessment of emotional functioning in brain-impaired individuals. *Psychological Assessment, 7*, 404–413.

Nelson, L.D., Satz, P., Mitrushina, M., Van Gorp, W., Cicchetti, D., Lewis, R., & Van Lancker, D. (1989). Development and validation of the Neuropsychology Behavior and Affect Profile. *Psychological Assessment: A Journal of Consulting and Clinical Psychology, 1*, 266–272.

O'Brien, K., & Lezak, M.D. (1988). Portland Adaptability Inventory. Cited in Lezak, M.D. (1995). *Neuropsychological Assessment* (p. 62). New York: Oxford University Press.

Oster, H., Hegley, D., & Nagel, L. (1992). Adult judgements and fine-grained analysis of infant facial expressions: Testing the validity of a priori coding formulas. *Developmental Psychology, 28*, 1115–1131.

Overall, J.E., & Gorham, D.R. (1962). The Brief Psychiatric Rating Scale. *Psychological Reports, 10*, 799–812.

Plutchik, R. (1984). Emotions: A general psychoevolutionary theory. In K.R. Scherer & P. Ekman (Eds.), *Approaches to Emotion* (pp. 197–219). Hillsdale, NJ: Erlbaum.

Reitan, R.M., & Wolfson, D. (1997). Emotional disturbances and their interaction with neuropsychological deficits. *Neuropsychology Review, 7*, 3–19.

Rorschach, H. (1942). *Psychodiagnostics: A Diagnostic Test Based on Perception*. Berne: Huber.

Rosenthal, R., Hall, J.A., Archer, D., Di Matteo, M., & Rogers, P.L. (1979). The PONS test: Measuring sensitivity to nonverbal cues. In S. Weitz (Ed.), *Nonverbal Communication* (pp. 357–370). New York: Oxford University Press.

Ross, E.D. (1981). The aprosodias: Functional–anatomic organization of the affective components of language in the right hemisphere. *Archives of Neurology, 38*, 561–569.

Ross, E.D. (1985). Modulation of affect and nonverbal communication by the right hemisphere. In M.-M. Mesulam (Ed.), *Principles of Behavioral Neurology* (pp. 239–257). Philadelphia: F.A. Davis.

Ross, E.D. (1997). Right hemisphere syndromes and the neurology of emotion. In S.C. Schacter & O. Devinsky (Eds.), *Behavioral Neurology and the Legacy of Norman Geschwind* (pp. 183–191). Philadelphia: Lippincott-Raven.

Ross, E.D., Edmondson, J.A., & Seibert, G.B. (1986). The effect of affect on various acoustic measures of prosody in tone and non-tone languages: A comparison based on computer analysis. *Journal of Phonetics, 14*, 283–302.

Ross, E.D., Edmondson, J.A., Seibert, G.B., & Homan, R.W. (1987). Acoustic analysis of affective prosody during right-sided Wada test: A within-subjects verification of the right hemisphere's role in language. *Brain and Language, 33*, 128–145.

Ross, E.D., & Mesulam, M.-M. (1979). Dominant language functions of the right hemisphere? Prosody and emotional gesturing. *Archives of Neurology, 36*, 144–148.

Ross, E.D., Thompson, R.D., & Yenkosky, J. (1997). Lateralization of affective prosody in brain and the callosal integration of hemispheric language functions. *Brain and Language, 56*, 27–54.

Ruckdeschel-Hibbard, M., Gordon, W.A., & Diller, L. (1986). Affective disturbances associated with brain damage. In S.B. Filskov & T.J. Boll (Eds.), *Handbook of Clinical Neuropsychology* (pp. 305–337). New York: John Wiley & Sons.

Santschi-Haywood, C., Perrine, K., Borod, J.C., Nelson, P.K., & Devinsky, O. (1996). Lateralization for prosodic emotional perception: Temporal lobe epilepsy and the intracarotid amobarbital procedure [abstract]. *Journal of the International Neuropsychological Society, 2*, 52.

Santschi-Haywood, C., Perrine, K., Borod, J.C., Nelson, P.K., & Devinsky, O. (1997). Prosodic emotional perception during the intracarotid amobarbital procedure (IAP): Effects of seizure variables [abstract]. *Epilepsia, 38* (Suppl. 8), 161.

Sarno, M.T. (1969). *The Functional Communication Profile Manual of Directions*. New York: Rusk Institute of Rehabilitation Medicine, New York University Medical Center.

Sbordone, R.J. (1996). Ecological validity: Some critical issues for the neuropsychologist. In R.J. Sbordone & C.J. Long (Eds.), *Ecological Validity of Neuropsychological Testing* (pp. 15–41). Delray Beach, FL: St. Lucie Press.

Schiff, B.B., & Lamon, M. (1989). Inducing emotion by unilateral contraction of facial muscles: A new look at hemispheric specialization and the experience of emotion. *Neuropsychologia, 27*, 923–935.

Schneider, F., Gur, R.E., Harper, M., Smith, R.J., Mozely, P.D., Censits, D.M., Alavi, A., & Gur., R.C. (1995). Mood effects on limbic blood flow correlate with emotional self-rating: A PET study with oxygen-15 labeled water. *Psychiatry Research: Neuroimaging, 61*, 265–283.

Scott, S., Caird, F., & Williams, B. (1984). Evidence for an apparent sensory speech disorder in Parkinson's disease. *Journal of Neurology, Neurosurgery, and Psychiatry, 47*, 840–843.

Semenza, C., Pasini, M., Zettin, M., Tonin, P., & Portolan, P. (1986). Right hemisphere patients' judgement on emotion. *Acta Neurologica Scandinavica, 74*, 43–50.

Shapiro, B.E., & Danly, M. (1985). The role of the right hemisphere in the control of speech prosody in propositional and affective contexts. *Brain and Language, 25*, 19–36.

Snyder, K.A., & Harrison, D.W. (1997). The Affective Auditory Verbal Learning Test. *Archives of Clinical Neuropsychology, 12*, 477–482.

Sobin, C., & Alpert, M. (1999). Emotions in speech: The acoustic attributes of fear, anger, sadness, and joy. *Journal of Psycholinguistic Research, 28*, 347–365.

Spreen, O., & Strauss, E. (1998). *A Compendium of Neuropsychological Tests*. New York: Oxford University Press.

St. Clair, J., Borod, J., Sliwinski, M., Cote, L., & Stern, Y. (1998). Cognitive and affective processing in Parkinson's disease patients with lateralized motor signs. *Journal of Clinical and Experimental Neuropsychology, 20*, 320–327.

Sweet, J.J., Newman, P., & Bell, B. (1992). Significance of depression in clinical neuropsychological assessment. *Clinical Psychology Review, 12*, 21–45.

Tabert, M.H., Borod, J.C., Schmidt, J.M., Grunwald, I., Shane, R., Obler, L.K., & Welkowitz, J. (1997). Word-type analysis of emotional lexical fluency data in aging normals [abstract]. *The Clinical Neuropsychologist, 11*, 309.

Tarter, R.E., & Edwards, K.L. (1986). Neuropsychological batteries. In T. Incagnoli, G. Goldstein, & C.J. Golden (Eds.), *Clinical Application of Neuropsychological Test Batteries* (pp. 135–153). New York: Plenum Press.

Tomarken, A.J., Davidson, R.J., & Henriques, J.B. (1990). Frontal brain asymmetry predicts affective responses to films. *Journal of Personality and Social Psychology, 59*, 791–801.

Tucker, D.M., Watson, R.T., & Heilman, K.M. (1977). Discrimination and evocation of affectively intoned speech in patients with right parietal disease. *Neurology, 27*, 947–950.

Velten, E. (1968). A laboratory task for induction of mood states. *Behavioral Research and Therapy, 6*, 473–482.

Weddell, R.A. (1989). Recognition memory for emotional facial expressions in patients with focal cerebral lesions. *Brain and Cognition, 11*, 1–17.

Weddell, R.A. (1994). Effects of subcortical lesion site on human emotional behavior. *Brain and Cognition, 25*, 161–193.

Weddell, R.A., Miller, J.D., & Trevarthen, C. (1990). Voluntary emotional facial expressions in patients with focal cerebral lesions. *Neuropsychologia, 28*, 49–60.

Weddell, R.A., Trevarthen, C., & Miller, J.D. (1988). Reactions of patients with focal cerebral lesions to success or failure. *Neuropsychologia, 26*, 373–385.

Weintraub, S., Mesulam, M.-M., & Kramer, L. (1981). Disturbances in prosody: A right-hemisphere contribution to language. *Archives of Neurology, 38*, 742–744.

Welkowitz, J., Bond, R.N., & Zelano, J. (1990). An automated system for the analysis of temporal speech patterns: Description of the hardware and software. *Journal of Communication Disorders, 23*, 347–364.

Williams, J.M., Matthews, A., & MacLeod, C. (1996). The emotional stroop task and psychopathology. *Psychological Bulletin, 120*, 3–24.

Yesavage, J.A., Brink, T.L., Rose, T.L., & Lum, O. (1983). Development and validation of a geriatric depression screening scale: Preliminary report. *Journal of Psychiatric Research, 17*, 37–49.

5

Neuroimaging Approaches to the Study of Emotion

MARK S. GEORGE, TERRENCE A. KETTER,
TIM A. KIMBRELL, ANDREW M. SPEER,
JEFF LORBERBAUM, CHRISTOPHER C. LIBERATOS,
ZIAD NAHAS, AND ROBERT M. POST

BACKGROUND

The recent technological revolution in functional neuroimaging has provided new insights into regional brain activity during normal and pathological emotions and has advanced understanding of several neuropsychiatric diseases. The list of different functional imaging tools can, however, be daunting for those not actively working in the area. Additionally, an incomplete knowledge of the nature of the source of the imaging signal can hinder complete understanding of the results of imaging studies. Therefore, in this chapter we outline several of the basic principles behind the use of functional imaging to study emotion. We then briefly describe the most commonly used functional imaging techniques and discuss some of the problems in most of the imaging research in this area. These introductory comments are illustrated with examples from the imaging literature as well as from the authors' primary work.

Common Paradigms in Functional Imaging Used To Examine the Neural Basis of Emotion

Recent advances in imaging techniques now enable direct examination of the working brain during episodes of clinical depression and during transient emotions in healthy controls, allowing for more direct testing of hypotheses concerning normal and abnormal neural mechanisms. Studies with these techniques have confirmed and refined some of the earlier models of how the brain regulates mood and emotion. Functional neuroimaging, however, a field with immense promise, is still in its infancy. Regardless of the imaging method used, most modern functional imaging studies applied to understanding emotion have one of the following basic approaches.

1. Single-case study. The classic single-case method involves finding a patient with a brain lesion who has some disorder related to emotion (e.g., pathological crying). With functional and structural imaging, one then attempts to understand how the brain regions that were damaged produce this disorderly change in behavior.

2. Between-group analysis. With between-group analysis, one images a group of subjects who have a mood disorder and compares them with one or two groups who vary on an important emotional feature or who were chosen to represent different ends of a continuous feature. For these analyses to work, attention must be paid to the activity at the time of the scan and whether there were differences between groups in the performance of this behavior (commonly used is an auditory continuous performance task). Also, because the sizes and shapes of different brains vary widely, attempts must be made to account for the differences in brain size for group comparisons. One approach is to measure activity in brain regions on each individual scan, typically guided by a template or magnetic resonance image (MRI) of the subject, and then compare (called a *region of interest* analysis). Alternatively, one can transform and reshape (called *stereotactically normalizing*) the images into a common brain space. The most common brain atlas used in functional neuroimaging is the Talairach atlas (Talairach & Tournoux, 1988). The most popular method of normalizing brain scans into Talairach Space is the statistical software package Statistical Parametric Mapping developed by Karl Friston and colleagues at the Hammersmith Hospital (currently at the National Hospital for Neurological Diseases at Queen's Square) (Friston et al., 1989, 1990).

3. Within-group analysis. In the within-group method, one commonly performs functional imaging on a group with a disorder of mood or emotion before and after a change in state (e.g., depressed patients before and after medication treatment). With nondiseased populations, subjects are imaged at rest and then during an emotional task, commonly either a mood state induced neuropsychologically or pharmacologically, or while performing a task related to processing emotion. Again, with this method one must transform the functional brain maps into a common space and then attempt to examine changes before and after and then reason back to the role of key brain region changes as a function of the behavior, treatment, or state change. Designing carefully constructed activation paradigms in which the control condition accounts for everything but the behavior

in question is challenging but vitally important (George, Ketter, & Post, 1994; Haxby et al., 1991; Ring et al., 1991) (see discussion below as well).

4. Within-individual analysis. The faster, nonradiation-based techniques like echoplanar blood oxygenation level–dependent (BOLD) functional MRI now allow for rapid acquisition of many brain images within an individual. For example, in the most common protocol in our laboratory, we acquire an entire brain volume every 3 seconds continuously over 6 minutes, generating 120 separate volumes of brain function. By subtly changing activity across these 6 minutes, one can test, within an individual, for regional brain changes associated with a specific behavior or emotion. This within-individual ability then eliminates the need for pooling of data across different individuals in a common brain space.

Certainly functional imaging is not limited to these paradigms or statistical analysis methods. The near future will likely see many more complex and dynamic uses of functional imaging to explore the regional brain basis of mood disorders and emotion. For example, several research groups have developed MRI sequences that can image regional brain perfusion without requiring paramagnetic contrast agents (serial perfusion MRI scanning) (Bohning et al., 1996, 1997b; Schwarzbauer, Morrisey, & Haase, 1996; Warach et al., 1994; Ye et al., 1996). Thus, unlike functional neuroimaging with single photon emission computed tomography (SPECT), positron emission tomography (PET), and traditional radioligands, MRI perfusion scanning is free of the yoke of radiation, allowing for repeated scanning as well as for scanning in previously excluded populations like healthy children. This technological advance will likely expand functional imaging from the binary pretreatment/post-treatment, snapshot mode of investigation commonly used today into a more dynamic serial tool able to provide longitudinal analyses of regional brain changes. This serial scanning ability will perhaps result in a shift of the language used in imaging studies from "on, off" and "ill, well" to the language of "half-lives" and directions and "vectors of change." We would argue that these new tools are shedding light on how different brain regions coordinate normal emotions and how regional brain dysfunction might cause mood dysregulation resulting in clinical depression and mania.

Another important imaging development that will likely reshape functional neuroimaging research into emotion is the new ability to noninvasively stimulate brain tissue with powerful hand-held electromagnets, a field called *transcranial magnetic stimulation* (TMS) (George, Lisanby, & Sackeim, 1999b; George, Wassermann, & Post, 1996c). One of the more profound difficulties with functional neuroimaging is determining whether a signal observed on an image is related to a behavior or disease in question. Noninvasive but direct stimulation of brain regions in awake human subjects while measuring changes in behavior or emotion is an important advance in emotion research. Later in this chapter we discuss several of the initial pilot studies using TMS to induce mood changes in healthy controls as well as in patients with depression. Furthermore, we describe developments in merging the new technology of transcranial magnetic stimulation with conventional neuroimaging. Combining transcranial magnetic stimulation with neuroimaging is an important new chapter in the evolution of the understanding of brain function, particularly the neural correlates of emotion (George et al., 1999c).

The Need for Understanding Above and Below the Level of the Regional Circuit

Several other concepts and caveats are important to bear in mind when assessing functional imaging studies. First, psychiatric conditions in general, and emotion research in particular, challenge researchers and clinicians to *simultaneously integrate information from multiple conceptual levels* to explain and understand these processes and illnesses. Models of mood and emotion regulation must account for genetic factors of disease susceptibility and temperament while also integrating knowledge about the effects of family, cognitive, and pharmacological therapies. Functional neuroimaging studies focus attention at the level of regional neuroanatomical defects. Obviously, this is not the total answer or method to understanding mood-related illnesses or even normal mood regulation in health. Eventually, modern psychiatry and psychology must integrate knowledge from diverse conceptual levels to fully understand the complexity of such behaviors as "emotion" and such neuropsychiatric conditions as "mood disorders."

Second, understanding *the distinction between overt brain structural abnormalities and brain dysfunction* is critical in conceptualizing mood regulation and dysregulation. In the 1860s, the British neurologist John Hughlings Jackson noted that abnormal brain function is not always associated with aberrant brain structure (Jackson, 1874). When dealing with patients with focal epilepsy, he noted that even when brain structure was grossly normal, abnormal seizure discharges could cause behaviors to temporarily disappear (e.g., the ability to move an extremity) or even bring out emergent properties (e.g., hallucinations or auras) (Jackson, 1873; Jackson & Stewart, 1899). Thus, problems in behavior (or function) could exist in the setting of grossly normal structure. In primary mood disorders, visually apparent structural abnormalities are generally absent in most individuals, although studies of groups of mood disorder patients have revealed structural differences in the prefrontal and temporal cortices (see Robinson & Manes, Chapter 10, this volume). Therefore, mood disorders, like primary generalized epilepsy (which lacks macroscopic cerebral lesions), may belong to a class of neuropsychiatric diseases with abnormal brain activity despite grossly normal structure. In epilepsy, the electroencephalogram has helped to legitimize the disease as a medical illness of the brain (Engel, 1989; Temkin, 1945). The new functional imaging tools discussed below (SPECT, PET, functional MRI [fMRI], and TMS) are now further destigmatizing the primary mood disorders by revealing abnormal regional brain function despite generally normal structure.

Finally, most functional imaging tools rely on the fact that *brain regions that are more active use more glucose for energy consumption and also receive more blood flow*. Most researchers also assume that *blood flow and energy metabolism are coupled* (Sokoloff, 1978). For example, while reading this chapter, the regions in your brain involved in processing visual information and synthesizing language are more active than they were before you began reading. Those activated regions thus use more glucose for energy than when you are not reading, and they receive more blood flow. These assumptions of increased blood flow and glucose use with greater neuronal activity serve as the background for most functional imaging studies. The functional image is, however, unable to determine exactly what a specific brain region is doing when it is activated. That is, is the brain region excitatory or inhibitory on other brain regions, and is it causing or inhibiting a behavior? In addition to this thorny issue, other problems are present in the interpretation of functional imaging studies.

What Does the Signal From Functional Imaging Actually Mean? Epistemological Caveats

Neuroscience operates under the assumption that behavioral events are mediated by neuronal events. This assumption is part of the larger assumption that characterizes modern science—that all events have physical causes (as opposed to nonmaterial causes, like ghosts, goblins, or souls). What follows from this is that every event occurs within a chain of events; every *cause* has a cause of its own. Notwithstanding the difficulties involved in determining that some neuronal activity is actually part of the causal chain of the behavior rather than being merely correlated with it (see, for example, the later discussion of TMS), there is still the problem of the appropriate level on which to assign causality. Often within the field of neuroscience, one assumes that a behavior is caused by some structural and/or functional problem with some neuronal group. For that behavior that has as its *cause* a neuronal event, however, we may still consider the cause of that neuronal event. Consider the causal chain: John pokes Mary, setting off a neuronal event that results in Mary's behavior of becoming angry. What is the cause of Mary's anger, the neuronal event or John's poking at her? The issue at stake is the appropriateness of stopping at the neuronal group in the chain of causality. The limitations we have in how to control behavior (i.e., where we can intervene in the causal chain) may help to answer this question, but at this point in interpreting signals in neuroimaging studies, one should be cautious in the assignment of causality.

Most neuroscientists using functional imaging skirt these philosophical issues by performing studies and then reporting the results in a strictly observational manner. For example, if we perform a PET study and the amygdala has increased blood flow during a drug-induced panic attack and we simply report these two things (increased amygdala signal and panic), then we have skirted the difficult but very important issue of exactly how the brain and the behavior relate. Most modern models of the brain basis of emotion assume that emotions are reflected in activity in a distributed neural network, comprised of several brain regions, with perhaps each module performing a subpart of the emotion (e.g., interpreting external events; see also Buck, Chapter 2; Ochsner & Schacter, Chapter 7; and Adolphs & Damasio, Chapter 8, this volume). Thus, within the realm of the philosophy of mind, most modern neuroscientists working with functional imaging would be classified as either functionalists or reductive materialists. *Functionalists* would say that the behavior arises from activity within the neural network (Churchland, 1984). They would allow for the possibility that complicated networks comprised of things other than neurons (e.g., computers) could also produce the behavior. In other areas of neuroscience, such as visual processing, this has largely happened as there are computers with complex pattern recognition capabilities. *Reductive materialists* would also say that the behavior arises from the activity within the network. Thus, in the example above, panic is caused by the activity in the amygdala. Emotions can be strictly mapped onto brain events, and only neurons can produce some behaviors such as emotions or consciousness.

Finally, there are *eliminative materialists*, who would agree that emotions and behaviors are strictly reducible to brain activity. They would add that, in many areas of science (e.g., physics, astronomy), as knowledge advanced, the descriptive language used was also radically changed (e.g., we no longer talk about the ether in the universe). In the field of emotion research, they would argue that as neuroscience advances, the terms we now use (happy, sad, fear) will likely be modified or discarded and replaced with more precise language (George, 1987; Rorty, 1971).

Thus, by interpreting functional imaging studies in a strictly observational mode, one can temporarily avoid complex issues of mind–brain function. In interpreting the results, however, most scientists are forced to grapple with the deeper issues of brain–behavior relationships. Most functional imaging studies today are performed within the paradigm of reductive materialism and attempt to determine the actual neural network associated with a behavior. Bearing these important concepts and assumptions in mind, one can properly begin to review the various techniques now available for noninvasively imaging the living, working human brain.

DESCRIPTIONS AND EXPLANATIONS OF FUNCTIONAL IMAGING TECHNIQUES, WITH BRIEF EXAMPLES

Structural Scans: Computed Tomography and Magnetic Resonance Imaging

The current revolution in neuroimaging technology began with the development by Hounsfield and others of the ability to sample gamma-ray emissions in a circular or tomographic way using the new power of computers. This key advance, sampling radioactivity in a circular way and then reconstructing it with computers to provide an image of the head, is the basis for computed tomography (CT), SPECT, PET, and, to some extent, MRI. CT scans are like traditional x-rays in that one emits a beam and then samples how it is distorted as it passes through the brain before being detected on the other side of the ring around the patient's head. This is done in a 360° arch around the head and then reconstructed. CT thus involves radiation, and is poor at resolving structures in the brain stem or posterior fossa. Conventional MRI involves sampling the degree to which hydrogen ions return to their normal configuration after a transient but powerful magnetic pulse (Cohen & Bookheimer, 1994). Thus, MRI involves no radiation and has remarkable resolving power (on the order of 1–2 mm). It is also very good at imaging structures surrounded by bone, such as the posterior fossa.

Functional Neuroimaging: Single Photon Emission Computed Tomography, Positron Emission Tomography, and Functional Magnetic Resonance Imaging

In contrast to CT and traditional MRI, which image the *structure* of the brain, several techniques have been developed recently with the power to look at brain *function*. As discussed above, brain structure does not equal function, and vice versa (Jackson, 1873; Taylor, 1958). That is, structural brain damage, such as a tumor, can produce either obliteration of the function normally subserved by that portion of the brain, or it can heighten the function of that portion of the brain (e.g., in the case of a seizure discharge [Jackson, 1874]). Additionally, one can have normal brain structure (at least to the limit of current technology) and have markedly abnormal function (i.e., areas of the brain that are normal structurally but are "off line" functionally). This commonly occurs following cortical strokes where the contralateral cerebellum is hypofunctional on PET or SPECT images even though it is structurally intact, a phenomenon referred to as *cerebellar diaschisis* (George et al., 1991). We now review these functional imaging tools (Table 5.1).

Quantitative Electroencephalograms

Electroencephalography (EEG) is perhaps the oldest of the techniques available for "imaging" brain function. An EEG records brain electrical activity, which

Table 5.1. Comparison of Several Functional Imaging Tools

METHOD	IMAGES	COST	AVAILABILITY	IONIZING RADIATION	SPATIAL RESOLUTION	TEMPORAL RESOLUTION
qEEG	Electrical activity	Low	Wide	No	Poor, 3–4 cm	Fast, milliseconds
PET	Flow (^{15}O), metabolism (FDG), or specific ligands	Expensive	Very limited	Yes	5–7 mm	1–3 minutes
SPECT	Flow (HMPAO) or specific ligands	Moderate	Wide	Yes	5–7 mm	1–2 minutes
fMRI	Flow or deoxyhemoglobin to oxyhemoglobin	Moderate	Limited	No	2–3 mm	Milliseconds
MR spectroscopy	H Li PO$_4$ Fl	Moderate	Limited	No	5–7 mm	Seconds
Magnetoencephalography	Magnetic activity	Expensive	Very limited	No	Poor	Fastest, milliseconds
TMS	Cortical representation	Low	Limited, but expanding rapidly	No	2–3 mm	Milliseconds

arises from the combined activity of brain neurons, at the level of the skull. The patterns of electrical activity over different brain regions reflect brain activity. EEG is temporally very precise (on the order of milliseconds) but is spatially very poor, even with many surface leads or electrodes. Furthermore, in addition to being spatially crude at the brain surface, it is unclear where the majority of the brain activity arises that comprises the EEG pattern. Several studies have now attempted to examine the relationship between surface EEG activity and regional brain activity (Parekh et al., 1995; Wheeler, Davidson, & Tomarken, 1993). Because of the problems with spatial resolution, many researchers have largely ignored EEG as an investigative probe. Several researchers, however, have used complex techniques to quantify the EEG patterns (quantitative EEG [qEEG]) and are using this as a tool for the study of emotion (Davidson, 1994; Leuchter et al., 1997; see also Davidson & Henriques, Chapter 11, this volume).

Single-Photon Emission Computed Tomography: Perfusion and Ligand

SPECT involves the peripheral injection into a vein of a radiotracer, which then travels into the brain and is deposited into neurons and glia (George et al., 1991). The gamma rays (or photons) that these radiotracers emit are then detected by rotating cameras and reconstructed into a three-dimensional image. Different SPECT radiotracers bind to brain structures and have different half-lives, which determine when the image can be acquired. A popular current tracer is ^{99m}Tc-hexamethyl propylene amine oxide (HMPAO), which distributes to the brain in a fashion roughly equivalent to blood flow (Devous et al., 1986; Ell, Cullum, & Costa, 1985). The tracer can be injected when the patient is anywhere in the hospital or in a research laboratory and then "sets" within the active brain regions within the next 2–5 minutes. Patients can then be transported to the nuclear medicine suite for actual image acquisition. If necessary, tranquilizing medications can be given to sedate the patient for scanning that will not affect the actual image acquired, as the perfusion pattern has already been deposited. This ability to inject while subjects are away from the nuclear medicine suite and outside of the actual camera makes SPECT imaging particularly useful for studying diseases such as epilepsy or mania or for injecting tracer in naturalistic settings for emotion activations. As reviewed above, those areas of the brain that are more active demand either more blood flow (the basis of perfusion SPECT, ^{15}O PET, and echoplanar BOLD fMRI) or more glucose (the basis of fluorodeoxyglucose [FDG] PET) (Sokoloff, 1977, 1978). Functional images thus change as a result of alterations in brain activity due to differences in the subjects' behavior during the scan.

Migliorelli, Starkstein, and colleagues have used SPECT injections in acutely manic patients who could not have been scanned without sedation (which would then unfortunately affect the functional image). They injected the tracer into the manic subjects when the subjects were away from the camera, and the tracer deposited in the brain. They were then able to sedate the subjects so that they could sit still for the scanning uptake without affecting the picture of brain activity, which reflected activity during the moments around injection. Consistent with a valence model of mood regulation, Migliorelli, Starkstein, and colleagues have found relative right temporal hypoactivity during mania (Migliorelli et al., 1993) (see also Robinson & Manes, Chapter 10, this volume). Recently in our laboratory at the Medical University of South Carolina, we used this ability of SPECT perfusion imaging to be injected when away from the camera to image brain activity while subjects were being stimulated with TMS over the left prefrontal cortex (George et al., 1999d; Stallings et al., 1997). Because of a concern that the presence of a TMS coil within a PET or SPECT camera might produce an artifact, we were able to stimulate when away from the camera and still image brain activity at that moment (Fig. 5.1) . This study demonstrates the possibility of perhaps using TMS to activate discrete neural circuits involved in emotion and then image the brain activity using SPECT.

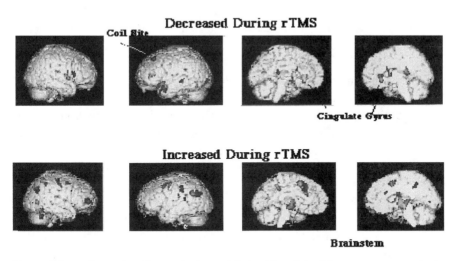

Figure 5.1. Perfusion SPECT results from eight healthy adults. The maps represent brain regions that were significantly different in activity from baseline to the task condition in which subjects were receiving intermittent high-frequency TMS over the left prefrontal cortex. The areas of peak significance ($P < 0.01$) are mapped onto a rendered MRI. During stimulation, there is decreased activity at the coil site and in the cingulate gyrus (top). There was increased activity in the brain stem during stimulation.

Positron Emission Tomography

Blood flow

Positron emission tomography involves the peripheral injection of radiotracers that, when they degrade, emit positrons. These are highly unstable particles that travel a short distance and then collide with an electron. This reaction releases two photons travelling in exactly the opposite direction (180° apart). These photons are then detected by rotating cameras outside of the head and computer reconstructed. In PET, as opposed to SPECT, the cameras are instructed to include for final analysis only those particles that are recorded simultaneously in a camera and in its 180° counterpart (called *coincidence detection*), thus enabling a more precise reconstruction of exactly where the photon originated. This, in general, gives PET a higher image resolution than SPECT (see Table 5.1). Most PET imaging in normal and pathological moods has been done with labeled glucose (^{18}FDG) or oxygen (^{15}O) in the form of water. These compounds have to be produced in a nearby cyclotron, which adds greatly to the cost as well as limits the availability of these types of scans. Additionally, both PET and SPECT offer the possibility of imaging more selective pharmacological systems in the brain with specific radiotracers. Examples with SPECT include dopamine receptors (George et al., 1994b; Ring et al., 1992), acetylcholine receptors, and benzodiazapine receptors with flumazenil. To date, PET studies with specific ligands have imaged dopamine, opiate, and acetylcholine receptors. PET radiotracers have also been made by attaching a labeled carbon to various neuroactive compounds such as labeled deprenyl or fluoxetine. PET ^{15}O image acquisition takes approximately 1–5 minutes, with FDG requiring on the order of 30 minutes. Thus, the differences between SPECT and PET are simply in their use of different tracers (photons, SPECT; positrons, PET) and cameras (photon collimaters, SPECT; coincidence detection, PET). The need for nearby production of positron-emitting tracers will likely continue to make PET more expensive and less available than SPECT. Advances in camera design may allow combined PET/SPECT cameras or SPECT cameras that can create metabolic images with FDG.

^{15}O PET has been used frequently in studies designed to elucidate the brain basis of emotion. ^{15}O deposits in the brain within 2–5 minutes in proportion to blood flow and then quickly washes out, leaving no radiation, so that another scan can be performed 12 minutes later with another injection. Depending on the camera and safety limits, one can acquire 12 or more separate scans in an individual within a 2-hour imaging session.

Using this technique, Pardo, Pardo, and Raichle (1993) initially found that left anterolateral prefrontal cortex activity increases when subjects are asked to think sad thoughts. As an added task at the end of a scanning session, subjects were asked to close their eyes and imagine a sad event. This initial study suffered from the lack of a control task with a memory component. Shortly thereafter, work in our own laboratory with 11 healthy adult women demonstrated that transient sadness is associated with increased activity in the left anterior cingulate, left medial frontal cortex, and the anterior temporal lobes bilaterally (George et al., 1995a) (Fig. 5.2). We employed a combined method of inducing the mood state neuropsychologically by having the subjects recall a personal emotional event and then having them examine mood-appropriate faces during ^{15}O injection. The control task involved the subjects remembering a neutral event and examining neutral faces. Others have now replicated and expanded on this work (Lane et al., 1997). Interestingly, the brain regions activated vary not only as a function of the mood (happy, sad, neutral) but also by how the mood state was achieved (Reiman et al., 1997). In general, emotional states achieved when subjects recall affectively laden past events involve more of the hippocampus, whereas externally generated emotions (e.g., with films, videos, or pharmacological challenges like procaine) are more likely to involve the amygdala.

Following up on our initial findings of sadness induction in adult women, we explored potential sex differences in the brain regions activated during emotional states. Men are less likely than women to experience disorders of mood or anxiety. We thus wondered if sex differences exist in the ability to self-induce transient emotional states (sadness or happiness) and also if regional cerebral blood

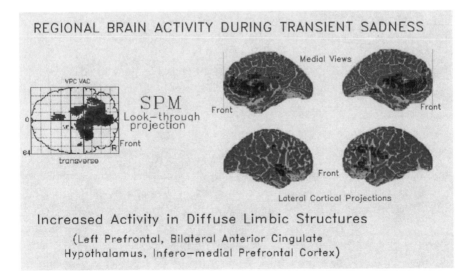

Figure 5.2. Statistical parametric maps of brain regions in 11 healthy adult women. Regions were activated during a state of self-induced transient sadness ($P < 0.01$ for display). Note the activity in the medial prefrontal cortex and other anterior paralimbic structures. SPM, statistical parametric mapping; VAC, anterior commisure; VPA, posterior commisure.

flow (rCBF) would differ between men and women either at rest or during transient emotional states. In a follow-up study, we scanned ten adult men and ten age-matched women, all healthy and never mentally ill, with PET and $H_2^{15}O$ at rest and during happy, sad, and neutral states self-induced by recalling affect-appropriate life events and looking at happy, sad, or neutral human faces (George et al., 1996a). There were no differences between men and women in the subjective ratings of difficulty, effort required, or degree of happiness or sadness induced. Women activated a significantly wider portion of their limbic system than did men during transient sadness, despite similar changes in mood. Although men self-induced transient emotional states to the same degree as women, women had more extensive rCBF changes than men (eight times as many voxels) in anterior limbic regions during transient sadness. The reason for these sex differences in rCBF, both at rest and during the transient emotional states, remains unclear. Potential sex differences with respect to emotion are, however, important and should be kept in mind in most functional imaging studies (Baxter et al., 1987; Shaywitz et al., 1995).

^{15}O PET can also be used to examine how our brains understand the emotional content of the external world. For example, important clues about the emotional states of others are conveyed in noncontent aspects of speech, referred to as *prosody*. In collaboration with Drs. Heilman, Bowers, and Bauer of Florida, we designed an ^{15}O PET study of 13 healthy volunteers. These subjects activated bilateral prefrontal cortex (left more than right) when listening for the emotional propositional content of a sentence. In contrast, when listening to the same set of sentences but responding based on the emotional prosodic content, they activated the right prefrontal cortex and insula. The results of this first PET study of emotional prosody agree with those in a substantial lesion and neuropsychological literature that implicates right lateralization of prosody (George et al., 1996b).

Metabolism

In addition to measuring blood flow, PET can be used to measure the metabolic activity of the brain by tagging glucose with a radiotracer (typically ^{18}FDG) and calculating how much of this tracer deposits in the brain. Like SPECT perfusion tracers, FDG can be infused away from the actual PET camera, allowing some flexibility. Because of the uptake time of 20–30 minutes and the long half-life, however, FDG PET is not an ideal instrument for activation studies, although some have used paired FDG in selected instances in which one scan serves as a baseline for comparison with a task in the second scan (Bremner et al., 1996; Wu et al., 1992). More typically, FDG PET has been used as a baseline measure to compare across groups of mood-disordered subjects (Baxter et al., 1985, 1989).

Functional Magnetic Resonance Imaging

The newest group of functional neuroimaging technologies is *functional MRI* (David, Blamire, & Breiter, 1994; Kwong et al., 1992; Rosen et al., 1994; Stehling, Turner, & Mansfield, 1991; Turner et al., 1991). Under this general heading are several techniques that use the power of MRI systems to image functional brain changes (rather than brain structure). One method is to inject a *bolus of a magnetic compound* and watch its distribution through the brain over a short time (generating a perfusion image of blood flow) (Rosen et al., 1991). This technique is easy to perform but requires an intravenous bolus injection, is limited in the number of boluses per individual due to kidney toxicity of the tracers, and only provides information about relative regional activity (not absolute flow). Alternatively, other groups are using a method of magnetically tagging hydrogen atoms in water as they course through the bloodstream and then imaging the same atoms as they perfuse through the brain (called *spin labelling and inversion recovery*) (Warach et al., 1994). This method is described in greater detail below.

Blood oxygen level–dependent functional magnetic resonance imaging

The most popular method of using MRI to image brain function capitalizes on the fact that oxyhemoglobin is nonmagnetic, whereas deoxyhemoglobin is paramagnetic. Thus brain areas with high demand will have a different ratio of oxyhemoglobin to deoxyhemoglobin and will thus give off a different magnetic signal (a technique that is blood oxygenation level dependent [BOLD]) (Turner et al., 1991). By taking very fast images (on the order of an image or more per second) using a rapid sampling technique (echoplanar acquisition) and high-performance magnetic gradients, one can rapidly image the differences between activity at rest and activity during a specific behavior and generate enough images to perform statistical analyses within a given individual. By acquiring structural MRI scans in the same slices as the functional data, one can precisely map regional brain changes without having to use morphing programs. This technique is ideally suited for tasks and behaviors that can be rapidly stopped and started, such as language, vision, and memory (David, Blamire, & Breiter, 1994). The use of this technique in studying emotion is hampered by the slow and variable onset of emotions as well as their inability to be quickly reversed. Some investigators have succeeded in using this tool to examine brain changes during emotional processing of stimuli such as faces (Breiter et al., 1996; Whalen et al., 1998).

Echoplanar BOLD fMRI is well suited to examining changes in cortical blood flow during precise cognitive tasks. When studying the brain basis of emotion, however, one is often interested in imaging structures at the base of the brain such as the orbitofrontal and medial temporal cortex. Echoplanar acquisition is susceptible to artifacts in areas where brain is near air, such as the air in the mastoid sinus. This is a perplexing problem with this technique in the study of the brain basis of emotion. Newer imaging sequences and the use of coronal slices has largely eliminated this susceptibility artifact; however, BOLD fMRI still requires precise on/off task cycling, which may be difficult in studies of induced emotions. The newest advances in BOLD fMRI are the use of a single event to generate the signal, which may expand this technique's use in emotion research by eliminating the need for on/off tasks as well as the concerns about movement during the task (for a general overview of this area, see Davidson & Irwin, 1998).

Serial perfusion magnetic resonance imaging scanning

One of the main impediments to serial functional imaging of mood disorders has been the limitation imposed by radiation safety limits with SPECT and PET. This radiation limit has severely hampered the ability to understand mood disorders not simply as episodes that clearly start and stop, but over time in regional brain activity through a mood cycle. Several groups have begun using the new imaging method of quantitative spin labeling and inversion recovery perfusion functional MRI (pfMRI) (Warach et al., 1994). This technique has been used in preclinical models studying cerebral perfusion or rCBF (Bohning et al., 1996) and has been shown in healthy controls to repeatedly and consistently measure cerebral perfusion (Bohning et al., 1997b). pfMRI involves neither an injection nor radiation exposure, and therefore multiple measures per subject can be done. Furthermore, it can quantitatively measure rCBF, which cannot be done with perfusion SPECT and requires an arterial line with PET scanning. The entire scanning sequence initially took about 30 minutes per slice, but we have recently reduced this to 5 minutes per slice, moving ever closer to achieving a scan time that will work in an acute clinical setting.

We have recently used pfMRI to serially scan rapid-cycling bipolar affective disorder (BPAD) patients as they progress through their mood cycle (Spur et al., 1997). As a comparison group, we have also scanned age-matched and sex-matched controls on the same day in the same scanner, using identical techniques. These studies are being used to test our hypothesis that BPAD mood disorder subjects, when depressed, have increased activity in the right anterior temporal and insular regions and that during mania the same areas are relatively hypoactive. We are also keenly interested in whether there is a temporal dissociation or lag between clinical symptoms or phenomenology and changes in regional rCBF. That is, clinical symptoms and improvement may precede rCBF changes. To date, we have found that there is a complex association between clinical mood state and global brain activity on the day of the scan (Speer et al., 1997).

Figure 5.3 shows the relationship between global gray matter perfusion and mood over time in one subject. Note that, although mood and global rCBF roughly correlate, there are exceptions when global perfusion precedes or lags behind

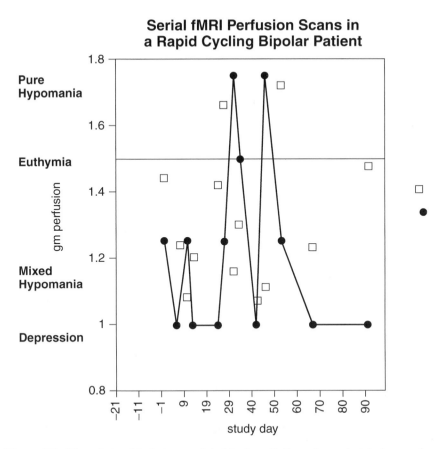

Figure 5.3. The relationship between global brain activity and mood state is complex, with several earlier reports indicating a positive correlation between global brain activity and mood (more activity in mania). Using the new technique of perfusion functional MRI, we have been directly addressing this issue. Shown are the global perfusion rates in the middle of the brain (horizontal line) (open squares) as a function of mood state.

clinical ratings. These pilot studies, with a novel noninvasive technology that permits measurement of absolute brain perfusion, are perhaps yet another window into the brain of BPAD subjects, allowing for the first time serial assessment of the regional brain changes associated with mood cycling. This advance hopefully will allow better examination of regional brain changes over time and of how they relate to clinical symptoms.

Magnetic resonance spectroscopy

Magnetic resonance spectroscopy (MRS) uses modified structural MRI scanners to study resonance spectra of compounds containing paramagnetic (odd atomic number) elements. Proton or ^{1}H MRS allows determination of lactate, glutamate, aspartate, gamma-aminobutyric acid, creatinine, choline, and N-acety-laspartate. Lithium (^{7}LI) and fluorine (^{19}F) MRS can assess cerebral concentrations of lithium and fluorinated drugs, respectively. Phosphorus (^{31}P) MRS allows determination of high-energy phosphates (ATP), intracellular pH, free magnesium, and some phospholipids, including phosphomonoesters (putative cell membrane "building blocks") and phosphodiesters (putative cell membrane breakdown products). Spectroscopy has to date been used by only a few groups to study mood or emotion (Cohen, Renshaw, & Yurgelun-Todd, 1995; Dager et al., 1995). Thus far, only a few groups interested in psychiatry or psychology have effectively tackled the daunting technological hurdles behind MRS, which range from radiofrequency coil designs to software packages. Theoretically, MRS, with the ability to noninvasively image chemical changes such as brain ATP, could prove to be the ultimate functional imaging tool.

Transcranial Magnetic Stimulation

Another recent technological development that will likely impact heavily on the field of functional imaging and emotion research is TMS. With the ability to non-invasively activate neurons, TMS offers the promise of overcoming the formidable barrier of the skull, with real-time noninvasive probing and testing of neuronal circuits and behavior. Transcranial magnetic stimulation uses the principle of inductance to convey electrical energy across the scalp and skull without the painful side effects of direct percutaneous electrical stimulation (for reviews, see George, Lisanby, & Sackeim, 1999b; George, Wassermann, & Post, 1996c). It involves placement of a small coil of wire on the scalp and a very powerful current passing through it (Barker, Jalinous, & Freeston, 1985; Roth et al., 1991; Saypol et al., 1991). A magnetic field is produced that moves unimpeded through the tissues of the head. The magnetic field, in turn, induces a much weaker electrical current in the brain.

The shape of the electromagnet coil is important because different coil shapes produce different magnetic fields (Cohen et al., 1990; Murro et al., 1992). The main differences are in the size and focality of the magnetic field. For instance, so-called butterfly or eight-shaped coils consist of two loops of windings that intersect in the middle. The magnetic field is maximal at the intersection and weaker elsewhere. This allows fairly focal stimulation of the brain and has allowed the technique to be used for cortical mapping (Bohning et al., 1997a; Pascual-Leone, Grafman, & Hallett, 1994; Pascual-Leone et al., 1995; Roberts et al., 1997; Wassermann et al., 1992; Wilson, Thickbroom, & Mastaglia, 1993). The stimulators and coils in production today develop about 1.5–2 Tesla at the face of the coil and are able to activate neurons 1.5–2 cm from the surface of the coil in the cortex (Epstein et al., 1990). Activation of neurons deeper in the brain may be possible with solid-core coils, formed by coiling wire around a bar of a paramagnetic material such as iron (Davey, Cheng, & Epstein, 1991; Weissman, Epstein, & Davey, 1992), or with other combinations of coils (Bohning, personal communication). Even though conventional TMS can directly activate only cortical neurons, it affects cells at some distance from the stimulation site through trans-synaptic connections. Preliminary evidence for trans-synaptic effects within the brain comes from changes in hormones induced by stimulation (George et al., 1996a) and widespread changes in brain activity during TMS detected with functional imaging techniques (discussed below) (Bohning et al., 1998a; George et al., 1995b; Kimbrell et al., 1997; Paus et al., 1997; Stallings et al., 1997; Wassermann et al., 1997).

Transcranial magnetic stimulation–induced changes in normal mood

One long-standing model of emotion regulation has been *the valence model of mood*, which postulates that whereas the left hemisphere mediates positive emotions (e.g., happiness), the right mediates negative emotions (anger, fear, disgust, anxiety, sadness) (Ross, Homan, & Buck, 1994; Sackeim & Gur, 1978; Sackeim, Gur, & Saucy, 1978). An individual's mood at any given time thus reflects the relative balance of the input of the two hemispheres. Either temporarily or permanently disabling one hemisphere would allow the other to act in an unbalanced manner (see Robinson & Manes, Chapter 10; Davidson & Henriques, Chapter 11; and Lisanby & Sackeim, Chapter 18, this volume). The valence hypothesis, while supported by many studies, is by no means proven, and several studies have yielded results inconsistent with this theory (House et al., 1990; Sharpe et al., 1990; for a critical review, see Sackeim, 1991). In addition, only a weak plurality of functional imaging studies in mood disorder patients support lateralized dysfunction.

We first sought to directly test the valence theory of mood by employing repetitive TMS (rTMS) to temporarily excite (and then disable) prefrontal cortex and observe the effects on mood (George et al., 1996d). Using rTMS over the right or left prefrontal cortex of ten adult healthy volunteers on different days, we discovered that left prefrontal stimulation caused an increase in self-rated sadness, while right stimulation caused increases in happiness (for stimulation, we used a figure-eight coil, 120% of motor threshold [MT], 5 Hz for 10 seconds, 2 minutes of rest, on and off ten times, a total of 20 minutes of stimulation, and 500 stimuli per session). This study confirmed and extended the initial study of Pascual-Leone, Catala, and Pascual (1996a), who had stimulated different brain regions within the same day and achieved roughly the same results, but significant mood effects were seen within 30 minutes of stimulation at higher frequency, shorter intertrain interval parameters (110% MT, 10 Hz for 5 seconds, 25 seconds apart, for ten trains). This TMS-induced mood effect appears to be specific to prefrontal stimulation, although active nonprefrontal sites were only explicitly tested in the initial study of George et al. (1996d).

In a recent follow-up study using a more fastidious design, we stimulated a different (from those in earlier study) group of controls with selective prefrontal stimulation on one day and entire hemisphere stimulation on another (Martin et al., 1997). During selective prefrontal stimulation in nine healthy controls over the right hemisphere, self-rated happiness increased, whereas left prefrontal stimulation resulted in increased sadness (80% MT, 20 Hz, 2 sec/min 20 times over 20 minutes). Entire hemisphere stimulation with a larger nonfocal coil and with identical parameters and ratings caused no significant change in mood (see Fig. 5.4). Interestingly, we also found that right stimulation caused significant increases in anxiety. Although the results are provocative, caution is clearly needed in the interpretation of these pilot studies in a new field with small sample sizes.

Use of repetitive transcranial magnetic stimulation as an antidepressant (a therapeutic probe of pathological mood)

Converging evidence from SPECT, PET, and qEEG points to hypofunction of the left prefrontal cortex in clinical depression (discussed above). Reasoning from these imaging studies, as well as from the rTMS mood effects in healthy controls and other initial pilot treatment studies (Grisaru et al., 1994; Hoflich et al., 1993; Kolbinger et al., 1995), we questioned whether daily prefrontal rTMS might improve mood in depressed subjects. We wondered whether one might be able to stimulate subconvulsively over prefrontal cortex and achieve an antidepressant effect. We initially studied the immediate effect of right versus left prefrontal rTMS in medication-resistant patients. Paradoxically and in direct contrast to the results obtained with healthy volunteers, in whom right prefrontal stimulation caused subtle but statistically significant increases in self-rated happiness, right prefrontal stimulation in the severely depressed adults resulted in marked increases of anxiety and worsening mood.

We therefore performed daily left prefrontal rTMS in six highly medication-resistant depressed inpatients. Depression scores significantly improved for the group as a whole (Hamilton Depression Scores decreased from 23.8 [4.2 SD at baseline] to 17.5 [8.4 SD] after treatment). Two subjects showed robust mood improvement, which occurred progressively over the course of several weeks. In one subject, depression symptoms completely remitted for the first time in 3 years. We concluded that daily left prefrontal rTMS was safe and well-tolerated and might alleviate depression (George et al., 1995b).

Dr. Pascual-Leone and colleagues (1996) next used a double-blind placebo-controlled design and reported that left prefrontal rTMS for 5 days (at 90% MT, 10 Hz, 10 seconds, 1 minute rest, 20 times each morning, 2000 stimuli per morning, 10,000 per site; 40,000 total per subject) significantly improved mood in 17 psychotically depressed subjects. Stimulation at other sites (e.g., right prefrontal, occipital) had no effect. Even at these high doses and numbers of stimuli, rTMS was well-tolerated (Pascual-Leone et al., 1996b).

Immediately after completing our open study in medication-refractory inpatients, we undertook a double-blind placebo-controlled crossover study of daily left prefrontal rTMS in depressed outpatients (20 Hz, 2 seconds, 1 minute rest, 80% MT, 200 times per day; 800 stimuli per morning; 8000 stimuli per site). There was a significant improvement in mood as a function of TMS treatment (George et al., 1997b), although the magnitude of change was not nearly as profound as in the study of Pascual-Leone et al. (1996b). There are now many groups in the United States and elsewhere using rTMS for investigating and treating depression and exploring the different rTMS parameters (location, intensity, frequency, dosing schedules, diagnostic groups) in rTMS depression treatment trials (for reviews, see George, Lisanby, & Sackeim, 1999b; George et al., 1999a; Lisanby & Sackeim, 1998). It is unclear what clinical role rTMS might have, if any, in the treatment of depression. Further work to elucidate normal mood regulation and how TMS affects different brain areas is crucial.

Combining transcranial magnetic stimulation with functional imaging to directly activate, visualize, and test neuronal circuits

As mentioned above, there are many technical issues associated with performing TMS in a PET, SPECT or MRI scanner. As a first step in this field, after performing a split FDG scan in a depressed patient in an early TMS treatment trial, we began using techniques in which the tracer uptake is removed from the actual scanner; the image can then be "developed" later, away from the TMS coil. In work at the National Institutes of Health, Kimbrell and colleagues (1997) have carried out a split-dose FDG PET study to look at the effects of low-frequency (1 Hz) TMS over prefrontal cortex. Some preliminary data from this study are shown in Figure 5.4, demonstrating that, compared with the resting scan, there are global decreases in brain metabolism and also regional *decreases* at the coil site and in the contralateral medial temporal region (perhaps the amygdala). Several other groups have also recently demonstrated local and trans-synaptic effects of rTMS (Bohning et al., 1998a,b; George et al., 1995b; Paus et al., 1997; Stallings et al., 1997; Wassermann et al., 1997). These studies demonstrate the power of coupling functional imaging with TMS to probe brain function (George et al., 1997a, 1999c).

GENERAL PROBLEMS COMMON TO MOST MODALITIES

Armed with a general understanding of the choice of imaging tools, one can now understand why different techniques are better suited for investigating different aspects of mood or emotion. Regardless of the imaging tool, there are several common problems that confront all researchers in this area. We discuss them briefly here.

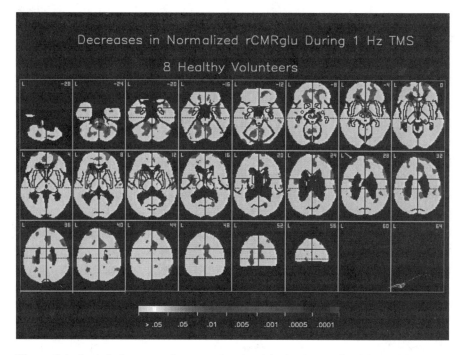

Figure 5.4. Statistical parametric maps of regional brain changes in eight healthy adults undergoing split-dose FDG PET. In the task condition, subjects received low-frequency TMS over the left prefrontal cortex. Compared with the control state, global brain metabolism significantly dropped during the prefrontal TMS, which was not seen in a parallel study with sham TMS over the same region. Note the decreases in normalized activity at the coil site, in the medial prefrontal cortex, and in the contralateral medial temporal cortex.

Monitoring of Emotion and Choice of an Appropriate Baseline

For any imaging study, measuring emotion is a thorny issue. One main problem is whether sampling disturbs the mood or emotion. That is, too frequent sampling of a subject's self-rated mood might interfere with the mood induction procedure. This issue is discussed in more detail elsewhere in this volume. The other issue is how to integrate psychophysiological measurements like heart rate and skin conductance into the imaging laboratory. In some environments, such as a SPECT study in a psychophysiology laboratory, this is trivial. In other situations, such as with an MRI scanner, this is very complex.

Just as measuring the emotion under study is difficult, it is not easy to determine the baseline for comparison with the emotional state. For studies with both healthy and mood-disordered individuals, the comparison is simple. In activation studies, however, the appropriate baseline is sometimes difficult to achieve. Even when comparing two groups, the choice of what mental task to have individuals focus on is also important. In general, groups now have subjects engage in a moderately difficult task, like an auditory continuous performance task, during "baseline scans." This ensures that the subjects are awake and alert and that the differences that are detected are less likely to have arisen from different cognitive tasks during the scan. This area is not settled, however, and there is no true consensus.

Study Design and Statistical Analysis

In general, imaging studies that build on hypotheses generated from other approaches (lesion studies, brain stimulation, the Wada procedure, and tachistoscopic studies) are the most straightforward. The statistical analysis can be limited to the region under question with a region of interest analysis. When researchers begin to perform more exploratory studies, however, both the choice of appropriate study design and the proper statistical analysis becomes less clear. Depending on the question, one can choose an event-related study (inject tracer during acute anxiety) or a block design (scan before and after an intervention or task, regardless of the subjective emotion).

A particularly perplexing problem within the field of functional imaging involves how to appropriately test for statistical significance within or between groups when numerous brain are compared. With limited comparisons and hypothesis-driven questions, traditional statistical analyses suffice. Once brain activity has been pooled and normalized into a common brain space, however, how can one effectively perform an exploratory analysis that accounts for the total number of comparisons (typically on the order of thousands)? An entire new branch of statistics has arisen within the field of functional imaging to deal with these thorny issues (Friston et al., 1990, 1994). Much as each of the separate imaging tools has particular advantages and disadvantages for a particular question, there are numerous approaches to statistical analysis. Common approaches to reduce the number of total comparisons involve smoothing of the data (thus decreasing the independence of each pixel and decreasing the total number of effectively discrete regions) (Friston et al., 1994), restriction of the initial search to key regions, or division of the group in half and two separate analyses, with the first half being exploratory in nature and the second half potentially confirming the results in the first half (Fox & Mintun, 1989). All approaches have their relative advantages and disadvantages.

SUMMARY AND CONCLUSIONS

Functional imaging has recently evolved into a complex area with multiple techniques for investigating brain function. Within the past 20 years, the field has gone from having only one functional imaging tool (EEG) with poor spatial resolution to now having a host of different techniques with a variety of specific advantages and drawbacks. In this chapter, we reviewed many of the common problems associated with performing imaging studies to examine the neural substrates of mood and then briefly described the more common imaging tools in use today. Other chapters in this volume expand on this introduction and provide more in-depth analyses of the work by many of the leading researchers in this area.

Thus, the field of functional neuroimaging offers much promise in elucidating the brain basis of mood and emotion. Functional imaging studies, constantly reminding us of the inextricable links between the mind and the brain, may finally put an end to dualistic concepts of mind and emotion separated from brain. They also offer the potential of forcing us to change our language about emotion into a more exact, neuroscientifically based discourse. As these techniques are refined and improved, they will undoubtedly help enhance our knowledge of the brain basis of emotion.

ACKNOWLEDGMENTS
Dr. George thanks NARSAD, the Stanley Foundation, NIAAA, NIDA, Dupont Pharma, Dantec International, Picker International, Solvay, Jansenn, and Lilly for financial support of many of the imaging projects discussed.

REFERENCES

Barker, A.T., Jalinous, R., & Freeston, I.L. (1985). Non-invasive magnetic stimulation of the human motor cortex. *Lancet, 1*, 1106–1107.

Baxter, L.R., Mazziotta, J.C., Phelps, M.E., Selin, C.E., et al. (1987). Cerebral glucose metabolic rates in normal human females versus normal males. *Psychiatry Research, 21*, 237–245.

Baxter, L.R., Jr., Phelps, M.E., Mazziotta, J.C., Schwartz, J.M., Gerner, R.H., Selin, C.E., & Sumida, R.M. (1985). Cerebral metabolic rates for glucose in mood disorders. Studies with positron emission tomography and fluorodeoxyglucose F 18. *Archives of General Psychiatry, 42*, 441–447.

Baxter, L.R., Jr., Schwartz, J.M., Phelps, M.E., Mazziotta, J.C., Guze, B.H., Selin, C.E., Gerner, R.H., & Sumida, R.M. (1989). Reduction of prefrontal cortex glucose metabolism common to three types of depression. *Archives of General Psychiatry, 46*, 243–250.

Bohning, D.E., Epstein, C.M., Vincent, D.J., & George, M.S. (1997a). Deconvolution of transcranial magnetic stimulation (TMS) maps [abstract]. *Neuroimage, 5*, S520.

Bohning, D.E., Shastri, A., McConnell, K., Nahas, Z., Lorberbaum, J., Roberts, D., Teneback, C., Vincent, D.J., & George, M.S. (1999). A combined TMS/fMRI study of intensity-dependent TMS over motor cortex. *Biological Psychiatry, 45*, 385–394.

Bohning, D.E., Shastri, A., Nahas, Z., Lorberbaum, J.P., Anderson, S.W., Dannels, W., Vincent, D.J., & George, M.S. (1998b). Echoplanar BOLD fMRI of brain activation induced by concurrent transcranial magnetic stimulation (TMS). *Investigative Radiology, 33(6)*, 336–340.

Bohning, D.E., Speer, A.M., Pecheny, A.P., Vincent, D.J., & George, M.S. (1997b). Acetazolamide-induced perfusion changes measured with MR spin-labelling [abstract]. *Neuroimage*, *5*, S380.

Bohning, D.E., Wright, A.C., Pecheny, A.P., & George, M.S. (1996). Repeatability of spin label–based in vivo perfusion maps [abstract]. *Neuroimage*, *3*, S128.

Breiter, H.C., Rauch, S.L., Kwong, K.K., Baker, J.R., Weisskoff, R.M., Kennedy, D.N., Kendrick, A.D., Davis, T.L., Jiang, A., Cohen, M.S., Stern, C.E., Belliveau, J.W., Baer, L., O'Sullivan, R.L., Savage, C.R., Jenike, M.A., & Rosen, B.R. (1996). Functional magnetic resonance imaging of symptom provocation in obsessive–compulsive disorder. *Archives of General Psychiatry*, *53*, 595–606.

Bremner, J.D., Innis, R.B., Salomon, R.M., Staib, L.H., Ng, C.K., Miller, H.L., Bronen, R.A., Krystal, J.H., Duncan, J., Rich, D., Price, L.H., Malison, R., Dey, H., Soufer, R., & Charney, D.S. (1997). Positron emission tomography measurement of cerebral metabolic correlates of tryptophan depletion-induced depressive relapse. *Archives of General Psychiatry*, *54*, 364–374.

Churchland, P.M. (1984). *Matter and Consciousness*. Cambridge, MA: MIT Press.

Cohen, B.M., Renshaw, P.F., & Yurgelun-Todd, D. (1995). Imaging the mind: Magnetic resonance spectroscopy and functional brain imaging. *American Journal of Psychiatry*, *152*, 655–658.

Cohen, L.G., Roth, B.J., Nilsson, J., Dang, N., Panizza, M., Bandinelli, S., Friauf, W., & Hallett, M. (1990). Effects of coil design on delivery of focal magnetic stimulation. Technical considerations. *Electroencephalography and Clinical Neurophysiology*, *75*, 350–357.

Cohen, M.S., & Bookheimer, S.Y. (1994). Localization of brain function using magnetic resonance imaging. *Trends in Neuroscience*, *17*, 268–277.

Dager, S.R., Strauss, W.L., Marro, K.I., Richards, T.L., Metzger, G.D., & Artru, A.A. (1995). Proton magnetic resonance spectroscopy investigation of hyperventilation in subjects with panic disorder and comparison subjects. *American Journal of Psychiatry*, *152*, 666–672.

Davey, K.R., Cheng, C.H., & Epstein, C.M. (1991). Prediction of magnetically induced electric fields in biologic tissue. *IEEE Transactions on Biomedical Engineering*, *38*, 418–422.

David, A., Blamire, A., & Breiter, H. (1994). Functional magnetic resonance imaging: A new technique with implications for psychology and psychiatry. *British Journal of Psychiatry*, *164*, 2–7.

Davidson, R.J. (1994). Asymmetric brain function, affective style, and psychpathology: The role of early experience and plasticity. *Development and Psychopathology*, *6*, 741–758.

Davidson, R.J., & Irwin, W. (1998). Functional MRI in the study of emotion. In C. Moonen & P.A. Bandettini (Eds.), *Medical Radiology—Diagnostic Imaging and Radiation Oncology: Functional MRI*. Heidelberg, Germany: Springer.

Devous, M.D., Stokely, E.M., Chehabi, H.H., & Bonte, F.J. (1986). Normal distribution of regional cerebral blood flow measured by dynamic single-photon emission tomography. *Journal of Cerebral Blood Flow and Metabolism*, *6*, 95–104.

Ell, P.J., Cullum, I., & Costa, D.C. (1985). Regional cerebral blood flow mapping with a new Tc-99m-labelled compound. *Lancet*, 50–51.

Engel, J. (1989). *Seizures and Epilepsy*. Philadelphia: FA Davis.

Epstein, C.M., Schwartzenberg, D.G., Davey, K.R., & Sudderth, D.B. (1990). Localizing the site of magnetic brain stimulation in humans. *Neurology*, *40*, 666–670.

Fox, P.T., & Mintun, M.A. (1989). Noninvasive functional brain mapping by change-distribution analysis of averaged PET images of $H_2^{15}O$ tissue activity. *Journal of Nuclear Medicine, 30*, 141–149.

Friston, K.J., Frith, C.D., Liddle, P.F., Dolan, R.J., Lammertsma, A.A., & Frackowiak, R.S.J. (1990). The relationship between global and local changes in PET scans. *Journal of Cerebral Blood Flow and Metabolism, 10*, 458–466.

Friston, K.J., Passingham, R.E., Nutt, J.G., Heather, J.D., Sawle, G.V., & Frackowiak, R.S.J. (1989). Localisation in PET images: Direct fitting of the intercommissural (AC-PC) line. *Journal of Cerebral Blood Flow and Metabolism, 9*, 690–695.

Friston, K.J., Worsley, K.J., Frackowiak, R.S.J., Mazziotta, J.C., & Evans, A.C. (1994). Assessing the significance of focal activations using their spatial extent. *Human Brain Mapping, 1*, 210–220.

George, M.S. (1987). Neuroscience and psychiatry. *American Journal of Psychiatry, 144*, 1103.

George, M.S., Avery, D., Nahas, Z., Molloy, M., Oliver, N.C., Risch, S.C., & Arana, G.W. (1999a). rTMS studies of mood and emotion. *Electroencephalography and Clinical Neurophysiology, 304*–314.

George, M.S., Ketter, T.A., Parekh, P.I., Herscovitch, P., & Post, R.M. (1996a). Gender differences in rCBF during transient self-induced sadness or happiness. *Biological Psychiatry, 40*, 859–871.

George, M.S., Ketter, T.A., Parekh, P.I., Horwitz, B., Herscovitch, P., & Post, R.M. (1995a). Brain activity during transient sadness and happiness in healthy women. *American Journal of Psychiatry, 152*, 341–351.

George, M.S., Ketter, T.A., & Post, R.M. (1994a). Activation studies in mood disorders. *Psychiatric Annals, 24(12)*, 648–652.

George, M.S., Lisanby, S.H., & Sackeim, H.A. (1999b). Transcranial magnetic stimulation: Applications in neuropsychiatry. *Archives of General Psychiatry, 56*, 300–311.

George, M.S., Nahas, Z., Bohning, D.E., Shastri, A., Teneback, C.C., Roberts, D., Speer, A.M., Lorberbaum, J., Vincent, D.J., Owens, S.D., Kozel, A.F., Molloy, M., & Risch, S.C. (1999c). Transcranial magnetic stimulation and neuroimaging. In M.S. George & R.H. Belmaker (Eds.), *Transcranial Magnetic Stimulation in Neuropsychiatry.* Washington, DC: American Psychiatric Press.

George, M.S., Parekh, P.I., Rosinsky, N., Ketter, T.A., Kimbrell, T.A., Heilman, K., Herscovitch, P., & Post, R.M. (1996b). Understanding emotional prosody activates right hemisphere regions. *Archives of Neurology, 53*, 665–670.

George, M.S., Ring, H.A., Costa, D.C., Ell, P.J., Kouris, K., & Jarritt, P. (1991). *Neuroactivation and Neuroimaging with SPECT.* London: Springer-Verlag.

George, M.S., Robertson, M.M., Costa, D.C., Ell, P.J., Trimble, M.R., Pilowsky, L., & Verhoeff, N.P.L.G. (1994b). Dopamine receptor availability in Tourette's syndrome. *Psychiatry Research, 55*, 193–203.

George, M.S., Stallings, L.E., Speer, A.M., Spicer, K.M., Vincent, D.J., Bohning, D.E., Cheng, K.T., Molloy, M., Teneback, C.C., & Risch, S.C. (1999d). Prefrontal repetitive transcranial magnetic stimulation (rTMS) reduces relative perfusion locally and remotely. *Human Psychopharmacology, 14*, 161–170.

George, M.S., Wassermann, E.M., Kimbrell, T.A., Little, J.T., Williams, W.E., Danielson, A.L., Greenberg, B.D., Hallett, M., & Post, R.M. (1997a). Daily left prefrontal rTMS improves mood in depression: A placebo-controlled crossover trial. *American Journal of Psychiatry, 154*, 1752–1756.

George, M.S., Wassermann, E.M., Kimbrell, T., Speer, A.M., Stallings, L., Roberts, D., Vincent, D.J., Beale, M., Cheng, K., & Spicer, K.M. (1997b). An overview of initial

studies combining conventional functional imaging (PET, SPECT, fMRI) with transcranial magnetic stimulation (TMS) to actively probe brain–behavior relationships [ab-
stract]. *Journal of Neuropsychiatry and Clinical Neurosciences*, 9, 131-#6.

George, M.S., Wassermann, E.M., & Post, R.M. (1996c). Transcranial magnetic stimulation: A neuropsychiatric tool for the 21st century. *Journal of Neuropsychiatry and
Clinical Neurosciences*, 8, 373–382.

George, M.S., Wassermann, E.M., Williams, W.A., Callahan, A., Ketter, T.A., Basser, P.,
Hallett, M., & Post, R.M. (1995b). Daily repetitive transcranial magnetic stimulation
(rTMS) improves mood in depression. *NeuroReport*, 6, 1853–1856.

George, M.S., Wassermann, E.M., Williams, W., Steppel, J., Pascual-Leone, A., Basser,
P., Hallett, M., & Post, R.M. (1996d). Changes in mood and hormone levels after
rapid-rate transcranial magnetic stimulation of the prefrontal cortex. *Journal of Neuropsychiatry and Clinical Neurosciences*, 8, 172–180.

Grisaru, N., Yarovslavsky, U., Abarbanel, J., Lamberg, T., & Belmaker, R.H. (1994).
Transcranial magnetic stimulation in depression and schizophrenia. *European Neuropsychopharmacology*, 4, 287–288.

Haxby, J.V., Grady, C.L., Ungerleider, L.G., & Horwitz, B. (1991). Mapping the functional neuroanatomy of the intact human brain with brain imaging. *Neuropsychologia*, 29, 539–555.

Hoflich, G., Kasper, S., Hufnagel, A., Ruhrmann, S., & Moller, H.J. (1993). Application
of transcranial magnetic stimulation in treatment of drug-resistant major depression—
A report of two cases. *Human Psychopharmacology*, 8, 361–365.

House, A., Dennis, M., Warlow, C., Hawton, K., & Molyneux, A. (1990). Mood disorders after stroke and their relation to lesion location. *Brain*, 113, 1113–1129.

Jackson, J.H. (1873). Observations on the localisation of movements in the cerebral hemispheres. *West Riding Lunatic Asylum Medical Reports*, 3, 175–190.

Jackson, J.H. (1874). On temporary mental disorders after epileptic paroxysms. *West Riding Lunatic Asylum Medical Reports*, 5, 103–129.

Jackson, J.H., & Stewart, P. (1899). Epileptic attacks with a warning of a crude sensation of
smell and with the intellectual aura (dreamy state) in a patient who had symptoms pointing to gross organic disease of the right temporo-sphenoidal lobe. *Brain*, 22, 534–549.

Kimbrell, T.A., George, M.S., Danielson, A.L., Dunn, R.T., Benson, B.E., Little, J.T.,
Herscovitch, P., Hallett, M., Post, R.M., & Wassermann, E.M. (1997). Changes in
cerebral metabolism during transcranial magnetic stimulation [abstract]. *Biological
Psychiatry*, 41, 108S-#374.

Kolbinger, H.M., Hoflich, G., Hufnagel, A., Moller, H.-J., & Kasper, S. (1995). Transcranial magnetic stimulation (TMS) in the treatment of major depression—A pilot
study. *Human Psychopharmacology*, 10, 305–310.

Kwong, K.K., Belliveau, J.W., Chesler, D.A., Goldberg, I.E., Weisskoff, R.M., Poncelet,
B.P., Kennedy, D.N., Hoppel, B.E., Cohen, M.S., & Turner, R. (1992). Dynamic magnetic resonance imaging of human brain activity during primary sensory stimulation.
Proceedings of the National Academy of Sciences of the United States of America, 89,
5675–5679.

Lane, R.D., Reiman, E.M., Ahern, G.L., Schwartz, G.E., & Davidson, R.J. (1997). Neuroanatomical correlates of happiness, sadness and disgust. *American Journal of Psychiatry*, 7, 926–933.

Leuchter, A.F., Cook, I.A., Uijtdehaage, S.H.J., O'Hara, R., Mandelkern, M., & Muten,
M. (1997). Noninvasive monitoring of brain function [abstract]. *APA New Research
Program*, 18-#45.

Lisanby, S.H., & Sackeim, H.A. (1999). TMS in major depression. In M.S. George & R.H. Belmaker (Eds.), *Transcranial Magnetic Stimulation in Neuropsychiatry*. Washington, DC: American Psychiatric Press.

Martin, J.D., George, M.S., Greenberg, B.D., Wassermann, E.M., Schlaepfer, T.E., Murphy, D.L., Hallett, M., & Post, R.M. (1997). Mood effects of prefrontal repetitive high-frequency TMS in healthy volunteers. *CNS Spectrums: The International Journal of Neuropsychiatric Medicine, 2*, 53–68.

Migliorelli, R., Starkstein, S.E., Teson, A., Quiros, G.D., Vazquez, S., Leiguarda, R., & Robinson, R.G. (1993). SPECT findings in patients with primary mania. *Journal of Neuropsychiatry and Clinical Neurosciences, 5*, 379–383.

Murro, A., Smith, J.R., King, D.W., & Gallagher, B.B. (1992). A model for focal magnetic brain stimulation. *International Journal of Bio-Med Computing, 31*, 37–43.

Pardo, J.V., Pardo, P.J., & Raichle, M.E. (1993). Neural correlates of self-induced dysphoria. *American Journal of Psychiatry, 150*, 713–719.

Parekh, P.I., Spencer, J.W., George, M.S., Gill, D.S., Ketter, T.A., Andreason, P.J., Herscovitch, P., & Post, R.M. (1995). Procaine-induced increases in limbic rcbf correlate positively with increases in occipital and temporal EEG fast activity. *Brain Topography, 7*, 209–216.

Pascual-Leone, A., Cammarota, A., Wassermann, E.M., Brasil-Neto, J., Cohen, L.G., & Hallett, M. (1995). Modulation of motor cortical outputs to the reading hand of braille readers. *Annals of Neurology, 34*, 33–37.

Pascual-Leone, A., Catala, M.D., & Pascual, A.P. (1996a). Lateralized effect of rapid-rate transcranial magnetic stimulation of the prefrontal cortex on mood. *Neurology, 46*, 499–502.

Pascual-Leone, A., Grafman, J., & Hallett, M. (1994). Modulation of cortical motor output maps during development of implicit and explicit knowledge. *Science, 263*, 1287–1289.

Pascual-Leone, A., Rubio, B., Pallardo, F., & Catala, M.D. (1996b). Beneficial effect of rapid-rate transcranial magnetic stimulation of the left dorsolateral prefrontal cortex in drug-resistant depression. *The Lancet, 348*, 233–237.

Paus, T., Jech, R., Thompson, C.J., Comeau, R., Peters, T., & Evans, A.C. (1997). Transcranial magnetic stimulation during positron emission tomography: A new method for studying connectivity of the human cerebral cortex. *Journal of Neuroscience, 17*, 3178–3184.

Reiman, E.M., Lane, R.D., Ahern, G.L., Schwartz, G.E., Davidson, R.J., Friston, K.J., Yun, L.S., & Chen, K. (1997). Neuroanatomical correlates of externally and internally generated human emotion. *American Journal of Psychiatry, 154*, 918–925.

Ring, H.A., George, M., Costa, D.C., & Ell, P.J. (1991). The use of cerebral activation procedures with single photon emission tomography. *European Journal of Nuclear Medicine, 18*, 133–141.

Ring, H.A., Trimble, M.R., Costa, D.C., George, M.S., Verhoeff, P., & Ell, P.J. (1992). Effect of vigabatrin on striatal dopamine receptors: Evidence for interactions of GABA and dopamine systems. *Journal of Neurology, Neurosurgery, and Psychiatry, 55*, 758–761.

Roberts, D.R., Vincent, D.J., Speer, A.M., Bohning, D.E., Cure, J., Young, J., & George, M.S. (1997). Multi-modality mapping of motor cortex: Comparing echoplanar BOLD fMRI and transcranial magnetic stimulation. *Journal of Neural Transmission, 104*, 833–843.

Rorty, R. (1971). In defense of eliminative materialism. In D.M. Rosenthal (Ed.), *Materialism and the Mind–Body Problem*. Englewood Cliffs, NJ: Prentice-Hall.

Rosen, B.R., Belliveau, J.W., Aronen, H.J., et al. (1991). Susceptibility contrast imaging of cerebral blood volume: Human experience. *Magnetic Resonance in Medicine*, 22, 293–299.

Rosen, B.R., Belliveau, J.W., Aronen, H.J., Hamberg, L.M., Kwong, K.K., & Fordham, J.A. (1994). Functional neuroimaging. In J. Kucharczyk, M. Moseley, & A.J. Barkovich (Eds.), *Magnetic Resonance Neuroimaging*. Boca Raton, FL: CRC Press.

Ross, E.D., Homan, R.W., & Buck, R. (1994). Differential hemispheric lateralization of primary and social emotions: Implications for developing a comprehensive neurology for emotions, repression and the subconscious. *Neuropsychiatry, Neuropsychology, and Behavioral Neurology*, 7, 1–19.

Roth, B.J., Saypol, J.M., Hallett, M., & Cohen, L.G. (1991). A theoretical calculation of the electric field induced in the cortex during magnetic stimulation. *Electroencephalography and Clinical Neurophysiology*, 81, 47–56.

Sackeim, H.A. (1991). Emotion, disorders of mood, and hemispheric functional specialization. In B.J. Carroll & J.E. Barrett (Eds.), *Psychopathology and the Brain* (pp. 209–242). New York: Raven Press.

Sackeim, H.A., & Gur, R.C. (1978). Lateral asymmetry in intensity of emotional expression. *Neuropsychologia*, 163, 473–481.

Sackeim, H.A., Gur, R.C., & Saucy, M.C. (1978). Emotions are expressed more intensely on the left side of the face. *Science*, 202, 434–436.

Saypol, J.M., Roth, B.J., Cohen, L.G., & Hallett, M. (1991). A theoretical comparison of electric and magnetic stimulation of the brain. *Annals of Biomedical Engineering*, 19, 317–328.

Schwarzbauer, C., Morrisey, S.P., & Haase, A. (1996). Quantitative magnetic resonance imaging of perfusion using magnetic labeling of water proton spins within the detection slice. *Magnetic Resonance in Medicine*, 35, 540–546.

Sharpe, M., Hawton, K., House, A., Molyneux, A., Sandercock, P., Bamford, J., & Warlow, C. (1990). Mood disorders in long-term survivors of stroke: Associations with brain lesion location and volume. *Psychological Medicine*, 20, 815–828.

Shaywitz, B.A., Shaywitz, S.E., Pugh, K.R., Constable, R.T., Skudlarski, P., Fulbright, R.K., Bronen, R.A., Fletcher, J.M., Shankweller, D.P., Katz, L., & Gores, J.C. (1995). Sex differences in the functional organization of the brain for language. *Nature*, 373, 607–609.

Sokoloff, L. (1977). Relation between physiological function and energy metabolism in the central nervous system. *Journal of Neurochemistry*, 29, 13–26.

Sokoloff, L. (1978). Local energy metabolism: Its relationship to local functional activity and blood flow. In M.J. Purves & L. Elliott (Eds.), *Cerebral Vascular Smooth Muscle and Its Control* (pp. 171–197). Amsterdam: Elsevier.

Speer, A.M., Upadhyaya, V.H., Bohning, D.E., Risch, S.C., Vincent, D.J., & George, M.S. (1997). New windows into bipolar illness: Serial perfusion MRI scanning in rapid-cycling bipolar patients [abstract]. *APA New Research Abstracts*, 111.

Stallings, L.E, Speer, A.M., Spicer, K.M., Cheng, K.T., & George, M.S. (1997). Combining SPECT and repetitive transcranial magnetic stimulation (rTMS)—left prefrontal stimulation decreases relative perfusion locally in a dose dependent manner [abstract]. *Neuroimage*, 5, S521.

Stehling, M.K., Turner, R., & Mansfield, P. (1991). Echo-planar imaging: Magnetic resonance imaging in a fraction of a second. *Science*, 254, 43–50.

Talairach, J., & Tournoux, P. (1988). *Co-Planar Stereotaxic Atlas of the Human Brain: 3-Dimensional Proportional System: An Approach to Cerebral Imaging*. New York: Thieme.

Taylor, J. (1958). *Selected Writings of John Hughlings Jackson*. New York: Basic Books.

Temkin, O. (1945). *The Falling Sickness: A History of Epilepsy from the Greeks to the Beginnings of Modern Neurology*. Baltimore: Johns Hopkins Press.

Turner, R., Le Bihan, D., Moonen, C.T., Despres, D., & Frank, J. (1991). Echo-planar time course MRI of cat brain oxygenation changes. *Magnetic Resonance in Medicine, 22*, 159–166.

Warach, S., Sievert, B., Darby, D., Thangaraj, V., & Edelman, R. (1994). EPISTAR perfusion echo-planar imaging of human brain tumors. *Journal of Magnetic Resonance Imaging, 4*, S8.

Wassermann, E.M., Kimbrell, T.A., George, M.S., Danielson, A.L., Herscovitch, P., Hallett, M., & Post, R.M. (1997). Local and distant changes in cerebral glucose metabolism during repetitive transcranial magnetic stimulation (rTMS) [abstract]. *Neurology, 48*, A107–P02.049.

Wassermann, E.M., McShane, L.M., Hallett, M., & Cohen, L.G. (1992). Noninvasive mapping of muscle representations in human motor cortex. *Electroencephalography and Clinical Neurophysiology, 85*, 1–8.

Weissman, J.D., Epstein, C.M., & Davey, K.R. (1992). Magnetic brain stimulation and brain size: Relevance to animal studies. *Electroencephalography and Clinical Neurophysiology, 85*, 215–219.

Whalen, P.J., Rauch, S.L., Etcoff, N.L., McInerney, S.C., Lee, M.B., & Jenike, M.A. (1998). Masked presentations of emotional facial expressions modulate amygdala activity without explicit knowledge. *The Journal of Neuroscience, 18*, 411–418.

Wheeler, R.E., Davidson, R.J., & Tomarken, A.J. (1993). Frontal brain asymmetry and emotional reactivity: A biological substrate of affective style. *Psychophysiology, 30*, 82–89.

Wilson, S.A., Thickbroom, G.W., & Mastaglia, F.L. (1993). Transcranial magnetic stimulation mapping of the motor cortex in normal subjects. The representation of two intrinsic hand muscles. *Journal of Neurological Sciences, 118*, 134–144.

Wu, J.C., Gillin, J.C., Buchsbaum, M.S., Hershey, T., Johnson, J.C., & Bunney, W.E. (1992). Effect of sleep deprivation on brain metabolism of depressed patients. *American Journal of Psychiatry, 149*, 538–543.

Ye, F.Q., Pejar, J.J., Jezzard, P., Duyn, J., Frank, J.A., & McLaughlin, A.C. (1996). Perfusion imaging of the human brain at 1.5 T using a single-shot EPI spin tagging approach. *Magnetic Resonance in Medicine, 36*, 219–224.

III

THEORETICAL PERSPECTIVES

6

Psychological Models of Emotion

KLAUS R. SCHERER

This chapter provides an overview of theories currently discussed in the psychology of emotion and the controversies and research issues they generate. As should become obvious in this review, many of the fundamental differences among the models relate to the thorny issue of the definition of the phenomenon called *emotion* and its conceptualization and operationalization. Not surprisingly, the disagreement as to the nature of emotion extends to the problem of delimitation of the psychological states or processes to be studied under this label from other affective phenomena. We first review the elements of the definition of emotion that seem to show at least some degree of convergence between different theorists.

DEFINITION AND DELIMITATION OF EMOTION

Although one occasionally encounters the position that organisms are always emotional, only more or less so, a sizeable number of emotion psychologists stress the *episodic* nature of emotion (Ekman, 1992a; Frijda et al., 1991; Scherer, 1993). The fundamental assumption of this position is that a noticeable change in the functioning of the organism is brought about by some triggering event, which can be external (such as the behavior of others, a change in a current situation, or an encounter with novel stimuli) or internal (such as thoughts, memories, or sensations). The emotion episode is supposed to last for a certain duration and then, with decreasing intensity, to more or less fade away. Therefore, it is normally easier to identify the onset than the offset of the changed state. The abruptness of both onset and offset of the episodes are expected to systematically vary for different kinds of emotion.

One of the major definitional issues is the question of what changes in different modalities are necessary and sufficient elements or components of the emotional episode. Although there are theorists who would restrict the use of the term *emotion* to a single modality (e.g., Clore [1994] would restrict it to conscious feelings of changed states), most current theorists subscribe to a multicomponential definition. These components generally include what has been called the "reaction triad" of emotion, namely, physiological arousal, motor expression, and subjective feeling. Some theorists extend the scope of necessary components to include motivational factors such as action tendencies and the cognitive processes that are involved in evaluating the eliciting events and the regulation of ongoing emotional processes (Buck, 1985, 1993; Ellsworth, 1991; Frijda, 1986, 1987; Scherer, 1984a,b, 1993).

Another point of definitional convergence is the assumption that emotions are normally triggered by internal or external stimuli or events that are of major significance to an organism. Thus, emotions have been called *relevance detectors* (Frijda, 1986). Relevance detectors require, of course, an evaluation of stimuli and events with respect to their *meaning* for the organism. Many theorists agree that the nature of this evaluation determines both the functional response of the organism—whether it is directed toward adaptation to or mastery of the event or situation—and the nature of the organismic and mental changes that will occur during the emotional episode.

Although there is much discussion of emotions as processes, which implies rapid changes over time, most theories and research still implicitly refer to *emotional states*, suggesting relative stability over time. This is mainly because few theorists have thus far attempted to directly address the nature of the changes occurring in the reaction modalities or in the emotion components during an emotional episode. To underline the unitary character of the emotional episode, I suggest that *interdependent and synchronized changes* in component processes are required as a necessary condition for the definition of emotion (Scherer, 1987, 1993).

Combining these elements of a definition of emotion (for which one finds increasing consensus in the literature) yields a working definition for the purposes of this chapter: emotions are episodes of coordinated changes in several components (including at least neurophysiological activation, motor expression, and subjective feeling but possibly also action tendencies and cognitive processes) in response to external or internal events of major significance to the organism. This working definition demarcates the coverage of emotion in this chapter from other affective phenomena that are not dealt with by the models reviewed here. Table 6.1 contrasts emotions thus defined with other affective phenomena on a number of essential design features (see also Frijda, 1993). It provides a brief definition with examples of five different types of affective states and traits. The different constructs are then compared on the basis of a matrix of design features that typically include intensity and duration, the degree of coordination or synchronization of different organismic systems during the state, the extent to which the change in state is triggered by or focused on an event or a situation, the extent to which the differentiated nature of the state is due to a process of antecedent evaluation or appraisal, the rapidity of change in the nature of the state, and the degree to which the state affects behavior.

Many of the controversies in emotion psychology can be traced to a failure to clearly distinguish between the different classes of phenomena. General affective valence or preference should not be treated in the same manner as emotional episodes, nor should more enduring affective states such as attitudes. For example, it is hardly helpful to use the study of simple preferences, such as liking for certain types of stimuli, to address theoretical issues with respect to the *emotion* construct as defined above.[1] The confusion between different types of affective phenomena, rampant in discussions of the psychology of emotion, has unfortunately spilled over into other areas such as neuropsychological approaches where the label *emotion* is often used for positive/negative valence of different types of stimulation. Clearly, one cannot hope to discover the underlying mechanisms unless one has first clearly delimited the phenomena one is trying to explain.

Another frequently encountered source of confusion relates to the tendency, based on popular usage of the terms, to treat *emotion* and *feeling* as synonyms. Although this is standard philosophical practice, it becomes extremely dangerous once one attempts to dissect the nature of the *components* of emotion. In such attempts it is helpful to define the subjective experiential component of the emotional reaction as "feeling" or "sentiment." As shown below, confusion between the phenomenon of emotion as a whole, consisting of several components, and one individual component, conscious subjective feeling, is responsible for much of the controversy surrounding the classic James-Lange theory.

This discussion of the definition and delimitation of emotion is concluded with a strong plea for researchers to avoid definitional confusion of this sort in future work. The linguistic labels attached to specific types of affective states are not always helpful. As is true for many other areas of psychology, popular usage of

---

[1]In this sense, Zajonc's insistence (1986) on the independence of affective preferences from "cognitive" processing does not appear to be very pertinent for theories of emotion.

Table 6.1. Design Feature Delimitation of Different Affective States*

BRIEF DEFINITIONS OF AFFECTIVE STATES	INTENSITY	DURATION	SYNCHRONIZATION	EVENT FOCUS	APPRAISAL ELICITATION	RAPIDITY OF CHANGE	BEHAVIORAL IMPACT
Emotion: relatively brief episode of synchronized responses by all or most organismic subsystems to the evaluation of an external or internal event as being of major significance (e.g., anger, sadness, joy, fear, shame, pride, elation, desperation)	$++ \rightarrow +++$	+	+++	+++	+++	+++	+++
Mood: diffuse affect state, most pronounced as change in subjective feeling, of low intensity but relatively long duration, often without apparent cause (e.g., cheerful, gloomy, irritable, listless, depressed, buoyant)	$+ \rightarrow ++$	++	+	+	+	++	+

Interpersonal stances: affective stance taken toward another person in a specific interaction, coloring the interpersonal exchange in that situation (e.g., distant, cold, warm, supportive, contemptuous)	+ → ++	+ → ++	+	++	+	+++	++
Attitudes: relatively enduring, affectively colored beliefs, preferences, and predispositions toward objects or persons (e.g., liking, loving, hating, valuing, desiring)	0 → ++	++ → +++	0	0	+	0 → +	+
Personality traits: emotionally laden, stable personality dispositions and behavior tendencies, typical for a person (e.g., nervous, anxious, reckless, morose, hostile, envious, jealous)	0 → +	+++	0	0	0	0	+

*Symbols indicate the degree to which the features are present, with 0 indicating the lowest (absence) and +++ indicating the highest; arrows indicate hypothetical ranges.

some terms has created semantic constructs that are less than optimal for exact scientific description. The use of a clearly identified design feature approach, as exemplified in Table 6.1, seems to be more promising in the long run.

HISTORICAL ROOTS OF CURRENT PSYCHOLOGICAL MODELS OF EMOTION

It is difficult to understand current theories and research objectives in the psychology of emotion—in particular the controversies in the field—without understanding the historical development of the current models. More than in other areas of psychology, the work on emotion has been strongly marked by the theorizing of a few major thinkers. A few examples of the continuity of some of the strands of argumentation that are used currently in debates about emotion are highlighted here.

Plato and the Cognition–Emotion Debate

Plato's suggestion that the soul has a tripartite structure, composed of the separate and opposing areas of cognition, emotion, and motivation, has influenced philosophers and psychologists for over two millennia. Aided by the "faculty" doctrines of eighteenth and nineteenth century philosophy, the urge to postulate separate systems for cognition, emotion, and motivation has been a near-constant source of controversy in the psychology of emotion (Hilgard, 1980). This ancient debate has been revitalized in recent years under the name of "cognition–emotion debate" (Lazarus, 1984a,b; Leventhal & Scherer, 1987; Zajonc, 1980, 1984a,b). Fifty years after Plato formulated the doctrine of the tripartite soul, Aristotle argued for the impossibility of such a separation and for the assumption of an interaction between the different levels of psychological functioning (Fortenbaugh, 1975). Echoing Aristotle, many modern theorists are trying to overcome thinking in separate systems and to highlight the interwovenness of cognitive, motivational, and emotional processes.

Descartes and the Mind–Body Debate

Descartes single handedly revolutionized the psychology and philosophy of emotion by insisting on dealing with mental and physiological processes at the same time. He thus laid the foundation for the mind–body debate about the relationships between mental and bodily phenomena, which continues unabated. Several current debates in emotion psychology, for example, about the nature of physiological patterning for specific emotional states or about the potential retroaction of expressive innervation of the muscles on mental states such as feeling, have generated heated controversy. Much of this is because the relationships between cognitive events and bodily changes remain uncharted and are often neglected. It has only been in recent years that theorists have attempted to link the antecedent evaluation of events (which was described by Aristotle, Descartes, Spinoza, Hume, and many other philosophers as the determinant of the nature of the ensuing emotion) to potentially stable patterns of adaptive responses in the central, peripheral, and somatic nervous systems of organisms (Scherer, 1984a, 1987; Smith, 1989; Smith & Ellsworth, 1985; Stemmler, 1996).

Darwin and the Biology versus Culture Debate

Of all historical works, Darwin's seminal book *The Expression of Emotion in Man and the Animals* (1872/1998) has probably had the most sweeping and enduring influence on modern psychology of emotion. He is responsible not only for the strong emphasis on the expression of emotion in face, body, and voice but also for many of the current concerns of emotion psychologists such as intercultural studies and developmental approaches. Most importantly, his observation of the widespread universality of a large number of emotional phenomena, particularly expression, has been the basis of a psychobiological current of theorizing that has long dominated the psychology of emotion (Ekman, 1972, 1973, 1984, 1992a; Izard, 1971, 1991, 1992; Tomkins, 1962, 1963, 1984). This tradition has been strongly attacked by anthropologists and social psychologists both early on (Mead, 1975) and, with renewed fervor, recently (Fridlund, 1994; Russell, 1994). As is often the case, the answer seems to lie in the middle. One can make a strong argument that emotion elicitation and emotion reaction are affected by *both* psychobiological and sociocultural factors (Ekman, 1972; 1992; Ellsworth, 1994; Mesquita, Frijda, & Scherer, 1997; Scherer & Wallbott, 1994).

James and the Center–Periphery Debate

William James's revolutionary suggestion (1884) that the emotion *is* the perception of differentiated bodily changes, specific for each emotion, has had a mixed impact on emotion psychology. While it catapulted the study of emotion to the forefront of the concerns of the young science of psychology at the time, it also led to a number of enduring confusions and quite sterile cul-de-sacs in research. As mentioned above, if one focuses on *feeling* as one of the components of emotion and as a reflection of what is happening in other components or modalities, James's suggestion that emotion is equal to feeling, as determined by the patterning of expressive and physiological reactions, is certainly acceptable, at least in part, to many modern psychologists. However, James' use of the term *emotion*, thereby referring to the complete process, including antecedent evaluation, while addressing only one component of the reaction, has muddled the issue. James himself became aware of this problem later and added that the bodily changes were determined by the overwhelming "idea" of the significance of the elements of a situation for the well-being of the organism (James, 1894, p. 518; see Scherer, 1996, pp. 282, 291–292).

The issue was further complicated by Schachter (1970), who proposed a theory of emotion that has dominated the textbooks for the last 30 years. Because there was little evidence for James's postulate of highly differentiated response patterning for specific emotions, Schachter suggested that an increase in general arousal would be sufficient to render the organism attentive to an emotion being experienced and to engage the organism in cognitive interpretations of the environment to find suitable emotion labels as justification for the increased arousal. Although this scenario might well happen under certain circumstances, it is highly improbable that this is the typical pattern for emotional processes. Consequently, the scenario is hardly a sufficient basis for a theory of emotion. Yet Schachter and Singer's ingenious experiment (1962), which has yet to be clearly replicated, plus Schachter's persuasive argumentation have maintained the popularity of this peripheral theory until quite recently.

These examples show to what extent the "giants" of the past have influenced theorizing and debate in emotion psychology and still do so today. They also indicate the necessity for current and future theorists to distance themselves from these early influences and to reevaluate the degree to which conceptualizations dating back hundreds of years provide a reasonable basis for present-day theorizing.

CURRENT PSYCHOLOGICAL MODELS OF EMOTION

Although there are several criteria with which to categorize the many current conceptualizations of emotion, the criterion of differentiation seems one of the most useful. Current emotion theories differ greatly with respect to both the number of emotions the theory is expected to explain and the principles that are evoked for the differentiation. In the following discussion, the currently used models are classified into four categories to highlight the principles that seem common to the respective approaches. Although there is obviously some variance between the models within each category, it is suggested that between-category variance is quite a bit larger than the within-category variance. It should be noted that both categorization and labeling are the result of the author's personal analysis of the bulk of theoretical work and may not be shared by other theorists.[2]

[2]In this discussion, the terms *theory* and *model* are used interchangeably and generously (in the sense that some of the approaches mentioned might fall short of the requirements for a theory in the full-fledged sense).

Dimensional Models

Unidimensional models

Proponents of unidimensional models, while acknowledging the existence of a multitude of fine distinctions between emotional states bearing different names, are convinced that one dimension is sufficient to make the important analytic distinctions. Depending on the theorist, this dimension is activation/arousal or valence, respectively. The idea that the major difference between emotional states is the relative degree of arousal from very little to very much was quite influential when general arousal models in physiology were popular. A pertinent example is the work of Duffy (1941), who is frequently cited as having advocated the abolishment of the term *emotion* in favor of the adoption of a continuum of terms to denote general excitation. Although such activation or arousal dimension models (with low versus high excitation poles) are no longer used much, the fundamental idea still permeates some of the theorizing and research in the area.

Many early psychologists argued that the pleasantness–unpleasantness dimension was the most important determinant of emotional feeling. This approach holds that the most important principle for emotion differentiation is valence, ranging from a bad, disagreeable, or unpleasant pole to a good, agreeable, or pleasant pole. This dimension allows one to distinguish between negative and positive emotions, a distinction that is intuitively appealing because it not only captures what is generally seen as the most important dimension of feeling but also reflects the two fundamental behavioral orientations of approach and avoidance (Schneirla, 1959). The distinction between positive and negative affect has been highly popular in sociopsychological treatments of emotional and affective states (e.g., Diener & Iran Nejad, 1986; Isen, Niedenthal, & Cantor, 1992) and it is currently one of the most accepted criteria for studying affect and mood states in social psychology, particularly social cognition (Clore & Parrot, 1991; Forgas, 1991; Schwarz, 1990) and personality. In the latter area, the idea of independent positive and negative dimensions, as in the so-called PANAS model (positive and negative affect scales) (Watson, Clark, & Tellegen, 1988) is increasingly popular.

Multidimensional models

One of the first suggestions for a multidimensional system was made by Wundt (1905), who advocated the use of both introspective and experimental methods, using physiological measurement, to study emotional feeling. He proposed that the nature of the emotional state was determined by its position on three independent dimensions: pleasantness–unpleasantness, rest–activation, and relaxation–attention. This three-dimensional model had a strong impact on early emotion psychology. Thus, Schlosberg (1954) propagated a three-dimensional model in American psychology, and he used two-dimensional models to study facial expression (Schlosberg, 1952). One of the attractions of this type of modeling is probably the fact that a multidimensional analysis of meaning transcends the study of emotion. Thus, Osgood and collaborators (see Osgood, May, & Miron, 1975; Osgood, Suci, & Tannenbaum, 1957) showed that virtually all linguistic and nonlinguistic concepts can be placed into such a three-dimensional space (valence, activation, and power) with respect to their meaning structure.

Multidimensional models have been popularized by Plutchik (1960, 1982) and Russell (1980, 1983). Both of these writers have postulated a two-dimensional scheme, with the standard emotions placed on a circle or circumplex in this space (valence, activation). Such two-dimensional models are appealing in that they allow one to graphically illustrate similarities and differences between emotions in terms of neighborhood in space.[3]

Dimensional models have been at the basis of much recent physiological and neuropsychological emotion research, which often emphasizes the valence dimension (e.g., Lang et al., 1993). Davidson (1992, 1993) has suggested a model that links the phylogenetically continuous approach–avoidance mechanism to positive–negative valence, postulating specific brain localizations for these functions. Borod (1992, 1993) has comprehensively reviewed the dimensional models that are currently used in the neuropsychology of emotion. In conclusion, although theorists adhering to dimensional models do not deny further differences between emotions, they remain fundamentally convinced that the functional distinction between approach tendencies in positive emotional states and the avoidance tendencies in negative emotional states is the basis of the neurophysiological and psychological affect differentiation.

Discrete Emotion Models

Circuit models

Circuit models, committed to a neuropsychological approach to emotion, suggest that the number of fundamental emotions and their differentiation are determined by evolutionarily developed neural circuits. The first such attempts to demonstrate emotional circuits in the brain were made by Cannon (1927), Papez (1937), and Arnold (1960). More recently, the two most prominent protagonists of this tradition have been Gray (1990) and Panksepp (1982, 1989).

---

[3]Evidence for a circumplex arrangement (Russell, 1980, 1983) is difficult to establish unequivocally because the spatial arrangement resulting from proximity analyses depends strongly on the selection of appropriate labels or expressions. Thus, one can demonstrate that by choosing a large array of verbal labels, one can fill the complete two-dimensional space with clouds rather than circumplex donuts (Gehm & Scherer, 1988; Scherer, 1984b).

Panksepp argues for four fundamental circuits, or emotive command "systems," which are expected to produce well-organized behavioral sequences elicited by neural stimulation: rage, fear, expectancy, and panic. Each of these neural circuits has very clear behavioral outputs. It is expected, however, that various interactions among these systems can lead to "second order emotive states" consisting of blended activities across the primary systems. This adjustment of a circuit model is obviously necessary once one moves from the emotional behaviors of lower mammals to primates, especially humans. In contrast, Gray (1990) highlights the biological mechanisms underlying attention and reinforcement.

Basic emotion models

Among the most popular conceptualizations of the nature of emotion have been theories suggesting the existence of basic or fundamental emotions such as anger, fear, joy, sadness, and disgust. The theorists in this tradition suggest that, during the course of evolution, a number of major adaptive emotional strategies developed (this is similar to the claims of circuit models). These strategies are thought to consist of a limited number, generally between 7 and 14, of basic or fundamental emotions each of which has its own specific eliciting conditions and its own specific physiological, expressive, and behavioral reaction patterns. Thus, Plutchik (1962, 1980) has proposed a set of basic emotions according to fundamental, phylogenetically continuous classes of motivation as identified by ethological research (Scott, 1969).

Many of the discrete emotion models are derived from Darwin's *The Expression of Emotion in Man and the Animals* (1872/1998). In this ground-breaking work, Darwin used a number of major emotion terms in the English language as chapter headings and demonstrated for each of these their functionality, evolutionary history, the universality across species, ontogenetic stages, and cultures. The theorist most responsible for the application of Darwin's seminal work to psychology was Tomkins (1962, 1963, 1984), who extended Darwin's theorizing to argue that a number of basic or fundamental emotions could be conceived of as phylogenetically stable *neuromotor programs*. Although Tomkins did not describe the nature of these programs in detail, the assumption was that specific eliciting conditions (which Tomkins sought in different gradients of neural firing) would automatically trigger a pattern of reactions ranging from peripheral physiological responses to muscular innervation, particularly in the face (which Tomkins considered as the primary differentiating effector system).

This concept has been popularized by two scholars strongly influenced by Tomkins, Ekman and Izard, who extended the theory and attempted to obtain pertinent empirical evidence, particularly with respect to early ontogenetic onset of the discrete emotion patterns (Izard, 1994; Izard et al., 1980, 1995), the discrete patterning of prototypical facial expressions for a number of basic emotions, and the universality of these patterns (Ekman 1972, 1973, 1980, 1992b, 1994; Ekman et al., 1987; Izard, 1971, 1990, 1994; Levenson et al., 1992). Given the limited number of such basic or discrete emotions, theorists in this tradition have had to postulate a mechanism of emotion mixing or *blending* to explain the large variety of emotional states that are popularly described by laymen and poets alike. In recent years, both Ekman and Izard have elaborated their theoretical ideas to account for both the large variety of emotional states (thus Ekman [1994] talks about "families of emotion") and the effects of the environment and culture on emotional development (Izard, 1994).

Given that the works of Tomkins, Izard, and Ekman have been responsible for the renaissance of work on emotion in post-war psychology, which was first dominated by behaviorism and then by cognitivism, much of present-day emotion psychology is in one way or another strongly influenced by the assumption of discrete fundamental emotions. Obviously, this idea is strongly supported by the existence of verbal labels with a very high frequency of usage, such as anger, fear, sadness, and joy, which serve to describe overarching concepts or prototypes.

Meaning Oriented Models

Lexical models

The structure of the semantic fields of emotion terms has often been used as the basis for model building in emotion psychology. The basic assumption is that the wisdom of the language somehow will help the theoretician to discover the underlying structure of a psychological phenomenon. Although it is debatable whether the denotative and connotative structures of the emotion lexicon in a particular language will neatly map to psychophysiological processes that are largely unconscious, this type of emotion modeling is intuitively appealing because it activates common cultural interpretation patterns. One such approach has been suggested by Oatley and Johnson-Laird (1987), focusing on goal structures. Ortony, Clore, and Collins (1988) performed a structural analysis of the emotion lexicon in order to demonstrate the underlying semantic implicational structure.

A different approach was used by Shaver and colleagues (1987), starting from work on conceptual structure (Rosch et al., 1976), to illustrate different levels of generality in the classification of emotional states. They used the method of cluster analysis to produce trees of emotion terms with differential degrees of generality. It is not always clear in the writings of the theorists in this tradition whether they are mostly interested in understanding the *labeling* of emotional states by lay persons, including the accompanying prototypical schemata, or whether they intend to extend the theoretical modeling to the emotion mechanism as a whole.

Social constructivist models

Another model of emotion claims that the meaning of emotion generally is constituted or constructed by socioculturally determined behavior and value patterns (Averill, 1980; Harré, 1986; Shweder, 1993). Although the proponents of this approach do not deny the psychobiological reaction components of emotion, they consider these secondary to the meaning conferred by the sociocultural context with respect to both the interpretation of the eliciting situation and the role of the emotion reaction in the person's sense-making and social interaction. Theorists in this tradition are also strongly interested in the emotion lexicon because they consider that the emotion labels available in a language reflect the emotional meaning structures in the respective culture.

Componential Models

Theorists of componential models start with the assumptions that emotions are elicited by a cognitive (but not necessarily conscious or controlled) evaluation of antecedent situations and events and that the patterning of the reactions in the different response domains (physiology, expression, action tendencies, and feeling) is determined by the outcome of this evaluation process. Although theorists in this tradition share these fundamental assumptions, their ideas diverge rather significantly with respect to both the conceptualization of emotion differentiation and the number of major emotions thus predicted.

One of the most restrictive of the componential models is that of Lazarus (1991). Together with Arnold (1960), Lazarus pioneered the notion of subjective appraisal, including the significance of an event for an organism and its ability to cope with the event, on the nature of the ensuing emotion (Lazarus, 1968, 1991). In his most recent modeling, Lazarus postulates a "theme"-based approach, which argues that a limited number of fundamental themes in appraisal generate a limited number of major emotions. While more explicitly modeling the elicitation process, this idea rejoins some of the fundamental assumptions of the discrete emotion theories, reviewed above.

At the other extreme of the componential models is the component process model proposed by Scherer (1982, 1984a,b, 1993), which assumes that there are as many different emotional states as there are differential patterns of appraisal results. Other theorists in this tradition (e.g., Ellsworth, 1991; Frijda, 1986, 1987; Roseman, 1984; Roseman, Wiest, & Swartz, 1994; Smith, 1989; Smith & Ellsworth, 1985; Smith & Lazarus, 1993) represent intermediate positions. Although these theorists generally do not endorse the idea of a small number of basic emotions, they tend to agree that there are overarching emotional prototypes or families. Thus, Scherer (1987, 1994) has suggested the concept of *modal* emotions, defined as frequently occurring patterns of appraisal or event types that are universally encountered by organisms, such as sadness in the case of loss or anger in the case of blocked goals.

One of the major features of componential theories is the effort to render the link between the elicitation of emotion and the response patterning more explicit. In many of the other types of models described above, the existence of differential patterning is either denied, as tends to be the case in dimensional models (which often still adhere to ideas of general arousal or valence), or ascribed to fixed neurophysiological circuits or neuromotor programs (as in the discrete emotion models). Theorists in the componential model category have started to work out detailed predictions of specific physiological, expressive, and motivational changes as consequences of specific appraisal results (Scherer, 1984a,b, 1986, 1987, 1992; Smith, 1989).

A SYNTHESIS OF THE MODELS

As is often the case in science, none of the classes of theories can be considered completely erroneous. Because the proponents of these theories are able to muster theoretical and empirical support for their claims, it is likely that each of the models captures and explains at least some aspects of reality. When comparing competing theories, one must determine exactly which of the many aspects of reality are highlighted by the respective theories and to what extent these aspects can be mapped onto each other given their relationships in reality. It seems useful to compare models with respect to their major focus. In doing so, it is appropriate to consider the need to rely on *verbal labels* of emotion to describe the phenomena to be modeled, something that all emotion models have in common.

The bases of verbal labels of emotional states are the changes in conscious subjective feeling states. Although the feeling states may reflect all the changes characterizing an emotion process in all of the organismic subsystems, verbal labels often represent only a salient part of those changes, those that reach awareness (see Kaiser & Scherer, 1997). In many cases, this process of becoming aware of a change and labeling it may be restricted to individual emotion components. For example, the term *tense*, which is frequently used as an affect descriptor, seems to refer almost exclusively to a special tonic state of the somatic nervous system, the striated musculature. If a certain set of terms is preferred in one theory of emotion and another set of terms with different referents in terms of component coverage is preferred in another theory, it is not surprising to find disagreements between the theories. It can be argued that because of this and related reasons the different classes of theories mentioned above tend to focus on different components of the emotion process.

Table 6.2 presents the unique profiles of each class of emotion model with respect to its main focus and to the way in which it deals with elicitation and re-

Table 6.2. Differential Foci of Several Psychological Models of Emotion

MODELS	MAJOR FOCUS	ELICITATION MECHANISM	DIFFERENTIATION MECHANISM
Dimensional	Subjective feeling	Rarely directly addressed; rudimentary approach–avoidance definition	Degree of similarity on feeling dimensions such as valence and activation
Discrete emotion	Motor expression or adaptive behavior patterns	Rarely directly addressed; typical situations or stimulus configurations	Phylogenetically continuous neuroanatomical circuits or motor programs
Meaning	Verbal descriptions of subjective feelings	Rarely directly addressed; cultural interpretation patterns	Socially shared, prototypical mental representations
Componential	Link between emotion-antecedent evaluation and differentiated reaction patterns	Appraisal mechanism based on a universally valid set of criteria, influenced by cultural and individual differences	Adaptive reactions in motor expression; physiological responses to appraisal results and the action tendencies generated by the results

sponse differentiation. It can be reasonably argued that the dimensional theories are almost exclusively concerned with the subjective feeling component and its verbal reflection, which, as described above, lends itself to dimensionalization. The large number of studies in this tradition that employ factor analysis, cluster analysis, or multidimensional scaling of emotion words underlines this tendency. The semantically oriented meaning theories, in constrast, are primarily concerned with studying the lexicon available for verbally labeling emotional states, an activity that, as semantic research tends to do generally, yields tree structures or taxonomy grids. Discrete emotion theories, historically linked to the study of facial expression, concentrate on the action system and particularly on the motor expression component. Because facial expression is the most discrete modality within the reaction component, it is not surprising to find that of discrete emotion models theorists postulate clearly differentiated patterns in the form of basic emotions.

These theories not only focus on different components of the emotion process but they also tend to be driven by different theoretical preoccupations. For example, while appraisal theorists are generally concerned with the cognitive front end, even though venturing predictions as to potential behavioral outcomes, circuit theorists and discrete emotion theorists mostly focus on the back end, the final response pattern subserving adaptational responses. The result of this, as one might expect, has been a remarkable confusion concerning the concept of emotion coupled with many fruitless debates on the nature of the phenomenon. If one considers emotion as a hypothetical construct referring to a process involving all of the above-mentioned components, few of the models described in this chapter can claim to explain emotion as a whole. At most, they can be considered subtheories, their range of validity being limited by the specific component processes they concentrate on. Because the components of emotion, and the underlying changes of the subsystems, can hardly be considered to be independent of each other, these partial theories need to be mapped onto each other. If one takes their respective foci of attention into account, they are actually much more compatible than is usually assumed.

The componential models, given the large number of facets of emotion that they encompass, might provide a suitable basis for such an attempt of mapping models onto each other. The dimensional structure of a "feeling space" as postulated by dimensional theorists does not contradict the postulate of component theorists that subjective feeling is one component of the total emotion process. On the contrary, one can even show ways in which major appraisal dimensions, such as goal conduciveness, urgency, and coping potential, map directly onto the feeling dimensions of valence, activation, and power/control (see Scherer, 1984b). As discussed above, componential models often acknowledge the existence of overarching emotion families or modal emotions, thus allowing one to bridge the gap to discrete emotion theories. Although component theories do not share the idea of a limited number of emotion-specific neuroanatomical circuits, they do postulate phylogenetically continuous, adaptive reaction patterns and action tendencies as produced by appraisal results.

With respect to meaning theories, component theorists share the social constructivists' insistence on the powerful role of sociocultural determinants of emotional experiences by assuming, for example, that cultural values can strongly affect appraisal, that the regulation of the emotion depends on norms and social context, and that the subjective experience reflects the sociocultural context. Component theorists do not, however, go as far as to maintain that emotional episodes are constituted entirely on the basis of cultural meaning structures. The findings of lexically oriented meaning theorists can also be easily integrated into component theories. Because the verbal labels can be expected to denote the conscious part of the feeling component (which is seen as reflecting the changes in all other components, including the cognitive, appraisal component), one would expect to find the semantic structure of the emotion lexicon to reveal both typical appraisal configurations and reaction prototypes.

CURRENT FOCI OF PSYCHOLOGICAL EMOTION RESEARCH

The current foci of interest in psychological theorizing and research on emotion can be grouped into three major categories: (*1*) the elicitation and differentiation of emotion through antecedent evaluation, (*2*) the emotion-specific response patterns of different modalities, and (*3*) the effects of emotion on other types of psychological functioning such as memory or judgment. These domains are briefly described here to demonstrate the ways that psychological models of emotion are put to use in research practice.

Emotion Elicitation and Differentiation

The issue of what determines whether an emotion is elicited and which kind of emotion will ensue can be approached from two different vantage points, an *exogenous* one, involving external events and situation changes outside of the organism or behaviors of self and others, and an *endogenous* one, based on the activation of memorized schemata or neurohormonal changes within the organism.

The exogenous point of view has been receiving renewed attention since the pioneering work of Arnold (1960) and Lazarus (1968) on the important role of the subjective appraisal of an event in emotion differentiation. Since the mid-1980s, many psychologists have proposed appraisal models of emotion (Ellsworth, 1991; Frijda, 1986; Oatley & Johnson-Laird, 1987; Roseman, 1984; Scherer, 1984a,b, 1986; Smith & Ellsworth, 1985), postulating that organisms evaluate events and situations in a number of given dimensions with the result of the appraisal process determining the nature of the ensuing emotion. This area has shown some remarkable convergence among the different appraisal theories that have received very strong and consistent support in experimental work designed to test the predictions (for a detailed review of this tradition, see Scherer, 1999).

One of the major criticisms leveled against appraisal theory is its presumed cognitive bias. Critics, however, have offered little with respect to alternative explanations of the elicitation and differentiation of the vast majority of emotional episodes. Appraisal theorists do not deny that emotions and particularly other affective states (as defined in Table 6.1) can be caused by other mechanisms, for example, the endogenous factors discussed below. Appraisal theorists have pointed out (Leventhal & Scherer, 1987; Scherer, 1984a) that the emotion-antecedent evaluation process can occur in a highly automatic fashion (for a discussion of the distinction between controlled and automatic processing, see Shiffrin & Schneider, 1977) and in a largely unconscious way. The idea of emotion-antecedent appraisal occurring at different levels of the central nervous system (e.g., the sensorimotor, schematic, or conceptual level) has been proposed

independently by a number of theorists approaching emotion from cognitive, clinical, and physiological perspectives (Mathews, 1988; Öhman, 1988). Several theorists are currently attempting to design experiments to more clearly distinguish
the underlying processes and their different levels and relationships (such as top-
down or bottom-up influences; see Van Reekum & Scherer, 1997). Given the
strong link between these traditions and work in the neuropsychology of emotion (e.g., the highly pertinent dual path model of emotion elicitation suggested
by LeDoux [1989]), the study of levels of processing is one of the most promising meeting points between psychologists and neuroscientists working on
emotion.

The study of the endogenous factors likely to elicit and differentiate emotions
is another such meeting point. The work done by Gray (1990) and Panksepp
(1982, 1989) on neuronal circuits involved in the generation and differentiation
of emotion and the potential effects of hormonal changes or drug intake are important examples of studies of endogenous factors. Another area of major interest is that of memory models that specify the mediating effects of neuropsychological mechanisms due to pathology (e.g., Damasio, 1994) or memory subsystems (Johnson & Multhaup, 1992). Another endogenous factor of interest,
largely unexplored (except for important work on temperament), concerns the
mediating effects of individual differences. For example, it is probable that specific features of an individual's central nervous system (e.g., cognitive speed or
varying neurohormonal states) can affect the cognitive evaluation of situations
or events (see Van Reekum & Scherer, 1997).

Patterning of Reaction Modalities

Much of the research on the psychology of emotion has been concerned with the
patterns of changes in motor expression, physiology, and subjective feeling (the
reaction triad described above). With respect to physiology and expression, one
of the major goals has been to demonstrate empirically the *specificity of patterning.* As discussed earlier, many of the psychological models described in this
chapter require at least some degree of specificity. The discrete emotion models
are located at one extreme of the specificity debate, suggesting a rather high degree of neuromotor and neurophysiological patterning. It has generally been the
work of the proponents of these models (such as Ekman, Davidson, Levenson,
and Izard) that has yielded empirical results showing a fairly high degree of
emotion-specific patterning. With respect to expression, the fact that judges are
reliably able to decode patterns of facial and vocal expressions of emotion produced by trained encoders (Ekman, 1984, 1992b; Scherer, 1989) suggests that
the assumption of specificity of patterning, even though somewhat difficult to
establish for actual facial movements (Gosselin, Kirouac, & Doré, 1995) or
acoustic features (Banse & Scherer, 1996), remains viable. Because similar

judgment approaches cannot be used to examine—even in an indirect fashion—physiological response patterning, researchers will need to demonstrate consistent configurations of physiological parameters characterizing specific emotional states. The degree to which the available evidence supports this assumption is strongly debated (Cacioppo et al., 1993; Levenson, 1992; Stemmler, 1996).

Surprisingly, the domain of subjective feeling states, which is the central response component for many emotion theorists, has received relatively little attention despite the burgeoning interest in consciousness. There have been few attempts to specify more clearly exactly how subjective feeling states could be conceptualized. Scherer (1987, 1993) has offered the definition of *subjective feeling* as a reflection in the central nervous system of all changes in both the central and peripheral systems during an emotional episode. This conceptualization does not require subjective feeling to be conscious. Rather, it can be assumed, as mentioned above, that only a small portion of the complete set of reflections of all ongoing changes reach the level of awareness or consciousness. An even smaller set of such aware reflections can in fact be verbalized (Kaiser & Scherer, 1997).

Traditionally, subjective feeling state has been measured exclusively via verbalization with a number of scales such as the Nowlis Mood Checklist or the Izard Differential Emotion Scale (DES). There has been very little effort to improve on the measurement of this important component of the emotion process (see Borod et al., Chapter 4, this volume). Some of the newer instruments, such as the positive-negative affect scales (PANAS; Watson & Tellegen, 1988) are directed toward valence rather than differentiated emotion states. It remains to be seen to what extent electroencephalography and neuroimaging methods will be used as nonverbal measures for subjective feeling (Davidson, 1992, 1993).

One of the major research issues in the domain of emotional reactions has been the interaction between different components. In particular, the question to what extent there is proprioceptive feedback from expressive innervation of the musculature about the quality and intensity of feeling states has been intensively studied (Cappella, 1993; Laird & Bresler, 1992; Leventhal & Tomarken, 1986; Matsumoto, 1987; Tourangeau & Ellsworth, 1979). Although the findings of some studies reporting feedback effects are hotly debated, the general pattern of the results suggests that a weak version of the proprioceptive feedback hypothesis might be viable.

Effects of Emotion on Other Psychological Functions

After a period of almost exclusive interest in emotion-free, cold cognition, there has been a remarkable surge of interest in hot cognition, that is, the way in which memory, learning, thinking, and judgment are affected by affective states. There is now rather consistent evidence showing that emotional states can have rather powerful effects on cognitive processing of various types, highlighting the need to focus on the interaction between cognition and emotion rather than trying to separate the two. The phenomena of particular interest to this new research are the effects of implicit or unconscious processing (Kihlstrom, 1987; Mathews et al., 1989; Niedenthal, 1990). Although most of this research has been driven by the valence-oriented dimensional theories, one might expect interesting findings from experiments in which other emotion conceptualizations are used to influence cognitive functioning. The specific effects of anger on cognitive processing, for example, are almost part of the popular lore. Clearly, research into hot cognition is a promising meeting point for emotion psychologists and neuropsychologists.

CONCLUSIONS

It remains to be seen which types of psychological models and research paradigms will best predict the responses of an individual to a particular stimulus or situation. It seems essential that any theoretical model of the response process will have to account for the nature of the antecedent processing, particularly the evaluation of events triggering the emotion and the relationships with the resulting pattern of reaction in different modalities. As argued above, it may well be possible to achieve convergence between the various psychological models discussed in this chapter after acknowledgment of their different foci and respective explanations for various aspects of the emotion process. The componential model might serve as a useful basis for such an attempt at convergence given the breadth of its focus with respect to the components of emotion and its attempt to theoretically predict the appraisal-reaction link in an explicit, detailed fashion. A final criterion for a psychological model of emotion is the degree to which it can be incorporated into the conceptual and empirical structures of adjoining disciplines such as neurophysiology, allowing easy transfer of concepts and findings.

REFERENCES

Arnold, M.B. (1960). *Emotion and Personality, Vols. 1, 2*. New York: Columbia University Press.

Averill, J.R. (1980). A constructivist view of emotion. In R. Plutchik & H. Kellerman (Eds.), *Emotion: Vol. 1. Theory, Research, and Experience* (pp. 305–340). New York: Academic Press.

Banse, R., & Scherer, K.R. (1996). Acoustic profiles in vocal emotion expression. *Journal of Personality and Social Psychology, 70*, 614–636.

Borod, J.C. (1992). Interhemispheric and intrahemispheric control of emotion: A focus on unilateral brain damage. *Journal of Consulting and Clinical Psychology, 60*, 339–348.

Borod, J.C. (1993). Emotion and the brain—Anatomy and theory: An introduction to the special section. *Neuropsychology, 7*, 427–432.

Buck, R. (1985). Prime theory: An integrated view of motivation and emotion. *Psychological Review, 92(3)*, 389–413.

Buck, R. (1993). What is this thing called subjective experience? Reflections on the neuropsychology of qualia. Special Section: Neuropsychological perspectives on components of emotional processing. *Neuropsychology, 7(4)*, 490–499.

Cacioppo, J.T., Klein, D.J., Berntson, G.C., & Hatfield, E. (1993). The psychophysiology of emotion. In M. Lewis & J.M. Haviland (Eds.), *Handbook of Emotions* (pp. 119–142). New York: Guilford Press.

Cannon, W.B. (1927). The James-Lange theory of emotion: A critical examination and an alternative theory. *American Journal of Psychology, 39*, 106–124.

Cappella, J.N. (1993). The facial feedback hypothesis in human interaction: Review and speculation. Special Issue: Emotional communication, culture, and power. *Journal of Language and Social Psychology, 12(1–2)*, 13–29.

Clore, G.L. (1994). Why emotions are never unconscious. In P. Ekman & R.J. Davidson (Eds.), *The Nature of Emotion: Fundamental Questions* (pp. 285–290). New York: Oxford University Press.

Clore, G.L., & Parrott, W.G. (1991). Moods and their vicissitudes: Thoughts and feelings as information. In J.P. Forgas (Ed.), *Emotion and Social Judgments. International Series in Experimental Social Psychology* (pp. 107–123). Oxford: Pergamon Press.

Damasio, A.R. (1994). *Descartes' Error: Emotion, Reason and the Human Brain*. New York: Avon.

Darwin, C. (1872). *The Expression of Emotions in Man and Animals*. London: John Murray. (3rd. edition, P. Ekman [Ed.]. London: HarperCollins, 1998.)

Davidson, R.J. (1992). Prolegomenon to the structure of emotion: Gleanings from neuropsychology. *Cognition and Emotion, 6(3–4)*, 245–268.

Davidson, R.J. (1993). Parsing affective space: Perspectives from neuropsychology and psychophysiology. Special Section: Neuropsychological perspectives on components of emotional processing. *Neuropsychology, 7(4)*, 464–475.

Diener, E., & Iran Nejad, A. (1986). The relationship in experience between various types of affect. *Journal of Personality and Social Psychology, 50(5)*, 1031–1038.

Duffy, E. (1941). An explanation of "emotional" phenomena without the use of the concept "emotion." *Journal of General Psychology, 25*, 283–293.

Ekman, P. (1972). Universals and cultural differences in facial expression of emotion. In J.R. Cole (Eds.), *Nebraska Symposium on Motivation* (pp. 207–283). Lincoln: University of Nebraska Press.

Ekman, P. (1973). Darwin and cross-cultural studies of facial expression. In P. Ekman (Ed.), *Darwin and Facial Expression* (pp. 1–83). New York: Academic Press.

Ekman, P. (1980). *The Face of Man: Universal Expression in a New Guinea Village*. New York: Garland.

Ekman, P. (1984). Expression and the nature of emotion. In K.R. Scherer & P. Ekman (Eds.), *Approaches to Emotion* (pp. 319–344). Hillsdale, NJ: Erlbaum.

Ekman, P. (1992a). An argument for basic emotions. *Cognition and Emotion, 6(3–4)*, 169–200.

Ekman, P. (1992b). Facial expression of emotion: New findings, new questions. *Psychological Science, 3*, 34–38.

Ekman, P., Friesen, W.V., O'Sullivan, M., Chan, A., et al. (1987). Universals and cultural differences in the judgments of facial expressions of emotion. *Journal of Personality and Social Psychology, 53(4)*, 712–717.

Ellsworth, P.C. (1991). Some implications of cognitive appraisal theories of emotion. In K. Strongman (Eds.), *International Review of Studies on Emotion* (pp. 143–161). New York: Wiley.

Ellsworth, P.C. (1994). Sense, culture, and sensibility. In S. Kitayama & M.R. Markus (Eds.), *Emotion and Culture. Empirical Studies of Mutual Influence* (pp. 23–50). Washington, DC: American Psychological Association.

Forgas, J.P. (1991). *Emotion and Social Judgments*. Oxford: Pergamon Press.

Fortenbaugh, W.W. (1975). *Aristotle on Emotion: A Contribution to Philosophical Psychology, Rhetoric, Poetics, Politics, and Ethics*. New York: Barnes & Noble Books.

Fridlund, A.J. (1994). *Human Facial Expression: An Evolutionary View*. New York: Academic Press.

Frijda, N.H. (1986). *The Emotions*. Cambridge and New York: Cambridge University Press.

Frijda, N.H. (1987). Emotion, cognitive structure, and action tendency. *Cognition and Emotion, 1*, 115–143.

Frijda, N.H. (1993). Moods, emotion episodes, and emotions. In M. Lewis & J.M. Haviland (Eds.), *Handbook of Emotions* (pp. 381–404). New York: Guilford Press.

Frijda, N.H., Mesquita, B., Sonnemans, J., & van Goozen, S. (1991). The duration of affective phenomena, or emotions, sentiments and passions. In K. Strongman (Ed.), *International Review of Emotion and Motivation* (pp. 187–225). New York: Wiley.

Gehm, T., & Scherer, K.R. (1988). Factors determining the dimensions of subjective emotional space. In K.R. Scherer (Ed.), *Facets of Emotion: Recent Research* (pp. 99–114). Hillsdale, NJ: Erlbaum.

Gosselin, P., Kirouac, G., & Doré, F.Y. (1995). Components and recognition of facial expression in the communication of emotion by actors. *Journal of Personality and Social Psychology, 68*, 1–14.

Gray, J.A. (1990). Brain systems that mediate both emotion and cognition. *Cognition and Emotion, 4(3)*, 269–288.

Harré, R.M. (Ed.) (1986). *The Social Construction of Emotions*. Oxford: Blackwell.

Hilgard, E.R. (1980). The trilogy of mind: Cognition, affection, and conation. *Journal of the History of the Behavioral Sciences, 16*, 107–117.

Isen, A.M., Niedenthal, P.M., & Cantor, N. (1992). An influence of positive affect on social categorization. *Motivation and Emotion, 16(1)*, 65–78.

Izard, C.E. (1971). *The Face of Emotion*. New York: Appleton-Century-Crofts.

Izard, C.E. (1990). Facial expressions and the regulation of emotions. *Journal of Personality and Social Psychology, 58(3)*, 487–498.

Izard, C.E. (1991). *The Psychology of Emotions*. New York: Plenum Press.

Izard, C.E. (1992). Basic emotions, relations among emotions, and emotion–cognition relations. *Psychological Review, 99*, 561–565.

Izard, C.E. (1994). Innate and universal facial expressions: Evidence from developmental and cross-cultural research. *Psychological Bulletin, 115*, 288–299.

Izard, C.E., Fantauzzo, C.A., Castle, J.M., Haynes, O.M., et al. (1995). The ontogeny and significance of infants' facial expressions in the first 9 months of life. *Developmental Psychology, 31(6)*, 997–1013.

Izard, C.E., Huebner, R.R., Risser, D., McGinnes, G.C., & Dougherty, L.M. (1980). The young infant's ability to produce discrete emotion expressions. *Developmental Psychology, 16(2)*, 132–140.

James, W. (1884). What is an emotion? *Mind, 9*, 188–205.

James, W. (1894). The physical basis of emotion. *Psychological Review, 1*, 516–529.

Johnson, M.K., & Multhaup, K.S. (1992). Emotion and MEM. In S.-A. Christianson (Ed.), *The Handbook of Emotion and Memory: Research and Theory* (pp. 33–66). Hillsdale, NJ: Erlbaum.

Kaiser, S., & Scherer, K.R. (1997). Models of "normal" emotions applied to facial and vocal expressions in clinical disorders. In W.F. Flack, Jr., & J.D. Laird (Eds.), *Emotions in Psychopathology* (pp. 81–98). New York: Oxford University Press.

Kihlstrom, J.F. (1987). The cognitive unconscious. *Science, 237,* 1445–1452.

Laird, J.D., & Bresler, C. (1992). The process of emotional experience: A self perception theory. In M.S. Clark (Ed.), *Review of Personality and Social Psychology.* Newbury Park, CA: Sage.

Lang, P.J., Greenwald, M.K., Bradley, M.M., & Hamm, A.O. (1993). Looking at pictures: Affective, facial, visceral, and behavioral reactions. *Psychophysiology, 30(3),* 261–273.

Lazarus, R.S. (1968). Emotions and adaptation: Conceptual and empirical relations. In W.J. Arnold (Ed.). *Nebraska Symposium on Motivation.* Lincoln, NE: University of Nebraska Press.

Lazarus, R.S. (1991). *Emotion and Adaptation.* New York and Oxford: Oxford University Press.

Lazarus, R.S. (1984a). On the primacy of cognition. *American Psychologist, 39,* 124–129.

Lazarus, R.S. (1984b). Thoughts on the relations between emotion and cognition. In K.R. Scherer & P. Ekman (Eds.), *Approaches to Emotion* (pp. 247–257). Hillsdale, NJ: Erlbaum.

LeDoux, J.E. (1989). Cognitive–emotional interactions in the brain. *Cognition and Emotion, 3,* 267–289.

Levenson, R.W. (1992). Autonomic nervous system differences among emotions. *Psychological Science, 3(1),* 23–27.

Levenson, R.W., Ekman, P., Heider, K., & Friesen, W.V. (1992). Emotion and autonomic nervous system activity in the Minangkabau of West Sumatra. *Journal of Personality and Social Psychology, 62(6),* 972–988.

Leventhal, H., & Scherer, K.R. (1987). The relationship of emotion to cognition: A functional approach to a semantic controversy. *Cognition and Emotion, 1,* 3–28.

Leventhal, H., & Tomarken, A.J. (1986). Emotion: Today's problems. *Annual Review of Psychology, 37,* 565–610.

Mathews, A. (1988). Anxiety and the processing of threatening information. In V. Hamilton, G.H. Bower, & N.H. Frijda (Eds.), *Cognitive Perspectives on Emotion and Motivation* (pp. 265–286). Dordrecht: Kluver Academic Publishers.

Mathews, A., Mogg, K., May, J., & Eysenck, M. (1989). Implicit and explicit memory bias in anxiety. *Journal of Abnormal Psychology, 98(3),* 236–240.

Matsumoto, D. (1987). The role of facial response in the experience of emotion: More methodological problems and a meta-analysis. *Journal of Personality and Social Psychology, 52(4),* 769–774.

Mead, M. (1975). Review of "P. Ekman: Darwin and facial expression." *Journal of Communication, 25,* 209–213.

Mesquita, B., Frijda, N.H., & Scherer, K.R. (1997). Culture and emotion. In J.E. Berry, P.B. Dasen, & T.S. Saraswathi (Eds.), *Handbook of Cross-Cultural Psychology: Vol. 2, Basic Processes and Developmental Psychology* (pp. 255–297). Boston: Allyn & Bacon.

Niedenthal, P.M. (1990). Implicit perception of affective information. *Journal of Experimental Social Psychology, 26(6),* 505–527.

Oatley, K., & Johnson-Laird, P.N. (1987). Towards a cognitive theory of emotions. *Cognition and Emotion, 1(1)*, 29–50.

Öhman, A. (1988). Preattentive processes in the generation of emotions. In V. Hamilton, G.H. Bower, & N.H. Frijda (Eds.), *Cognitive Perspectives on Emotion and Motivation* (pp. 127–144). Dordrecht: Kluwer Academic Publishers.

Ortony, A., Clore, G.L., & Collins, A. (1988). *The Cognitive Structure of Emotions*. New York: Cambridge University Press.

Osgood, C.E., May, W.H., & Miron, M.S. (1975). *Cross-Cultural Universals of Affective Meaning*. Urbana: University of Illinois Press.

Osgood, C.E., Suci, G.J., & Tannenbaum, P.H. (1957). *The Measurement of Meaning*. Urbana: University of Illinois Press.

Panksepp, J. (1982). Toward a general psychobiological theory of emotions. *Behavioral and Brain Sciences, 5(3)*, 407–467.

Panksepp, J. (1989). The neurobiology of emotions: Of animal brains and human feelings. In A. Manstead & H. Wagner (Eds.), *Handbook of Social Psychophysiology* (pp. 5–26). Chichester, England: Wiley.

Papez, J.W. (1937). A proposed mechanism of emotion. *Archives of Neurological Psychiatry, 38*, 725–743.

Plutchik, R. (1962). *The Emotions: Facts, Theories, and a New Model*. New York: Random House.

Plutchik, R. (1980). *Emotion: A Psychobioevolutionary Synthesis*. New York: Harper & Row.

Rosch, E., Mervis, C.B., Gray, W.D., Johnson, D.M., & Boyes-Braem, P. (1976). Basic objects in natural categories. *Cognitive Psychology, 8*, 382–439.

Roseman, I.J. (1984). Cognitive determinants of emotion: A structural theory. *Review of Personality and Social Psychology, 5*, 11–36.

Roseman, I.J., Wiest, C., & Swartz, T.S. (1994). Phenomenology, behaviors, and goals differentiate discrete emotions. *Journal of Personality and Social Psychology, 67(2)*, 206–221.

Russell, J.A. (1980). A circumplex model of affect. *Journal of Personality and Social Psychology, 39*, 1161–1178.

Russell, J.A. (1983). Pancultural aspects of the human conceptual organization of emotions. *Journal of Personality and Social Psychology, 45*, 1281–1288.

Russell, J.A. (1991). Culture and the categorization of emotions. *Psychological Bulletin, 110*, 426–450.

Russell, J.A. (1994). Is there universal recognition of emotion from facial expression? A review of the cross-cultural studies. *Psychological Bulletin, 115*, 102–141.

Schachter, S. (1970). The assumption of identity and peripheralist–centralist controversies in motivation and emotion. In M. B. Arnold (Eds.), *Feelings and Emotions: The Loyola Symposium* (pp. 111–121). New York: Academic Press.

Schachter, S., & Singer, J.E. (1962). Cognitive, social and physiological determinants of emotional states. *Psychological Review, 69*, 379–399.

Scherer, K.R. (1982). Emotion as a process: Function, origin, and regulation. *Social Science Information, 21*, 555–570.

Scherer, K.R. (1984a). On the nature and function of emotion: A component process approach. In K.R. Scherer & P. Ekman (Eds.), *Approaches to Emotion* (pp. 293–318). Hillsdale, NJ: Erlbaum.

Scherer, K.R. (1984b). Emotion as a multicomponent process: A model and some cross-cultural data. In P. Shaver (Ed.), *Review of Personality and Social Psychology*, Vol. 5 (pp. 37–63). Beverly Hills, CA: Sage.

Scherer, K.R. (1986). Vocal affect expression: A review and a model for future research. *Psychological Bulletin, 99*, 143–165.

Scherer, K.R. (1987). *Toward a Dynamic Theory of Emotion: The Component Process Model of Affective States.* University of Geneva, Geneva, Switzerland: Geneva Studies in Emotion.

Scherer, K.R. (1989). Vocal correlates of emotion. In A. Manstead & H. Wagner (Eds.), *Handbook of Psychophysiology: Emotion and Social Behavior* (pp. 165–197). London: Wiley.

Scherer, K.R. (1992). What does facial expression express? In K. Strongman (Ed.), *International Review of Studies on Emotion*, Vol. 2 (pp. 139–165). Chichester: Wiley.

Scherer, K.R. (1993). Neuroscience projections to current debates in emotion psychology. *Cognition and Emotion, 7*, 1–41.

Scherer, K.R. (1994). Toward a concept of "modal emotions". In P. Ekman & R.J. Davidson (Eds.), *The Nature of Emotion: Fundamental Questions* (pp. 25–31). New York: Oxford University Press.

Scherer, K.R. (1996). Emotion. In M. Hewstone, W. Stroebe, & G.M. Stephenson (Eds.). *Introduction to Social Psychology: A European Perspective* (2nd ed.). Oxford, England: Blackwell.

Scherer, K.R. (1999). Appraisal theories. In T. Dalgleish & M. Power (Eds.), *Handbook of Cognition and Emotion* (pp. 637–663). Chichester: Wiley.

Scherer, K.R., & Wallbott, H.G. (1994). Evidence for universality and cultural variation of differential emotion response patterning. *Journal of Personality and Social Psychology, 66*, 310–328.

Schlosberg, H.A. (1952). The description of facial expressions in terms of two dimensions. *Journal of Experimental Psychology, 44*, 229–237.

Schlosberg, H.A. (1954). Three dimensions of emotion. *Psychological Review, 61*, 81–88.

Schneirla, T.C. (1959). An evolutionary and developmental theory of biphasic processes underlying approach and withdrawal. In M.R. Jones (Ed.), *Nebraska Symposium on Motivation*, Vol. 7 (pp. 1–42). Lincoln: University of Nebraska Press.

Schwarz, N. (1990). Feelings as information: Informational and motivational functions of affective states. In R.M. Sorrentino & E.T. Higgins (Eds.), *Handbook of Motivation and Cognition: Foundations of Social Behavior*, Vol. 2 (pp. 527–561). New York: Guilford Press.

Scott, J.P. (1969). The emotional basis of social behavior. *Annals of the New York Academy of Sciences, 159*, 777–790.

Shaver, P., Schwartz, J., Kirson, D., & O'Connor, C. (1987). Emotion knowledge: Further exploration of a prototype approach. *Journal of Personality and Social Psychology, 52*, 1061–1086.

Shiffrin, R.M., & Schneider, W. (1977). Controlled and automatic human information processing: II. Perceptual learning, automatic attention and a general theory. *Psychological Review, 84*, 127–190.

Shweder, R.A. (1993). The cultural psychology of the emotions. In M. Lewis & J.M. Haviland (Eds.), *Handbook of Emotions* (pp. 417–434). New York: Guilford Press.

Smith, C.A. (1989). Dimensions of appraisal and physiological response in emotion. *Journal of Personality and Social Psychology, 56*, 339–353.

Smith, C.A., & Ellsworth, P.C. (1985). Patterns of cognitive appraisal in emotion. *Journal of Personality and Social Psychology, 48*, 813–838.

Smith, C.A., & Lazarus, R.S. (1993). Appraisal components, core relational themes, and the emotions. Special Issue: Appraisal and beyond: The issue of cognitive determinants of emotion. *Cognition and Emotion, 7(3–4)*, 233–269.

Stemmler, G. (1996). Psychophysiologie der Emotionen. [Psychophysiology of emotions]. *Zeitschrift für Psychosomatische Medizin und Psychoanalyse, 42(3)*, 235–260.

Tomkins, S.S. (1962). *Affect, Imagery, Consciousness, Vol. 1: The Positive Affects*. New York: Springer.

Tomkins, S.S. (1963). *Affect, Imagery, Consciousness, Vol. 2: The Negative Affects*. New York: Springer.

Tomkins, S.S. (1984). Affect theory. In K.R. Scherer & P. Ekman (Eds.), *Approaches to Emotion* (pp. 163–196). Hillsdale, NJ: Erlbaum.

Tourangeau, R., & Ellsworth, P.C. (1979). The role of facial response in the experience of emotion. *Journal of Personality and Social Psychology, 37(9)*, 1519–1531.

Van Reekum, C.M., & Scherer, K.R. (1997). Levels of processing for emotion-antecedent appraisal. In G. Matthews (Ed.), *Cognitive Science Perspectives on Personality and Emotion* (pp. 259–300). Amsterdam: Elsevier.

Watson, D., Clark, L.A., & Tellegen, A. (1988). Development and validation of brief measures of positive and negative affect: The PANAS scales. *Journal of Personality and Social Psychology, 54(6)*, 1063–1070.

Wundt, W. (1905). *Grundzüge der physiologischen Psychologie* (5th ed.) [Fundamentals of Physiological Psychology]. Leipzig: Engelmann.

Zajonc, R.B. (1980). Feeling and thinking: Preferences need no inferences. *American Psychologist, 2*, 151–176.

Zajonc, R.B. (1984a). On the primacy of affect. In K.R. Scherer & P. Ekman (Eds.), *Approaches to Emotion* (pp. 259–270). Hillsdale, NJ: Lawrence Erlbaum.

Zajonc, R.B. (1984b). The interaction of affect and cognition. In K. R. Scherer & P. Ekman (Eds.), *Approaches to Emotion* (pp. 239–246). Hillsdale, NJ: Erlbaum.

7

A Social Cognitive Neuroscience
Approach to Emotion and Memory

KEVIN N. OCHSNER AND DANIEL L. SCHACTER

In the movie *Blade Runner*, a woman named Rachel discovers that what she has always believed to be her most poignant childhood recollections are not her memories at all. Rachel learns that she is an artificially created, genetically engineered entity known as a *replicant*. She is physically indistinguishable from ordinary humans, and her psychological identity is based on memories taken from the life of her creator's niece. But if the personal past revealed in her recollections is imaginary, then who is Rachel? How can she think about herself in the present or plan for the future unless there is a past self to serve as a point of departure?

As one of us put it recently, "Memory's usefulness does not lie in its ability to replay the details of our lives with total accuracy, but in its power to recreate and sustain the important emotional experiences of our lives" (Schacter, 1996a). For Rachel, memories of childhood were certainly not accurate in the conventional sense, but they did provide her with an essential backdrop against which her present experiences could be evaluated. This backdrop is as essential for us as it is for replicants because memories, be they real or artificial, are an essential means of grounding our emotional lives; indeed, the behavior and reactions of replicants without a personal history was childlike and unpredictable, and they experienced life not as a coherent flow of comprehensible experience, but as a series of unexpected actions, consequences, and potential threats. This fictional example serves to illustrate that recreating emotional experiences is an essential means of making sense of who we were in the past, who we are now, and who we might become in the future (Ross & Conway, 1986).

In this chapter, we examine how emotion influences memory by exploring the functional role that the appraisal and encoding of emotional experiences, and subsequent recall of them, plays in everyday life. Rachel's story illustrates the importance of recalling emotional events for defining the self. But certainty of self is only one functional end that memory of the emotional past makes possible. Recalling significant events serves current goals and can aid in the regulation of moods, can motivate current actions, and can be used to predict the consequences of future ones.

Traditional approaches to the question of how emotion influences memory have framed the issue in absolute terms, asking whether emotion makes memory better or worse, whether emotional memories are indelible, whether pleasant or unpleasant experiences are recalled more readily, or whether emotion promotes memory for central or peripheral detail (e.g., Bradley, 1994; Christianson, 1992; Conway, 1997; Matlin & Stang, 1978). From our perspective, the answer to each of these questions would include an important qualifier: it depends (see also Ochsner & Schacter, in press). We include this qualification because, as we will argue, the exact manner in which emotion influences memory cannot be specified without reference to how, in a specific situation, memory of one's emotional reactions serves a specific goal.

In this context, emotion is viewed as a process that identifies significant persons, objects, or events (e.g., Frijda, 1986; Lazarus, 1991) and readies appropriate responses to them. Emotions are therefore constructions based on current, contextually bound evaluations of personal significance and are not enduring properties of stimuli; the bully I fear today I might embrace tomorrow if I discover that he is a blood relative. Remembering an emotional experience is also a constructive process, but one that involves appraisal with respect to past events rather than current ones, and is similarly shaped by the significance of a given memory to one's current goals and desires. To say that emotional appraisal or that remembering is constructive is not to say that the construction process is always conscious or deliberative; in fact, as we argue below, in both cases construction first involves the operation of quick and automatic processes, with more deliberative processes coming into play only if need be. Therefore, to understand the relationship between emotion and memory, we need to understand two kinds of constructive processes and their interaction: (1) how we determine what is emotionally significant; (2) how we encode, store, and retrieve information; and (3) how the former guides the latter. Encoding and retrieval of explicit memory for specific emotional, and primarily nontraumatic, life episodes are the focus of this chapter (for an excellent review of the effects of moods on cognition and judgment, see Bower & Forgas, 1999; for a review of the research and theory concerning memory for especially traumatic events, see Conway, 1997; for a review of emotion and implicit memory, see Tobias, Kihlstrom & Schacter, 1992).

APPROACH AND ORGANIZATION

The goal-oriented approach to understanding emotion and memory that we elaborate here draws on and integrates data from social cognition and cognitive neuroscience; we call it the *social cognitive neuroscience approach.* This approach is distinct from traditional cognitive neuroscience in that it attempts not just to elucidate abstract information processing mechanisms and their neural substrates (Ochsner & Kosslyn, 1999) but also aims to understand how these mechanisms function in the context of current goals and motivations. Cognitive psychology and neuroscience have impressively demonstrated that memory is an active process that involves interpretation and construction at all stages (e.g., Schacter, Norman, & Koutstaal, 1998); social psychology has shown that the memory distortions or biases produced by the constructive process are motivated and may be systematically guided by self-relevant goals (e.g., Ross, 1989; Ross & Conway, 1986; Singer & Salovey, 1996). In this chapter, we consider how data from social cognition and cognitive neuroscience together can provide a more complete account of how emotion determines the directions and paths that the construction process takes than could either approach taken alone.

This chapter is divided into three main sections. In the first, we discuss how appraisal of the emotional significance of information directs attention during encoding; in the second, we consider how the encoded information may be modified by subsequent rehearsal and consolidation; and in the third, we outline the ways in which goals and emotional cues in the retrieval environment help guide the construction of memories for these experiences.

EMOTION GUIDES ENCODING

Attention to incoming information enhances subsequent recollection of it (e.g., Craik et al., 1996), and attention is drawn to the information appraised as most significant to one's self in the context of current goals (Lazarus, 1991). These goals can be simple and global, such as the general goal to avoid physical or emotional harm, or they can be more specific, such as the desire to attain a particular promotion, make a good impression, or calm a frustrated friend. Appraising the significance of stimuli to one's self in the context of such current goals can evoke different emotions depending on the persons and objects involved and on which goals and needs are currently most important (Frijda, 1986;

Lazarus, 1991). Each emotion thus results from appraisals of different kinds of self-relevance: At turns, we might be sad if we think about the possible irrevocable loss of a loved one from illness, angry if we attribute responsibility for this outcome to a doctor's failure to give proper care, or hopeful if we feel that the medical care might result in a cure (Lazarus, 1991).

Although theorists differ in their specifications of which emotions result from which types of appraisal, most theories specify that appraisal involves the operation of fast, automatic, and mainly nonconscious processes, as well as conscious and more deliberate ones (Frijda, 1986; Lazarus, 1991; Ohman, Flykt, & Lundqvist, 1999; Zajonc, 1998). The fast and automatic processes seem adapted to making a quick bottom-up evaluation of a stimulus in terms of its valence, indicating that it is good or bad, to be approached or avoided. The slower and more deliberate processes involve memory retrieval and reasoning to counteract, augment, or reshape the more diffuse bottom-up signals. Both steps in the appraisal process can influence what is encoded and later remembered, and we consider the contributions of each in turn.

Automatic Capture of Attention by Emotion

If benefits the rabbit to be able to identify the hungry fox as quickly as possible. Indeed, the more quickly an organism can determine if an event or object should be approached or avoided, the more likely that organism is to survive (Davidson, 1992). Evolutionary survival pressures have served us well: There is good evidence that merely looking at a stimulus leads to evaluation of it, and once a stimulus is identified as emotionally self-relevant, it may be difficult to ignore (Ohman et al., 1999).

Studies of the *automatic evaluation effect* indicate that bottom-up perception of a stimulus may reflexively activate information in memory about its affective properties, thereby providing the first source of information about how to respond to it (Bargh et al., 1992). In these studies, subjects judge the valence of a target word that has been preceded by a prime word of similar or different valence. Speeding or facilitation of this judgment for prime-target pairs that have similar valence appears to occur automatically and has been found across a variety of conditions that vary awareness of the prime-target relation (e.g., Bargh et al., 1992; Fazio, Sambonmatsu, Powell, & Kardes, 1986).

Emotional information also attracts and holds attention, as revealed by studies employing the emotional *Stroop* paradigm. In the standard Stroop task, subjects must attend to the color of a word and ignore its identity; the task is difficult because the relatively automatic process of reading the word interferes with the relatively controlled process of naming its color. In the emotional Stroop paradigm, it takes longer to name the color of emotional stimuli than it takes to name the color of neutral stimuli, and this difference is taken to reflect a perceptual bias favoring the automatic encoding of affective information (for review, see Williams, Mathews, & MacLeod, 1996). In a prototypical experiment, Pratto and John (1991) found that normal subjects took longer to name the colors of positive and negative words than it took them to name the colors of neutral words, suggesting that attention was indeed captured by the emotional significance of these stimuli. What is positive or negative may differ from person to person, however, depending on their current goals and concerns. Consistent with this suggestion, Riemann and McNally (1995) found interference effects only for emotionally valenced words that were relevant to topics of current concern to their subjects (as assessed by pre-experimental questionnaires). Importantly, emotion-specific interference effects may disappear when clinical symptoms go into remission (Matthews et al., 1995), suggesting that it is the emotional salience of words specific to the presence of the disorder—not just greater experience with these words—that underlies the interference effects.

The ability of emotional, and especially threatening, information to attract and hold attention may help explain why people tend to recall best information that is most relevant to extracting the affective significance of a stimulus (often referred to as *central details*), causing memory for other kinds of information (often referred to as *peripheral details*) to suffer. Thus, for example, Loftus and Burns (1982) found that subjects who watched a videotape of a staged bank robbery in which the escaping robbers shot a small boy in the face had impaired memory for the events immediately preceding the attack compared with subjects who viewed a tape in which the robbers simply ran past the boy. This phenomenon is sometimes referred to as "weapon focus" in which witnesses to an actual or simulated crime tend to recall information about the weapons at the expense of other details about the setting and (Loftus, Loftus, & Messo, 1987).

It is possible that information central to appraising a stimulus is remembered more accurately simply because subjects look at it longer. A series of studies by Christianson et al. (1991) suggest, however, that improved memory for emotional information can occur even when the amount of viewing time for emotional and neutral information is equated. In studies with either tachistoscopic presentations or records of eye movements and fixation duration to equate looking time across emotional and neutral slides, memory was consistently more accurate for information central to the content of a set of emotional images. It seems that more information per unit time can be extracted about central, emotional details, and heightened attention to these details may be the mechanism that facilitates this process.

Guidance of Deliberative, Elaborative Encoding by Emotion

In some situations, the quick and automatic classification of a stimulus as good or bad may be all that is needed to guide our behavior in the most appropriate way. But in many instances, we need more information about the events we are reacting to, including why they have happened. For example, suppose you are bumped roughly while waiting in line at the supermarket. Your quick appraisal might be negative, perhaps initiating a rush of anger, but it would be smart to check this reaction if you realize that the bump was accidental, was not a threat, and was not intended to cause harm. Drawing inferences about the nature of our feelings in light of additional inferences about the causes of the events that elicited them, including the intentions and motivations of others, enables us to have greater complexity of emotional experience and expression (Lazarus, 1991; Stein, Wade, & Liwag, 1997).

Although there is debate about exactly which parts of the appraisal process (or which kinds of appraisals) are conscious and controlled as opposed to nonconscious and automatic, it seems clear that making inferences about causality and intentionality relies on the look-up of information in memory (Lazarus, 1991; Zajonc, 1998). Depending on the emotion elicited, different emotion-specific scripts or schemas will be accessed, each of which specifies what kinds of information are important to identify and evaluate (Lazarus, 1991). This knowledge then can be used effortfully to guide attention to the emotionally relevant internal (e.g., feelings, goals, and plans) and external (e.g., goal-relevant actors and events) stimuli specific to a given situation (Lazarus, 1991; Stein, Wade, & Liwag, 1997). In contrast to early accounts of emotion, which suggested that arousal results in a global disruption of attentional control (Easterbrook, 1959), this approach suggests that emotion directs attention in a specific way: Schema-relevant information will be noted and remembered well, whereas schema-irrelevant information will not be noted and will be remembered poorly (Levine & Burgess, 1997; Stein, Wade, & Liwag, 1997).

For most emotional schemas or scripts, the actions of others are more relevant than their appearance. Thus, people recall actions more often than the appearance of perpetrators of real (Yuille & Cutshall, 1986) or simulated (Clifford & Scott, 1978) attacks and recall themes better than perceptual detail in films depicting either a bank robbery or a boy being hit by a car (Christianson & Loftus, 1987). Studies that have compared memory for central and peripheral details generally have found increased memory for central, thematic, and appraisal-relevant information, including weapons (Burke, Heuer, & Reisberg, 1992; Loftus et al., 1987). It is possible that "weapon focus" may result in part from an effortful direction of attention.

Although schemas may help guide attention to important information, they may also limit our ability to draw accurate inferences about the causes of others' behavior. One way this can happen is when schema-guided encoding leads us to fill in missing or unattended information as an emotional event unfolds. Thus, we may recall feelings, motivations, and reactions that were inferred and not stated explicitly (Heuer & Reisberg, 1990). The need to fill in information could be made greater if we attempt to divide our limited attentional resources between internal sensations and external actors and events. This may explain why Wahler and Afton (1980) found that highly stressed mothers who were having problems with their children tended to describe their children's behaviors in general, dispositional terms (e.g., malicious or naughty) and did not recall situational antecedents of the behaviors in question.

Dispositional attributions following from schema-driven emotional appraisals also can have negative consequences for one's perception of self and recall of personal experiences. A vivid example is found in people who have suffered from depression or who have attempted suicide. Depressed persons tend to evaluate events in terms of their relevance to an abstract negative self-concept, thereby encoding their personal experiences in an overly general way. As suggested by Williams and Dritschel (1988), these individuals may focus internally, appraising the significance of an event in ways that confirm a global, stable, and negative disposition (e.g., "I have always been a failure") and fail to adequately consider the situational antecedents and aspects of their experiences. By turning otherwise neutral happenings into events diagnostic of their negative self-view, they can later retrieve only very general, and mostly negative, accounts of their lives (Williams, 1996). Repetition of this cycle may be an important contributor to the etiology and perpetuation of depression (Nolen-Hoeksema, 1991).

A tendency to selectively elaborate emotional information relevant to a disposition or self-concept may also explain why most people who usually have very positive self-views (Taylor, 1989) tend to recall (Denny & Hunt, 1992) or recognize (Mogg, Mathews, & Weinman, 1987) positive words more accurately than negative or neutral ones after having been asked to judge their self-relevance during encoding (for a meta-analysis, see Matt, Vasquez, & Campbell, 1992). Similarly, depressed people tend to recall or recognize depression-relevant words more often than other word types (e.g., Watkins et al., 1992). An interesting exception to this self-referential rule is exhibited by patients with generalized anxiety disorder, who tend to recall anxiety-relevant words either no more often than, or even less frequently than, other word types (see Mineka & Nugent, 1995). In contrast to depressed and normal people, who readily encode information that confirms their pre-existing self-views, it seems that anxious individuals try to avoid elaboration of self-threatening information (Mineka & Nugent, 1995).

Special Neural Mechanisms for Encoding Emotion

Data from neuropsychology, neuroimaging, and animal learning studies provide converging support for the idea that separate processes are responsible for the automatic and deliberative encoding of affective information and suggest further that each may depend on discrete, but interacting, neural systems (see Ochsner

& Felman-Barrett, in press, for complete discussion; see also Reiman, Lane, Ahern, Schwartz & Davidson, 1996). Support for the existence of a separate processing pathway for the quick affective evaluation of objects and events comes primarily from studies of conditioned emotional responses and functional neuroimaging studies of responses to emotional stimuli. In extensive research with rats, LeDoux and colleagues have shown that learning to associate a light or a tone with the fearful anticipation of a shock requires only a direct and fast connection between a sensory organ and the amygdala, and the connection can completely bypass a longer route that sensory percepts take through the neocortex (see LeDoux, 1995). Research measuring classic conditioning of galvanic skin responses in humans has also indicated that the amygdala is necessary for learning to associate aversive physical states with specific visual stimuli (LaBar, LeDoux, Spencer, & Phelps, 1995).

In humans, functional neuroimaging studies and studies of patients with brain damage have shown the amygdala to be linked to the encoding of emotional information. For example, amygdala lesions will disrupt recognition of the emotions conveyed through facial expression, especially fear (e.g., Adolphs et al., 1994; Calder et al., 1996; for review of lesion studies, see Borod, 1992), and fear but not happy faces activate the amygdala, even when presented subliminally (Whalen et al., 1998). Similarly, amygdala activity measured during presentation of an emotional story has been found to be highly correlated with greater subsequent recall of the emotional elements of the story (Cahill et al., 1996), whereas patients with degenerative decay of the amygdala show impairments in their memory of these elements (Cahill et al., 1995). The selective importance of the amygdala for encoding emotional memories also has been demonstrated by studies of amnesic patients with an intact amygdala. Such patients can acquire affective preferences for music (Johnson, Kim, & Risse, 1985), can develop valenced attitudes toward people based on their experience with them (Johnson, Kim, & Risse, 1985), and can acquire conditional fear responses (Bechara et al., 1995) even though they cannot consciously remember their experiences with these various sorts of stimuli. Release of the neurotransmitter norepinephrine within the amygdala appears to be the mechanism by which the amygdala "stamps" in emotional memories, as shown by the memory-impairing effects of drugs that block norepinephrine in animals and humans alike (Cahill et al., 1994; McGaugh & Cahill, 1997). LeDoux (1995) has suggested that a neural "significance code" is quickly computed and stored by the amygdala and may provide a template for further, more complex stimulus evaluation.

The system responsible for this more complex and deliberative control of affective appraisals seems to involve aspects of the frontal lobe (Damasio, 1994; Stuss, Eskes, & Foster, 1994). The ability to generate top-down plans, revise or inhibit habitual responses, and monitor the task relevance of information is impaired by lesions of the lateral and dorsal prefrontal cortices (Shimamura, 1995;

Stuss, Eskes, & Foster, 1994). Furthermore, functional neuroimaging studies show that frontal cortices are activated during effortful, attention-demanding, perceptual or memory tasks that require strategic uses of attention and transformation of information in working memory (Schacter et al., 1996a; Tulving et al., 1994; for review of frontal contributions to memory and imagery, see Ochsner & Kosslyn, 1999). Interestingly, increased activation of the left inferior prefrontal lobe is associated with amount, or depth, of elaborative semantic processing during encoding (Tulving et al., 1994), and this area is hypofunctional in individuals with depression (Davidson, 1992; Drevets & Raichle, 1995). This hypofunctionality could play a role in the over-general encoding of experience exhibited by depressed people (Williams, Mathews, & MacLeod, 1986).

In contrast, the ventral medial frontal (VMF) and orbital frontal (OF) cortices have unique and strong reciprocal connections with the amygdala and are important for evaluating the affective, personal significance of choices and using that information to guide reasoning and action (Damasio, 1994). VMF and OF lesions may produce deficits in motivation, can result in poor control of affective impulses, and have been shown to eliminate the anticipatory, "anxious" autonomic response that precedes personally important decisions, thereby rendering patients unable to use their feelings to guide actions (Bechara et al., 1996; Damasio, 1994; Damasio, Tranel, & Damasio, 1990). The mechanism by which the ventral and medial frontal areas influence the amygdala may involve inhibition of the stimulus–visceral response associations that the amygdala codes. In both animals and humans, lesions to these areas may impair inhibition of conditioned responses that are no longer appropriate and limit the recoding of stimulus significance when it has changed (LeDoux, 1995; Rolls, 1995). Furthermore, using functional magnetic resonance imaging, Davidson and colleagues (Davidson, personal communication) have recently shown that an area of the left medial frontal lobe may tonically inhibit activity in the amygdala and that dysfunction of this connection may be a marker for depression. There have been few studies in humans that have examined VMF and OF contributions to memory for emotional information.

Summary

The preceding analysis suggests that emotion is a product of the process by which we appraise the significance of stimuli and that the interaction of at least two types of appraisal processes can explain the results of many studies of memory for emotional events. Quick, automatic processes evaluate the valence of stimuli and maintain attention on them, while more deliberate, reflective processes modify, amplify, or inhibit this initial response, depending on how the significance of the given stimulus is appraised relative to current goals and needs. Each process may involve the action of distinct, but highly interactive neural systems:

The amygdala helps to evaluate stimulus significance quickly, and the prefrontal cortex can modify an initial appraisal and generate new ones if necessary.

POSTEVENT ELABORATION AND CONSOLIDATION OF EMOTIONAL INFORMATION

Role of Rehearsal

Every time we ask ourselves about the appearance of the attacker who stole our wallet, or wonder how our last court case ended in a disappointing loss, we are rehearsing and re-encoding our memories of those events. Emotional events by their very nature are significant and self-defining, with our major successes and failures denoting milestones in our personal development (Ross & Conway, 1986; Singer & Salovey, 1996). Except for very traumatic experiences (e.g., Christianson & Nilsson, 1984), in many cases our emotional memories are more often thought about and recounted to others than are their pallid, nonemotional cousins (Schacter, 1996b). Public events of personal emotional consequence, such as the assassination of President Kennedy or the explosion of the space shuttle Challenger, afford additional opportunities for recoding and rehearsal through further selective exposure to the event through media, friends, and relatives (Neisser & Harsch, 1992; Schacter, 1996b).

Negative events are especially likely to be rehearsed, as one repeatedly attempts to understand their significance and why they occurred (Skowronski & Carlston, 1989); as discussed earlier, if this process becomes habitual and self-critical, such reappraisals can fuel a ruminative cycle of negative-self evaluation that may foster depression (Nolen-Hoeksema, 1991). Unfortunately, however, it may be difficult to avoid rehearsal of negative events, even when one wants not to do so, because emotional memories may be difficult to ignore or suppress (Wentzlaff, 1993).

Not surprisingly, therefore, the amount of rehearsal an emotional event receives generally has been found to influence subsequent memory for it. Thomas and Diener (1990) asked subjects to record daily experiences in diaries and found that subjects had a tendency to rehearse and remember more negative than positive events. Interestingly, we might later overestimate the frequency with which we experienced negative events, perhaps mistaking frequency of rehearsal for frequency of occurrence (Singer & Salovey, 1996; Thomas & Diener, 1990). Broadly consistent results have been obtained by other researchers in studies showing a modestly positive relationship between affect, rehearsal, and memory in both old subjects (Cohen, Conway, & Maylor, 1994) and young subjects (Cohen, Conway, & Maylor, 1994; Conway & Bekerian, 1988; Rubin & Kozin, 1984; see, however, Christianson & Loftus, 1990; Pillemer, 1984). Repeatedly thinking about an unpleasant experience may enhance memory for it by increasing the depth with which it is processed (Wagenaar, 1994).

Reminiscence Effects

When tested immediately after encoding, memory for arousing stimuli may be worse than memory for neutral stimuli, although if memory is tested again hours or days later, recall of the emotional material may have a distinct advantage (for review, see Revelle & Loftus, 1992). This rebound in memory for emotional material as a function of retention interval is known as a *reminiscence effect*, and, although at first it appeared to be reliably demonstrable using both words (Kleinsmith & Kaplan, 1963) and pictures (Kaplan & Kaplan, 1969), some later failures to replicate under conditions that used slightly different stimuli and procedures cast doubt on the reliability of the phenomenon (e.g., Corteen, 1969). Christianson (1992) suggested that the effect is most reliable with paired associate learning and might reflect some idiosyncrasies particular to that paradigm.

More recent research has produced similarly conflicting results. On the positive side, Bradley and Baddeley (1990) found a reminiscence-like effect for associations generated to positive, negative, or neutral words after a 1 month delay, although this result may be more attributable to forgetting of neutral words than to enhanced memory for emotional ones. On the negative side, Burke, Heuer, and Reisberg (1992) found only a very small effect of retention interval in recall of both central and peripheral details of an emotional slide sequence. Despite these inconsistencies, however, a recent meta-analysis of many of the older studies concluded that the effect is reliable, if not especially large (Park & Banaji, 1996).

An initial account of the reminiscence effect postulated that arousal leads to temporary inhibition during memory consolidation (Walker & Tarte, 1963). Exactly why this should be the case was, however, never adequately specified. A more likely explanation has been suggested by Revelle and Loftus (1992). According to their "tick-rate" hypothesis, emotional arousal increases the rate at which information is encoded, and more information is encoded per unit time from an emotional than a neutral event (cf. Christianson et al., 1991). In the short term, it may be more difficult to find any one specific detail among the many that have been encoded. The increased rate of processing also promotes the rapid integration and assimilation of encoded details into pre-existing knowledge structures. In the long term, this means that emotional experiences will have undergone more consolidation per unit time than nonemotional experiences, resulting in relatively greater recall of them

A recent study by LaBar and Phelps (1998) has shown that the amydala is responsible for this consolidation effect. Patients with unilateral temporal lobectomies were aroused by emotional pictures, but failed to show an improvement in memory for them over time.

Summary

The appraised emotional significance of objects, persons, or events influences how much attention is paid to them and how much one elaborates on their significance both when they were first encountered and subsequently as their significance is reappraised. Emotion thus influences the nature and distinctiveness of what is encoded and stored and therefore strongly determines what information is potentially available for subsequent recall. In the next section, we consider how emotion guides the retrieval of these memory traces.

EMOTION INFLUENCES/GUIDES RETRIEVAL PROCESSES

Constructing a record of a past experience seems to involve at least two steps (for a more complete discussion, see Schacter, Norman, & Koutstaal, 1998). First, stored traces interact with retrieval cues either from the external environment or from those generated internally, and the product of this interaction provides the "raw material" for recollection (Norman & Schacter, 1996; Schacter, Norman, & Koutstaal, 1998; Tulving, 1983). Second, decision and reasoning processes operate on this raw material to help refine, reconsider, and supplement what has been "served up" in response to the initial retrieval query, and, if further information is required, the search can begin all over again by constructing new cues to retrieve additional specific past episodes (e.g., Schacter, Norman, & Koutstaal, 1998). Appraisal of one's current emotional state, the significance of cues in the current retrieval environment, and their relationship to goals and the self may strongly influence the operation of both of these processes.

Affective Retrieval Cues Can Bias Retrieval

The synergistic combination of cue and trace information has been called the *ecphoric* process (Schacter, 1982; Semon, 1909/1923; Tulving, 1983), and the output of the ecphoric interaction is substantially determined by the nature of the retrieval cue itself. An incomplete, poorly specified, or incorrectly specified cue may retrieve a memory that is related to, but not an exact match for, the episode that was desired (Schacter, Norman, & Koustaal, 1998). In the absence of criteria that clearly identify that such close matches are incorrect, these false memories may be experienced as accurate (e.g., Roediger & McDermott, 1995; Schacter, Israel, & Racine, 1999; Schacter et al., 1996b). This seamless blending of present and past experience may be a powerful route by which emotion can bias retrospection.

Sometimes the cues that bias the retrieval process are one's own current affective reactions. For example, Eich et al. (1985) found that individuals currently experiencing high levels of headache pain tended to recall the pain they experienced in the past as having been more severe than it actually was. For these patients, present pain cues may have combined with traces of past painful experiences, thereby systematically shifting estimates of past pain to be more like the level of the pain currently being felt. Although other studies on memory for pain (e.g., Linton & Mellin, 1982) and memory for mood (Matt, Vasquez, & Campbell, 1992) are compatible with this view, the exact way in which ecphory may lead to a recall bias in these studies is difficult to assess. Painful experiences and diffuse moods may have many components, both positive and negative, and it is difficult to specify exactly which aspects will synergistically combine with exactly what stored information. Furthermore, recall could be influenced by current pain levels not because the ecphoric process has been biased but because current pain and affect primes memories for past experiences with similar levels of pain or affect, making them more easily accessible (Bower & Forgas, 1999; Salovey & Smith, 1997).

The power of ecphoric processes to bias recall of affective information was examined by Ochsner, Schacter, and Edwards (1997) using a procedure that escapes the above-noted problems of studying memory for pain and mood. Subjects studied photographs of faces while listening to a corresponding voice speaking in a happy and excited or angry and frustrated tone. When subjects later were presented with photos of the same people as cues in a recall test for tone of voice, they tended to recall the pictured person as having spoken in a tone of voice consistent with the affect conveyed by the retrieval cue in front of them: If the face had a slightly positive expression, they tended to recall that the person had spoken happily; if the face had a slightly negative expression, they recalled the person as having spoken angrily. This recall bias was quite robust, did not depend on overall level of recall accuracy, and was accompanied by high confidence that recall was correct. In these experiments, the ecphoric process seems to have been dominated by the affect present in the retrieval cue rather than the affect present in the memory trace, and this effect may be related to the dominance of visual over auditory cues in the perception of nonverbal affective information (Rosenthal et al., 1979). This method of controlling the exact nature and valence of cue and trace information may allow further examination of the specific ways in which ecphoric processes can bias memory for emotional experiences.

Evaluations of and Judgments About Past Episodes Are Guided by Current Emotion

If the ecphoric process may occasionally produce information that is systematically biased by retrieval cues, the second step of the memory construction process may be subject to even greater influence by emotion. Current goals may set the occasion for remembering emotional experiences by guiding people to recall episodes that enhance or preserve a self-concept or help regulate moods and may even help fill in memories for affective feelings that were not well encoded in the first place. Furthermore, the emotional nature of what is recalled may also influence judgments people make about various attributes of their memories.

Retrieval as self-regulation

The constructive recall of affective events may at times be led by the desire to remember the emotional past in a way that helps create a particular view of the self in the present (Conway & Ross, 1984; Ross, 1989). For most people, this view is quite rosy, which suggests that, by and large, people are good at using recall of past experiences to bolster positive self-regard (Taylor, 1989). This does not mean that everyone will have a generalized bias to recall more positive than negative experiences (although this may be the case for happy people; see Seidlitz & Diener, 1993), but it does suggest that if it is costly or inconsistent with a current schematic self-view to recall a past mistake or negative experience, we may distort memory of it in the present. Indeed, examples of this phenomenon abound: Good students tend to recall poor grades as having been better than they were (Bahrick, Hall, & Berger, 1996), gamblers tend to recall unsuccessful wagers as exceptions rather than the rule (Gilovich, 1983), and married men whose emotions toward their wives sour over time may recall feeling less positive about early marital interactions than they initially reported (Holmberg & Holmes, 1994, cited by Levine, 1997).

How we remember positive and negative events will be determined by differences in the individual nature of the self-concept that we are chronically trying to regulate. Thus, Higgins and Tykocinski (1992) found that individuals who are motivated by the attainment of positive experiences will better recall information related to the presence or absence of positive outcomes (e.g., finding a $20 bill or going to see an eagerly anticipated film that turns out to no longer be playing), whereas individuals motivated to avoid negative experience will better recall information related to the presence or absence of negative outcomes (e.g., being stuck in the subway or getting a break from a hectic work schedule). An important aspect of these data is that recall was driven by the focus of the subjects on positive or negative outcomes as defined relative to their enduring self-goals—and not by the absolute valence of the events. Thus an individual motivated toward achieving positive experiences might remember more about the failure to achieve a good grade on a test than she will remember about the fact that her parents did not scold her afterwards, even though the former experience was aversive and the latter unexpectedly positive (cf. Singer, 1990).

The ability to re-evaluate past experience as congruent with one's self concept may have important implications for mental health. Indeed, the tendency to give even stressful life events a positive spin may lead to happiness (Seidlitz & Diener, 1993), whereas a bias to initially interpret situations as confirmations of a negative self-concept may lead to depression (Nolen-Hoeksema, 1991). The gradual accumulation of positive life experiences, guided by self-enhancing interpretation of events, may be one of the most significant contributors to a stable sense of subjective well-being (Seidlitz & Diener, 1993; Taylor, 1989).

Retrieval as mood regulation

A powerful way to build and maintain a positive self-concept is to develop the ability to regulate one's current emotional state. Recall of past personal experiences often occurs in the service of this goal (Erber, 1996). Quite often, this goal manifests itself in the desire to transform negative feeling states into positive ones, as shown in 1994 by Josephson, Singer, and Salovey (cited by Singer & Salovey, 1996), who found that induction of a sad mood can lead to conscious attempts to boost mood through the recall of positive personal experiences (cf. McFarland & Buehler, 1997). Positive moods may not always be desirable, however, and Parrott and Sabini (1990) have suggested that people sometimes use memory to deflate positive moods in order to motivate themselves to work rather than play, maintain a realistic self-concept, or temper undue optimism. The ability to regulate mood using memory may be related to one's self-concept: When in a bad mood, individuals high in self-esteem are more likely than individuals low in self-esteem to recall positive memories and, in so doing, feel better (Smith & Petty, 1995).

Importantly, whether or not retrieval of a particular positive or negative memory has a mood-depressing or mood-elevating effect may depend in large part on the perspective one takes when evaluating its personal significance during recall. On the one hand, it is true that replaying an unpleasant experience in one's mind can depress mood and may prime retrieval of further negative memories (Bower & Forgas, 1999; Smith & Petty, 1995; Strack, Schwarz, & Gschneidinger, 1985). For example, recall of recent events can boost mood if the events were positive and depress mood if they were negative (Strack, Schwarz, & Gschneidinger, 1985), and this effect may be increased if one believes that the recalled events are indicative of one's current abilities to cope with stresses and seek out enjoyable experiences (Janoff-Bulman, 1992).

On the other hand, recall of a negative event can actually enhance mood if one's life can be judged as having improved subsequently (Strack, Schwarz, & Gschneidinger, 1985). This process can be seen particularly clearly in studies of recall of past painful or traumatic experiences. To feel that one has control over pain, especially if it is chronic and enduring, it may be important to believe that one's level of pain has changed over time (Salovey & Smith, 1997). Toward this end, we may recall past pain as having been more or less intense than it actually was, depending on which pain level is most adaptive and is most likely to foster a sense of well-being, control, and hope in the present. Thus, people with high but not low levels of dental anxiety will recall a trip to the dentist as having been more painful than it actually was (Kent, 1985), and mothers tend to rate labor pain as having been less intense 2 weeks after birth than they did during delivery (Norvell, Gaston-Johansson, & Fridh, 1987). Importantly, current levels of pain may bias memory for past pain only if current pain influences one's emotional state (Eich, Rachman, & Lopatka, 1990). This suggests that, if current pain is not aversive enough to affect mood, it will not lead people to recall their past pain inaccurately.

Whether we view an important, self-defining event as a success or failure can determine whether it makes us happy or sad (Moffitt & Singer, 1994; Strack, Schwarz, & Gschneidinger, 1985). In general, reinterpretation of the past can promote coping and emotional change and may improve mood by allowing people to feel that they have learned, grown, and gained control over the factors that influence their happiness (Folkman & Lazarus, 1984; Janoff-Bulman, 1992). Our construals of the past are not, however, infinitely malleable: If an experience has positive or negative effects that are too far-reaching, it may serve as a weighty anchor that constrains the way we evaluate subsequent life events. In such situations, a sense of control may be hard to come by. For example, Brickman, Coates, and Janoff-Bulman (1978) found that lottery winners took less pleasure than controls in mundane everyday activities, presumably because the extremely positive experience of winning the lottery had changed the scale against which they measured the quality of their present experience. Accident victims who had been rendered paraplegic showed a similar effect, though not because they had actually experienced a greatly positive event in the past but because they idealized the past relative to their current state. Paraplegics thus took less pleasure than controls in daily activities, but did so because they were comparing the present to a past that was made more positive in retrospect than it actually was.

Nevertheless, with some limits, recall and causal thinking about even very traumatic experiences can benefit mental and physical health. Pennebaker and colleagues have shown that systematic writing or talking about traumatic personal experiences such as the death of a loved one, or instances of physical or sexual abuse, may boost immune system functioning, reduce anxiety, and improve grades and work performance (for a brief summary, see Pennebaker, 1997). Importantly, a significant predictor of these effects appears to be how often the narratives of traumatic episodes include reference to their causes and eliciting circumstances (Pennebaker, 1997).

These studies illustrate an important point about the way in which we recall emotional events: Our initial interpretation of a given event's emotional significance need not be the last one we ever have, and how we encoded it initially need not determine how we react to it at recall. Re-evaluation of the significance of an event in the context of one's current circumstances, with the goal of unearthing the factors that lead us to experience maladaptive emotions, can be a powerful tool for building a happy life (Janoff-Bulman, 1992; Seidlitz & Diener, 1993).

Current appraisals may bias the content of emotional memories

A particularly compelling illustration of the power of current appraisals to alter memory of past appraisals was recently reported by Levine (1997), who studied the attitudes of supporters of candidate Ross Perot during the 1992 presidential campaign. She first assessed their emotions of hope, anger, and sadness following from Perot's withdrawal from the race in mid-July. Perot re-entered the race in early October, and after the election in November, Levine again assessed current feelings about Perot's candidacy and asked the supporters to recall how they had initially felt about Perot's withdrawal a few months before. Although memory for these past feelings generally was fairly accurate, it was systematically biased to be consistent with current feelings about the desirability and implications of a Perot presidency. The key finding was that specific past emotions were recalled accurately or were overestimated when they were consistent with current appraisals, but were underestimated when they were inconsistent with them (cf. Conway & Ross, 1984).

Such systematic distortions in memory for emotions may also occur because people have theories about how memory for emotions or attitudes change over time (Ross, 1989). Depending on the emotion involved, these theories might dictate whether feelings increase, decrease, or stay the same across time. Although they may be transmitted through personal and cultural experience, we may be unaware that implicit theories are guiding the assumptions we make about the accuracy of our memories. For example, although research provides only equivocal support for an increase in anxiety and distress during menstruation, there is a widely held cultural belief that such distress is prevalent and powerful (McFarland, Ross, & DeCourville, 1989). McFarland, Ross, and DeCourville (1989) suggest that adherence to this belief may guide women to recall past menstrual cycles as having been more aversive than they actually were.

Current appraisals can fill in missing information

In our efforts to remember the emotional past in a way that helps make adaptive sense in the present, current emotional concerns can sometimes find their way into memories of our past feelings simply because these past feelings were not well encoded in the first place. Consider, for example, Levine's study (1997) of Perot supporters. In that study, recall of past feelings could have been used by Perot supporters to justify their current beliefs, as when a "loyal" supporter who wanted Perot to win in November recalls that he was always hopeful that Perot would re-enter the campaign. It is also possible, however, that the supporters' initial emotional reactions were not well encoded and that current appraisals helped to "fill in the gaps" in their spotty memories. Thus, when Perot withdrew, the feelings experienced by a loyal supporter may not have been strongly encoded, and thus their postelection feelings in November served as a template for fleshing out their incompletely stored feelings from the past.

Researchers on pain and the affect associated with body states have also suggested that affective reactions may not be stored well in memory: When trying to recall them, we have no recourse other than to use our current feelings as a starting point and to use theories about how our feelings may have changed to revise our initial estimate accordingly (Ross & Buehler, 1993; Salovey & Smith, 1997).

Duration is another dimension of emotional experience that may be poorly encoded. Consequently, overall duration of an event may not influence our retrospective evaluations of the pleasantness of an experience. Frederickson and Kahneman (1993) found that retrospective liking judgments for films were determined entirely by their positive and negative content and not at all by how long they lasted. If duration is not well encoded, when asked to explicitly recall the duration of an emotional episode, we may use memory of its intensity as a guide. Loftus et al. (1987) found that, as the violent content of film clips increased, so did subjects' retrospective evaluations of their durations.

We may fail to encode the duration of emotional episodes in part because the peaks and valleys of pain and pleasure capture and hold our attention so that a given experience is encoded in terms of its most salient or most recent emotional aspect. Noting changes in the emotional qualities of a situation could have great survival value: Knowing when guilt slips into shame, frustration into anger, or sadness into depression can help us to predict and better understand our own and others' emotional reactions in the future. In keeping with this idea, Varey and Kahneman (1992) found that memory for extended emotional experiences was determined by the rise or fall of pleasant and unpleasant sensation and not by how long each kind of feeling lasted. In further research, they found that this bias may even lead people to prefer painful stimulation that lasts for a longer amount of time as long as it tapers off at the end. Kahneman et al. (1993) had subjects hold their hand in an unpleasant cold water bath for 60 seconds in one trial and in another had them hold their hand in the bath for 60 seconds plus an additional 30 seconds during which the water temperature slowly rose 1°C. Most of the subjects preferred to repeat the longer trial even though it produced a greater amount of total painful stimulation.

Finally, it is worth noting that poor memory for perceptual details that are peripheral and not relevant to extracting the central emotional theme of an evolving emotion episode (Frijda, 1986) may be due in part to reconstruction of these details during retrieval because they were not well encoded initially. Attention does tend to be inwardly directed during emotional experiences (Lazarus, 1991; Stein, Wade, & Liwag, 1997), and subjects may infer the nature of perceptual details on the basis of stored knowledge of similar events or from cues in the environment.

Emotion influences the subjective experience of remembering

As discussed earlier, emotion tends to shift one's focus inward, toward regulation and interpretation of one's internal state (Stein, Wade, & Liwag, 1997). Focusing inward on one's emotions may lead to recollection of memories from a first-person *field* perspective in which events unfold in one's field of view just as they did initially. In contrast, a more abstract focus during recall may lead one to recall an event from an *observer* perspective in which one watches himself or herself from a third-person point of view (Robinson & Swanson, 1993).

Which perspective we adopt during recall may importantly determine how we think about the causes of an event and consequently how we appraise the emotional significance of it in the future. Frank and Gilovich (1989) instructed subjects to recall past conversations from either a third-person, observer perspective or from a first-person, field perspective. When in the observer mode, subjects tended to make more dispositional attributions for their own and their conversation partner's actions. This suggests that a detached, emotionally flat focus during recall can foster interpretation of past behaviors in terms of stable dispositions, which could have important implications for individuals with depression. Flat affect during retrieval could lead depressed persons to recall events from an observer perspective, which may only foster their tendency to encode and think about past behaviors in terms of stable, dysfunctional dispositions (Nolen-Hoeksema, 1991).

Subjective ratings of the vividness of a memory may also be related to the emotion experienced during its encoding. When asked to recall significant (Conway & Bekerian, 1988), exceptionally clear (Rubin & Kozin, 1984), or consequential and traumatic (Christianson & Loftus, 1990) personal memories, the experiences recalled are typically rated as highly vivid and emotional. Only a single study has examined the relation between vividness and recall of both positive and negative personal experiences. Reisberg et al. (1988) asked subjects either to recall and rate memories from positive and negative event cues (e.g., "passing a major examination in school") or to provide narrative descriptions of such memories in an interview. In both cases, rated vividness of the memories was highly correlated with the intensity but not the valence of the emotions experienced.

Some problems arise, however, with the interpretation of these different studies of vividness in autobiographical memory. First, the instructions used to elicit memories or to guide ratings of vividness may sometimes have biased the results. For example, Rubin and Kozin (1984) told subjects to recall memories with a flashbulb-like vivid character (Brown & Kulik, 1977), which may have led them to rate any clear memory as being more vivid. Second, and more importantly, it is not clear what memory attributes drive ratings of vividness: Memories could have been rated as vivid because the subjects were confident in the memories, because the subjects felt they re-experienced the memories, or because the subjects thought the memories were intense. Whatever the reason for the relationship, the correlation between emotional intensity and vividness does not mean the former caused the latter.

A more reliable means for assessing the relationship between recollective experience and emotion involves what has come to be known as the remember/know procedure (Gardiner & Java, 1993; Tulving, 1985). In this procedure, when an item is recognized on a memory test, participants are asked to decide if they "remember" that item with attendant sensory, semantic, and/or emotional detail or if they just "know" that it was seen previously but cannot recollect anything specific about its prior occurrence. "Remember" responses are sensitive to factors influencing explicit memory, and, given that judged personal emotional significance and self-relevance may boost recall, we would expect that these factors would make one more likely to "remember" an event as well. Indeed, Conway and Dewhurst (1995) found that self-referential encoding selectively increases the prevalence of "remember" recollective experiences. Similarly, Ochsner (2000) found that highly negative and arousing photographs were more likely to be "remembered" than were neutral or positive photos (cf. Mogg et al., 1992). This finding is important because it runs counter to previous failures to find a difference in memory for positive and negative events (Bradley et al., 1992; Reisberg et al., 1988). The previous studies tested only recognition memory, a quantitative measure that may not be sensitive to the qualitative effects that emotion may have on memory.

Neural Mechanisms Involved in Retrieval of Emotional Information

The neural structures involved in retrieving emotional memories include some that are generally involved in retrieving memories regardless of their emotional content, plus some of the same structures that are used to encode and evaluate the initial emotional significance of an experience. The former areas include the right prefrontal cortex and hippocampus. Both neuropsychological and functional neuroimaging studies of the recollection of episodic memories have shown that the right frontal lobe may play an important role in generating effortful retrieval strategies (e.g., Schacter et al., 1996a,b; Tulving et al., 1994), whereas the hippocampus may help locate stored memory traces and support recollective experience (Schacter et al., 1996a; for reviews, see Cabeza & Nyberg, 1997; Schacter & Wagner, 1999).

Unfortunately, information concerning neural structures that may be involved specifically in the retrieval of emotional memories is limited because only a very few studies have examined emotional memory in neuropsychological populations, and even fewer have studied emotional memory using functional neuroimaging. A few studies have shown that right-hemisphere but not left-hemisphere lesions selectively impair the expression of emotion (Borod et al., 1996), as well as decrease the specificity of events reported during autobiographical recall. This is consistent with evidence that the right hemisphere is preferentially involved in the perception and expression of emotional behavior more generally (Borod, 1992; Borod et al., 1996). Given the consistent finding of right frontal involvement in retrieval of episodic memories, these data suggest that there may be some linkage between the mechanisms that govern the retrieval of episodic memories and the mechanisms that imbue them with emotional flavor. It is interesting to speculate that one reason the right frontal lobe is specifically involved in episodic memory is because it may help to re-instantiate the emotional context present during encoding (Cimino, Verfaellie, Bowers, & Heilman, 1991).

A larger body of data come from animal and human studies that support involvement of the amygdala in the encoding of affectively significant information but demonstrate that the amygdala is necessary for the storage and retrieval of these associations as well. In studies of fear conditioning, for example, the amygdala appears to be the site where the critical stimulus–visceral response association is coded, so if the amygdala is lesioned after training, expression of conditioned fear is prevented (LeDoux, 1995). Studies of rats (Phillips & LeDoux, 1992), monkeys (Zola-Morgan et al., 1991), and human patients with amygdala or hippocampal lesions have suggested that, although it is the hippocampus and not the amygdala that is critical for storing the perceptual or conceptual aspects of an event, the coding of visceral reactions by the amygdala gives a boost to memory for emotional information (Bechara et al., 1995; Cahill et al., 1994, 1995; Hamann, Cahill, & Squire, 1997; Johnson, Kim, & Risse, 1985).

A handful of neuorimaging studies involving recall of emotional events have also revealed the activation of structures involved in the encoding and generation of one's initial emotional reactions to the recollected events. This may be due, at least in part, to the fact that these studies have been concerned primarily with identifying the neural structures that support the generation and experience of emotion and elicit emotion by asking subjects both to recall specific personal emotional episodes and to view emotionally evocative pictures. These studies have consistently revealed activation of medial prefrontal cortex and thalamus (George et al., 1995; Lane et al., 1997a,b), regardless of the kind of emotion being recalled. As discussed earlier, these areas are also involved in learning and modulating the expression of emotional responses (e.g., Damasio, 1994). Some areas of activation specific to the recall of individual emotions have been observed (e.g., the insula has been associated with sadness; Lane et al., 1997b), but, given the small number of studies conducted thus far, no consistent patterns have yet emerged.

Interestingly, although amygdala activation has been observed during perception of emotionally evocative stimuli (e.g., Reiman et al., 1997), greater amygdala activity has not been consistently observed when subjects also are asked to recall personal, emotional episodes. This could be because the emotion-related physiological responses that the amygdala coordinates occur only when an emotion is being experienced strongly, and subjects' recollections may not have been sufficiently vivid to elicit additional amygdala activity. Alternatively, current neuroimaging methodology may not be sensitive to small changes in amygdala activity that could be generated by recall as opposed to perception of emotional events (cf. Kosslyn & Ochsner, 1994).

Summary

The preceding analysis suggests that retrieving a memory of an emotional experience can be biased in two ways. First, cues in the retrieval environment can combine with stored traces to produce a memory that is consciously experienced as accurate, even though its affective qualities may be more a product of current than past feelings. Second, effortful search for, and evaluation of, past emotional experiences may be shaped by current goals to justify, further, or explain current self-beliefs or to alter current moods. In some cases, because the emotions experienced during a given event were not well encoded, current feelings can serve to fill gaps in memory; the use of implicit theories of how emotions—and memory of them—change over time may guide this process. Retrieval of emotional memories may involve the same neural structures used to retrieve neutral ones, but there is as of yet little evidence to support this claim directly. It is clear, however, that retrieving past emotional experiences does require the action of the neural systems used to encode and store specifically affective information.

CONCLUSION

This chapter has drawn from research in both social psychology and cognitive neuroscience to inform an account of the relationship between emotion and memory that converges on three important principles: (1) Encoding of emotional experiences is guided by both automatic and deliberative appraisal processes that capture and guide attention to, and promote elaboration of, information that is judged to be most personally significant in the context of current goals and desires. (2) Retrieval of past emotional experiences is often biased such that memories of them make sense when evaluated from the perspective of one's current goals and feelings about them. (3) Separate but interacting neural systems are involved in the quick and automatic, or more effortful and reflective, encoding and retrieval of these memories.

Hamlet said, "nothing is either good nor bad, but thinking makes it so," and this review has outlined some ways that people make use of this ability to reinterpret their past in order to serve current and future-looking goals. In doing so, we have not offered specific directives about exactly which types of details, emotions, or events will be remembered most accurately. Instead, we have attempted to highlight the individualized nature of emotional processes and the importance of understanding the reasons why an emotional event is recalled in order to understand the content of subjective reports about the past. As noted at the outset, this emphasis reflects our contention that research on emotion and memory should move beyond questions such as whether emotional memories are indelible or highly fallible or which kinds of emotion make memory better or worse (e.g., see Bradley, 1994; Christianson, 1992; Conway, 1997; Matlin & Stang, 1978). These questions often are ill-posed, seek absolute answers that cannot be obtained (Tulving, 1985), and overlook the constructive, goal-driven nature of emotional encoding and recollection (Ochsner & Schacter, in press).

In closing, it is important to note that the work reviewed in this chapter was weighted most heavily toward the social and cognitive end of the social–cognitive–neuroscience spectrum. This bias stems from the fact that researchers only now are beginning to explore the neural bases of emotion and memory, and as future work maps the structures involved in motivated remembering of emotional experiences, the scales should balance out. Our thinking suggests that this balancing act will be most successful if researchers remember that remembering begins with a goal in mind and that feelings follow after.

REFERENCES

Adolphs, R., Tranel, D., Damasio, H., & Damasio, A. (1994). Impaired recognition of emotion in facial expressions following bilateral damage to the human amygdala. *Nature*, *372*, 669–672.

Bahrick, H.P., Hall, L.K., & Berger, S.A. (1996). Accuracy and distortion in memory for high-school grades. *Psychological Science*, *7*, 265–271.

Bargh, J.A., Chaiken, S., Govender, R., & Pratto, F. (1992). The generality of the attitude activation effect. *Journal of Personality and Social Psychology*, *62*, 893–912.

Bechara, A., Damasio, H., Tranel, D., & Damasio, A.R. (1996). Failure to respond autonomically to anticipated future outcomes following damage to prefrontal cortex. *Cerebral Cortex*, *6*, 215–225.

Bechara, A., Tranel, D., Damasio, H., & Adolphs, R. (1995). Double dissociation of conditioning and declarative knowledge relative to the amygdala and hippocampus in humans. *Science*, *269*, 1115–1118.

Borod, J.C. (1992). Interhemispheric and intrahemispheric control of emotion: A focus on unilateral brain damage. *Journal of Consulting and Clinical Psychology*, *60*, 339–348.

Borod, J.C, Rorie, K.D., Haywood, C.S., Andelman, F., Obler, L.K., Welkowitz, J., Bloom,

R.L., & Tweedy, J.R. (1996). Hemispheric specialization for discourse reports of emotional experiences: Relationships to demographic, neurological, and perceptual variables. *Neuropsychologia, 34*, 351–359.

Bower, G.H., & Forgas, J.P. (in press). Affect, memory, and social cognition. In E.E. Eich (Ed.), *Counter-Points: Cognition and Emotion*. Oxford: Oxford University Press.

Bradley, B.P., & Baddeley, A.D. (1990). Emotional factors in forgetting. *Psychological Medicine, 20*, 351–355.

Bradley, M.M. (1994). Emotional memory: A dimensional analysis. In S.H.M.v. Goozen, N.E.V.d. Poll, & J.A. Sergeant (Eds.), *Emotions: Essays on Emotion Theory* (pp. 97–134). Hillsdale, NJ: Lawrence Erlbaum Associates.

Bradley, M.M., Greenwald, M.K., Petry, M.C., & Lang, P.J. (1992). Remembering pictures: Pleasure and arousal in memory. *Journal of Experimental Psychology: Learning, Memory, & Cognition, 18*, 379–390.

Brickman, P., Coates, D., & Janoff-Bulman, R. (1978). Lottery winners and accident victims: Is happiness relative? *Journal of Personality and Social Psychology, 36(8)*, 917–927.

Brown, R., & Kulik, J. (1977). Flashbulb memories. *Cognition, 5*, 73–99.

Burke, A., Heuer, F., & Reisberg, D. (1992). Remembering emotional events. *Memory & Cognition, 20*, 277–290.

Cabeza, R., & Nyberg, L. (1997). Imaging cognition: An empirical review of PET studies with normals subjects. *Journal of Cognitive Neuroscience, 9*, 1–25.

Cahill, L., Babinsky, R., Markowitsch, H.J., & McGaugh, J.L. (1995). The amygdala and emotional memory. *Nature, 377*, 295–296.

Cahill, L., Haier, R.J., Fallon, J., Alkire, M., Tang, C., Keator, D., Wu, J., & McGaugh, J.L. (1996). Amygdala activity at encoding correlated with long-term, free recall of emotional information. *Proceedings of the National Academy of Sciences of the United States of America, 93*, 8016–8021.

Cahill, L., Prins, B., Weber, M., & McGaugh, J.L. (1994). β-Adrenergic activation and memory for emotional events. *Nature, 371*, 702–704.

Calder, A.J., Young, A.W., Rowland, D., & Perrett, D.I. (1996). Facial emotion recognition after bilateral amygdala damage: Differentially severe impairment of fear. *Cognitive Neuropsychology, 13*, 699–745.

Christianson, S.-A. (1992). Emotional stress and eyewitness memory: A critical review. *Psychological Bulletin, 112*, 284–309.

Christianson, S.-A., & Loftus, E.F. (1987). Memory for traumatic events. *Applied Cognitive Psychology, 1*, 225–239.

Christianson, S.-A., & Loftus, E.F. (1990). Some characteristics of people's traumatic memories. *Bulletin of the Psychonomic Society, 28*, 195–198.

Christianson, S.-A., Loftus, E.F., Hoffmann, H., & Loftus, G.R. (1991). Eye fixations and memory for emotional events. *Journal of Experimental Psychology: Learning, Memory, and Cognition, 17*, 693–701.

Christianson, S.-A., & Nilsson, L.-G. (1984). Functional amnesia as induced by psychological trauma. *Memory and Cognition, 12*, 142–155.

Cimino, C.R., Verfaellie, M., Bowers, D., & Heilman, K.M. (1991). Autobiographical memory: Influence of right hemisphere damage on emotionality and specificity. *Brain and Cognition, 15*, 106–118.

Clifford, B.R., & Scott, J. (1978). Individual and situational factors in eyewitness testimony. *Journal of Applied Psychology, 63*, 352–359.

Cohen, G., Conway, M.A., & Maylor, E.A. (1994). Flashbulb memories in older adults. *Psychology and Aging, 9*, 454–463.

Conway, M.A. (1997). *Recovered and False Memories*. Oxford: Oxford University Press.

Conway, M.A., & Bekerian, D.A. (1988). Characteristics of vivid memories. In M.M. Grunebeg, P. Morris, & R.N. Sykes (Eds.), *Practical Aspects of Memory: Current Research and Issues*, Vol. 1 (pp. 519–524). Chichester, England: Wiley.

Conway, M.A., & Dewhurst, S.A. (1995). The self and recollective experience. *Applied Cognitive Psychology, 9*, 1–19.

Conway, M.A., & Ross, M. (1984). Getting what you want by revising what you had. *Journal of Personality and Social Psychology, 47*, 738–748.

Corteen, R.S. (1969). Skin conductance changes and word recall. *British Journal of Psychology, 60*, 81–84.

Craik, F.I.M., Govoni, R., Naveh-Benjamin, M., & Anderson, N.D. (1997). The effect of divided attention on encoding and retrieval processes in human memory. *Journal of Experimental Psychology: General, 125*, 159–180.

Damasio, A.R. (1994). *Descartes' Error: Emotion, Reason, and the Human Brain*. New York: G.P. Putnam's Sons.

Damasio, A.R., Tranel, D., & Damasio, H. (1990). Individuals with sociopathic behavior caused by frontal damage fail to respond autonomically to social stimuli. *Behavioural Brain Research, 41*, 81–94.

Davidson, R.J. (1992). Anterior cerebral asymmetry and the nature of emotion. Special issue: The role of frontal lobe maturation in cognitive and social development. *Brain and Cognition, 20*, 125–151.

Denny, E.B., & Hunt, R.R. (1992). Affective valence and memory in depression. *Journal of Abnormal Psychology, 101*, 575–580.

Drevets, W.C., & Raichle, M.E. (1995). Positron emission tomographic imaging studies of human emotional disorders. In M.S. Gazzaniga (Ed.), *The Cognitive Neurosciences* (pp. 1153–1164). Cambridge, MA: MIT Press.

Easterbrook, J.A. (1959). The effect of emotion on cue utilization and the organization of behavior. *Psychological Review, 66*, 183–201.

Eich, E., Rachman, S., & Lopatka, C. (1990). Affect, pain, and autobiographical memory. *Journal of Abnormal Psychology, 99*, 174–178.

Eich, E., Reeves, J.L., Jaeger, B., & Graff-Radford, S.B. (1985). Memory for pain: Relation between past and present pain intensity. *Pain, 23*, 375–380.

Erber, R. (1996). The self-regulation of moods. In L.L. Martin & A. Tesser (Eds.), *Striving and Feeling: Interactions Among Goals, Affect, and Self-Regulation* (pp. 251–275). Mahwah, NJ: Lawrence Erlbaum Associates.

Fazio, R.H., Sanbonmatsu, D.M., Powell, M.C., & Kardes, F.R. (1986). On the automatic activation of attitudes. *Journal of Personality and Social Psychology, 50*, 229–238.

Folkman, S., & Lazarus, R. (1984). Personal control and stress and coping processes: A theoretical analysis. *Journal of Personality and Social Psychology, 46*, 839–852.

Frank, M.G., & Gilovich, T. (1989). Effect of memory perspective on retrospective causal attributions. *Journal of Personality and Social Psychology, 57*, 399–403.

Fredrickson, B.L., & Kahneman, D. (1993). Duration neglect in retrospective evaluations of affective episodes. *Journal of Personality and Social Psychology, 65*, 45–55.

Frijda, N. (1986). *The Emotions*. Cambridge: Cambridge University Press.

Gardiner, J.M., & Java, R.I. (1993). Recognising and remembering. In A.F. Collins, S.E. Gathercole, M.A. Conway, & P.E. Morris (Eds.), *Theories of Memory* (pp. 163–188). Hove, United Kingdom: Erlbaum.

George, M.S., Ketter, T.A., Parekh, P.I., & Horwitz, B. (1995). Brain activity during transient sadness and happiness in healthy women. *American Journal of Psychiatry, 152*, 341–351.

Gilovich, T. (1983). Biased evaluation and persistence in gambling. *Journal of Personality and Social Psychology, 44*, 1110–1126.

Hamann, S.B., Cahill, L., & Squire, L.R. (1997). Emotional perception and memory in amnesia. *Neuropsychology, 11*, 104–113.

Heuer, F., & Reisberg, D. (1990). Vivid memories of emotional events: The accuracy of remembered minutiae. *Memory and Cognition, 18*, 496–506.

Higgins, E.T., & Tykocinski, O. (1992). Self-discrepancies and biographical memory: Personality and cognition at the level of psychological situation. *Personality and Social Psychology Bulletin, 18*, 527–535.

Janoff-Bulman, R. (1992). *Shattered Assumptions: Towards a New Psychology of Trauma*. New York: Free Press.

Johnson, M.K., Kim, J.K., & Risse, G. (1985). Do alcoholic Korsakoff's syndrome patients acquire affective reactions? *Journal of Experimental Psychology: Learning, Memory, and Cognition, 11*, 27–36.

Kahneman, D., Fredrickson, B.L., Schreiber, C.A., & Redelmeier, D.A. (1993). When more pain is preferred to less: Adding a better end. *Psychological Science, 4*, 401–405.

Kaplan, R., & Kaplan, S. (1969). The arousal–retention interval revisited: The effects of some procedural changes. *Psychonomic Science, 15*, 84–85.

Kent, G. (1985). Memory of dental pain. *Pain, 21*, 187–194.

Kleinsmith, L.J., & Kaplan, S. (1963). Paired-associate learning as a function of arousal and interpolated interval. *Journal of Experimental Psychology, 65*, 190–193.

Kosslyn, S.M., & Ochsner, K.N. (1994). In search of occipital activation during mental imagery. *Trends in Neurosciences, 17*, 290–292.

LaBar, K.S., LeDoux, J.E., Spencer, D.D., & Phelps, E.A. (1995). Impaired fear conditioning following unilateral temporal lobectomy in humans. *Journal of Neuroscience, 15*, 6846–6855.

LaBar, K.S., & Phelps, E.A. (1998). Arousal-mediated memory consolidation: Role of the medial temporal lobe in humans. *Psychological Science, 9*, 490–493.

Lane, R.D. Reiman, E.M., Ahern, G.L., & Schwartz, G.E. (1997a). Neuroanatomical correlates of happiness, sadness, and disgust. *American Journal of Psychiatry, 154*, 926–933.

Lane, R.D., Reiman, E.M., Bradley, M.M., Lang, P.J., Ahern, G.L., Davidson, R.J., & Schwartz, G.E. (1997b). Neuroanatomical correlates of pleasant and unpleasant emotion. *Neuropsychologia, 35*, 1437–1444.

Lazarus, R.S. (1991). *Emotion and Adaptation*. New York: Oxford University Press.

LeDoux, J.E. (1995). Emotion: Clues from the brain. *Annual Review of Psychology, 46*, 209–235.

Levine, L.J. (1997). Reconstructing memory for emotions. *Journal of Experimental Psychology: General, 126*, 165–177.

Levine, L.J., & Burgess, S.L. (1997). Beyond general arousal: Effects of specific emotions on memory. *Social Cognition, 15*, 157–181.

Linton, S.J., & Mellin, L. (1982). The accuracy of remembering chronic pain. *Pain, 13*, 281–285.

Loftus, E.F., & Burns, T. (1982). Mental shock can produce retrograde amnesia. *Memory and Cognition, 10*, 318–323.

Loftus, E.F., Loftus, G., & Messo, J. (1987). Some facts about "weapon focus." *Law and Human Behavior, 11*, 55–62.

Loftus, E.F., Schooler, J.W., Boone, S.M., & Kline, D. (1987). Time went by so slowly: Overestimation of event duration by males and females. *Applied Cognitive Psychology*, *1*, 3–13.

Mathews, A., Mogg, K., Kentish, J., & Eysenck, M. (1995). Effect of psychological treatment on cognitive bias in generalized anxiety disorder. *Behaviour Research and Therapy*, *33*, 293–303.

Matlin, M.W., & Stang, D.J. (1978). *The Pollyanna Principle*. Cambridge, MA: Schenkman.

Matt, G.E., Vasquez, C., & Campbell, W.K. (1992). Mood-congruent recall of affectively toned stimuli: A meta-analytic review. *Clinical Psychology Review*, *12*, 227–255.

McFarland, C., & Buehler, R. (1997). Negative affective states and the motivated retrieval of positive life events: The role of affect acknowledgment. *Journal of Personality and Social Psychology*, *73*, 200–214.

McFarland, C., Ross, M., & DeCourville, N. (1989). Women's theories of menstruation and biases in recall of menstrual symptoms. *Journal of Personality and Social Psychology*, *57*, 522–531.

McGaugh, J.L., & Cahill, L. (1997). Interaction of neuromodulatory systems in modulating memory storage. *Behavioural Brain Research*, *83*, 31–38.

Mineka, S., & Nugent, K. (1995). Mood-congruent memory biases in anxiety and depression. In D.L. Schacter, J.T. Coyle, G.D. Fischbach, M.-M. Mesulam, & L.E. Sullivan (Eds.), *Memory Distortion: How Minds, Brains, and Societies Reconstruct the Past* (pp. 173–196). Cambridge, MA: Harvard University Press.

Moffitt, K.H., & Singer, J.A. (1994). Continuity in the life story: Self-defining memories, affect, and approach/avoidance personal strivings. *Journal of Personality*, *62*, 21–43.

Mogg, K., Gardiner, J.M., Stavrou, A., & Golombok, S. (1992). Recollective experience and recognition memory for threat in clinical anxiety states. *Psychonomic Bulletin and Review*, *30*, 109–112.

Mogg, K., Mathews, A., & Weinman, J. (1987). Memory bias in clinical anxiety. *Journal of Abnormal Psychology*, *96*, 94–98.

Neisser, U., & Harsch, N. (1992). Phantom flashbulbs: False recollections of hearing the news about Challenger. In E. Winograd & U. Neisser (Eds.), *Affect and Accuracy in Recall: Studies of "Flashbulb Memories"* (pp. 9–31). Cambridge: Cambridge University Press.

Nolen-Hoeksema, S. (1991). Responses to depression and their effects on the duration of depressive episodes. *Journal of Abnormal Psychology*, *100*, 569–582.

Norman, K.A., & Schacter, D.L. (1996). Implicit memory, explicit memory, and false recognition: A cognitive neuroscience perspective. In L.M. Reder (Ed.), *Implicit Memory and Metacognition*. Hillsdale, NJ: Erlbaum.

Norvell, K.T., Gaston-Johansson, F., & Fridh, G. (1987). Remembrance of labor pain: How valid are retrospective pain measurements? *Pain*, *31*, 77–86.

Ochsner, K.N. (2000). Are affective events richly remembered or simply familiar? The experience and process of recollecting affective events. *Journal of Experimental Psychology: General* (in press).

Ochsner, K.N., & Feldman-Barrett, L. (in press). The neuroscience of emotion. To appear in T.J. Mayne & G. Bonnano (Eds.), *Emotion: Current Issues and Future Directions*. Guilford Press: New York.

Ochsner, K.N., & Kosslyn, S.M. (1999). The cognitive neuroscience approach. In D.E. Rumelhart & B. Martin-Bly (Eds.), *Handbook of Cognition and Perception*, Vol. 10 (pp. 319–365). San Diego: Academic Press.

Ochsner, K.N., & Schacter, D.L. (in press). Remembering emotional events: A social cognitive neuroscience approach. To appear in R.J. Davidson, H. Goldsmith, & K.R. Scherer (Eds.), *Handbook of the Affective Sciences*. New York: Oxford University Press.

Ochsner, K.N., Schacter, D.L., & Edwards, K. (1997). Illusory recall of vocal affect. *Memory, 5*, 433–455.

Ohman, A., Flykt, A., & Lundqvist, D. (1999). Unconscious emotion: Evolutionary perspectives, psychophysiological data, and neuropsychological mechanisms. In R. Lane & L. Nadel (Eds.), *Cognitive Neuroscience of Emotion* (pp. 296–327). Oxford, UK: Oxford University Press.

Park, J., & Banaji, M. (1996). *The Effect of Arousal and Retention Delay on Memory: A Meta-Analysis*. Paper presented at the Eighth Annual Convention of the American Psychological Society, San Francisco.

Parrott, W.G., & Sabini, J. (1990). Mood and memory under natural conditions: Evidence for mood incongruent recall. *Journal of Personality and Social Psychology, 59*, 321–336.

Pennebaker, J.W. (1997). Writing about emotional experiences as a therapeutic process. *Psychological Science, 8*, 162–166.

Phillips, R.G., & LeDoux, J.E. (1992). Differential contribution of amygdala and hippocampus to cued and contextual fear conditioning. *Behavioral Neuroscience, 106*, 274–285.

Pillemer, D.B. (1984). Flashbulb memories of the assassination attempt on President Reagan. *Cognition, 16*, 63–80.

Pratto, F., & John, O.P. (1991). Automatic vigilance: The attention-grabbing power of negative social information. *Journal of Personality and Social Psychology, 61*, 380–391.

Reiman, E.M., Lane, R.D., Ahern, G.L., & Schwartz, G.E. (1997). Neuroanatomical correlates of externally and internally generated human emotion. *American Journal of Psychiatry, 154*, 918–925.

Reiman, E.M., Lane, R.D., Ahern, G.L., Schwartz, G.E., & Davidson, R.J. (1996). Positron emission tomography, emotion, and consciousness. In S.R. Hameroff, A.W. Kaszniak, & A.C. Scott (Eds.), *Toward a Science of Consciousness: The First Tucson Discussions and Debates* (pp. 311–320). Cambridge, MA: MIT Press.

Reisberg, D., Heuer, F., McLean, J., & O'Shaughnessy, M. (1988). The quantity, not the quality, of affect predicts memory vividness. *Bulletin of the Psychonomic Society, 26*, 100–103.

Revelle, W., & Loftus, D.A. (1992). The implications of arousal effects for the study of affect and memory. In S.-Å. Christianson (Ed.), *The Handbook of Emotion and Memory: Research and Theory* (pp. 113–149). Hillsdale, NJ: Erlbaum.

Riemann, B., & McNally, R.J. (1995). Cognitive processing of personally relevant information. *Cognition and Emotion, 9*, 325–340.

Robinson, J.A., & Swanson, K.L. (1993). Field and observer modes of remembering. *Memory, 1*, 169–184.

Roediger, H.L. III., & McDermott, K.B. (1995). Creating false memories: Remembering words not presented in lists. *Journal of Experimental Psychology: Learning, Memory, and Cognition, 21*, 803–814.

Rolls, E.T. (1995). A theory of emotion and consciousness, and its application to understanding the neural basis of emotion. In M. Gazzaniga (Ed.), *The Cognitive Neurosciences* (pp. 1091–1106). Cambridge, MA: MIT Press.

Rosenthal, R., Hall, J.A., DiMatteo, M.R., Rogers, P.L., & Archer, D. (1979). *Sensitivity to Nonverbal Communication: The PONS Test*. Baltimore: The Johns Hopkins University Press.

Ross, M. (1989). Relation of implicit theories to the construction of personal histories. *Psychological Review, 96*, 341–357.

Ross, M., & Buehler, R. (1994). Creative remembering. In U. Neisser & R. Fivush (Eds.), *The Remembering Self: Construction and Accuracy in the Self-Narrative*, Vol. 6 (pp. 205–235). New York: Cambridge University Press.

Ross, M., & Conway, M. (1986). Remembering one's own past: The construction of personal histories. In R.M. Sorrentino & E.T. Higgins (Eds.), *Handbook of Motivation and Cognition: Foundations of Social Behavior* (pp. 122–144). New York: Guilford Press.

Rubin, D.C., & Kozin, M. (1984). Vivid memories. *Cognition, 16*, 81–95.

Salovey, P., & Smith, A.F. (1997). Memory for the experience of physical pain. In N.L. Stein, P.A. Ornstein, B. Tversky, & C. Brainerd (Eds.), *Memory for Emotional and Everyday Events* (pp. 295–314). Mahwah, NJ: Erlbaum and Associates.

Schacter, D.L. (1982). *Stranger Behind the Engram: Theories of Memory and the Psychology of Science*. Hillsdale, NJ: Erlbaum.

Schacter, D.L. (1996a). Memory serves as a link, not an instant replay. *Los Angeles Times*, August 21.

Schacter, D.L. (1996b). *Searching for Memory: The Brain, the Mind, and the Past*. New York: Basic Books.

Schacter, D.L., Alpert, N.M., Savage, C.R., Rauch, S.L., & Albert, M.S. (1996a). Conscious recollection and the human hippocampal formation: Evidence from positron emission tomography. *Proceedings of the National Academy of Sciences of the United States of America, 93*, 321–325.

Schacter, D.L., Curran, T., Galluccio, L., Milberg, W., & Bates, J. (1996b). False recognition and the right frontal lobe: A case study. *Neuropsychologia, 34*, 793–808.

Schacter, D.L., Israel, L., & Racine, C. (1999). Suppressing false recognition in younger and older adults: The distinctiveness heuristic. *Journal of Memory and Language, 40*, 1–24.

Schacter, D.L., Norman, K.A., & Koutstaal, W. (1998). The cognitive neuroscience of constructive memory. *Annual Review of Psychology, 49*, 289–318.

Schacter, D.L., & Wagner, A.D. (1999). Medial temporal lobe activations in fMRI and PET studies of episodic encoding and retrieval. *Hippocampus, 9*, 7–24.

Seidlitz, L., & Diener, E. (1993). Memory for positive versus negative life events: Theories for the differences between happy and unhappy persons. *Journal of Personality and Social Psychology, 64*, 654–663.

Semon, R. (1909/1923). *Mnemic Psychology*. London: George Allen & Unwin.

Shimamura, A.P. (1995). Memory and frontal lobe function. In M. Gazzaniga (Ed.), *The Cognitive Neurosciences* (pp. 803–813). Cambridge, MA: MIT Press.

Singer, J.A. (1990). Affective responses to autobiographical memories and their relationship to long-term goals. *Journal of Personality, 58*, 535–563.

Singer, J.A., & Salovey, P. (1996). Motivated memory: Self-defining memories, goals, and affect regulation. In L.L. Martin & A. Tesser (Eds.), *Striving and Feeling: Interactions Among Goals, Affect, and Self-Regulation* (pp. 229–250). Mahwah, NJ: Erlbaum Associates.

Skowronski, J.J., & Carlston, D.E. (1989). Negativity and extremity biases in impression formation: A review of explanations. *Psychological Bulletin, 105*, 131–142.

Smith, S.M., & Petty, R.E. (1995). Personality moderators of mood congruency effects on cognition: The role of self-esteem and negative mood regulation. *Journal of Personality and Social Psychology, 68,* 1092–1107.

Stein, N.L., Wade, E., & Liwag, M.D. (1997). A theoretical approach to understanding and remembering emotional events. In N.L. Stein, P.A. Ornstein, B. Tversky, & C. Brainerd (Eds.), *Memory for Emotional and Everyday Events* (pp. 15–47). Mahwah, NJ: Erlbaum and Associates.

Strack, F., Schwarz, N., & Gschneidinger, E. (1985). Happiness and reminiscing: The role of time perspective, affect, and mode of thinking. *Journal of Personality and Social Psychology, 49,* 1460–1469.

Stuss, D.T., Eskes, G.A., & Foster, J.K. (1994). Experimental neuropsychological studies of frontal lobe functions. In F. Boller & J. Grafman (Eds.), *Handbook of Neuropsychology*. Amsterdam: Elsevier.

Taylor, S. (1989). *Positive Illusions: Creative Self-Deception and the Healthy Mind*. New York: Basic Books.

Thomas, D.L., & Diener, E. (1990). Memory accuracy in the recall of emotions. *Journal of Personality and Social Psychology, 59,* 291–297.

Tobias, B., Kihlstrom, J.F., & Schacter, D.L. (1992). Emotion and implicit memory. In S.A. Christianson (Ed.), *Handbook of Emotion and Memory* (pp. 67–92). Hillsdale, NJ: Erlbaum Associates.

Tulving, E. (1983). *Elements of Episodic Memory*. Oxford, England: Clarendon Press.

Tulving, E. (1985). Varieties of consciousness and levels of awareness in memory. In A. Baddeley & L. Weiskrantz (Eds.), *Attention: Selection, Awareness and Control: A Tribute to Donald Broadbent*. Oxford: Oxford University Press.

Tulving, E., Kapur, S., Craik, F.I.M., Moscovitch, M., & Houle, S. (1994). Hemispheric encoding/retrieval asymmetry in episodic memory: Positron emission tomography findings. *Proceedings of the National Academy of Science of the United States of America, 91,* 2016–2020.

Varey, C.A., & Kahneman, D. (1992). Experiences extended across time: Evaluation of moments and episodes. *Journal of Behavioral Decision Making, 5,* 169–185.

Wagenaar, W.A. (1994). Is memory self-serving? In U. Neisser & R. Fivush (Eds.), *The Remembering Self: Construction and Accuracy in the Self-Narrative*, Vol. 6 (pp. 191–204). New York: Cambridge University Press.

Wahler, R.G., & Afton, A.D. (1980). Attentional processes in insular and non-insular mothers: Some differences in their summary reports about child problem behaviors. *Child Behavior Therapy, 2,* 25–41.

Walker, E.L., & Tarte, R.D. (1963). Memory storage as a function of arousal and retention interval. *Journal of Verbal Learning and Verbal Behavior, 2,* 113–119.

Watkins, P.C., Mathews, A., Williamson, D.A., & Fuller, R.D. (1992). Mood congruent memory in depression: Emotional priming or elaboration. *Journal of Abnormal Psychology, 101,* 581–586.

Wentzlaff, R.M. (1993). The mental control of depression: Psychological obstacles to emotional well-being. In D.M. Wegner & J.W. Pennebaker (Eds.), *Handbook of Mental Control* (pp. 239–257). Engelwood Cliffs, NJ: Prentice Hall.

Whalen, P.J., Rauch, S.L., Etcoff, N.L., McInerney, S.C., Lee, M.B., & Jenike, M.A. (1998). Masked presentations of emotional facial expressions modulate amygdala activity without explicit knowledge. *Journal of Neuroscience, 181,* 411–418.

Williams, J.M.G., & Dritschel, B.H. (1988). Emotional disturbance and the specificity of autobiographical memory. *Cognition and Emotion, 2,* 221–234.

Williams, J.M.G. (1996). Depression and the specificity of autobiographical memory. In

D.C. Rubin (Ed.), *Remembering Our Past*: *Studies in Autobiographical Memory* (p$_t$ 244–267). New York: Cambridge University Press.

Williams, J.M.G., Mathews, A., & MacLeod, C. (1996). The emotional Stroop task and psychopathology. *Psychological Bulletin, 120,* 3–24.

Yuille, J.C., & Cutshall, J.L. (1986). A case study of eyewitness memory of a crime. *Journal of Applied Psychology, 71,* 291–301.

Zajonc, R. (1998). Emotions. In D.T. Gilbert, S.T. Fiske, & G. Lindzey (Eds.), *Handbook of Social Psychology*, 4th ed. New York: McGraw Hill.

Zola-Morgan, S., Squire, L.R., Alverez-Royo, P., & Clower, R.P. (1991). Independence of memory functions and emotional behavior: Separate contributions of the hippocampal formation and the amygdala. *Hippocampus, 1,* 207–220.

8

...y of Emotion at a Systems Level

RALPH ADOLPHS AND ANTONIO R. DAMASIO

Our understanding of emotion has lagged behind our knowledge of most other domains of cognition, both theoretically and empirically. In large part, this can be attributed to the fact that emotion was not considered part of cognition until very recently. In fact, adherents of both behaviorism and cognitivism made it a point to exclude emotion and motivation from the study of the mind. Ironically, it was work in computer intelligence that perhaps first pointed to the impossibility of cognition without emotion. The problem is that information processing, devoid of emotion and motivation, is without any intrinsic value. Given a constrained task, or a specific piece of information to process, a system without emotion can be designed to perform the task or to process the information (as modern "expert systems" do). But how, in the real world, would such a system ever decide what to do? Attention, memory, and decision-making all require selectivity; the system must be able to distinguish between inputs and outputs that are important and those that are irrelevant out of the vast multitude of stimuli and of behaviors available. Emotion provides such guidance and is indispensable for the adaptive functioning of higher organisms.

In this chapter, we survey the field from the perspective of large-scale neural systems that provide the underpinnings of cognitive functions. Our goal is to provide a modern framework for thinking about emotion that is consistent with studies in animals and humans and that suggests specific testable hypotheses. Given the constraints of this chapter, our emphasis is on the neural systems responsible for *retrieval of knowledge* about emotions, and we focus on two neural structures: *amygdala* and *right somatosensory cortices*.

THEORETICAL OVERVIEW

Damasio (1994, 1995) has articulated a systems-level theory of emotion that is motivated by an understanding at the levels of evolutionary and ecological description and that proposes specific neuroanatomical hypotheses for experimental studies. Fundamental to this view is the idea that the subject matter of emotion is a relation between organism and environment, namely, the effect that interaction between the two has on the organism's survival and well-being. Emotions thus pertain to the *value* that stimuli and situations have for the organism. Survival value ultimately translates into the ability to maintain homeostasis, bodily integrity, and adaptive brain state. Such a biologically motivated view is consonant with several other theoretical treatments of emotion (e.g., Frijda, 1986; Lazarus, 1991; Plutchik, 1980).

Extending ideas first developed by the psychologist William James over a century ago, we propose that an emotion comprises a collective change in body and brain states in response to the evaluation of a particular event or entity (or in response to the memory of a particular event or entity) with respect to its importance for the organism's survival (Damasio, 1994, 1995). These state changes produce, respectively, somatic changes (including motor behavior, facial expression, autonomic changes, and endocrine changes) and changes in the processing mode of neural systems (changes in the way the brain processes information). Emotions additionally pertain to neural representations of body state changes (which may be the direct result of actual changes in body state or which may be centrally generated without any actual body state changes). Emotions would thus engage those neural structures that represent body states and those structures that link perception of external stimuli to body states. This would encompass somatosensory cortices and components of basal ganglia and structures such as ventral frontal cortex and amygdala, respectively. Aspects of emotion involving changes in global neural processing modes (as are evident, for instance, during intense emotional arousal or during states such as depression) would involve neuromodulatory structures such as the basal forebrain cholinergic system, the noradrenergic locus coeruleus, dopaminergic midbrain and brain stem systems, and the serotonergic raphe nuclei, among others.

The above framework may seem too inclusive. What are we to make of states such as hunger, thirst, and pain, which are not normally considered emotions? In our view, there is no principle difference between these states and emotions, except that hunger, thirst, and pain are more primitive, play a lesser role in social communication, and can be found in a larger number of organisms. Our folk psychological concept of emotion may not acknowledge the continuity, at the level of neural systems, between hunger, thirst, pain, and emotions. This does not, however, mean that they are not fundamentally similar; it just means that our concept of emotion has some arbitrary boundaries (see Griffiths [1997] for an extended treatment of this issue, although we do not endorse his eliminativism).

The topic of emotion subsumes several distinct processes, which can be operationalized in different ways. Three useful domains in which emotion can be studied are knowledge about emotion (including recognition, naming, evaluation, and appraisal), experience of emotion (a domain that we have labeled *feelings* (Damasio, 1995), and expression of emotion (through language, facial expression, and other behaviors related to social communication).

While recognition, experience, and expression of emotion are all dissociable, they are also closely linked (for review, see Borod, 1993a). Several lines of evidence bear this out. Perhaps expectedly, the experience and expression of emotion are highly correlated (Rosenberg & Ekman, 1994), although such correlation will depend on the circumstances under which the emotion is expressed (Fridlund, 1994). Production of emotional facial expressions (Adelman & Zajonc, 1989) and other somatovisceral responses (Cacioppo, Berntson, & Klein, 1992) directly cause changes in emotional experience, brain activity (Ekman & Davidson, 1993), and autonomic state (Levenson, Ekman, & Friesen, 1990). Viewing emotional expressions on others' faces causes systematic changes in one's own facial expression (Dimberg, 1982) and emotional experience (Schneider et al., 1994).

KNOWLEDGE OF EMOTION

When we speak of "happiness" or "fear," we are using a verbal label as shorthand for a cluster of phenomena (experiences, behaviors, body states, and so forth), knowledge of which comprises the concept of happiness or fear. When we attempt to assess recognition of emotions by subjects, the particular tasks we use may engage the subject in retrieving various of these knowledge components.

The retrieval of conceptual knowledge is perhaps most easily understood with regard to lexical stimuli, such as words. In such an experiment, a subject would read or hear a word denoting an emotion, for example, the word *anger*, and would then be asked to retrieve knowledge regarding the emotion denoted by the word *anger*. One could ask, for instance, if this is a pleasant or an unpleasant emotion, if anger is more similar to disgust than it is to happiness, if anger is arousing or relaxing, and so on. All of these items of knowledge are components of the normal concept of the emotion of "anger." One could perform the same experiment without using the lexical label and instead show subjects a facial expression of anger, asking the same questions about it as one might ask about the label.

THE AMYGDALA

Arguably, the brain structure that has received the most attention with regard to its role in emotion is the amygdala. The amygdala is a collection of nuclei situated in the anterior mesial temporal lobe that receive highly processed sensory information from all modalities (although the amygdala receives direct olfactory input from the olfactory bulb) and that have extensive, reciprocal connections with a large number of other brain structures whose function can be modulated by emotion (for review, see Amaral et al., 1992). Thus, the amygdala has massive connections, both direct and via the thalamus, with the ventromedial frontal cortices, known to play a key role in planning and decision-making. The amygdala connects with hippocampus, basal ganglia, and basal forebrain, all structures that participate in various aspects of memory and attention. Of course, the amygdala also projects to structures, such as the hypothalamus, that are involved in controlling homeostasis and visceral and neuroendocrine output. Consequently, the amygdala is situated so as to link information about external stimuli conveyed by sensory cortices, on the one hand, with modulation of decision-making, memory, attention, and somatic, visceral, and endocrine processes, on the other hand. All the latter processes will be influenced by the emotional significance of the external stimulus that is being processed. Thus, our decisions, our memory, our attention, and our somatic responses depend in part on the emotion associated with, or elicited by, a stimulus or event.

Insights into the function of the amygdala date back to lesion studies in animals that focused on abnormal behavioral responses to emotional and social stimuli (Kling & Brothers, 1992; Weiskrantz, 1956). The most consistent finding from these studies resembled an agnosia for the emotional and social significance of stimuli, often resulting in pathological tameness and placidity of the animal, together with a tendency to approach stimuli that normal animals would avoid. Although some broadly similar results have been reported after lesions of the amygdala in humans (Aggleton, 1992; Davis, 1992b), several cases of bilateral amygdala damage have been reported without the obvious placidity that is typically found in animal studies (Markowitsch et al., 1994; Tranel & Hyman, 1990). We have conjectured that amygdala damage may have less obvious consequences on social behavior in humans than it does in monkeys or rats because humans possess special compensatory mechanisms, such as language and much greater general problem-solving skills (Adolphs et al., 1995). Nonetheless, recent data have confirmed a critical role for the human amygdala in making social judgments about other people, in particular in judging whether another individual is trustworthy or should be approached. The findings here have been consonant with those from animal studies: Humans with bilateral amygdala damage tend to approach and to trust other people who normal individuals judge to be unapproachable and untrustworthy (Adolphs, Tranel, & Damasio, 1998).

Insights into the functions of the human amygdala have come also from studies in which the amygdala was stimulated electrically. Although such experiments are rare, they have found that experiences or behaviors associated with fear and anger can be elicited by such stimulation (Gloor et al., 1982; Halgren et al., 1978). The interpretation that the amygdala plays an important role in the *experience* of emotions is not presently warranted, however, because a number of studies with functional imaging have failed to find activation of the amygdala during the experience of emotions (e.g., Cahill et al., 1996; Fredrikson et al.,1995).

The Amygdala's Role in Recognizing Emotional Facial Expressions

Neurophysiological recording of neurons in the amygdala of animals has shown that neuronal reponses are modulated by the affective significance of sensory stimuli (Muramoto et al., 1993; Nishijo, Ono, & Nishino, 1988) and can be selective for the sight of faces (Leonard et al., 1985; Nakamura, Mikami, & Kubota, 1992; Rolls, 1992). We have studied a rare human subject (subject SM) who has selective bilateral damage to the amygdala (Tranel & Hyman, 1990) performing tasks that involved facial expressions of emotion as stimuli. Detailed analyses of data from magnetic resonance (MR) scans of SM's brain confirmed complete bilateral lesion of the amygdala, with some minor damage to the adjacent anterior entorhinal cortex; all other structures were undamaged (Fig. 8.1). These findings were corroborated by functional imaging: A resting ^{18}F-deoxyglucose positron emission tomography (PET) study showed essentially no glucose uptake by the tissue of the amygdala. When shown facial expressions of fear, SM often mislabeled the emotion (usually as anger, surprise, or disgust) and on several occasions was unable to generate any label to describe facial expressions of fear (stating that she had no idea what the face was expressing) (Fig. 8.2). The impairment was verified with a quantitative task in which the subject was asked to rate the intensity of different emotions signaled by facial expressions. SM gave facial expressions of fear abnormally low ratings of the intensity of fear expressed, and she also endorsed somewhat low ratings when judging facial expressions that are similar to fear, such as anger and surprise (Adolphs et al., 1994, 1995) (Fig. 8.3).

In addition, SM was unable to judge normally the similarity between different emotional facial expressions. Whereas normal subjects recognize a continuum of emotions, SM tended to lump all expressions of the same emotion to-

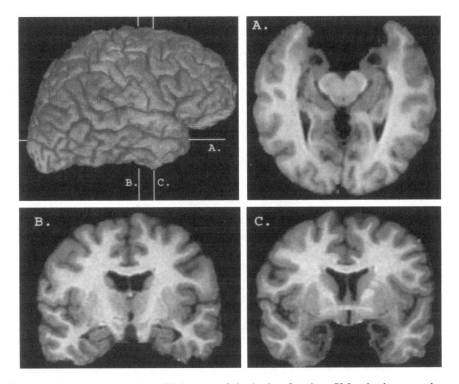

Figure 8.1. High-resolution MR images of the brain of patient SM, who has complete and selective bilateral amygdala damage. There is minor damage to the anterior entorhinal cortex. All other brain structures are normal. (**Top left**): Three-dimensional reconstruction of SM's brain, showing planes of sections. (**A**) Horizontal section at the level of the amygdala. (**B**) Coronal section at the level of the hippocampus. (**C**) Coronal section at the level of the amygdala. All images were obtained by computing an average from three separate MR scans of SM's brain, providing superior resolution. (Images provided by H. Damasio, Human Neuroimaging and Neuroanatomy Laboratory.)

gether (they all received nearly identical ratings on a variety of tasks) and judged different emotions to be very dissimilar (Adolphs et al., 1994). The above results could not be accounted for by visuoperceptual impairments because the subject performed normally on a large number of visuoperceptual tasks, including discrimination among unfamiliar faces (Tranel & Hyman, 1990), ability to recognize people's identity from their faces (Adolphs et al., 1994), and ability to discriminate between subtly different expressions on the same face or between sexes. The finding that the amygdala is important to process facial expressions of fear has now been replicated in several other studies with both the lesion method (Calder et al., 1996; Young et al., 1995, 1996) and functional imaging (Breiter et al., 1996; Morris et al., 1996).

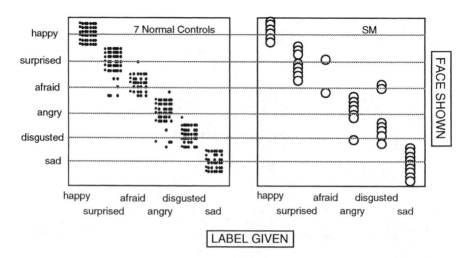

Figure 8.2. Impaired labeling of facial expressions of fear following amygdala damage. Seven normal control subjects and SM were shown 39 facial expressions of emotion from Ekman & Friesen (1976) (six of each of the basic emotions, and three neutral faces) and asked to provide a label of the emotion spontaneously. SM was impaired in labeling faces expressing fear (she only labeled a single face of fear correctly in the figure). Subjects' labels are shown as data points when synonymous with the words in the figure (e.g., when calling angry faces "mad"); labels that are not clear synonyms (e.g., calling a sad face "guilty") were omitted from the figure (accounting for the absent data points for some of the control subjects).

Additional studies with subject SM have revealed that the impairment extends to the retrieval of conceptual knowledge regarding emotions in tasks that do not involve facial expressions as stimuli. She was unable to draw facial expressions of fear from memory (Adolphs et al., 1995), and she was also impaired in retrieving some conceptual knowledge of emotions when given lexical stimuli, such as words or stories denoting emotions (Adolphs, Russell, & Tranel, 1999); again, the impairment was most striking with regard to fear.

We have attempted to decompose SM's impaired retrieval of knowledge of some facial expressions of emotion by asking her to judge specific components of knowledge. In one recent experiment, we found that SM was severely impaired in knowing that negatively valenced emotions (notably fear and anger) were highly arousing, while she was entirely normal in knowing that they were unpleasant (Adolphs, Russell, & Tranel, 1999) (Fig. 8.4).

It is not obvious how to characterize SM's impaired performance on the above tasks. Interpretations that clearly *cannot* be made are to conclude that she has no fear or that she does not know what fear is. The impairment is more specific and appears to consist of an inability to access *some* knowledge regarding the emotion signaled by external sensory stimuli, such as facial expressions. This sug-

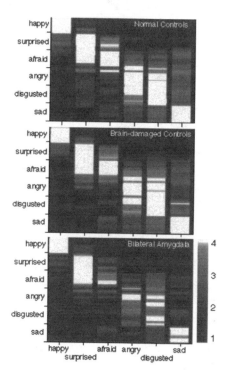

Figure 8.3. Impaired recognition of fear in facial expressions following amygdala damage. Raw rating scores of facial expressions of emotion are shown from seven normal controls (*top panel*), 16 brain-damaged controls without damage to amygdala (*middle panel*), and eight subjects with bilateral amygdala damage (*bottom panel*). (From Adolphs et al., 1999.) The emotional stimuli (36 faces; six each of each of the six basic emotions indicated) are ordered on the y-axis according to their perceived similarity (stimuli perceived to be similar, e.g., happy and surprised faces, are adjacent; stimuli perceived to be dissimilar, e.g., happy and sad faces, are distant; cf. Adolphs et al., 1995). The six emotion labels on which subjects rated the faces are displayed on the x-axis. Greyscale brightness encodes the mean rating given to each face by a group of subjects, as indicated in the scale. Thus, a darker line would indicate a lower mean rating than a brighter line for a given face; and a thin bright line for a given emotion category would indicate that few stimuli of that emotion received a high rating, whereas a thick bright line would indicate that many or all stimuli within that emotion category received high ratings. Because very few mean ratings were < 1 or > 4, the graphs were truncated outside these values. Data from subjects with bilateral amygdala damage indicate abnormally low ratings of negative emotions (thinner bright bands across any horizontal position corresponding to an expression of a negative emotion). (From Adolphs et al., 1999; copyright Elsevier Science Publishers, 1999.)

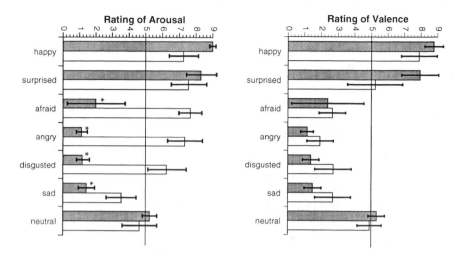

Figure 8.4. Mean ratings of arousal and valence for 39 facial expressions of emotion. Subjects were asked to explicitly rate the same 39 stimuli used in the studies shown in Figures 8.2 and 8.3 with respect to the valence (pleasantness) and arousal depicted. Data were averaged for all faces that express the same emotion (six of each basic emotion; three neutral). Means and standard deviations are shown for 24 normal controls (white bars) and for subject SM (three experiments; gray bars). SM's ratings of arousal of negative emotions were more than 2 SD below the control mean (*). (Data are from Adolphs, Russell, & Tranel, 1999. Reproduced from Adolphs, Russell, & Tranel, 1999.)

gests a role for the amygdala not in storage of knowledge about fear, or in the experience of fear, but rather in linking external sensory stimuli to systems into which knowledge about fear is acquired during learning and from which such knowledge can be subsequently retrieved. The amygdala thus connects percepts of emotional sensory stimuli, on the one hand, with a variety of neural systems involved in acquisition of, response to, and knowledge about such stimuli, on the other. Taken together, the above data support the idea that the amygdala is important in order to link perception of stimuli that signal potential threat/danger with behaviors, or with knowledge, related to emotional arousal.

This interpretation makes some specific predictions. First, amygdala damage should impair the ability to acquire associations between emotional sensory stimuli and some components of the normal response to such stimuli. Second, the amygdala's role in the acquisition of knowledge regarding emotion would predict that damage to the amygdala early in life would result in more severe impairments in such knowledge (because it would not have been acquired normally during development), whereas damage to the amygdala later in life might result in less severe impairments. Third, there should be neural structures other than the amygdala that are important for the retrieval of knowledge about emotions, if appropriately triggered. All three of these predictions have been recently tested and found to be supported. We discuss each in turn below.

The Amygdala's Role in Conditioning

The best studied function of the amygdala concerns its role in associative memory for aversive stimuli. A large number of studies, primarily in rats, have shown that the amygdala is required for the acquisition and expression of conditioned behavioral responses to stimuli that have been previously paired with an intrinsically aversive event, a paradigm called *fear conditioning* (Davis, 1992a; Le Doux, 1996). The role of the amygdala in fear conditioning as demonstrated in animals is consonant with recent data from humans: Subjects with amygdala lesions fail to show conditioned skin-conductance responses to stimuli that have been paired with an aversive, loud noise (Bechara et al., 1995; LaBar et al., 1995), and functional imaging studies in normal subjects have shown amygdala activation to aversively conditioned stimuli (Buechel et al., 1998). These and other studies have suggested that the amygdala specifically mediates behaviors and responses correlated with arousal and stress (Davis, 1992b; Kesner, 1992), including a key role in the acquisition of information during emotionally arousing situations or regarding emotionally arousing stimuli (Phelps & Anderson, 1997).

In one study, we tested the ability of a subject with bilateral amygdala damage (subject SM) to acquire conditioned autonomic responses to stimuli that had been paired with an aversive startle stimulus. This experiment was very similar to fear conditioning experiments with animals (Davis, 1992a; Le Doux, 1996). Briefly, subjects were presented with a startling, aversive loud auditory stimulus, which reliably evoked skin-conductance responses both in normal subjects and in SM. This startle stimulus was paired with slides of a certain color: Blue slides were accompanied by the startle stimulus, whereas slides of other colors were not. Normal subjects soon acquired conditioned autonomic responses: The presentation of a blue slide alone (without the startle stimulus) now evoked conditioned skin-conductance changes. We found that these conditioned autonomic responses were independent of the acquisition of declarative knowledge because amnesic subjects also acquired conditioned skin-conductance responses, even though they did not remember which slides had been paired with the startle stimulus. Subject SM, on the other hand, did not acquire conditioned skin-conductance responses on this task, even though she was able to remember which slides had been paired with the startle stimulus (Bechara et al., 1995). These studies suggest that in humans, as in animals, the amygdala plays a key role in acquiring conditioned responses to stimuli that have been paired with aversive emotional stimuli in the past.

It should be noted that the amygdala appears not to be essential for acquiring all types of nondeclarative knowledge associated with emotion. In an experiment with an amnesic patient who had complete bilateral amygdala damage, it was found that the patient could acquire covert behavioral preferences with regard to other people: He would develop a positive bias toward people who had been kind to him in the past and a negative bias toward those who had not (Tranel & Damasio, 1993).

The Amygdala's Role in Learning and Development

Although the above studies provide strong support for the idea that the amygdala is important to acquire responses associated with emotionally arousing stimuli, the amygdala's role in acquisition of declarative knowledge regarding emotion has remained controversial. Studies with animals suggested that the amygdala itself does not contribute to declarative memory and that surrounding white matter and cortex are instead important in this regard. Recent studies in humans, however, argue that the amygdala does play a role in declarative knowledge, although this role is modulatory rather than essential, parallel with its modulatory role in emotionally motivated learning in animals (Cahill & McGaugh, 1998).

In a study of two subjects with complete and relatively selective bilateral amygdala damage, we found a specific impairment in long-term declarative memory for emotional but not for neutral material. While normal subjects remembered emotional material better than neutral material, subjects with bilateral amygdala damage remembered emotional material only as well as neutral material (Adolphs et al., 1997a). These findings are consonant with a PET study that found that amygdala activation at the time emotional material was encoded into declarative memory correlated with how well it could be later recalled (Cahill et al., 1996).

Summary

The findings reviewed above would predict that damage to amygdala might cause the most severe impairments in declarative memory regarding emotions when it has occurred early in life, blocking the normal acquisition of such knowledge during development. Furthermore, the evidence points to a specific role in acquisition of knowledge linked to high emotional arousal, consistent with the amygdala's importance in knowledge regarding fear, a highly arousing emotion. Consonant with this idea, we found impaired recognition of facial expressions of fear in a subject who had sustained amygdala damage early in life (Adolphs et al., 1994) but not in two subjects who sustained amygdala damage as adults (Hamann et al., 1996). In an additional study, we probed the knowledge of emotional arousal signaled by facial expressions, words, and stories in three subjects who had sustained complete bilateral amygdala damage early in life and in two subjects who had sustained such damage as adults. As predicted, we found that early-onset amygdala damage caused disproportionately severe impairments in knowledge of the arousal signaled by emotional stimuli (Adolphs et al., 1997b). Interestingly, knowledge of the valence (pleasantness/unpleasantness) was normal in all amygdala subjects in this study (see also Adolphs, Russell, & Tranel, 1999).

Although these studies argue for an important role for the amygdala in the acquisition of knowledge about emotion during development, other lesion studies (Adolphs, Tranel, & Damasio, 1998; Broks et al., 1998), as well as functional imaging studies (Breiter et al., 1996; Morris et al., 1996), suggest that the amygdala may serve a more general role in processing emotions and is important for recognizing emotional and social information in adults without developmental damage.

THE SOMATOSENSORY CORTICES

Clinical and experimental studies have suggested that the right hemisphere is preferentially involved in processing emotion in both humans (e.g., Blonder, Bowers, & Heilman, 1991; Borod, 1993b; Borod et al., 1992; Bowers et al., 1987, 1991; Ross, 1985; Silberman & Weingartner, 1986; Van Strien & Morpurgo, 1992) and nonhuman primates (Hamilton & Vermeire, 1988; Hauser, 1993; Morris & Hopkins, 1993). Lesions in right temporal and parietal cortices have been shown to impair emotional experience, arousal (Heller, 1993), and imagery (Blonder, Bowers, & Heilman, 1991; Bowers et al., 1991) for emotion. It has been proposed that the right hemisphere contains modules for nonverbal affect computation (Bowers, Bauer, & Heilman, 1993), which may have evolved to subserve aspects of social cognition (Borod, 1993b). There is currently some argument over the extent to which the right hemisphere participates in emotion: Is it specialized to process all emotions, or is it specialized only for processing emotions of negative valence (Borod, 1992; Davidson, 1992; Silberman & Weingartner, 1986)? It may well be that an answer to this issue will depend on more precise specification of which components of emotion are under consideration (Borod, 1993a; Davidson, 1993).

Selective impairments in recognizing facial expressions, with sparing of the ability to recognize identity, can occur following right temporoparietal lesions (Bowers et al., 1985). Specific anomia for emotional facial expressions has been reported following right middle temporal gyrus lesions (Rapcsak, Kaszniak, & Rubens, 1989). The evidence that the right temporoparietal cortex is important in processing emotional facial expressions is corroborated by data from PET imaging (Gur, Skolnick, & Gur, 1994) and neuronal recording (Ojemann, Ojemann, & Lettich, 1992) in humans. Additionally, anthropological analyses of the depiction of faces in art and painting support the idea that the right hemisphere is specialized to process the emotional and social signals that faces can signal (Grusser, 1984).

A prediction made by the hypothesis that the human amygdala is critical for the acquisition of knowledge regarding emotion is that structures other than the amygdala would play a key role in the storage and retrieval of such knowledge. In this view, the amygdala's contribution to memory is in some ways analogous to that of the hippocampal formation: Both structures are important during acquisition and/or consolidation of new information but are not structures where such knowledge is ultimately stored. The storage and retrieval of knowledge is presumed to rely on neocortical sectors.

On the basis of our framework regarding emotion and on the basis of the studies reviewed at the beginning of this section, we hypothesized that somatosensory cortices in the right hemisphere would be important for the retrieval of knowledge regarding emotions. We tested this hypothesis in a group of 25 subjects with neocortical lesions performing a task of recognition of emotion in facial expressions. A detailed analysis of the overlaps of lesions in these subjects revealed that sectors in right parietal cortex, when lesioned, reliably caused impairments in the retrieval of knowledge about emotions depicted in facial expressions (Adolphs et al., 1996a). A recent study extended these methods to three-dimensional analysis of the overlaps of lesions that correlated with the most impaired performances. The analysis showed that lesions encompassing the face representation of right primary somatosensory cortex, possibly including SII, insula, and anterior supramarginal gyrus, as well as underlying white matter, most reliably correlated with impaired recognition of emotional facial expressions (Adolphs et al., 1996b). The results of this study are shown in Figure 8.5.

The question arises as to why the processing of emotion, much like the processing of language, should be notably lateralized. One possibility is that both language and emotion serve an important role in communication, with a premium on processing speed. In the case of language, this has been clear for some time: Both the comprehension and production of language require neural processing with high temporal acuity. In the case of emotion, ecological considerations would similarly suggest that signals need to be processed rapidly. The consolidation of all neural components required to process language, or facial expression, in one hemisphere would enable such rapid processing. Intrahemispheric delay, on the other hand, would introduce an unacceptable lag. This constraint would be expected to be all the more acute the larger the brain, and one would expect lateralization of function to be especially prominent in human brains, where spatial proximity of processing components will be a major factor in processing speed (Ringo et al., 1994).

One interpretation of the right hemisphere's demonstrated specialization in many tasks involving emotion situates the processing of emotion in relation to the processing of somatic information. This view (Damasio, 1994, 1995) stresses that emotion involves output to, and input from, the body (including visceral and

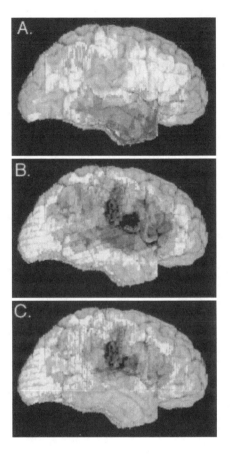

Figure 8.5. Right somatosensory sectors involved in retrieval of knowledge of the emotion signaled by facial expressions. We asked 25 subjects with focal right cortical lesions to rate facial expressions of emotion, and compared their ratings with those given by 15 normal controls. Data were mapped onto a normal reference brain, using a technique called MAP-3. Briefly, each subject's lesion was mapped onto the corresponding spatial location in the normal reference brain, and greyscale was used to encode the number of lesions from different subjects that overlapped at a given volumetric location. Overlaps from more subjects correspond to a darker shade of grey, whereas overlaps from only one or a few subjects correspond to lighter shades of grey. All computations were done using the software BRAINVOX (Frank, Damasio, & Grabowski, 1997) on Silicon Graphics workstations. (**A**) Lesions of all subjects who were normal in rating facial expressions of emotion. (**B**) Lesions of all subjects who were impaired in rating facial expressions of emotion. (**C**) Subtraction image (B–A) showing the difference in the lesion overlaps between all impaired subjects and all normal subjects. The subtraction revealed a focal, three-dimensional region that when damaged, always correlated with impaired task performance (dark region centered on somatosensory cortex). We thus infer that lesions that include this region result in impairments due to damage to this specific region. Detailed anatomical analyses showed that this region comprised the face representation of primary somatosensory cortex (SI), some of SII, possibly some insula and supramarginal gyrus, as well as considerable white matter, which may serve to connect visual cortical regions with somatosensory cortical regions. (Data are from Adolphs et al., 1996b.)

endocrine aspects). There is evidence that the right hemisphere is specialized for representing the body, as borne out by the finding that right hemisphere lesions, more often than left, can cause lack of awareness of one's own body state. It is quite conceivable that emotion and representation of the body co-evolved and that both are aspects of the same integrative, homeostatic function, which is relatively lateralized to the right hemisphere.

We can apply this framework to the interpretation of the results given in Figure 8.5: that lesions in the area of face representation in the right somatosensory cortex impair recognition of emotion in visually presented facial expressions. Briefly, we believe that subjects asked to perform the task of recognizing facial expressions of emotion will normally utilize a somatic image of the face. Given a facial expression to judge, a subject's normal strategy will include the central generation of a somatosensory image of the face corresponding to the expression seen. In essence, the subject approaches the task by asking, "how would I feel if I had this facial expression" (i.e., how would this face feel)? An apparently critical component of this strategy is the ability to form a mental somatosensory image that in turn can be used to trigger other knowledge in both image form and encoded in language that together permit normal responses on the task.

OTHER STRUCTURES

Several other neural structures are involved in knowledge about emotions, although discussion of these structures falls outside the scope of this chapter. There is considerable evidence that the frontal lobes, particularly their ventral sectors, are important to recognize emotions. Lesions in these regions impair the recognition of emotions in facial expressions and prosody (Hornak, Rolls, & Wade, 1996), and ventral frontal cortex and amygdala have been shown to operate as two components of a neural system for processing the reinforcing properties of stimuli (Gaffan, Murray, & Fabre-Thorpe, 1993). Additional structures important to emotion include the cingulate cortices, sectors of the basal ganglia, and monoaminergic/cholinergic nuclei that we mentioned at the beginning of this chapter. The interested reader is referred to Damasio (1995) for further discussion of other neural structures.

GOING BEYOND THE BRAIN

In closing, we wish to return to comments we made at the beginning: The subject matter of emotion pertains fundamentally to the survival value of interactions between organism and environment. The environment, in the case of higher vertebrates, includes the social environment. Emotions thus involve not only the survival of the organism in life and death situations, but also social survival among members of a group. In the case of humans, the social aspect assumes great importance, and it is impossible to do full justice to the topic of emotion without thinking about social development, social communication, and culture. These topics have been explored in detail by social psychologists and anthropologists, but, at this time, very little is known about the neural systems that are involved in social and cultural aspects of emotion (e.g., next to nothing is known about the neural underpinnings of so-called social emotions, such as jealousy, pride, and embarrassment).

One important direction for the future will be to expand our current account of emotion. We have a working framework of what emotion shares in common in all animals; the next task will be to elucidate what distinguishes emotion in humans from emotion in other animals. We consider it probable that regions of neocortex, especially in prefrontal cortex, will turn out to play a key role in those aspects of emotion that are uniquely human (Damasio, 1994). Ultimately, however, emotions, like other domains of the human mind, may be explained not solely as properties of individuals, but will be seen to arise from relations between multiple brains and their external environments, embedded in the context of a particular culture.

ACKNOWLEDGMENTS
This work was supported by a Sloan Research Fellowship and a FIRST award from NIMH to R.A. and by a program project grant from NINDS and a grant from the Mathers Foundation to A.R.D.

REFERENCES

Adelman, P.K., & Zajonc, R.B. (1989). Facial efference and the experience of emotion. *Annual Review of Psychology, 40,* 249–280.

Adolphs, R., Damasio, H., Tranel, D., & Damasio, A.R. (1996a). Cortical systems for the recognition of emotion in facial expressions. *Journal of Neuroscience, 16,* 7678–7687.

Adolphs, R., Damasio, H., Tranel, D., Frank, R., & Damasio, A.R. (1996b). The right second somatosensory cortex (S-II) is required to recognize emotional facial expressions in humans. *Society for Neuroscience Abstracts, 22,* 1854.

Adolphs, R., Cahill, L., Schul, R., & Babinsky, R. (1997a). Impaired declarative memory for emotional material following bilateral amygdala damage in humans. *Learning and Memory, 4,* 291–300.

Adolphs, R., Lee, G.P., Tranel, D., & Damasio, A.R. (1997b). Bilateral damage to the human amygdala early in life impairs knowledge of emotional arousal. *Society for Neuroscience Abstracts, 23,* 1582.

Adolphs, R., Russell, J.A., & Tranel, D. (1999). A role for the human amygdala in recognizing emotional arousal. *Psychological Science, 10,* 167–171.

Adolphs, R., Tranel, D., & Damasio, A.R. (1998). The human amygdala in social judgment. *Nature, 393,* 470–474.

Adolphs, R., Tranel, D., Damasio, H., & Damasio, A. (1994). Impaired recognition of emotion in facial expressions following bilateral damage to the human amygdala. *Nature*, *372*, 669–672.

Adolphs, R., Tranel, D., Damasio, H., & Damasio, A.R. (1995). Fear and the human amygdala. *Journal of Neuroscience*, *15*, 5879–5892.

Aggleton, J.P. (1992). The functional effects of amygdala lesions in humans: A comparison with findings from monkeys. In J.P. Aggleton (Ed.), *The Amygdala: Neurobiological Aspects of Emotion, Memory, and Mental Dysfunction* (pp. 485–504). New York: Wiley-Liss.

Amaral, D.G., Price, J.L., Pitkanen, A., & Carmichael, S.T. (1992). Anatomical organization of the primate amygdaloid complex. In J.P. Aggleton (Ed.), *The Amygdala: Neurobiological Aspects of Emotion, Memory, and Mental Dysfunction* (pp. 1–66). New York: Wiley-Liss.

Bechara, A., Tranel, D., Damasio, H., Adolphs, R., Rockland, C., & Damasio, A.R. (1995). Double dissociation of conditioning and declarative knowledge relative to the amygdala and hippocampus in humans. *Science*, *269*, 1115–1118.

Blonder, L.X., Bowers, D., & Heilman, K. (1991). The role of the right hemisphere in emotional communication. *Brain*, *114*, 1115–1127.

Borod, J.C. (1992). Interhemispheric and intrahemispheric control of emotion: A focus on unilateral brain damage. *Journal of Consulting and Clinical Psychology*, *60*, 339–348.

Borod, J.C. (1993a). Emotion and the brain—Anatomy and theory: An introduction to the special section. *Neuropsychology*, *7*, 427–432.

Borod, J.C. (1993b). Cerebral mechanisms underlying facial, prosodic, and lexical emotional expression: A review of neuropsychological studies and methodological issues. *Neuropsychology*, *7*, 445–463.

Borod, J.C., Andelman, F., Obler, L.K., Tweedy, J.R., & Welkowitz, J. (1992). Right hemisphere specializations for the identification of emotional words and sentences: Evidence from stroke patients. *Neuropsychologia*, *30*, 827–844.

Bowers, D., Bauer, R.M., Coslett, H.B., & Heilman, K.M. (1985). Processing of faces by patients with unilateral hemisphere lesions. *Brain and Cognition*, *4*, 258–272.

Bowers, D., Bauer, R.M., & Heilman, K.M. (1993). The nonverbal affect lexicon: Theoretical perspectives from neuropsychological studies of affect perception. *Neuropsychology*, *7*, 433–444.

Bowers, D., Blonder, L.X., Feinberg, T., & Heilman, K.M. (1991). Differential impact of right and left hemisphere lesions on facial emotion and object imagery. *Brain*, *114*, 2593–2609.

Bowers, D., Coslett, H.B., Bauer, R.M., Speedie, L.J., & Heilman, K.H. (1987). Comprehension of emotional prosody following unilateral hemispheric lesions: Processing defect versus distraction defect. *Neuropsychologia*, *25*, 317–328.

Breiter, H.C., Etcoff, N.L., et al. (1996). Response and habituation of the human amygdala during visual processing of facial expression. *Neuron*, *17*, 875–887.

Broks, P., Young, A.W., Maratos, E.J., Coffey, P.J., Calder, A.J., Isaac, C., Mayes, A.R., Hodges, J.R., Montaldi, D., Cezayirli, E., Roberts, N., & Hadley, D. (1998). Face processing impairments after encephalitis: Amygdala damage and recognition of fear. *Neuropsychologia*, *36*, 59–70.

Buechel, C., Morris, J., Dolan, R.J., & Friston, K.J. (1998). Brain systems mediating aversive conditioning: An event-related fMRI study. *Neuron*, *20*, 947–957.

Cacioppo, J.T., Berntson, G.G., & Klein, D.J. (1992). What is an emotion? The role of somatovisceral afference, with special emphasis on somatovisceral "illusions." In M.S. Clark (Ed.), *Emotion and Social Behavior*, Vol. 14 (pp. 63–98). Newbury Park, CA: Sage Publications.

Cahill, L., Haier, R.J., Fallon, J., Alkire, M.T., Tang, C., Keator, D., Wu, J., & McGaugh, J.L. (1996). Amygdala activity at encoding correlated with long-term, free recall of emotional information. *Proceedings of the National Academy of Sciences of the United States of America, 93*, 8016–8021.

Cahill, L., & McGaugh, J.L. (1998). Mechanisms of emotional arousal and lasting declarative memory. *Trends in Neuroscience, 21*, 294–299.

Calder, A.J., Young, A.W., Rowland, D., Perrett, D.I., Hodges, J.R., & Etcoff, N.L. (1996). Facial emotion recognition after bilateral amygdala damage: Differentially severe impairment of fear. *Cognitive Neuropsychology, 13*, 699–745.

Damasio, A.R. (1994). *Descartes' Error: Emotion, Reason, and the Human Brain*. New York: Grosset/Putnam.

Damasio, A.R. (1995). Toward a neurobiology of emotion and feeling: Operational concepts and hypotheses. *The Neuroscientist, 1*, 19–25.

Davidson, R.J. (1992). Anterior cerebral asymmetry and the nature of emotion. *Brain and Cognition, 6*, 245–268.

Davidson, R.J. (1993). Cerebral asymmetry and emotion: Conceptual and methodological conundrums. *Cognition and Emotion, 7*, 115–138.

Davis, M. (1992a). The role of the amygdala in conditioned fear. In J.P. Aggleton (Ed.), *The Amygdala: Neurobiological Aspects of Emotion, Memory, and Mental Dysfunction*, (pp. 255–306). New York: Wiley-Liss.

Davis, M. (1992b). The role of the amygdala in fear and anxiety. *Annual Review of Neuroscience, 15*, 353–375.

Dimberg, U. (1982). Facial reactions to facial expressions. *Psychophysiology, 19*, 643–647.

Ekman, P., & Davidson, R.J. (1993). Voluntary smiling changes regional brain activity. *Psychological Science, 4*, 342–345.

Ekman, P., & Friesen, W. (1976). *Pictures of Facial Affect*. Palo Alto, CA: Consulting Psychologists Press.

Frank, R.J., Damasio, H., & Grabowski, T.J. (1997). Brainvox: An interactive, multimodal visualization and analysis system for neuroanatomical imaging. *NeuroImage, 5*, 13–30.

Fredrikson, M., Wik, G., Annas, P., Ericson, K., & Stone-Elander, S. (1995). Functional neuroanatomy of visually elicited simple phobic fear: Additional data and theoretical analysis. *Psychophysiology, 32*, 43–48.

Fridlund, A.J. (1994). *Human Facial Expression*. New York: Academic Press.

Frijda, N.H. (1986). *The Emotions*. New York: Cambridge University Press.

Gaffan, D., Murray, E.A., & Fabre-Thorpe, M. (1993). Interaction of the amygdala with the frontal lobe in reward memory. *European Journal of Neuroscience, 5*, 968–975.

Gloor, P., Olivier, A., Quesney, L.F., Andermann, F., & Horowitz, S. (1982). The role of the limbic system in experiential phenomena of temporal lobe epilepsy. *Annals of Neurology, 12*, 129–144.

Griffiths, P.E. (1997). *What Emotions Really Are*. Chicago: University of Chicago Press.

Grusser, O.-J. (1984). Face recognition within the reach of neurobiology and beyond it. *Human Neurobiology, 3*, 183–190.

Gur, R.C., Skolnick, B.E., & Gur, R.E. (1994). Effects of emotional discrimination tasks on cerebral blood flow: Regional activation and its relation to performance. *Brain and Cognition, 25*, 271–286.

Halgren, E., Walter, R.D., Cherlow, D.G., & Crandall, P.H. (1978). Mental phenomena evoked by electrical stimulation of the human hippocampal formation and amygdala. *Brain, 101*, 83–117.

Hamann, S.B., Stefanacci, L., Squire, L.R., Adolphs, R., Tranel, D., Damasio, H., & Damasio, A. (1996). Recognizing facial emotion. *Nature, 379*, 497.

Hamilton, C.R., & Vermeire, B.A. (1988). Complementary hemispheric specialization in monkeys. *Science, 242*, 1691–1694.

Hauser, M.D. (1993). Right hemisphere dominance for the production of facial expression in monkeys. *Science, 261*, 475–477.

Heller, W. (1993). Neuropsychological mechanisms of individual differences in emotion, personality, and arousal. *Neuropsychology, 7*, 476–489.

Hornak, J., Rolls, E.T., & Wade, D. (1996). Face and voice expression identification in patients with emotional and behavioral changes following ventral frontal lobe damage. *Neuropsychologia, 34*, 247–261.

Kesner, R.P. (1992). Learning and memory in rats with an emphasis on the role of the amygdala. In J.P. Aggleton (Ed.), *The Amygdala: Neurobiological Aspects of Emotion, Memory, and Mental Dysfunction* (pp. 379–400). New York: Wiley.

Kling, A.S., & Brothers, L.A. (1992). The amygdala and social behavior. In J. P. Aggleton (Ed.), *The Amygdala: Neurobiological Aspects of Emotion, Memory, and Mental Dysfunction* (pp. 353–378). New York: Wiley-Liss.

LaBar, K.S., LeDoux, J.E., Spencer, D.D., & Phelps, E.A. (1995). Impaired fear conditioning following unilateral temporal lobectomy in humans. *Journal of Neuroscience, 15*, 6846–6855.

Lazarus, R.S. (1991). *Emotion and Adaptation.* New York: Oxford University Press.

Le Doux, J. (1996). *The Emotional Brain.* New York: Simon and Schuster.

Leonard, C.M., Rolls, E.T., Wilson, F.A.W., & Baylis, G.C. (1985). Neurons in the amygdala of the monkey with responses selective for faces. *Behavioral Brain Research, 15*, 159–176.

Levenson, R.W., Ekman, P., & Friesen, W.V. (1990). Voluntary facial action generates emotion-specific autonomic nervous system activity. *Psychophysiology, 27*, 363–384.

Markowitsch, H.J., Calabrese, P., Wuerker, M., Durwen, H.F., Kessler, J., Babinsky, R., Brechtelsbauer, D., Heuser, L., & Gehlen, W. (1994). The amygdala's contribution to memory—A study on two patients with Urbach-Wiethe disease. *NeuroReport, 5*, 1349–1352.

Morris, J.S., Frith, C.D., Perrett, D.I., Rowland, D., Young, A.W., Calder, A.J., & Dolan, R.J. (1996). A differential neural response in the human amygdala to fearful and happy facial expressions. *Nature, 383*, 812–815.

Morris, R.D., & Hopkins, W.D. (1993). Perception of human chimeric faces by chimpanzees: Evidence for a right hemisphere advantage. *Brain and Cognition, 21*, 111–122.

Muramoto, K., Ono, T., Nishijo, H., & Fukuda, M. (1993). Rat amygdaloid neuron responses during auditory discrimination. *Neuroscience, 52*, 621–636.

Nakamura, K., Mikami, A., & Kubota, K. (1992). Activity of single neurons in the monkey amygdala during performance of a visual discrimination task. *Journal of Neurophysiology, 67*, 1447–1463.

Nishijo, H., Ono, T., & Nishino, H. (1988). Single neuron responses in amygdala of alert monkey during complex sensory stimulation with affective significance. *Journal of Neurosciences, 8*, 3570–3583.

Ojemann, J.G., Ojemann, G.A., & Lettich, E. (1992). Neuronal activity related to faces and matching in human right nondominant temporal cortex. *Brain, 115*, 1–13.

Phelps, E.A., & Anderson, A.K. (1997). What does the amygdala do? *Current Biology, 7*, R311–R314.

Plutchik, R. (1980). *Emotion: A Psychoevolutionary Synthesis*. New York: Harper and Row.

Rapcsak, S.Z., Kaszniak, A.W., & Rubens, A.B. (1989). Anomia for facial expressions: Evidence for a category specific visual–verbal disconnection syndrome. *Neuropsychologia, 27*, 1031–1041.

Ringo, J.L., Doty, R.W., Demeter, S., & Simard, P.Y. (1994). Time is of the essence: A conjecture that hemispheric specialization arises from interhemispheric conduction delay. *Cerebral Cortex, 4*, 331–343.

Rolls, E.T. (1992). Neurophysiology and functions of the primate amygdala. In J.P. Aggleton (Ed.), *The Amygdala: Neurobiological Aspects of Emotion, Memory, and Mental Dysfunction*. New York: John Wiley.

Rosenberg, E.L., & Ekman, P. (1994). Coherence between expressive and experiential systems in emotion. *Cognition and Emotion, 8*, 201–230.

Ross, E.D. (1985). Modulation of affect and nonverbal communication by the right hemisphere. In M.-M. Mesulam (Ed.), *Principles of Behavioral Neurology* (pp. 239–258). Philadelphia: F.A. Davis.

Schneider, F., Gur, R.C., Gur, R.E., & Muenz, L.R. (1994). Standardized mood induction with happy and sad facial expressions. *Psychiatry Research, 51*, 19–31.

Silberman, E.K., & Weingartner, H. (1986). Hemispheric lateralization of functions related to emotion. *Brain and Cognition, 5*, 322–353.

Tranel, D., & Damasio, A.R. (1993). The covert learning of affective valence does not require structures in hippocampal system or amygdala. *Journal of Cognitive Neuroscience, 5*, 79–88.

Tranel, D., & Hyman, B.T. (1990). Neuropsychological correlates of bilateral amygdala damage. *Archives of Neurology, 47*, 349–355.

Van Strien, J.W., & Morpurgo, M. (1992). Opposite hemispheric activations as a result of emotionally threatening and non-threatening words. *Neuropsychologia, 30*, 845–848.

Weiskrantz, L. (1956). Behavioral changes associated with ablation of the amygdaloid complex in monkeys. *Journal of Comparative Physiology and Psychology, 49*, 381–391.

Young, A.W., Aggleton, J.P., Hellawell, D.J., Johnson, M., Broks, P., & Hanley, J.R. (1995). Face processing impairments after amygdalotomy. *Brain, 118*, 15–24.

Young, A.W., Hellawell, D.J., Van de Wal, C., & Johnson, M. (1996). Facial expression processing after amygdalotomy. *Neuropsychologia, 34*, 31–39.

9

Neuropsychological Theories of Emotion

GUIDO GAINOTTI

HISTORICAL DEVELOPMENT

The expression "neuropsychological theories of emotion" refers to the set of theoretical models that have accompanied and oriented clinical and experimental studies aiming to clarify the relationships between emotions and the brain. Neuropsychological theories of emotion have been largely influenced by two factors, on the one hand, by more general psychological and neurobiological models, and on the other hand, by the characteristicts of emotions and of brain structures taken as models in studies conducted on specific subjects in a given historical period.

As for psychological theories of emotion (analyzed in detail in this volume by Scherer, Chapter 6), they have always influenced from two complementary points of view studies aiming to clarify the problem of the representation and organization of emotions in the human brain. From the first viewpoint, the representation of emotions is considered as a loosely organized and fuzzily demarcated behavioral system. Studies conducted along this line have basically tried to determine if data obtained by neuropsychological investigations can be better explained by making reference to the organizing principle of the emotional dimensions (arousal level, emotional valence, motoric direction, and so on) or to that of the discrete emotional categories. The second viewpoint focuses on the componential nature of emotions, aiming to determine whether the clinical data point to the existence of a "central processor" of emotions or whether instead lesions tend to selectively affect one or another of a set of emotional components (e.g., emotional computation of sensory data, emotional expression, autonomic response, emotional experience, and so on), showing that they are subserved by different parts of the brain.

As for the kinds of emotions and brain structures used as models in different historical periods, the first studies conducted in this area by Goltz (1892), Woodworth and Sherrington (1904), Dusser de Barenne (1920), Bazett and Penfield (1922), and others were directed at rather primitive emotions, such as rage and fear, and at the contrasting effects on cognitive and emotional functions produced by a lesion of cortical versus subcortical structures. The underlying model was, therefore, that of substantial independence between emotional and cognitive functions in the animal brain. Furthermore, the anatomicoclinical observation that involuntary and uncontrollable emotional outbursts can be observed in patients with multiple lesions of the corticodiencephalic pathways allowed two further conclusions: (1) that this model may also apply to humans, and (2) that in both animals and humans, cortical areas control the subcortical structures subserving the basic emotional mechanisms.

Studies Focused on Subcortical Structures Subserving the Basic Emotional Mechanisms

In an effort to identify the subcortical structures that are crucially involved in emotional expression, Bard (1928, 1929) proposed that the hypothalamus may play a critical role in emotions. It must be acknowledged, indeed, that his model was influenced by experiments showing that electrical stimulation of the hypothalamus produces a sustained sympathetic arousal (Karplus & Kreidl, 1909, 1927) and by the fact that the emotion considered by Bard, namely rage, is characterized by a strong sympathetic arousal. Nevertheless, Bard's model was considered valid for emotions in general and oriented the attention of investigators toward the arousal dimension of emotion. The discovery by Moruzzi and Magoun (1949) that the ascending reticular activating system plays a crucial role in arousal functions had, therefore, a profound influence not only on neurobiological models of the mind in general but also on more specific neuropsychological theories of emotion.

Several authors (e.g., Duffy, 1962; Lindsey, 1951) were, in fact, led to assume that the structures subserving the arousal mechanisms also subserve the central and peripheral components of emotions. In contrast, the much more complex and articulated anatomical model of emotions proposed by Papez (1937) suggested that different parts of the brain may mediate different components of emotions. To be sure, Papez proposed (1) that the hypothalamus, the anterior thalamic nuclei, the cingulate gyrus, the hippocampus, and their interconnections may constitute a harmonious mechanism that elaborates the functions of central emotions and participate in emotional expression; and (2) that the hypothalamic component of the circuit might be mainly involved in functions of emotional evaluation and of emotional expression, whereas the cortical component (namely, the cingulate gyrus) might be involved in the elaboration of emotional experience.

The Papez model, suggesting that the psychological complexity of emotions should correspond to an equally complex anatomical organization, was further developed by McLean (1949, 1961), who coined the term "limbic system" to denote a highly interconnected set of subcortical and cortical structures, mainly involved in vegetative and emotional functions. McLean (1986) further pushed the analogy between the intrinsic organization of the emotional system and the anatomical organization of the limbic system by suggesting that both systems may be characterized by a phylogenetically determined hierarchical organization. According to McLean (1986), the most primitive, drive-related forms of behavior (such as the fight–flight reactions), which are present in phylogenetically old species such as the reptilians, would be subsumed by the hypothalamus and by the related parts of the paleostriatum. In contrast, the family-related patterns of behavior (namely, nursing in connection with maternal care, audiovocal communication for maternal–offspring contact, and play), which are characteristic only of mammals, would be subserved by the cingulate gyrus, which is the phylogenetically more recent part of the limbic system.

Studies on Hemispheric Asymmetries in Emotional Representation

A set of different neuropsychological models have been advanced more recently based on data suggesting that not only the cortical/subcortical (or the limbic/nonlimbic) dichotomy, but also the right hemisphere/left hemisphere distinction, could be relevant to understanding the cerebral organization of emotions. Some of these models (influenced in part by the importance attributed to cognitive factors in contemporary psychological theories of emotions) propose that the different cognitive styles of the right and left hemispheres may subserve this interhemispheric difference. Tucker (1981, 1989) has suggested, for example, that two cognitive features could favor the right, rather than the left, hemisphere in the processing of emotional information: (1) the tendency to represent experience in an analogical (rather than in an arbitrary verbal) code; and (2) the ability to integrate information in a syncretic and holistic manner rather than treating it in a sequential, analytical fashion.

Following a similar line of thought, Ross (1981, 1984) has proposed that the right hemisphere dominance for emotions (documented by many clinical and experimental data) may basically concern the communicative (rather than other more elementary) components of emotions.

Other interpretations of the hemispheric asymmetries in emotional processing have, on the contrary, been suggested by the different emotional behaviors shown by patients subjected to pharmacological inactivation of the right and left hemisphere (Alemà & Donini, 1960; Perria, Rosadini, & Rossi, 1961; Terzian & Cecotto, 1959). The earliest proponents of these models (Davidson et al., 1979; Davidson & Fox, 1982; Rossi & Rosadini, 1967; Sackeim et al., 1982; Terzian & Ceccotto, 1959) argued that a neuropsychological model of emotional valence could explain many clinical and experimental data assuming a left-hemisphere dominance for "positive" emotions and a right-hemisphere prevalence for "negative" emotions. More recent formulations of the same theory (Davidson, 1984, 1992; Davidson & Tomarken, 1989; Davidson et al., 1990) have shifted attention from the positive–negative to the approach–withdrawal dimension, which is considered to be similar to the pleasantness dimension but could actually be more consistent with some clinical and experimental data (for detailed accounts of the various formulations of the "valence hypothesis," see Borod, 1992; Davidson, 1993; Heller, 1993).

Other more biologically oriented neuropsychological theories of emotion have recently assumed that a phylogenetically determined hierarchical principle might explain the different representations of emotions at the levels of the right and left hemispheres. Thus, Ross et al. (1994) have proposed that the most primitive forms of emotions, which usually have a negative valence, might be more strongly represented in the right hemisphere, whereas the most phylogenetically advanced social forms of emotion might be mostly represented in the left hemisphere. In contrast, Gainotti, Caltagirone, and Zoccolotti (1993; see also Gainotti, 1994, 1997) have proposed that the hierarchical principle that regulates the different representations of emotion in the right and left hemispheres may concern different levels of emotional processing rather than different categories of emotions.

The psychological model taken as reference by Gainotti et al. was Leventhal's view (see Leventhal, 1979, 1984; Leventhal & Scherer, 1987) of emotions as a hierarchically organized multilevel processing system. According to Leventhal, this system has at bottom a basic set of innate neuromotor programs, at an intermediate level a set of learned automatic emotional schemata, and at the top a processing system subserving functions of emotional conceptualization and emotional control. Gainotti et al. suggested that the schematic level of emotional processing may be mainly subserved by the right hemisphere and that the level of emotional conceptualization and control might be mostly subsumed by the left hemisphere.

Although space does not allow me to develop all the problems sketched in this short historical introduction, I do dwell in more detail on some of them in ensuing sections of this chapter. In particular, the issues that I take into account, because they play a critical role in neuropsychological theories of emotions, concern (1) the relationships between the emotional and the cognitive systems, (2) the main features that distinguish the emotional from the cognitive system, (3) the componential nature of emotions, and (4) the hierarchical organization of the emotional processing system. In my attempt to discuss these basic issues, I try to focus attention more on human than on animal studies and to consider most of the brain structures (or the main anatomical variables) that have attracted the attention of authors interested in the study of the brain–emotion relationships instead of focusing on just one.

CURRENT NEUROPSYCHOLOGICAL THEORIES OF HUMAN EMOTION

Shifts in Basic Assumptions About the Relationships Between Emotional and Cognitive Systems

Implicit or explicit assumptions about the relationships between emotional and cognitive systems changed considerably as studies of brain–emotions relationships developed. In the earliest studies two sets of data had attracted the investigators' attention: (1) the contrast between cognitive disorders resulting from lesions of cortical areas and emotional disorders resulting from lesions of subcortical structures, and (2) the observation that integrated emotional outbursts can be observed after disconnection of subcortical structures (subserving emotional expression) from the influence of cortical inhibitory areas. The neuropsychological models underlying these observations assumed that emotional and cognitive functions are subserved by different brain structures and that the cognitive system usually keeps the emotional system under control so that impulsive and socially disruptive forms of emotional response do not assume control of overt behavior.

During several decades, the assumption that elementary emotional mechanisms may be subserved by some subcortical brain structures seemed to be confirmed by the observation that behavioral manifestations of emotions can be obtained by stimulation of subcortical structures, such as the hypothalamus, the septal nuclei, and the amygdala (for reviews, see Brodal, 1981; Buck, 1976; Macchi, 1989). The fact that similar expressive emotional displays could be obtained by stimulation of cortical areas (such as the cingulate or the parahippocampal gyrus) was not considered to be inconsistent with the hypothesis of subcortical localization of the basic emotional mechanisms because these emotional manifestations were interpreted as due to the afterdischarge provoked by the cortical stimulation over the above-mentioned subcortical structures. Thus, the only change in this general model until the 1970s was a progressive increase in the importance attributed to the amygdala for various aspects of emotional behavior, with a correlative decrease in the role attributed to the hypothalamus for these functions (but see Panksepp [1982] for a different viewpoint).

Furthermore, results of animal studies showing that electrical stimulation of the amygdala usually provokes strong fear and anger reactions (Delgado, 1960; Kaada, 1951; McLean & Delgado, 1953; Ursin & Kaada, 1960) were extrapolated to humans, due to the observation that patients with epileptic foci localized in the mesial parts of the temporal lobe often experience critical emotional phenomena characterized by fear.

The neuropsychological model assuming that the basic command systems for primitive fear–anger emotions are located in the amygdala became very popular and had important medical and social implications. It was, in fact, assumed that many instances of aggressive behavior were due, in epileptic patients, to the direct action of a focus firing within the amygdala (Falconer et al., 1958; Geschwind, 1974; Treffert, 1964; Walker, 1973) and that even non-ictal manifestations of aggression or of sociopathic behavior could result from a chronic stimulation of the amygdala from a patent or covert epileptic focus (Walker, 1973). Even though more carefully controlled investigations by Gloor (1967), Ounstead (1969), Gunn and Bonn (1971), and Rodin (1973) failed to confirm the relationship between temporal lobe epilepsy and ictal or interictal aggressive behavior, the model survived, leading to the development of neurosurgical strategies for treatment and control of aggressive behavior (Valenstein, 1973).

In more recent years, the model assuming that emotional and cognitive functions must be subserved by quite different anatomical structures (and that the amygdala may house elementary emotional mechanisms) has been in part reconsidered and substituted with the assumption that, at least in humans, emotional and cognitive functions must be strongly reciprocally interconnected.

This new theoretical approach has been motivated by several factors. The most important of these is the influence exerted by psychological theories of emotion (Frijda, 1986, 1987; Lazarus, 1982, 1984; Scherer, 1984; see also Scherer, Chapter 6, this volume) which have consistently claimed that a process of cognitive appraisal constitutes the necessary prerequisite of any emotional event. A second factor, discussed earlier, is the discovery that emotions are not equally represented in the right and left hemispheres and the hypothesis that this asymmetrical representation of emotions may be basically due to cognitive factors. Finally, the hypothesis of an integrated, rather than of an independent, representation of the emotional and cognitive systems has been strengthened by more careful analyses of the effects of amygdala stimulation in humans. These studies, recently reviewed by Halgren (1991) and Gloor (1990), have consistently shown that the quality of experiential phenomena provoked by stimulation of the amygdala or other temporolimbic structures is not related to the exact electrode position but rather to the personality and the ongoing psychological problems of the patient.

The amygdala is, therefore, considered by some researchers to be an essential point of integration of cognitive representations with affective significance rather than as a structure subserving basic emotional mechanisms. On the other hand, if in our search for structures in humans that house these basic emotional mechanisms, we come back from the amygdala to the hypothalamus, we see that lesions of this structure do not disrupt proper emotional functions. In a well-controlled neuropsychological investigation, Weddell (1994) has, in fact, recently shown that in patients with hypothalamic tumors, autonomic and endocrinological disorders are very common, survival–appetitive disorders (concerning eating, drinking, and sexual behavior) are less frequent, but still common, whereas personality disturbances and disorders of social–emotional communication are very rare.

Both the amygdala and the hypothalamus seem, therefore, to subserve only some fragments of the complex repertoire of physiological and behavioral patterns that characterize the emotional schemata. To be sure, in humans, the amygdala seems to play a prominent role in complex situations that require the integration of emotional and cognitive functions, whereas the hypothalamus seems to regulate much more elementary autonomic and endocrinological functions as well as basic survival–appetitive behaviors that are usually considered apart from the properly emotional system.

Taken together, these data seem to suggest that emotions must be considered as a multicomponent adaptive system spanning from very primitive and hard-wired survival-related behavioral schemata to much more complex and learned behavioral patterns, highly integrated with the cognitive system. The points, that play a crucial role in this tentative general interpretation of the emotional system and that, I intend to discuss in the next sections of this chapter mainly concern (1) the defining features of emotions, with special emphasis on the distinction between emotional and cognitive systems; (2) the componential nature of the emotional processing system; and (3) the hierarchical organization of emotions and the integration between emotional and cognitive systems.

The Defining Features of Emotions and the Distinction Between Emotional and Cognitive Systems

Several authors have tried to identify some points of reference with which to differentiate the behavioral schemata belonging to the conceptual field of emotions from those belonging to contiguous but different conceptual areas. One very simple reference axis could be the duration of the behavioral pattern at issue. According to Ekman (1984), who has tried to analyze the problem with reference to this axis, emotions are reactions that last several seconds and must be differentiated from both very brief responses (such as the reflex reactions) and long-lasting behavioral schemata (such as affects or personality traits).

A second important reference axis, which is more clearly linked with the main line of thought followed in this chapter, refers to the complexity and the level of phylogenetic development typical of the behavioral pattern taken into account. From this point of view, emotions are behavioral reactions with an intermediate level of complexity and can, therefore, be distinguished by (1) very simple, primitive, and hard-wired behavioral patterns (such as reflex responses or some basic survival-related appetitive behaviors), and (2) more complex and learned cognitive activities.

Because the most important controversies regarding human emotion, such as the debate between Zajonc (1980, 1984) and Lazarus (1982, 1984), have concerned the interface between the emotional system and the cognitive system, I discuss here the main similarities and differences between the two. For simplicity, it could be said that the general architectures of the two systems are similar, but their specific scopes are different. As for the structural similarities, most authors (e.g., Ekman, 1984; Gainotti, 1989, 1994; Leventhal, 1984; Oatley & Johnson-Laird, 1985, 1987; Scherer, 1984) consider both the emotional and the cognitive system as phylogenetically advanced adaptive systems based on integrated work with several components aimed at (1) scanning the external milieu, (2) selecting and analyzing the most relevant stimuli, (3) providing an appropriate response to these stimuli, and (4) learning to give a subjective (emotional) or objective (cognitive) meaning to these stimuli. As for the different scopes of the emotional and cognitive systems, they will be considered first by looking at the general logic of each system. The model proposed by Oatley and Johnson-Laird (1985, 1987) is appropriate from this point of view because it suggests that the organism has at its disposal two operative (the emotional and the cognitive) systems to face a partially unpredictable environment. The emotional system is viewed, within this model, as an emergency system capable of interrupting ongoing action with an urgency procedure to rapidly select a new operative scheme. The cognitive system is considered, on the contrary, to be a more complex and advanced adaptive system, capable of exhaustively processing complicated situations and elaborating the strategies required to solve the problems raised by the situations but needing much more time to carry out its work. According to Oatley and Johnson-Laird (1985, 1987), the emotional system is based on a certain number of modules (automata) that rapidly and automatically process a restricted number of signals and trigger an immediate response, whereas the cognitive system is based on more sophisticated modules and is supported by a propositional structure, which allows a conscious and controlled analysis of information and the selection of appropriate strategies. The major characteristics that distinguish the emotional from the cognitive system are listed in Table 9.1.

The Componential Nature of the Emotional Processing System

The data in Table 9.1 introduce the problem of the componential nature of emotions by showing that the specific scope of the emotional system strongly influences the manner in which this system processes ongoing information, selects the most appropriate behavioral responses, learns to attribute meaning to a stimulus category, and so on.

Table 9.1. Main Differences Existing Between the Emotional and the
Cognitive Systems

BEHAVIORAL OR COGNITIVE DOMAIN	EMOTIONAL SYSTEM	COGNITIVE SYSTEM
Scanning of the external milieu and orientation of attention	Automatic orientation elicited by external stimuli	Intentional orientation of attention at least, in part, determined by internal representations
Analysis of sensory data and computation of stimulus significance	Quick computation of crude, poorly processed sensory data leading to a direct motor response	Exhaustive but slower computation of highly processed information; leads to gathering of further information about the stimulus
Behavioral motor response	Immediately selected from a small number of innate operative patterns corresponding to the basic needs of the species in question; intervenes with an emergency procedure, making very probable the achievement of the operative pattern selected	The selection of the operative strategy results from a thorough analysis of the external situation and of information stored in long-term memory; often requires the inhibition of the most spontaneous motor response
Learning mechanisms	Based on conditioned, automatic, and unconscious learning	Based on controlled and conscious acquisition of information in declarative memory
Level of autonomic activation	A high activation of the autonomic nervous system is a basic component of emotions	A high level of autonomic activation can disturb the good functioning of the cognitive system

From the neuropsychological point of view, this functional architecture of the emotional system raises the problem of the relationships between specific components of emotions and underlying brain structures. Some efforts have therefore been made, in both animal and human studies, to map the main components of emotion to discrete brain structures, and some of these studies have yielded convincing results. In particular, several authors (e.g., Adolphs et al., 1994, 1995; Calder et al., 1996; Downer, 1961; Fuster & Uyeda, 1971; Jones & Mishkin, 1972; Nishijo, Ono, & Nishino, 1988; Ono et al., 1973; Young et al., 1995) have shown that the amygdala could be the structure where the external stimuli are computed by the emotional system. Furthermore, LeDoux (1986, 1987, 1989, 1993) has convincingly shown that the qualitative features of the emotional computation of sensory data reported in Table 9.1 could be explained on the basis of anatomical reasons, namely, the direct links existing between the thalamus and the amygdala. Even the strongest supporters of the "cognitive" theories of emotions, such as Mandler (1980) and Lazarus (1982, 1984), agree that a global, rapid, and unconscious computation is sufficient to evaluate if an external situation can have a dangerous or a pleasant meaning for the individual. The subcortical route directly linking the thalamus with the amygdala could transmit to this structure the crude, poorly processed sensory data needed to make this sort of computation immediately.

Other authors have shown that the hypothalamus could be crucially involved in the regulation of the autonomic components of emotions (for reviews, see LeDoux, 1987; Smith & DeVito, 1984), and these data have been recently confirmed by the study of Weddell (1994) on patients with brain tumors selectively involving the hypothalamus or other brain structures, discussed earlier.

Less clear-cut are data concerning other structures usually considered to be involved in the expression of emotions or in the control of their spontaneous expression. Thus, the ventral striatum, the ventral pallidum, and more generally the basal ganglia have been considered to be involved in the execution of the emotional responses for both anatomical and clinical reasons. From the anatomical point of view, these structures receive strong afferents from the amygdala, the hippocampus, and other limbic structures and send projections to cortical, subcortical, and brain stem components of the motor system (De Long et al., 1984; Graybiel, 1984; Krettek & Price, 1978; Mogenson, 1987; Nauta & Domesick, 1984). From the clinical point of view, patients with a degenerative disease of the basal ganglia (e.g., Parkinson's disease) typically have "masked facies," that is, a reduced propensity to make spontaneous facial emotional expressions (Brozgold et al., 1998; Buck & Duffy, 1980; Katsikitis & Pilowsky, 1991; Smith, Smith, & Ellgring, 1996) and a similar inability to communicate affects with the prosodic contours of speech (Borod et al., 1990; Critchley, 1981). Furthermore, analogous defects in facial and vocal expression of emotions have been reported by some authors (e.g., Cancelliere & Kertesz, 1990; Cohen, Riccio, & Flannery, 1994) in stroke patients with lesions involving the basal ganglia. The specificity of these expressive emotional disturbances, however, has been questioned by studies showing that not only the expression but also the comprehension of emotional stimuli is impaired in patients with vascular (Cancelliere & Kertesz, 1990), neoplastic (Weddell, 1994), or degenerative (Blonder, Gur, & Gur, 1989; Speedie et al., 1990) disease of the basal ganglia.

A very similar picture can be obtained if we pass from the basal ganglia to the frontal lobes (and in particular to the fronto-orbital cortex), which, according to most authors, play a major role in the intentional control of the emotional expressive apparatus and in the inhibition of socially unacceptable emotional displays (for review, see Stuss & Benson, 1986).

Recent neuropsychological investigations have, in fact, confirmed that patients with frontal lobe damage are very impaired in the production of facial emotional expressions, both intentionally (Caltagirone et al., 1989a; Weddell, Miller, & Trevarthen, 1990) and in response to emotional stimuli (Borod et al., 1985; Weddell, Miller, & Trevarthen, 1988). As in the case of studies conducted on patients with lesions involving the basal ganglia, however, the specificity of expressive emotional defects resulting from frontal lobe injury is at present also controversial. Although some studies have shown that a lesion of the frontal lobes does not significantly affect the comprehension of facial emotional expressions (Kolb & Taylor, 1981; Prigatano & Pribram, 1982), other authors have shown that frontal lesions may influence not only the production but also the comprehension of facial emotional expressions (Hornak, Rolls, & Wade, 1996; Weddell, 1989, 1994). The theoretical problem raised by these data could be very important because both the frontal lobes and the basal ganglia are usually considered to be components of the motor/executive system rather than of other systems involved in the processing of (emotional or cognitive) information.

A conservative position could, therefore, consist of assuming that methodological reasons (concerning either the patients or the material used to test the comprehension of emotional material), in part, explain these unexpected data. As a matter of fact, a methodological problem common to all the tasks used to investigate the comprehension of emotional stimuli in brain-damaged patients is the fact that the kind of information processing requested by these tasks corresponds much more to a cognitive than to an emotional computation. Almost all these tasks, in fact, require one to decide if the emotion expressed by a given face or a given voice belongs, for example, to the category "fear" or to the category "anger," but this kind of computation of the sensory data can hardly be considered as emotional if we refer to the criteria reported in Table 9.1. Furthermore, because the expressive features that allow this sort of categorization are generally unknown to the patients, emotional comprehension tasks often are both perceptually and cognitively demanding. Taken together, these reasons suggest that results obtained from emotional comprehension tasks performed by brain-damaged patients be interpreted with caution.

The Hierarchical Organization of the Emotional System

I have repeatedly made a number of assumptions in this chapter based implicitly on a neurobiological model of emotion whose main points can be summarized as follows:

(1) Emotion must be considered as a nonhomogeneous, hierarchically organized, multicomponent adaptive system. (2) This system has partly changed its

nature during phylogenetic evolution because it originally had the functions of an automatic emergency system but later developed more and more important links with the propositional cognitive system. (*3*) Behavioral patterns included under the heading of "emotion" span, accordingly, from a small set of hard-wired survival-related behavioral schemata, mainly related to social interactions, to a large number of learned complex behavioral patterns, highly integrated with the cognitive system. (*4*) The neuropsychological theories of emotion discussed in this chapter often differ as a function of the lower (automatic) or higher (more cognitive) part of the emotional system taken into account by different authors.

This neurobiological model of emotion finds its psychological counterpart in the perceptual-motor theory of emotion developed by Leventhal (1974, 1979, 1984), which makes the following assumptions: (*1*) Every emotion is formed by different components and is based on operations arising at various levels. (2) The emotional processing system is hierarchically organized. (*3*) This hierarchical organization is the result of a construction made by the individual during his developmental history. According to Leventhal, the lowest level of the system is formed by a set of innate neuromotor programs. Each of these programs corresponds to a basic emotion and generates a specific pattern of expressive (behavioral and autonomic) reactions and of concomitant subjective feelings in response to specific releasing stimuli. With the individual's ontogenetic development, this basic sensorimotor structure becomes incorporated into two different memory systems corresponding to two different levels of emotional processing: the schematic level and the conceptual level. The schematic level is based on a mechanism of conditioned learning and is formed by the analog records of the conditions in which a given environmental situation has been associated with the generation of a given neuromotor program (and of the corresponding emotional experience). Memories stored in this system are, therefore, formed by the syncretic association between a given stimulus and the resulting expressive reaction, including the concomitant subjective feelings. These memories are automatically reactivated during a new encounter with the eliciting situation, generating a spontaneous, felt emotion.

The conceptual level, on the other hand, is based on the functioning of the semantic declarative memory system and contains a set of abstract propositions about emotions rather than a set of felt memories. These abstract propositions mainly concern stored knowledge about emotion-provoking situations and social rules stating how to respond appropriately (i.e., deliberately rather than spontaneously) to these situations. This system is, therefore, involved in the cognitive evaluation of the emotional meaning of complex situations and in the development of intentional control over the emotional expressive apparatus. Even if, according to Leventhal, both the schematic and the conceptual levels are involved in each emotional response and only the degree of their involvement varies according to individual and sociocultural factors, the neuroanatomical substrates of these two levels should be different. The schematic level should mainly rely on

subcortical circuits and structures (and in particular on the interconnections between the hypothalamus and amygdala), whereas the conceptual level should be
mostly based on the cortical functions of cognitive appraisal and of behavioral
control. Some authors have, however, suggested that this could not be the whole
story and that, in addition to the distinction between subcortical and cortical structures, one should also consider the differences between the right and left hemispheres in this search for the neuroanatomical substrates of the schematic and
conceptual levels of emotional processing.

To be sure, Buck (1984), Gainotti, Caltagirone, and Zoccolotti (1993), and
Lamendella (1977) have suggested that the two sides of the brain could play a
complementary role in emotional behavior, the right hemisphere being more involved in the automatic (expressive and autonomic) components of emotion and
the left hemisphere in functions of control and of modulation of spontaneous
emotional expression.

Data suggesting that the right hemisphere may have a prominent role in various aspects of emotional behavior, and in particular in the generation of the expressive and autonomic components of spontaneous emotions, have been reviewed
elsewhere (e.g., Borod, 1993; Borod, Santschi Haywood, & Koff, 1997; Gainotti,
1996, 1997; Gainotti, Caltagirone, & Zoccolotti, 1993; Wittling, 1995). I therefore do not think it necessary to take them into account here. I think it useful, on
the contrary, to briefly discuss the complementary hypothesis that assumes that
the left hemisphere may play a critical role in functions of emotional control.

Three independent lines of evidence seem to support this hypothesis. The first
is the observation that left brain–damaged patients (and in particular those with
Broca's aphasia) often show an excess of emotional reactivity, which renders them
at least, in part, similar to patients with bilateral corticobulbar lesions. This similarity has been pointed out by Horenstein (1970) and by Gainotti (1972, 1983).
The former stressed the emotional lability of aphasic patients, noting that they easily cry when exposed to (happy or sad) emotionally laden stimuli. The latter noted
that the sudden crying spells of patients with Broca's aphasia resemble in some
ways the paroxysmal outbursts of crying of patients with a pseudobulbar state. This
clinical impression has been studied more thoroughly by House et al. (1989), who
focused on the manifestations of emotionalism in stroke patients. These authors
showed that sudden episodes of uncontrollable outbursts of crying are often observed in patients with left frontal lesions, suggesting that the anterior regions of
the left hemisphere may play a critical role in functions of emotional control.

The second line of evidence consists of the observation, reported by Heilman,
Schwartz, and Watson (1978) and by Meadows and Kaplan (1994), that the vegetative (electrodermal) response to emotional stimuli is higher in left brain–
damaged patients than in normal controls. Although these data have not been
confirmed by other authors (e.g., Caltagirone et al., 1989b, Morrow et al., 1981;
Zoccolotti et al., 1986), they suggest that, at least in certain groups of left

brain–damaged patients, the defect of cortical control may provoke not only an accentuation of the expressive behavioral reaction but also an increased vegetative response to emotional stimuli.

Finally, a third group of data that could be compatible with the hypothesis of left hemisphere dominance for the intentional control of the facial expressive apparatus is the difference between the right and left halves of the face in the production of positive and negative emotional expressions. Although most authors who have studied this problem have shown a greater expressivity of the left hemiface for all types of emotions (for reviews, see Borod & Koff, 1984; Borod, Santschi Haywood, & Koff, 1997; Gainotti, 1989), some authors have shown greater expressivity of the left (with respect to the right) hemiface for negative emotions but not for smiling or for other positive emotions (Borod & Caron, 1980; Sackeim & Gur, 1978; Schwartz, Ahern, & Brown, 1979). The literature dealing with normal adult facial asymmetry during emotional expression and with the stronger asymmetries found for negative emotions has been reviewed in detail by Borod, Santschi Haywood, and Koff (1997).

These data have generally been discussed in the context of the hypothesis that assumes different hemispheric specialization for positive and negative emotions, but Etcoff (1986) has rightly noted that there are other possible interpretative contexts. Smiling differs, in fact, from other emotional facial expressions not only because of the positive polarity of the emotion it usually expresses but also because it represents the emotional facial expression easiest to reproduce voluntarily and most currently used for approach and for social communication. A dominance of the left hemisphere in the intentional control of the expressive facial apparatus could, therefore, counterbalance the "natural" expressivity of the left hemiface, resulting from the general superiority of the right hemisphere in the spontaneous expression of emotions. A very similar interpretation of the differences between the right and left halves of the face in the expressions of positive and negative emotions has been advanced by Buck (1984) and by Rinn (1984) in a model that also stresses the possible dominance of the left hemisphere for functions of emotional control. According to these authors, the greater asymmetry between the left and right halves of the face in the expression of negative emotions could be due to the greater inhibition exerted in this case on the right half of the face by the left hemisphere to attenuate the overt expression of socially censurable negative emotions. The lesser degree of asymmetry presented by smiling could be due to the fact that this form of "emotional" expression is used for social purposes and is not inhibited by the left hemisphere.

Possible Relationships Between the Left/Right and the Cortical/Subcortical Dichotomies in the Study of Human Emotion

Studies of hemispheric asymmetries in representation and control of emotions (and in particular the model assuming right-hemisphere dominance for automatic, spontaneous emotions and left-hemisphere prevalence for emotional control) raise some important questions about the relationships between hemispheric and sub-cortical levels of emotional representation. With reference to the excellent chapter of Tucker, Derryberry, and Luu (Chapter 6, this volume), which underlines the strong interactions that develop between cortical and subcortical mechanisms during the process of encephalization, we could ask if hemispheric asymmetries in representation and control of emotions are mostly due to asymmetrical bottom-up or top-down processes.

In the first case, the hemispheric asymmetries for emotional functions could be due to a greater emotional involvement of the right-hemisphere subcortical structures, whereas in the second case, they could be due to a left-hemisphere cortical dominance for cognitive and control functions. To test the first hypothesis experimentally, some authors have tried to generate data from animal studies to support a greater role of the right-hemisphere subcortical structures, and in particular of the amygdala, in emotional function. These data are, however, controversial because Coleman-Mesches, Salinas, and McGaugh (1996; see also Coleman-Mesches & McGauch, 1995a–c) have obtained results suggesting a prevalence of the right amygdala for emotional functions in the rat, but other studies (Coleman-Mesches, West, & McGaugh, 1997; LaBar & LeDoux, 1996; LaBar et al., 1995) have found no difference between the right and left amygdala for other aspects of emotional functioning.

The second hypothesis is perhaps more speculative and difficult to submit to strong empirical control, but it is substantially accepted by most authors and supported by clinical and experimental data. This hypothesis, which assumes that the development of language in the left hemisphere may have greatly increased the capacity of intentional control of this hemisphere, is consistent with Luria's views (1966) on the regulatory role of language on various aspects of human behavior and with Gazzaniga's studies (1995) on the cognitive capacities of the isolated right and left hemispheres in split-brain patients. This author has, in fact, shown that the left hemisphere is surprisingly superior to the right hemisphere not only in linguistic tasks but also in apparently nonverbal tasks requiring organization and control functions.

Finally, the hypothesis of greater involvement of the left hemisphere in functions of intentional control is consistent with the interpretation recently proposed by Gainotti (1993, 1996) of the unilateral neglect syndrome, very typical of right-hemisphere lesions. Drawing on evidence suggesting that the neglect syndrome may be due to a selective disruption of the automatic components of the spatial orienting of attention, Gainotti (1993, 1996) proposed that the automatic and the controlled components of the spatial orienting mechanisms may be subserved respectively by the right and the left hemispheres. Both in attention-orienting and in emotional functions, automaticity could, therefore, be a main feature of the right hemisphere and intentional control the hallmark left hemisphere functioning. The hypothesis that the right hemisphere may preferentially subserve the automatic "schematic level" and the left hemisphere the controlled "conceptual level" of emotional processing seems, therefore, consistent with the basic requirement of an internal coherence between the principles of organization underlying respectively the emotional system and the right and left hemispheres.

REFERENCES

Adolphs, R., Tranel, D., Damasio, H., & Damasio, A.R. (1994). Impaired recognition of emotion in facial expressions following bilateral damage to the human amygdala. *Nature, 372,* 669–672.

Adolphs, R., Tranel, D., Damasio, H., & Damasio, A.R. (1995). Fear and the human amygdala. *Journal of Neuroscience, 15,* 5879–5891.

Alemà, G., & Donini, G. (1960). Sulle modificazioni cliniche ed elettroencefalografiche da introduzione intracarotidea di iso-amil-etil-barbiturato di sodio nell'uomo. *Bollettino della Società Italiana di Biologia Sperimentale, 36,* 900–904.

Bard, P. (1928). A diencephalic mechanism for the expression of rage with special reference to the sympathetic nervous system. *American Journal of Physiology, 84,* 490–515.

Bard, P. (1929). The central representation of the sympathetic system. *Archives of Neurology and Psychiatry, 22,* 230–246.

Bazett, H.C., & Penfield, W.G. (1922). A study of the Sherrington decerebrate animal in the chronic as well as the acute condition. *Brain, 45,* 185–265.

Blonder, L.X., Gur, R.E., & Gur, R.C. (1989). The effects of right and left hemiparkinsonism on prosody. *Brain and Language, 36,* 193–207.

Borod, J.C. (1992). Interhemispheric and intrahemispheric control of emotion: A focus on unilateral brain damage. *Journal of Consulting and Clinical Psychology, 60,* 339–348.

Borod, J.C. (1993). Cerebral mechanisms underlying facial, prosodic, and lexical emotional expression: A review of neuropsychological studies and methodological issues. *Neuropsychology, 7,* 445–463.

Borod, J.C., & Caron, H. (1980). Facedness and emotion related to lateral dominance, sex, and expression type. *Neuropsychologia, 18,* 237–241.

Borod, J.C., Kent, J., Koff, E., Martin, C., & Alpert, M. (1988). Facial asymmetry while posing positive and negative emotions: Support for the right hemisphere hypothesis. *Neuropsychologia, 26,* 759–764.

Borod, J.C., & Koff, E. (1984). Asymmetries in affective facial expression: Behavior and anatomy. In N. Fox & R. Davidson (Eds.), *The Psychobiology of Affective Development* (pp. 293–323). Hillsdale, NJ: Lawrence Erlbaum.

Borod, J.C., Koff, E., Perlman, M., & Nicholas, M. (1985). Channels of emotional expression in patients with unilateral brain damage. *Archives of Neurology, 42,* 345–348.

Borod, J.C., Santschi Haywood, C., & Koff, E. (1997). Neuropsychological aspects of facial asymmetry during emotional expression: A review of the normal adult literature. *Neuropsychology Review, 7,* 41–60.

Borod, J.C., Welkowitz, J., Alpert, M., Brozgold, A.Z., Martin, C., Peselow, E., & Diller, L. (1990). Parameters of emotional processing in neuropsychiatric disorders: Conceptual issues and a battery of tests. *Journal of Communication Disorders, 23,* 247–271.

Brodal, A. (1981). *Neurological Anatomy in Relation to Clinical Medicine*, 3rd Ed. New York: Oxford University Press.

Brozgold, A.Z., Borod, J.C., Martin, C.C., Pick, L.H., Alpert, M., & Welkowitz, J. (1998). Social functioning and facial emotional expression in neurological and psychiatric disorders. *Applied Neuropsychology*, *5*, 15–23.

Buck, R. (1976), *Human Motivation and Emotion*. New York: Wiley.

Buck, R. (1984). *The Communication of Emotion*. New York: Guilford Press.

Buck, R., & Duffy, R.J. (1980). Nonverbal communication of affect in brain-damaged patients. *Cortex*, *16*, 351–362.

Calder, A.J., Young, A.W., Rowland, D., Perret, D.I., Hodges, J.R., & Etcoff, N.L. (1996). Facial emotion recognition after bilateral amygdala damage: Differentially severe impairment of fear. *Cognitive Neuropsychology*, *13*, 699–745.

Caltagirone, C., Ekman, P., Friesen, W., Gainotti, G., Mammucari, A., Pizzamiglio, L., & Zoccolotti, P. (1989a). Posed emotional expression in unilateral brain damaged patients. *Cortex*, *25*, 653–663.

Caltagirone, C., Zoccolotti, P., Originale, G., Daniele, A., & Mammucari, A. (1989b). Autonomic reactivity and facial expression of emotions in brain-damaged patients. In G. Gainotti & C. Caltagirone (Eds.), *Emotions and the Dual Brain* (pp. 204–221). Heidelberg: Springer.

Cancelliere, A.E.B., & Kertesz, A. (1990). Lesion localization in acquired deficits of emotional expression and comprehension. *Brain and Cognition*, *13*, 133–147.

Cohen, M.J., Riccio, C.A., & Flannery, A.M. (1994). Expressive aprosodia following stroke to the right basal ganglia: A case report. *Neuropsychology*, *8*, 242–245.

Coleman-Mesches, K., & McGaugh, J.L. (1995a). Differential of pre-training inactivation of the right and left amygdalae on retention of inhibitory avoidance training. *Behavioral Neuroscience*, *109*, 642–647.

Coleman-Mesches, K., & McGaugh, J.L. (1995b). Differential involvement of the right and left amygdalae in expression of memory for aversively motivated training. *Brain Research*, *670*, 75–81.

Coleman-Mesches, K., & McGaugh, J.L. (1995c). Muscimol injected into the right or left amygdaloid complex differentially affects retention performance following aversively motivated training. *Brain Research*, *676*, 183–188.

Coleman-Mesches, K., Salinas, J.A., & McGaugh, J.L. (1996). Unilateral amygdala inactivation after training attenuates memory for reduced reward. *Behavioral Brain Research*, *77*, 175–178.

Coleman-Mesches, K., West, M.A., & McGaugh, J.L. (1997). Opposite effects on two different measures of retention following unilateral inactivation of the amygdala. *Behavioral Brain Research*, *86*, 17–23.

Critchley, E.M.R. (1981). Speech disorders of Parkinsonism: A review. *Journal of Neurology, Neurosurgery, and Psychiatry*, *44*, 751–758.

Davidson, R.J. (1984). Affect, cognition, and hemispheric specialization. In C.E. Izard, J. Kagan & R. Zajonc (Eds.) *Emotions, Cognition, and Behavior*. Cambridge: Cambridge University Press.

Davidson, R.J. (1992). Emotion and affective style: Hemispheric substrates. *Psychological Science*, *3*, 39–43.

Davidson, R.J (1993). Parsing affective space: Perspectives from neuropsychology and psychophysiology. *Neuropsychology*, *7*, 464–475.

Davidson, R.J., Ekman, P., Saron, C.D., Senulis, J.A., & Friesen, W.V. (1990). Approach–withdrawal and cerebral asymmetry: Emotional expression and brain pathology. *Journal of Personality and Social Psychology*, *58*, 330–341.

Davidson, R.J., & Fox, N.A. (1982). Asymmetrical brain activity discriminates between positive versus negative stimuli in ten month old human infants. *Science, 218*, 1235–1237.

Davidson, R.J., Schwartz, G.E., Saron, C., Bennett, J., & Goleman, D.J. (1979). Frontal versus parietal EEG asymmetry during positive and negative affect. *Psychophysiology, 16*, 202–203.

Davidson, R.J., & Tomarken, A.J. (1989). Laterality and emotion: An electrophysiological approach. In F. Boller & J. Grafman (Eds.), *Handbook of Neuropsychology*, Vol. 3 (pp. 419–441). Amsterdam: Elsevier North Holland.

Delgado, J.M.R. (1960). Emotional behavior in animals and human. *Psychiatric Research Reports, 12*, 259–266.

DeLong, M.R., Georgopoulos, A.P., Crutcher, M.D., Mitchell, S.J., Richardson, R.T., & Alexander, G.E. (1984). Functional organization of the basal ganglia: Contribution of single-cell recording studies. *CIBA Foundation Symposium, 107*, 64–78.

Downer, J.C.D. (1961). Changes in visual gnostic function and emotional behavior following unilateral temporal lobe damage in the "split-brain" monkey. *Nature, 191*, 50–51.

Duffy, E. (1962). *Activation and Behavior*. New York: Wiley.

Dusser de Barenne, J.G. (1920). Recherches expérimentales sur les fonctions du système nerveux central, faites en particulier sur deux chats dont le néopallium a été enlevé. *Archives de Neurologie et Physiologie, 4*, 31–123.

Ekman, P. (1984). Expression and the nature of emotion. In K. Scherer & P. Ekman (Eds.), *Approaches to Emotion* (pp. 319–344). Hillsdale, NJ: Erlbaum.

Etcoff, N. (1986). The neuropsychology of emotional expression. In G. Goldstein & R.E. Tarter (Eds.), *Advances in Clinical Neuropsychology* (pp. 127–179). New York: Plenum Press.

Falconer, M.A., Hill, D., Meyer, A., Wilson, J.L., & Wilson, J.L. (1958). Clinical, radiological, and EEG correlations with pathological changes in temporal lobe epilepsy and their significance in surgical treatment. In M. Baldwin & P. Bailey (Eds.), *Temporal Lobe Epilepsy* (pp. 396–405). Springfield, IL: C.C. Thomas.

Frijda, N.H. (1986). *The Emotions*. New York: Cambridge University.

Frijda, N.H. (1987). Emotions, cognitive structures, and action tendency. *Cognition and Emotion, 1*, 115–143.

Fuster, J.M., & Uyeda, A.A. (1971). Reactivity of limbic neurons of the monkey to appetitive and aversive signals. *Electroencephalography and Clinical Neurophysiology, 30*, 281–293.

Gainotti, G. (1972). Emotional behavior and hemispheric side of lesion. *Cortex, 8*, 41–55.

Gainotti, G. (1983). Laterality of affect: The emotional behavior of right and left brain-damaged patients. In M.S. Myslobodsky (Ed.), *Hemisyndromes: Psychobiology, Neurology, and Psychiatry* (pp. 175–192). New York: Academic Press.

Gainotti, G. (1989). Features of emotional behavior relevant to neurobiology and theories of emotions. In G. Gainotti & C. Caltagirone (Eds.), *Emotions and the Dual Brain* (pp. 9–27). Heidelberg: Springer.

Gainotti, G. (1993). The role of spontaneous eye movements in orienting attention and in unilateral neglect. In I.H. Robertson & J.C. Marshall (Eds.), *Unilateral Neglect: Clinical and Experimental Studies* (pp. 107–122). Hove: Erlbaum.

Gainotti, G. (1994). Bases neurobiologiques et contrôle des émotions. In X. Seron & M. Jeannerod (Eds.), *Neuropsychologie Humaine* (pp. 471–486). Liège: Mardaga.

Gainotti, G. (1996). Lateralization of brain mechanisms underlying automatic and controlled forms of spatial orienting of attention. *Neuroscience and Biobehavioral Reviews, 20(4)*, 617–622.

Gainotti, G. (1997). Emotional disorders in relation to unilateral brain damage. In T.E. Feinberg & M. Farah (Eds.), *Behavioral Neurology and Neuropsychology*. New York: McGraw-Hill.

Gainotti, G., Caltagirone, C., & Zoccolotti, P. (1993). Left/right and cortical/subcortical dichotomies in the neuropsychological study of human emotions. *Cognition and Emotion, 7*, 71–93

Gazzaniga, M.S. (1995). Principles of human brain organization derived from split-brain studies. *Neuron, 14*, 217–228.

Geschwind, N. (1974). The clinical setting of aggression in temporal lobe epilepsy. In W.S. Field & W.H. Sweet (Eds.), *The Neurobiology of Violence* (pp. 64–72). St. Louis: Warren H. Green.

Gloor, P. (1967). Discussion. *UCLA Forensic Medical Science, 7*, 95–133.

Gloor, P. (1990). Experiential phenomena of temporal lobe epilepsy. *Brain, 113*, 1673–1694.

Goltz, F. (1892). Der Hund ohne Grosshirn. *Pfluegers Archiv für die Gesamte Physiologischen Menschen Tiere, 51*, 570–614.

Graybiel, A.M. (1984). Neurochemically specified subsystems in the basal ganglia. *CIBA Foundation Symposium, 107*, 114–144.

Gunn, J., & Bonn, J. (1971). Criminality and violence in epileptic prisoners. *British Journal of Psychiatry, 118*, 337–343.

Halgren, E. (1991). Emotional neurophysiology of the amygdala within the context of human cognition. In J.P. Aggleton (Ed.), *The Amygdala: Neurobiological Aspects of Emotion, Memory, and Mental Dysfunction* (pp. 191–228). New York: Wiley-Liss.

Heilman, K.M., Schwartz, H.D., & Watson, R.T. (1978). Hypoarousal in patients with neglect and emotional indifference. *Neurology, 28*, 229–232.

Heller, W. (1993). Neuropsychological mechanisms of individual differences in emotion, personality and arousal. *Neuropsychology, 7*, 476–489.

Horenstein, S. (1970). Effects of cerebrovascular disease on personality and emotionality. In A.L. Benton (Ed.), *Behavioral change in cerebrovascular disease* (pp. 121–137). New York: Harper.

Hornak, J., Rolls, E.T., & Wade, D. (1996). Face and voice expression identification in patients with emotional and behavioral changes following ventral frontal damage. *Neuropsychologia, 34*, 247–61.

House, A., Dennis, M., Molyneux, A., Warlow, C., & Hawton, K. (1989). Emotionalism after stroke. *British Medical Journal, 298*, 991–994.

Jones, B., & Mishkin, M. (1972). Limbic lesions and the problem of stimulus-reinforcement associations. *Experimental Neurology, 36*, 362–377.

Kaada, B.R. (1951). Somato-motor, autonomic, and electrocorticographic responses to electrical stimulation of "rhinencephalic" and other forebrain structures in primates, cat and dog. *Acta Physiologica Scandinavica, 24*, 1–285.

Karplus, J.P., & Kreidl, A. (1909). Gehirn und Sympathicus. I Zwischenhirnbasis und Halssympathicus. *Pfluegers Archiv für die Gesamte Physiologischen Menschen Tiere, 129*, 138–144.

Karplus, J.P., & Kreidl, A. (1927). Gehirn und Sympathicus. VII Uber Beziehungen der Hypothalamuszentren zu Blutdruck und innerer Sekretion. *Pfluegers Archiv für Gesamte Physiologischen Menschen Tiere, 215*, 667–670.

Katsikitis, M., & Pilowsky, I. (1991). A controlled study of facial expression in Parkinson's disease and depression. *Journal of Nervous and Mental Disease, 179*, 683–688.

Kolb, B., & Taylor, D.C. (1981). Affective behavior in patients with localized cortical excision: Role of lesion site and side. *Science, 214,* 89–91.

Krettek, J.E., & Price, J.L. (1978). Amygdaloid projections to subcortical structures within the basal forebrain and brainstem in the rat and cat. *Journal of Comparative Neurology, 178,* 225–254.

LaBar, K.S., & LeDoux, J.E. (1996). Partial disruption of fear conditioning in rats with unilateral amygdala damage: Correspondence with unilateral temporal lobectomy in humans. *Behavioral Neuroscience, 110,* 991–997.

LaBar, K.S., LeDoux, J.E., Spencer, D.D., & Phelps, E.A. (1995). Impaired fear conditioning following unilateral temporal lobectomy in humans. *Journal of Neuroscience, 15,* 6846–6855.

Lamendella, J.T. (1977). The limbic system in human communication. In H. Whitaker & H.A. Whitaker (Eds.), *Studies in Neurolinguistics,* Vol. 3 (pp. 157–222). New York: Academic Press.

Lazarus, R.S. (1982). Thoughts on relations between emotion and cognition. *American Psychologist, 37,* 1019–1024.

Lazarus, R.S. (1984). On the primacy of cognition. *American Psychologist, 39,* 124–129.

LeDoux, J.E. (1986). Neurobiology of emotion. In J.E. LeDoux & W. Hirst (Eds.), *Mind and Brain* (pp. 301–358). Cambridge: Cambridge University Press.

LeDoux, J.E. (1987). Emotion. In V.B. Mountcastle, R. Plum, & S.T. Geiser (Eds.), *Handbook of Physiology* (*pp. 419–459*). *Section I, The Nervous System,* Vol. V, *Higher Functions of the Brain, Part I.* Bethesda, MD: American Physiological Society.

LeDoux, J.E. (1989). Cognitive–emotional interactions in the brain. *Cognition and Emotion, 3,* 267–289.

LeDoux, J.E. (1993). Cognition versus emotion again. This time in the brain. A response to Parrot and Schulkin. *Cognition and Emotion, 7,* 61–64.

Leventhal, H. (1974). *Emotions: A Basic Problem for Social Psychology: Classic and Contemporary Integrations.* Chicago: McNally.

Leventhal, H. (1979). A Perceptual-motor processing model of emotion. In P. Pliner, K. Blankestein, & I.M. Spiegel (Eds.), *Perception of Emotion in Self and Others,* Vol. 5 (pp. 1–46). New York: Plenum.

Leventhal, H. (1984). A perceptual motor theory of emotion. In L. Berkowitz (Ed.), *Advances in Experimental Social Psychology,* Vol. 17 (pp. 117–182). New York: Academic Press.

Leventhal, H., & Scherer, K. (1987). The relationship of emotion to cognition: A functional approach to a semantic controversy. *Cognition and Emotion, 1,* 3–28.

Lindsley, D.B. (1951). Emotions. In S.S. Stevens (Ed.), *Handbook of Experimental Psychology* (pp. 473–516). New York: Wiley.

Luria, A.R. (1966). *Higher Cortical Functions in Man.* New York: Basic Books.

Macchi, G. (1989). Anatomical substrates of emotional reactions. In F. Boller & J. Grafman (Eds.), *Handbook of Neuropsychology* (pp. 283–303). Amsterdam: Elsevier/North Holland.

Mandler, G. (1980). The generation of emotion: A psychological theory. In R. Plutchick & H. Kellerman (Eds.), *Emotion, 1: Theories of Emotion* (pp. 219–243). New York: Academic Press.

McLean, P.D. (1949). Psychosomatic disease and the visceral brain: Recent developments bearing on the Papez theory of emotion. *Psychosomatic Medicine, 1,* 338–353.

McLean, P.D. (1961). Le système limbique du point de vue de la self-protection et de la conservation de l'espèce. In T. Alajouanine (Ed.), *Physiologie et pathologie du rhinencéphale* (pp. 111–126). Paris: Masson.

McLean, P.D. (1986). Culmination developments in the evolution of the limbic system: The thalamo-cingulate division. In B.K. Doane & K.E. Livingstone (Eds.), *The Limbic System: Functional Organization and Clinical Disorders* (pp. 58–76). New York: Raven.

McLean, P.D., & Delgado, J.M.R. (1953). Electrical and chemical stimulation of fronto-temporal portion of limbic system in the waking animal. *Electroencephalography and Clinical Neurophysiology, 5*, 91–100.

Meadows, M.E., & Kaplan, R.F. (1994). Dissociation of autonomic and subjective responses to emotional slides in right hemisphere damaged patients. *Neuropsychologia, 32*, 847–856.

Mogenson, G.J. (1987). Limbic–motor integration. *Progress in Psychobiology and Physiological Psychology, 12*, 117–170.

Morrow, L., Vrtunski, B., Kim, Y., & Boller, F. (1981). Arousal responses to emotional stimuli and laterality of lesion. *Neuropsychologia, 19*, 65–71.

Moruzzi, G., & Magoun, H.W. (1949). Brain stem reticular formation and activation of the EEG. *EEG and Clinical Neurophysiology, 1*, 455–473.

Nauta, W.J.H., & Domesick, V.B. (1984). Afferent and efferent relationships of the basal ganglia. *CIBA Foundation Symposium, 107*, 3–23.

Nishijo, H., Ono, T., & Nishino, H. (1988). Single neuron responses in amygdala of alert monkey during complex sensory stimulation with affective significance. *Journal of Neuroscience, 8*, 3570–3583.

Oatley, K., & Johnson-Laird, P. (1985). Sketch for a cognitive theory of the emotion. *University of Sussex, Cognitive Sciences*, Research Paper No. 45.

Oatley, K., & Johnson-Laird, P. (1987). Toward a cognitive theory of emotions. *Cognition and Emotion, 1*, 29–50.

Ono, T., Fukuda, M., Nishino, H., Sasaki, K., & Muramoto, K.I. (1983). Amygdaloid neural responses to complex visual stimuli in an operant feeding situation in the monkey. *Brain Research Bulletin, 11*, 515–518.

Ounstead, C. (1969). Aggression and epilepsy: Rage in children with temporal lobe epilepsy. *Journal of Psychosomatic Research, 13*, 237–242.

Panksepp, J. (1969). Toward a general psychobiological theory of emotions. *Behavioral and Brain Sciences, 5*, 407–467.

Papez, J.W. (1937). A proposed mechanism of emotion. *Archives of Neurology and Psychiatry, 79*, 217–224.

Perria, L., Rosadini, G., & Rossi, G.F. (1961). Determination of side of cerebral dominance with amobarbital. *Archives of Neurology, 4*, 173–181.

Prigatano, G.P., & Pribam, K.H. (1982). Perception and memory of facial affects following brain injury. *Perceptual and Motor Skills, 54*, 859.

Rinn, W.E. (1984). The neuropsychology of facial expression: A review of the neurological and psychological mechanisms for producing facial expression. *Psychological Bulletin, 95*, 52–77.

Rodin, E.A. (1973). Psychomotor epilepsy and aggressive behavior. *Archives of General Psychiatry, 28*, 210–213.

Ross, E.D. (1981). The prosodias: Functional-anatomical organization of the affective components of language in the right hemisphere. *Archives of Neurology, 38*, 561–569.

Ross, E.D. (1984). Right hemisphere's role in language, affective behavior, and emotion. *Trends in Neuroscience, 7*, 342–346.

Ross, E.D., Homan, R.W., & Buck, R. (1994). Differential hemispheric lateralization of primary and social emotions. *Neuropsychiatry, Neuropsychology, and Behavioral Neurology, 7*, 1–19.

Rossi, G.F., & Rosadini, G. (1967). Experimental analysis of cerebral dominance in man. In C.J. Millikan & F.L. Darley (Eds.), *Brain Mechanisms Underlying Speech and Language* (pp. 167–174). New York: Grune & Stratton.

Sackeim, H.A., Greenberg, M.S., Weimar, A.L., Gur, R.C., Hungerbuhler, J.P., & Geschwind, N. (1982). Hemispheric asymmetry in the expression of positive and negative emotions. *Archives of Neurology, 39*, 210–218.

Sackeim, H.A., & Gur, R.C. (1978). Lateral asymmetry in intensity of emotional expression. *Neuropsychologia, 16*, 473–481.

Scherer, K.R. (1984). On the nature and function of emotion: A component process approach. In K.R. Scherer & P. Ekman (Eds.), *Approaches to Emotion* (pp. 293–318). Hillsdale, NJ: Erlbaum.

Schwartz, G.E., Ahern, G.L., & Brown, S.L. (1979). Lateralized facial muscle response to positive and negative emotional stimuli. *Psychophysiology, 16*, 561–571.

Smith, M.C., Smith, M.K., & Ellgring, H. (1996). Spontaneous and posed facial expression in Parkinson's disease. *Journal of the International Neuropsychological Society, 2*, 383–391.

Smith, O.A., & DeVito, J.L. (1984). Central neural integration for the control of autonomic responses associated with emotion. *Annual Review of Neurosciences, 7*, 43–65.

Speedie, L.J., Brake, N., Folstein, S.E., Bowers, D., & Heilman, K.M. (1990). Comprehension of prosody in Huntington's disease. *Journal of Neurology, Neurosurgery, and Psychiatry, 53*, 607–610.

Stuss, D.T., & Benson, D.F. (1986). *The Frontal Lobes.* New York: Raven

Terzian, H., & Cecotto, S. (1959). Su un nuovo metodo per la determinazione e lo studio della dominanza emisferica. *Giornale di Psichiatria e Neuropatologia, 87*, 889–924.

Treffert, D.A. (1964). The psychiatric patient with an EEG temporal lobe focus. *American Journal of Psychiatry, 120*, 765–771.

Tucker, D.M. (1981). Lateral brain function, emotion, and conceptualization. *Psychological Bulletin, 89*, 19–46.

Tucker, D.M. (1989). Neural substrates of thought and affective disorders. In G. Gainotti & C. Caltagirone (Eds.), *Emotions and the Dual Brain* (pp. 225–234). Heidelberg: Springer.

Ursin, H., & Kaada, B.R. (1960). Function localization within the amygdaloid complex in the cat. *Electroencephalography and Clinical Neurophysiology, 12*, 1–20.

Valenstein, E. (1973). *Brain Control.* New York: Wiley & Sons.

Walker, A.E. (1973). Man and his temporal lobes (John Hughlings Jackson Lecture). *Surgical Neurology, 1*, 69–79.

Weddell, R.A. (1989). Recognition memory for emotional facial expressions in patients with focal cerebral lesions. *Brain and Cognition, 11*, 1–17.

Weddell, R.A. (1994). Effects of subcortical lesion site on human emotional behavior. *Brain and Cognition, 25*, 161–193.

Weddell, R.A., Miller, D.J., & Trevarthen, C. (1988). Reactions of patients with focal cerebral lesions to success or failure. *Neuropsychologia, 26*, 373–385.

Weddell, R.A., Miller, D.J., & Trevarthen, C. (1990). Voluntary emotional facial expression in patients with focal cerebral lesions. *Neuropsychologia, 28*, 49–60.

Wittling, W. (1995). Brain asymmetry in the control of autonomic-physiologic activity. In R.J. Davidson & K. Hugdahl (Eds.), *Brain Asymmetry* (pp. 305–357). Cambridge: MIT Press.

Woodworth, R.S., & Sherrington, C.S. (1904). A pseudoaffective reflex and its spinal path. *Journal of Physiology, 31*, 234–243.

Young, A.W., Aggleton, J.P., Hellawell, D.J., Johnson, M., Broks, P., & Hanley, J.R. (1995). Face processing impairments after amygdalotomy. *Brain, 118*, 15–24.

Zajonc, R.B. (1980). Feeling and thinking: Preferences need no inferences. *American Psychologist, 2*, 151–176.

Zajonc, R.B. (1984). On the primacy of affect. In K.R. Scherer & P. Ekman (Eds.), *Approaches to Emotion* (pp. 259–270). Hillsdale, NJ: Lawrence Erlbaum.

Zoccolotti, P., Caltagirone, C., Benedetti, N., & Gainotti, G. (1986). Perturbation des réponses végétatives aux stimuli émotionnels au cours des lésions hémisphériques unilatérales. *Encéphale, 12*, 263–268.

IV

EMOTIONAL DISORDERS

10

Elation, Mania, and Mood Disorders: Evidence from Neurological Disease

ROBERT G. ROBINSON AND
FACUNDO MANES

The first reports of emotional disorders associated with brain damage (usually caused by cerebrovascular disease) were made by neurologists and psychiatrists in case descriptions. Meyer (1904), for example, wrote that mood disorders following brain injury were probably the result of a combination of social, psychological, and biological factors. He proposed that in some cases there may be relationships between particular "traumatic insanities," such as delirium or dementia, and specific locations and causes of brain injury. Babinski (1914) noted that patients with right-hemisphere disease frequently displayed the symptoms of anosognosia, euphoria, and indifference. Bleuler (1951) wrote that, after stroke, "melancholic moods lasting for months and sometimes longer appear frequently." Kraepelin (1921) recognized a frequent association between manic depressive insanity and cerebrovascular disease and thought that, in some cases, the atherosclerotic disease produced the mood disorder.

Goldstein (1939) was the first to describe an emotional mood disorder thought to be uniquely associated with brain disease: the catastrophic reaction. The catastrophic reaction is an emotional outburst involving various degrees of anger, frustration, depression, tearfulness, refusal, shouting, swearing, and sometimes aggressive behavior. Goldstein (1939) ascribed this reaction to the inability of the organism to cope when faced with a serious defect in its physical or cognitive functions. In his extensive studies of brain injury in war, Goldstein (1942) described two symptom clusters: those related directly to physical damage of a circumscribed area of the brain and those related secondarily to the organism's psychological response to the injury. Emotional symptoms, therefore, represented the latter category (i.e., the psychological response of an organism struggling with physical or cognitive impairments).

A second abnormality unique to brain injury, also involving a disturbance (this time an absence) of mood, was the indifference reaction described by Hécaen, deAjuriaguerra, and Massonet (1951) and Denny-Brown, Meyer, and Horsenstein (1952). The indifference reaction associated with right-hemisphere lesions consists of symptoms of indifference toward failures, lack of interest in family and friends, enjoyment of foolish jokes, and minimization of physical difficulties. It is associated with neglect of the left half of the body and space.

A third "mood" disorder uniquely associated with brain injury is pathological laughing or crying. Ironside (1956) described the clinical manifestations of this disorder. Such patients' emotional displays were characteristically unrelated to their inner emotional state. Crying, for example, may occur spontaneously or after some seemingly minor provocation. This phenomenon has been given various names, such as *emotional incontinence*, *emotional lability*, *pseudobulbar affect*, and *pathological emotionalism*.

The first systematic study to contrast the mood disorders of patients with right- and left-hemisphere brain damage was done by Gainotti (1972). He reported that depressive catastrophic reactions were more frequent among patients with left-hemisphere brain damage, particularly those with aphasia, than among patients with right-hemisphere lesions. Gainotti agreed with Goldstein's explanation (1942) that it was a desperate reaction of the organism when confronted with a severe physical disability. The indifference reaction, on the other hand, was not easy to understand. Gainotti (1972) suggested that denial of illness and organization of the nonverbal type of synthesis may play an important role in this emotional disorder.

In conclusion, there have been two primary lines of thought in the study of emotional disorders that are associated with structural brain disease. One attributes mood disorders to an understandable psychological reaction to the associated impairment; the other, based on a lack of association between severity of impairment and severity of emotional disorder, suggests a direct causal connection between emotional disorders and structural brain damage.

ELATION AND MANIA ASSOCIATED WITH STROKE

Mania is a relatively rare consequence of acute stroke lesions. Although prevalence studies have not been conducted, Robinson et al. (1988) reported that less than 1% of patients with acute stroke have mania. Most of the patients included in studies of mania following stroke present with manic symptoms and are only secondarily found to have brain injury. These patients, however, have typical manic syndromes, and their symptoms are not significantly different from those of patients with mania who do not have brain injury (Starkstein et al., 1987a).

Relationship to Lesion Location

Cummings and Mendez (1984) reported two patients who developed mania after right thalamic infarcts and reviewed the case literature, which suggested an association of mania with right-hemisphere lesions. Based on a series of 17 patients with post-brain-injury mania, Robinson et al. (1988) reported a significantly increased frequency of right-hemisphere lesions compared with 31 major depressed patients and 28 nonmood-disordered controls (Fig. 10.1). These lesions involved the basal and polar areas of the right temporal lobe as well as subcortical areas of the right hemisphere, such as the head of the caudate and right thalamus.

In another study, Starkstein et al. (1990b) used positron emission tomography (PET) with 18-fluorodeoxyglucose to examine the metabolic abnormalities in

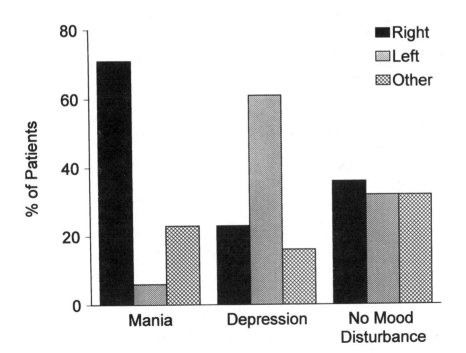

Figure 10.1. The percentage of patients with mania, major depression, or no mood disorder after brain injury, divided by lesion location as visualized on CT scan. Mania was strongly associated with right-hemisphere lesions and major depression with left-hemisphere injury. (Data are from Robinson et al., 1988.)

three patients with mania following right basal ganglia strokes. These patients were found to have focal hypometabolic deficits in the right basotemporal cortex. This finding suggested that lesions that lead to secondary mania may do so through their distant effects on the right basotemporal cortex. This phenomenon, called *diaschisis* (i.e., lesions producing distant effects), is a well-recognized consequence of brain injury.

Risk Factors for Mania Following Stroke

Because not every patient with a right orbitofrontal or basotemporal lesion develops a manic syndrome, the question arises as to whether there are potential predisposing factors for secondary mania (Robinson et al., 1988; Starkstein et al., 1987a). Patients with secondary mania were found to have a significantly higher frequency of familial history of psychiatric disorders, as well as significantly more subcortical brain atrophy (as determined by increased ventricular to brain ratios) than did patients with similar brain lesions but without mania. Interestingly, secondary mania patients without a genetic predisposition had significantly more subcortical atrophy than secondary mania patients with a family history of mood disorder, suggesting that subcortical atrophy and genetic predisposition may be independent risk factors for mania following brain injury (Starkstein et al., 1987a).

Mechanism

To postulate a mechanism for secondary mania, two clinicopathological correlations need to be explained. First, most lesions associated with secondary mania involved (directly or indirectly) a limbic or limbic-related area of the brain. Second, virtually all of these lesions were localized to the right hemisphere.

Several studies have demonstrated that the amygdala (located in the limbic portion of the temporal lobe) plays an important role in the production of instinctive reactions and the association between stimulus and emotional response (Gloor, 1986). The amygdala receives its main afferents from the basal diencephalon (which in turn receives psychosensory and psychomotor information from the reticular formation), and the temporopolar and basolateral cortices (which receive main their afferents from heteromodal association areas) (Beck, 1949; Crosby, Humphrey, & Laner, 1962). The basotemporal cortex receives afferents from associated cortical areas and the orbitofrontal cortex, and it sends efferent projections to the entorhinal cortex, hippocampus, and amygdala. By virtue of these connections, the basotemporal cortex may represent a cortical link between sensory afferents and instinctive reactions (Goldar & Outes, 1972).

The orbitofrontal cortex can be subdivided into two regions: a posterior one, which is restricted to the limbic functions and should be considered part of the limbic system; and an anterior one, which exerts a tonic inhibitory control over the amygdala by means of its connection through the uncinate fasciculus with the basotemporal cortex (Nauta, 1971). Lesions or dysfunction of these areas may result in motor disinhibition (e.g., hyperactivity, pressured speech), intellectual disinhibition (e.g., flight of ideas, grandiose delusions), and instinctive disinhibition (e.g., hyperphagia and hypersexuality).

The second finding that needs to be incorporated into an explanation of mania following stroke is that it almost always occurs following right-hemisphere lesions. Laboratory studies of the neurochemical and behavioral effects of brain lesions in rats found that small suction lesions in the right (but not the left) frontal cortex of rats produced a significant increase in locomotor activity (Robinson, 1979). Similar abnormal behavior was also found after electrolytic lesions were made in the right (but not left) nucleus accumbens (which is considered part of the ventral striatum) (Kubos, Moran, & Robinson, 1987). Moreover, right frontocortical suction lesions also produced a significant increment in dopaminergic turnover in the nucleus accumbens that was not seen with left-hemisphere lesions (Starkstein et al., 1988). Thus, it is possible that in the presence of predisposing factors, such as a genetic burden or subcortical atrophy, a significant increment in biogenic amine turnover in the nucleus accumbens produced by specific right-hemisphere lesions may be part of the mechanism that results in manic syndrome.

A case report (Berthier et al., 1990) suggested that the mechanism of secondary mania was not related to the release of transcallosal inhibitory fibers (i.e., the release of left limbic areas from tonic inhibition due to a right-hemisphere lesion). A patient who developed secondary mania after bleeding from a right basotemporal arteriovenous malformation underwent a Wada test before the therapeutic embolization of the malformation. Amytal injection in the left carotid artery did not abolish the manic symptoms (which would be the expected finding if the "release" theory were correct).

In conclusion, secondary mania is a rare complication of stroke lesions. Three risk factors for mania following stroke have been identified: (*1*) a family history of psychiatric disorders (Robinson et al., 1988), (*2*) increased subcortical atrophy (Starkstein et al., 1987a), and (*3*) seizure disorder (Shukla et al., 1987). Most patients with secondary mania have right-hemisphere lesions, which involve the orbitofrontal and/or basotemporal cortex, or subcortical structures such as the thalamus or head of the caudate. Secondary mania may result from disinhibition of dorsal cortical and limbic areas, dysfunction of asymmetrical biogenic amine pathways, or both.

Treatment

Although no systematic treatment studies of secondary mania have been conducted, one report suggests several potentially useful treatment modalities. Bakchine et al. (1989) carried out a double-blind, placebo-controlled treatment study of a single patient with secondary mania. Clonidine (600 μg/day) rapidly reversed the manic symptoms, whereas carbamazepine (1200 mg/day) was associated with no mood changes, and levodopa (375 mg/day) was associated with increased manic symptoms. Other treatment modalities, such as antiepileptic drugs (valproate and carbamazepine), neuroleptics, and lithium, have been reported to be useful for secondary mania (Robinson et al., 1988). None of these treatments has been evaluated in double-blind, placebo-controlled studies.

MANIA ASSOCIATED WITH TRAUMATIC BRAIN INJURY

Prevalence

Mania is more frequent among patients with traumatic brain injury (TBI) than among patients with stroke lesions (Jorge et al., 1993c; Robinson et al., 1988; Shukla et al., 1987). In a study of 66 patients with acute TBI, 6 (9%) had secondary mania (Jorge et al., 1993c). One of these patients (17%) presented a bipolar course. The manic episodes, however, were short-lived, with a mean duration of 2 months. The mean duration of the elevated mood (i.e., elation), without meeting other diagnostic criteria for mania, however, was 5.7 months. In addition, three of the six secondary mania patients developed brief episodes of violent behavior at some point during the 1-year follow-up period. Aggressive behavior was significantly more frequent in the secondary mania group than among patients who did not experience an affective disorder. At the time of the diagnosis, three patients were receiving drug treatment (two patients received lorazepam, and one patient, haloperidol); however, the duration of mania did not appear to be significantly different between those who were and were not treated.

Relationship to Impairment Variables

In the study of six patients with mania following TBI, the severity of mania was not associated with severity of brain injury, degree of physical or cognitive impairment, frequency of personal or family history of psychiatric disorder, or quality of social functioning (Jorge et al., 1993c). Shukla et al. (1987) reported on 20 patients who developed mania following TBI. The clinical correlates were severe head trauma in 13 of 20, partial seizures in 8 patients and generalized seizures in 2, and irritable mood in 17 of 20. There was no family history of bipolar disorder, and 14 of the 20 had recurrent mania without depression. Thus, although further studies of the relationships between impairment or risk factors and the development of mania need to be conducted, the present data suggest that mania is not a response to the associated impairments and that seizure disorder may play a role in the etiology of post-TBI mania.

Relationship to Lesion Location

The Jorge et al. (1993c) study of secondary mania syndromes found that the major correlate of mania was the presence of anterior temporal lesions. This finding was consistent with the finding in patients with stroke that mania was associated with right basotemporal lesions. The trauma study did not have sufficient numbers of patients with unilateral lesions to examine the right-hemisphere versus left-hemisphere effect. Factors such as personal history of mood disorders or post-traumatic epilepsy did not appear to significantly influence the frequency of secondary mania in this group of patients. Furthermore, although Shukla et al. (1987) did not find a lateralized effect of seizure disorder on mania, the electroencephalographic abnormalities had a temporal lobe focus in nine of ten seizure patients.

Mechanism

It has been suggested that the development of abnormal electrical activation patterns in limbic networks, functional changes in aminergic inhibitory systems, and the presence of aberrant regeneration pathways may play important roles in the genesis of mania (Csernansky et al., 1988; Stevens, 1990).

BIPOLAR DISORDER ASSOCIATED WITH STROKE OR TRAUMA

Starkstein et al. (1991) studied 19 patients with a diagnosis of secondary mania. Seven of these patients had previously met *Diagnostic and Statistical Manual of Mental Disorders*, Third Edition, Revised (DSM-III-R), criteria for the organic mood syndrome of depression. The remaining 12 patients had mania without prior depression. All the patients had computed tomographic (CT) scan evidence of vascular, neoplastic, or traumatic brain lesion and no history of other neurological, toxic, or metabolic conditions.

There were no significant between-group differences in age, sex, race, education, handedness, or personal history of psychiatric disease. Also, no significant differences were found on neurological examination. On psychiatric examination, which was carried out during the index manic episode, no significant differences were observed in the types or frequencies of manic symptoms. The bipolar group, however, showed significantly greater intellectual impairment as measured by Mini-Mental State Examination scores ($P < 0.05$). Patients with bipolar disorder also had lesions restricted to the right hemisphere, which involved subcortical structures including the head of the caudate or thalamus. One patient developed a bipolar illness after surgical removal of a pituitary adenoma. In contrast to these subcortical lesions, most of those in the unipolar mania group had lesions involving the right basotemporal and orbitofrontal cortex (Fig. 10.2).

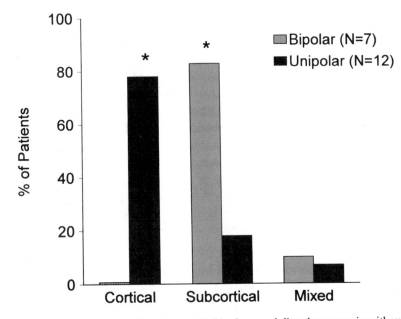

Figure 10.2. Lesion location in patients with bipolar mood disorder or mania without depression after stroke, traumatic brain injury, or surgical lesions. Patients with bipolar disorder had a significantly greater frequency of subcortical (basal ganglia or thalamus) lesions than did patients with mania alone, who had more cortical lesions. Only two patients had mixed cortical and subcortical lesions.

Shukla et al. (1987) did not examine cortical versus subcortical lesion location, but the fact that 70% of the 20 patients had only manic episodes is consistent with the hypothesis that cortical lesions lead to unipolar disorder (manic unipolar) because TBI tends to be predominantly cortical in location.

The causes of both bipolar and unipolar mood disorder remain unknown. Pappata et al. (1987) reported that subcortical lesions induce hypometabolic effects in many regions, including contralateral brain areas (i.e., crossed-hemisphere and crossed-cerebellar diaschisis). It is, therefore, possible that subcortical lesions may induce metabolic changes in left frontocortical regions, which are associated with depression. Mania may develop at a later stage, when these changes become restricted to the orbitofrontal and basotemporal cortices of the right hemisphere.

DEPRESSION ASSOCIATED WITH STROKE

Depression is probably the most common emotional disorder associated with stroke. Utilizing structured psychiatric interviews and established diagnostic criteria, researchers have usually identified two forms of depressive disorder associated with brain disease. One type is major depression as defined by the DSM-IV criteria for depression due to stroke with major depressive-like episode. The second type of depression is dysthymic depression as defined by the DSM-III (excluding the 2 year duration criterion and the exclusionary organic factor) or the DSM-IV research criteria for minor depression.

The prevalences of these depressions vary, depending on the setting in which patients are studied as well as on the nature and location of the brain injury. In a study of 103 consecutive patients admitted to the hospital with acute cerebrovascular lesions, we found that 27% met symptom criteria for major depression, and 20% met symptom criteria for dysthymic (minor) depression (Robinson et al., 1983b). Most other studies of patients hospitalized (in acute care or rehabilitation hospitals) with cerebrovascular lesions have reported similar frequencies of major depression (range 11%-27%) and minor depression (range 20%-40%). The frequency of depression in community settings, however, appears to be lower. House et al. (1990b) found that 11% had major and 12% had other types of depression among 89 community patients examined during the first month post-stroke. Burvill et al. (1995) found that 15% of 294 community patients with acute stroke had major depression and 8% had minor depression.

Longitudinal Course of Depression

The longitudinal course of post-stroke depression has been investigated by our group (Robinson, Bolduc, & Price, 1987) as well as by Morris, Robinson, and Raphael (1990) and Astrom, Adolfsson, and Asplund (1993). In our study, all patients with major depression recovered fully 1–2 years post-stroke. Minor depression, however, had a less favorable prognosis, with only 30% having recovered by 2 years post-stroke (half of the minor depressed patients had developed major depression). In addition, about 30% of patients who were not depressed at the initial hospital evaluation became depressed after discharge. Morris, Robinson, and Raphael (1990) found that, among a group of 99 patients in a stroke rehabilitation hospital, those with major depression had a duration of illness of 40 weeks, whereas those with adjustment disorders (minor depression) had a duration of depression of only 12 weeks. Astrom, Adolfsson, and Asplund (1993) showed that the majority of patients with acute-onset major depression recovered by 1 year (8 of 14), but, among those who were still depressed, only one of the six had recovered by 3 years.

In summary, the available data suggest that post-stroke depression is not a transient but a long-standing disorder with a usual natural course of somewhat less than 1 year for major depression and perhaps a more variable course for minor depression. Some major depressions last more than 3 years, and some minor depressions evolve into major depression and may last for several years.

Relationship to Impairment

Although many clinicians have assumed that the most powerful determinant of depression after stroke was the severity of associated physical impairment, empirical studies have consistently failed to find a strong relationship between severity of depression and severity of physical impairment (Eastwood et al., 1989, Morris, Robinson, & Raphael, 1990; Robinson et al., 1983b). This is not to say, however, that there is no relationship. Numerous studies have demonstrated that severity of physical impairment correlates with severity of depression and, in some subpopulations, may be an important contributing factor to depression (Astrom, Adolfsson, & Asplund, 1993; Eastwood et al., 1989; Morris et al., 1992b; Robinson et al., 1983b).

Although the effect of impairment on depression appears to be fairly weak in most patients, there is considerable evidence that depression adversely affects post-stroke recovery in activities of daily living (ADL). Parikh et al. (1990) compared 25 patients with post-stroke depression (either major or minor depression) and 38 stroke patients with no mood disorders who were matched for severity of ADL impairments in the hospital. After controlling for many of the variables that have been shown to influence stroke outcome (such as acute treatment on a stroke unit; size, nature, and location of brain injury; age; education; recurrent stroke or other medical illness; and duration of rehabilitation services), patients with in-hospital post-stroke depression were found to have a significantly poorer recovery than nondepressed stroke patients at 2 years follow-up (Fig. 10.3).

Several studies have found that patients with major depression after left-hemisphere stroke lesions had significantly greater cognitive deficits than non-depressed patients with brain lesions of a similar size and location (House et al., 1991; Robinson et al., 1986; Starkstein et al., 1988). These cognitive deficits were observed in a wide range of neuropsychological tests, including orientation, language, visuoconstructional ability, executive motor functions, and frontal lobe tasks (Bolla-Wilson et al., 1989). In contrast, among patients with right-hemisphere lesions, patients with major depression did not differ from nondepressed patients on any of the measures of cognitive impairment. These findings suggest that left-hemisphere lesions (particularly left frontal and left basal ganglia) associated with major depression may produce a different kind of depression than right-hemisphere lesions. Although there are several reports of improved intellectual function in stroke patients treated with antidepressants (Fogel & Sparadeo, 1985; Gonzalez-Torrecillas, Mendlewicz, & Lobo, 1995) these studies did not use double-blind controls.

It is difficult to confidently diagnose depression in a patient with severe comprehension deficits, and most investigators have excluded such patients from studies of post-stroke depression. Some investigators (Ross & Rush, 1981) have suggested that a diagnosis of depression should be based on behavioral observations

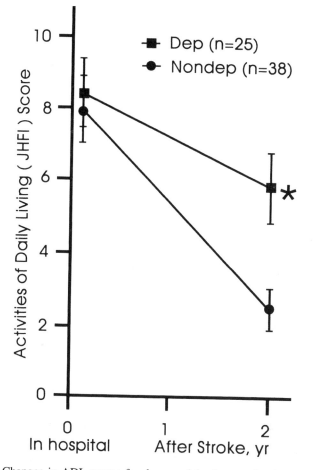

Figure 10.3. Changes in ADL scores for depressed (major or minor) patients and non-depressed patients at the time of the in-hospital evaluation and again 2 years later. Depressed patients show less recovery than nondepressed patients. (Reprinted with permission from Parikh et al., 1990.)

(i.e., diminished sleep and food intake, restlessness and agitation, and retarded or tearful behavior). The reliability as well as sensitivity and specificity of these criteria for detecting depression have not yet, however, been demonstrated.

Robinson and Benson (1981), in a study of depression in patients with fluent or nonfluent aphasia, found that patients with nonfluent aphasia had a significantly higher frequency of depression than did patients with fluent aphasia.

Although the higher frequency of depression among nonfluent aphasic patients might be attributed to greater awareness of language impairment, we found that the frequency of depression was no higher in aphasic patients than in nonaphasic patients and was variable, which accounted best for frequency of depression. In their study, however, Starkstein and Robinson (1988) concluded that the most important variable was lesion location. This finding suggests that nonfluent language impairment and depression may not be causally related but may be independent outcomes of the same lesion.

Relationship to Lesion Location

Robinson et al. (1983a) and Starkstein, Robinson, and Price (1987b) found among patients with acute stroke that major depression was significantly associated with lesions in anterior areas of the left hemisphere, including the left lateral frontal cortex and the left basal ganglia (Fig. 10.4) (Starkstein et al., 1987a). Basal ganglia lesions (caudate and/or putamen) were associated with major depression in seven of eight patients with left-sided lesions, while only one of seven patients with right-sided lesions and none of the patients with left or right thalamic lesions had major depression. The association of acute left-hemisphere stroke with major depression has also been reported by Astrom, Adolfsson, and Asplund (1993) and Herrmann et al. (1995), but not by House et al. (1990a).

Among patients with right-hemisphere stroke, we found that those with frontal or parietal damage showed the highest frequency of depression (Starkstein et al.,

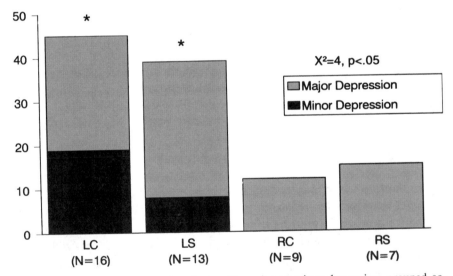

Figure 10.4. The percentage of patients with major or minor depression, grouped according to stroke lesion location. LC, left cortical; LS, left subcortical; RC, right cortical; and RS, right subcortical. Patients with either left cortical or left subcortical lesions had a significantly greater frequency of major depression during the acute stroke period than patients with right hemisphere lesions. (Data from Starkstein et al., 1987b.)

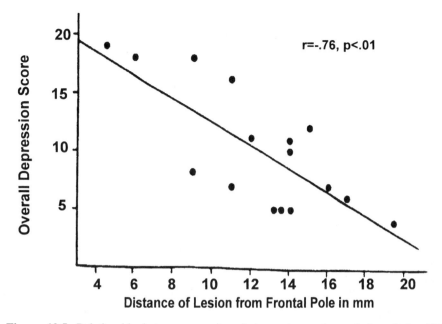

Figure 10.5. Relationship between severity of depression and proximity of the CT scan–visualized lesion to the frontal pole for patients with stroke or TBI involving the left hemisphere. Lesions whose anterior border was closer to the frontal pole were associated with more depressive symptoms. (Reprinted with permission from Robinson & Szetela, 1981.)

1989c). Similar results were reported by Finset (1988), who found that patients with lesions in the right parietal white matter had a higher frequency of depression than did patients with lesions involving other locations in the right hemisphere.

Perhaps the most consistent finding in post-stroke depression, however, has been the association of depressive symptoms with intrahemispheric lesion location. In 1981, we reported that among a group of 29 patients with left-hemisphere lesions produced by trauma or stroke, there was an inverse correlation between severity of depression and distance of the anterior border of the lesion from the frontal pole as measured on CT scan ($r = 0.76$, $P < 0.001$) (Fig. 10.5) (Robinson & Szetela, 1981). In 1983, we reported the same phenomenon in another group of 10 patients with single-stroke lesions of the left anterior hemisphere ($r = -0.92$, $P < .001$). When patients with left posterior lesions were added ($N = 18$), the correlation decreased to $r = -0.54$, $P < 0.05$. This phenomenon was also found in other groups of patients with purely cortical lesions of the left hemisphere ($N = 16$; $r = -0.52$, $P < 0.05$) (Starkstein, Robinson, & Price, 1987b), purely left subcortical lesions ($N = 13$; $r = -0.68$, $P < 0.01$) (Starkstein, Robinson, & Price, 1987b), and left-handed patients (Robinson et al., 1985). This phenomenon has now been replicated by five different groups of investigators studying patients from Canada (Eastwood et al., 1989; Sinyor et al., 1986), England (House et al., 1990b), Germany (Herrmann, Bartles, & Wallesch, 1993), and Australia (Morris et al., 1992a). Some found a correlation between severity of depression and proximity of the lesion to the frontal pole in combined right- and left-hemisphere lesion groups (House et al., 1990b; Sinyor et al., 1986), while others found it only with left-sided lesions (Eastwood et al., 1989; Morris, Robinson, & Raphael, 1992a). Longitudinal studies have found that proximity of the lesion to the frontal pole is significantly associated with severity of depression most strongly during the first 6 months post-stroke (Astrom, Adolfsson, & Asplund, 1993; Parikh et al., 1987), suggesting that the pathophysiology is a dynamic one that changes over time.

Although there is some difference in the strength of this correlation (and, therefore, the amount of variance in severity of depression explained by lesion location), this phenomenon has emerged as one of the most consistent and robust clinicopathological correlations ever described in neuropsychiatry. In summary, several studies conducted by different investigators support the hypothesis that major depressive disorder after acute stroke is more frequent following lesions in the left anterior hemisphere than lesions at any other lesion location and that depressive symptoms are more severe if the lesion is closer to the frontal pole.

Comparison of Cortical and Subcortical Lesions in the Production of Post-Stroke Mood Disorders

Patients with CT-verified single-stroke lesions involving either cortical tissue or restricted entirely to subcortical structures were examined for mood disorders (Starkestein et al., 1987b). Those with left anterior lesions, either cortical or subcortical, had significantly greater frequency and severity of depression than did patients with any other lesion location. A strong correlation between the severity of the depression and the proximity of the lesion to the frontal pole was observed for both left cortical and subcortical groups. Right-hemisphere lesions did not show the same correlation with depression but were associated with a significantly higher incidence of undue cheerfulness. These findings demonstrate the importance of the location of subcortical lesions in post-stroke mood disorders and suggest that anterior subcortical structures may play an important but lateralized role in the production or regulation of mood.

Mechanism of Depression Following Stroke

Although the cause of post-stroke depression is not known, it has been hypothesized that disruption of the biogenic amine–containing pathways by the stroke lesion may play an etiological role (Robinson et al., 1983a). The noradrenergic and serotonergic cell bodies are located in the brain stem and send ascending projections through the medial forebrain bundle to the frontal cortex. The ascending axons then arc posteriorly and run longitudinally through the deep layers of the cortex, arborizing and sending terminal projections into the superficial cortical layers (Morrison, Molliver, & Grzanna, 1979). Lesions that disrupt these pathways in the frontal cortex or the basal ganglia may affect many downstream fibers. Based on these neuroanatomical facts and on the clinical finding that the severity of depression correlates with the proximity of the lesion to the frontal pole, we have suggested that post-stroke depression may be the consequence of severe depletion of norepinephrine, serotonin, or both produced by frontal or basal ganglia lesions (Robinson et al., 1983a).

Supporting this hypothesis, some investigations have shown (in rats) that biogenic amines are depleted in response to ischemic lesions. This biochemical response to ischemia is also lateralized (Robinson, 1979). Right-hemisphere lesions produce depletions of norepinephrine and an accompanying behavior change of locomotor hyperactivity, whereas lesions of the left hemisphere do not (Robinson, 1979).

Treatment of Depression Following Stroke

Although relatively few studies have examined the effectiveness of the treatment of depression among patients with brain disease, there are three randomized, double-blind studies of the efficacy of antidepressant treatment. Lipsey et al. (1984) examined 14 patients treated with nortriptyline and 20 patients given placebo. Patients received 25 mg for 1 week, 50 mg for 2 weeks, 75 mg for 1 week, and 100 mg for 2 weeks. The group taking the active drug (11 completed the study) showed a significant decrease in depression scores compared with the placebo group (15 completed the study) (Fig. 10.6). Side effects were observed in 3 of 14 nortriptyline treated patients; two developed delirium, and one had sudden syncope of unknown cause. Patients receiving nortriptyline showed a significantly greater improvement in depression as measured by the Hamilton Depression Rating Scale and the Zung Self-Rating Depression Scale. Active and placebo groups, however, did not differ significantly in their mean Hamilton Depression Scores until weeks 4 and 6 of treatment.

The second controlled study, carried out by Reding et al. (1986), demonstrated the usefulness of another antidepressant drug (trazodone) for post-stroke depression. In this study, 27 patients participating in a stroke rehabilitation program were randomly assigned to treatment. Depressed patients taking trazodone were found to have greater improvements in ADL scores than patients treated with placebo. This trend became statistically significant when the treatment groups were restricted to patients with abnormal dexamethasone tests.

The third treatment study was conducted by Andersen, Vestergaard, and Riis, (1993), who used the specific serotonin-reuptake inhibitor (SSRI) citalopram.

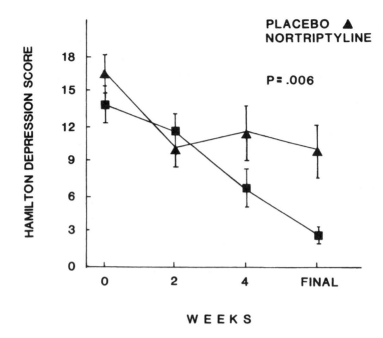

Figure 10.6. Hamilton Depression scores during a 6 week double-blind treatment trial of nortriptyline versus placebo for patients with depression (major or minor) after stroke. Patients receiving acute treatment improved significantly more than those receiving placebo. (Reprinted with permission from Lipsey et al., 1984.)

The Hamilton Depression scores of stroke patients taking citalopram ($N = 27$) were significantly more improved at both 3 and 6 weeks after beginning treatment compared with those of patients taking placebo ($N = 32$).

In summary, although additional controlled treatment trials with a variety of antidepressant medications need to be conducted, current data support the efficacy of antidepressant medication, including the SSRIs, in the treatment of poststroke depression.

DEPRESSION ASSOCIATED WITH PARKINSON'S DISEASE

As with stroke, depression is a frequent finding in patients with Parkinson's disease (PD). Although the frequent association of emotional disorders with PD was recognized more than 70 years ago (Lewy, 1923), it has only been within the past several years that investigators have begun to empirically examine the nature of the relationship. Some investigators have suggested that the high frequency of depression in PD is the understandable consequence of progressive physical impairment (Mindham, 1970). Other investigators have not, however, found a significant correlation between the severity of depression and the severity of physical impairment and have suggested that depression may be a consequence of neurochemical changes in specific brain areas (Mayeux, Stern, & Williams, 1986; Mayeux, Williams, & Stern, 1984).

Prevalence

In several studies, the frequency of depression was reported to be around 40% (Celesia & Wanamaker, 1972; Gothan, Brown, & Marsden, 1986; Mayeux, Williams, & Stern, 1984). In a recent prospective study of a consecutive series of 105 patients, Starkstein et al. (1990a) found that 21% met DSM-III criteria for major depression, while 20% met DSM-III criteria for dysthymic (minor) depression. The highest frequency of depression was found in the early and late stages of PD (Fig. 10.7).

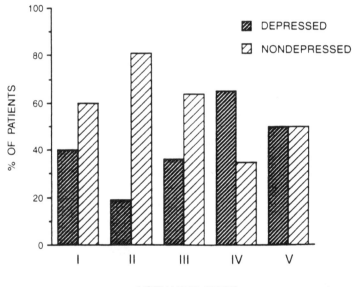

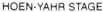

Figure 10.7. The percentage of patients ($N = 105$) at each stage (I–V) of Parkinson's disease who were depressed. All patients were attending an outpatient care clinic whose disease ranged in duration from a few months to more than 15 years. The relative frequency of depression was higher in both the early and late stages of the illness than in the middle stages. We have hypothesized that the early depressions may be associated with left-hemisphere dysfunction, whereas the late depression may be a psychological response to impairment (Starkstein, Robinson, & Preziosi, 1990b). (Reprinted with permission from Robinson & Travella, 1996.)

Relationship to Cognitive Impairment

In PD, cognitive impairments may range from subtle deficits in frontal lobe–related tasks to an overt dementia (El-Awar, Bekcer, & Hammond, 1987). Mayeux, Stern, and Rose (1981), using a modified Mini-Mental State Examination, reported a significant correlation between cognitive deficits and severity of depression (i.e., severe depression was associated with severe cognitive impairments).

This relationship was also reported by Starkstein et al. in three studies. In the first study, the association between depression, cognitive impairments, and stage of PD was examined (Starkstein, Bolduc, & Preziosi, 1989a). Patients in the late stages showed significantly greater overall cognitive impairments than did patients in the early stages, and those impairments were restricted to tasks involving motor-related functions (Fig. 10.8). Depressed patients in the late stages of the disease showed the most significant impairment (Starkstein et al., 1989b). Taken together, these findings suggest that cognitive deficits may primarily be a result of motor impairments, but, when depression also occurs, the cognitive deficits are greater and increase in severity as the PD progresses (Starkstein, Bolduc, & Preziosi, 1989a).

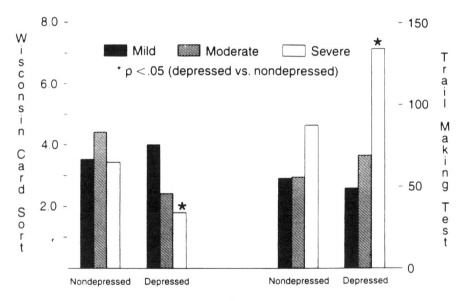

Figure 10.8. Cognitive performance as measured by the number of correctly selected categories on the Wisconsin Card Sorting Task and seconds to complete the Trail Making Test by Parkinson's disease patients with and without depression. Depressed patients were significantly ($P < 0.05$) more impaired than nondepressed patients during the moderate and severe stages of PD. Among the depressed patients, performance on these "frontal lobe" tasks declined with advancing stages of PD. (Reprinted with permission from Robinson & Travella, 1996.)

In the second study, the association between cognitive impairments and type of severity of depression (major or minor) among patients with PD was examined. No differences were found on cognitive tasks between minor depressed and non-depressed patients, but patients with major depression showed the worst cognitive performance. This impairment was greatest on frontal lobe–related tasks, such as the Wisconsin Card Sorting test (Starkstein et al., 1989b). In the third study, the influence of depression on the longitudinal evolution of cognitive deficits was examined in a 3–4 year follow-up. Both groups, depressed and nondepressed patients, showed significant declines in Mini-Mental State Examination scores over time, but the depressed patients had significantly greater cognitive decline than did nondepressed subjects (Starkstein, Bolduc, & Preziosi, 1989a).

These findings demonstrate that depression may be associated not only with cognitive impairments at the time depression is present but also with more rapid cognitive deterioration. These findings support the speculation of Sano, Stern, and William (1989) that depression may be an early finding in patients with PD who later show dementia.

Mechanism

Several studies have demonstrated that patients with PD and dementia may show senile plaques and neurofibrillary tangles compatible with the diagnosis of Alzheimer's disease (AD) as well as severe depletion of cholinergic neurons in the nucleus basalis of Meynert or Lewy bodies in cortical regions (Perry, Curtis, & Dick, 1985). Few neuropathological studies have, however, been carried out in patients with PD and depression. Depression in PD may also be related to changes in other biogenic amines. Mayeux, Williams, and Stern (1984) showed that patients with PD and depression had significantly lower 5-HIAA (a metabolite of serotonin) levels in the cerebrospinal fluid than did patients with PD without depression. However, patients with PD and both dementia and depression had the lowest 5-HIAA cerebrospinal fluid values (Sano, Stern, & William, 1989).

In a recent study, the metabolic abnormalities associated with depression in PD were examined with neuroimaging techniques (Mayberg et al., 1990). Regional cerebral glucose metabolism was determined in depressed ($N = 5$) and nondepressed ($N = 4$) patients with PD using [^{18}F]-fluoro-1-deoxy-D-glucose (FDG) PET. Patients with PD and major depression had significantly lower metabolic activities in the head of the caudate and the inferior frontal cortex than did nondepressed PD patients of comparable age, duration, and stage of illness. Moreover, there was a significant correlation between Hamilton Depression Scale scores and the relative regional metabolism in the inferior frontal cortex ($r = 0.73$, $P < 0.05$) (i.e., the lower the relative regional metabolic activity in the inferior frontal cortex, the more severe the depression).

Treatment

A question that remains unanswered is whether the treatment of depression may influence the progression of intellectual impairments in patients with PD. In the longitudinal 3–4 year follow-up study (Starkstein et al., 1990a), six patients in the depressed group who had received treatment for depression had only an 11% decrease in cognitive scores compared with a 23% decrement in cognitive scores among non-treated depressed patients. Moreover, the two patients who were receiving the highest doses of tricyclics did not show a decline in their Mini-Mental State Examination scores. These preliminary findings are very encouraging, and further prospective double-blind treatment studies are needed to determine whether the use of antidepressants may delay the progression of cognitive impairment in patients with PD.

DEPRESSION ASSOCIATED WITH TRAUMATIC BRAIN INJURY

Kinsella, Moran, and Ford (1988) reported that, in a series of 39 patients, 33% were classified as depressed and 26% as suffering from anxiety within 2 years of severe head injury. Fedoroff et al. (1992) and Jorge et al. (1993b) found that 28 of 66 patients (42%) admitted to a head trauma unit developed major depression at some point during a 1-year follow-up period. Of 66 patients admitted to the hospital with acute closed head injury without significant spinal cord or other organ system injury, 17 (26%) met diagnostic criteria for major depression at the time of the initial in-hospital evaluation. In addition, 3% met criteria for minor (dysthymic) depressive disorder. This frequency is consistent with that found by several other investigators (Brooks, Campsie, & Symington, 1986; Gualtieri & Cox, 1991).

Longitudinal Course of Depression

Mood disorders following TBI may be transient syndromes lasting for a few weeks, or they may be persistent disorders lasting for many months (Grant & Alwes, 1987). Other authors have suggested that transient disorders may be the result of neurochemical changes provoked by brain injury, whereas prolonged depressive disorders may be of a more complex nature and may be reactive to physical or cognitive impairment (Lishman, 1988; Prigatano, 1987; VanZomeren & Saan, 1990).

We have reported empirical data to support these suggestions (Jorge et al., 1993b). Diagnoses of depression were based on a semistructured psychiatric interview (Wing, Cooper, & Sartorius, 1974). Of the original 66 patients evaluated with acute TBI, 54 were re-evaluated at 3 months, 43 at 6 months, and 43 at 1 year. The prevalence of depression was 30% at 3 months, 26% at 6 months, and 26% at 1 year (Jorge et al., 1993a). The mean duration of major depression was 4.7 months. There was, however, a group of seven patients (41% of the depressed group) who had transient depressions lasting 1.5 months, while the nine remaining patients' depression had a mean duration of 7 months. The patients with transient depression showed a strong association with left anterior lesion location (Fischer exact $P =$ 0.006). Prolonged depressions, on the other hand, were associated with impaired social functioning, suggesting that biological factors may lead to transient depression, whereas prolonged depressions may result from psychological factors.

Risk Factors for Depression Following Traumatic Brain Injury

Several premorbid factors may influence patients' emotional responses to acute TBI and may, therefore, be relevant to the etiology of depressive disorder following TBI (Lishman, 1973). In the study of 66 patients with acute TBI, there was a significantly greater frequency of previous personal history of psychiatric disorder in the major depressed group than in the nondepressed patients (Fedoroff et al., 1992). In addition, the depressed patients had significantly more impaired social functioning as measured by the Social Functioning Examination (SFE) (Starr, Robinson, & Price, 1983) (Fig. 10.9). The SFE, during the initial

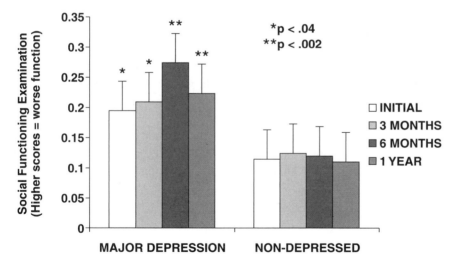

Figure 10.9. Social functioning exam (SFE) scores for patients either with major depression or without depression during 1 year after traumatic brain injury (TBI). The SFE scores reflect function during the month before evaluation. Therefore, the initial score indicates social functioning before TBI. Both before and after head injury, patients with depression had significantly more impaired social functioning than nondepressed patients. This probably reflects the effect of depression on social functioning and vice versa. (Reprinted with permission from Robinson & Travella, 1996.)

evaluation, measured the quality and personal satisfaction with social functioning during the period before brain injury. This suggests, as other investigators have reported, that patients with poor social adjustment and social dissatisfaction before the brain injury were more prone to develop depression.

Relationship to Lesion Location

Some empirical evidence supports an association between post-TBI depression and specific lesion locations. Lishman (1968) reported that several years after penetrating brain injury, depressive symptoms were more common among patients with right-hemisphere lesions. Depressive symptoms were also more frequent among patients with frontal and parietal lesions than among those with lesions at other locations. Grafman, Vance, and Swingartner (1986) also reported that, several years after head injury, depressive symptoms were more frequently associated with penetrating injuries involving right-hemisphere (right orbitofrontal) lesions than lesions at other locations.

Traumatic brain injury is characterized by the presence of diffuse and focal lesions that may be the direct result of traumatic shear injury or secondary to ischemic complications (Katz, 1992). Of the 66 patients previous described, 42 (64%) had a diffuse pattern of brain injury on their CT scans, and 24 (36%) presented with focal lesions. There were no significant differences between major depressed and nondepressed groups in the frequencies of diffuse or focal patterns of injury. In addition, no significant differences were found in the frequencies of extraparenchymal hemorrhages, contusions, intracerebral or intraventricular hemorrhages, hydrocephalus, or CT findings suggestive of brain atrophy. There was, however, a significant association between lesion location and the development of major depression. The presence of left anterior hemisphere lesions (i.e., left dorsolateral frontal cortex or left basal ganglia) was the strongest correlate of major depression (Fig. 10.10). In contrast, other frontal lesions (i.e., left, right, or bilateral frontal lesions, including orbitofrontal cortex) were associated with a lesser probability of development of major depression (Fedoroff et al., 1992). These results are consistent with previous findings in stroke patients of an increased frequency of depression among patients with left dorsolateral cortical and left basal ganglia lesions (Starkstein, Robinson, & Price, 1987b).

Relationship to Impairment Variables

Empirical studies have reported conflicting findings with regard to the relationship between impairment and depressive symptoms following TBI (Bornstein, Miller, & VanSchoor, 1989; Prigatano, 1986). In the previously described study of 66 patients with TBI, there was no significant association between depression and severity of intellectual impairment (i.e., Mini-Mental State Examination) or

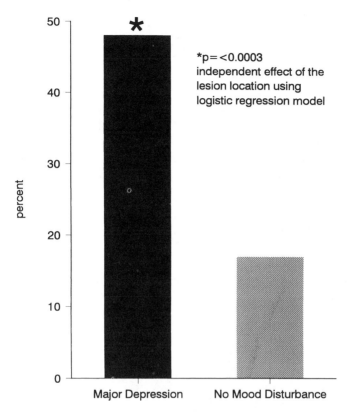

*p=<0.0003
independent effect of the
lesion location using
logistic regression model

Figure 10.10. The proportion of patients with major depression or no mood disturbance at 1 month after traumatic brain injury (TBI) who had evidence on CT scan of injury involving the left dorsal lateral frontal cortex and/or left basal ganglia. Because patients with TBI frequently have multiple areas of injury, a logistic regression analysis was used to examine the independent effects of each area of injury. The strongest independent effect of lesions on depression was found in this left anterior brain region. (Reprinted with permission from Robinson & Travella, 1996.)

ADL (Fedoroff et al., 1992). Social functioning, however, was the clinical variable that had the most consistent relationship with depression throughout the follow-up period (Jorge et al., 1993b). One might infer from these findings that social intervention as well as the treatment of depression may be necessary to alleviate these severe and long-lasting mood disorders.

Treatment

There have been no double-blind, placebo-controlled studies of the efficacy of pharmacological treatments of depression in TBI patients. The selection of antidepressant drugs for the treatment of post-TBI depression is usually guided by their side-effect profiles. Mild anticholinergic activity, minimal lowering of seizure threshold, and low sedative effect are the most important factors to be considered in the choice of an antidepressant drug for this population (Silver, Hales, & Yudofsky, 1990).

There are case reports of successful treatments of post-TBI depression with psychostimulants (Gualtieri, 1988). These include dextroamphetamine (8–60 mg/day), methylphenidate (10–60 mg/day), and pemoline (56–75 mg/day). They are prescribed twice a day, with the last dose at least 6 hours before sleep to prevent initial insomnia. Treatment is begun at lower doses, which are then gradually increased. Patients taking stimulants need close medical monitoring to prevent abuse or toxic effects.

Electroconvulsive therapy is not contraindicated in TBI patients. It may be considered when other methods of treatment are unsuccessful.

Finally, the role of social interventions and adequate psychotherapeutic support should be considered in the treatment of depression. Psychological and pharmacological treatments, however, need to be examined in controlled treatment trials.

SUMMARY AND CONCLUSIONS

Emotional and mood disorders are commonly associated with brain injury. Insights into the causes of these disorders may be gained by investigation of their similarities and differences in several different neurological disorders. This chapter has focused on mood disorders associated with stroke, PD, and TBI.

There are numerous emotional and behavioral disorders that occur after cerebrovascular lesions. Mania is a rare complication of stroke and is strongly associated with right-hemisphere damage involving the orbitofrontal cortex, basal temporal cortex, thalamus, or basal ganglia. Risk factors for mania include a family history of psychiatric disorders and subcortical atrophy. Although patients with secondary mania are usually treated with medications with proven efficacy in primary mania, the most effective treatment modality remains to be determined. Bipolar disorders are associated with subcortical lesions of the right hemisphere, whereas right cortical lesions lead to mania without depression. Depression occurs in about 40% of stroke patients. Depression is significantly associated with left frontal and left basal ganglia lesions during the acute post-stroke period and may be successfully treated with nortriptyline.

Major depression and dysthymic disorders are frequent in PD. Depression may be associated not only with cognitive impairments at the time depression is present but also with more rapid cognitive deterioration. Further studies are needed to determine whether the use of antidepressants may delay the progression of cognitive impairment in patients with PD.

Among patients with acute TBI, 25% of those studied fulfilled criteria for major depressive disorders. The mean duration of major depression was 4.7 months, and a total of 42% developed major depression at some time during the first year after injury. Patients with generalized anxiety disorder and comorbid major depression had longer lasting mood problems than did patients with depression and no anxiety.

There are many areas that are ripe for future research. The most important elements of social functioning that contribute to depression need to be explored, as well as the effect of social intervention. The role of antidepressants in treating these depressive disorders has not been systemically explored and deserves study.

Finally, the mechanism of these depressions, both those associated with psychosocial factors and those associated with neurobiological factors (e.g., strategic lesion locations), need to be investigated. It is only through the discovery of their mechanism that specific and rational treatment strategies for these disorders will be developed.

ACKNOWLEDGMENTS
The authors are indebted to Drs. Sergio E. Starkstein, Thomas R. Price, John R. Lipsey, Rajesh M. Parikh, J. Paul Fedoroff, Helen S. Mayberg, and Karen Bolla, who participated in many of these studies. This work was supported by the following NIMH grants: Research Scientist Award MH00163, MH52879, and MH53592.

REFERENCES

Andersen, G., Vestergaard, K., & Riis, J. (1993). Citalopram for post-stroke pathological crying. *Lancet, 342(8875)*, 837–839.

Astrom, M., Adolfsson, R., & Asplund, K. (1993). Major depression in stroke patients: A 3-year longitudinal study. *Stroke, 24*, 976–982.

Babinski, J. (1914). Contribution a l'étude des troubles mentaux dans l'hemiplégie organique cerebrale (anosognosie). *Revue Neurologique (Paris), 27*, 845–848.

Bakchine, S., Lacomblez, L., Benoit, N., Parisot, F., Chain, F., & Lhermitte, F. (1989). Manic-like state after orbitofrontal and right temporoparietal injury: Efficacy of clonidine. *Neurology, 39*, 778–781.

Beck, E. (1949). A cytoarchitectural investigation into the boundaries of cortical areas 13 and 14 in the human brain. *Journal of Anatomy, 83*, 145–147.

Berthier, M.L., Starkstein, S.E., Robinson, R.G., & Leiguarda, R. (1990). Limbic lesions in a patient with recurrent mania. *Journal of Neuropsychiatry and Clinical Neurosciences, 2*, 235–236.

Bleuler, E.P. (1951). *Textbook of Psychiatry*. New York: Macmillan.

Bolla-Wilson, K., Robinson, R.G., Starkstein, S.E., Boston, J., & Price, T.R. (1989). Lateralization of dementia of depression in stroke patients. *American Journal of Psychiatry, 146*, 627–634.

Bornstein, R.A., Miller, H.B., & VanSchoor, J.T. (1989). Neuropsychological deficit and emotional disturbance in head injured patients. *Journal of Neurosurgery, 70*, 509–513.

Brooks, N., Campsie, L., & Symington, C. (1986). The five-year outcome of severe blunt head injury: A relative's view. *Journal of Neurology, Neurosurgery, and Psychiatry, 49*, 764–770.

Burvill, P.W., Johnson, G.A., Jamrozik, K.D., Anderson, C.S., Stewart-Wynne, E.G., & Chakera, T.M.H. (1995). Prevalence of depression after stroke: The Perth Community Stroke Study. *British Journal of Psychiatry, 166*, 320–327.

Celesia, G.G., & Wanamaker, W.M. (1972). Psychiatric disturbances in Parkinson's disease. *Diseases of the Nervous System, 33*, 577–583.

Crosby, E., Humphrey, T., & Laner, E. (1962). *Correlative Anatomy of the Nervous System*. New York: MacMillan.

Csernansky, J.G., Mellentin, J., Beauclair, L., & Lombrozo, L. (1988). Mesolimbic dopaminergic supersensitivity following electrical kindling of the amygdala. *Biological Psychiatry, 23*, 285–294.

Cummings, J.L., & Mendez, M.F. (1984). Secondary mania with focal cerebrovascular lesions. *American Journal of Psychiatry, 141*, 1084–1087.

Denny-Brown, D., Meyer, J.S., & Horenstein, S. (1952). The significance of perceptual rivalry resulting from parietal lesions. *Brain, 75*, 434–471.

Eastwood, M.R., Rifat, S.L., Nobbs, H., & Ruderman, J. (1989). Mood disorder following cerebrovascular accident. *British Journal of Psychiatry, 154*, 195–200.

El-Awar, M., Bekcer, J.T., & Hammond, K.M. (1987). Learning deficits in Parkinson's disease: Comparison with Alzheimer's disease and normal aging. *Archives of Neurology, 44*, 180–184.

Fedoroff, J.P., Starkstein, S.E., Forrester, A.W., Geisler, F.H., Jorge, R.E., Arndt, S.V., & Robinson, R.G. (1992). Depression in patients with acute traumatic brain injury. *American Journal of Psychiatry, 149*, 918–923.

Finset, A. (1988). Depressed mood and reduced emotionality after right hemisphere brain damage. In M. Kinsbourne (Ed.), *Cerebral Hemisphere Function in Depression* (pp. 49–64). Washington, DC: American Psychiatric Press.

Fogel, B.S., & Sparadeo, F.R. (1985). Focal cognitive deficits accentuated by depression. *Journal of Nervous and Mental Disease, 173*, 129–134.

Gainotti, G. (1972). Emotional behavior and hemispheric side of the brain. *Cortex, 8*, 41–55.

Gloor, P. (1986). Role of the human limbic system in perception, memory and affect: Lessons for temporal lobe epilepsy. In B.K. Doane & K.E. Livingston (Eds.), *The Limbic System: Functional Organization and Clinical Disorders*. New York: Raven Press.

Goldar, J.C., & Outes, D.L. (1972). Fisiopatología de la desinhibición instintiva. *Acta Psiquiátrica y Psicológica de América Latina, 18*, 177–185.

Goldstein, K. (1939). *The Organism: A Holistic Approach to Biology Derived from Pathological Data in Man*. New York: American Books.

Goldstein, K. (1942). *After Effects of Brain Injuries in War*. New York: Grune & Stratton.

Gonzalez-Torrecillas, J.L., Mendlewicz, J., & Lobo, A. (1995). Repercussion of early treatment of post-stroke depression on neuropsychological rehabilitation. *International Psychogeriatrics, 7*, 547–560.

Gothan, A.M., Brown, R.G., & Marsden, C.D. (1986). Depression in Parkinson's disease: A quantitative and qualitative analysis. *Journal of Neurology, Neurosurgery, and Psychiatry, 49*, 381–389.

Grafman, J., Vance, S.C., & Swingartner, H. (1986). The effects of lateralized frontal lesions on mood regulation. *Brain*, *109*, 1127–1148.

Grant, I., & Alwes, W. (1987). Psychiatric and psychological disturbances in head injury. In H.S. Levin, J. Grafman, & H.M. Eisenberg (Eds.), *Neurobehavioral Recovery from Head Injury* (pp. 215–232). London: Oxford University Press.

Gualtieri, C.T. (1988). Pharmacotherapy and the neurobehavioral sequelae of traumatic brain injury. *Brain Injury*, *2*, 101–129.

Gualtieri, C.T., & Cox, D.R. (1991). The delayed neurobehavioral sequelae of traumatic brain injury. *Brain Injury*, *5*, 219–232.

Hécaen, H., de Ajuriaguerra, J., & Massonet, J. (1951). Les troubles visuoconstructifs par lésion parieto occipitale droit. *Encéphale*, *40*, 122–179.

Herrmann, M., Bartels, C., Schumacher, M., & Wallesch, C.-W. (1995). Poststroke depression: Is there a pathoanatomic correlate for depression in the postacute stage of stroke? *Stroke*, *26*, 850–856.

Herrmann, M., Bartles, C., & Wallesch, C.-W. (1993). Depression in acute and chronic aphasia: Symptoms, pathoanatomical–clinical correlations, and functional implications. *Journal of Neurology, Neurosurgery, and Psychiatry*, *56*, 672–678.

House, A., Dennis, M., Mogridge, L., Warlow, C., Hawton, K., & Jones, L. (1991). Mood disorders in the year after stroke. *British Journal of Psychiatry*, *158*, 83–92.

House, A., Dennis, M., Warlow, C., Hawton, K., & Molyneaux, A. (1990a). The relationship between intellectual impairment and mood disorder in the first year after stroke. *Psychological Medicine*, *20*, 805–814.

House, A., Dennis, M., Warlow, C., Hawton, K., & Molyneux, K. (1990b). Mood disorders after stroke and their relation to lesion location. A CT scan study. *Brain*, *113*, 1113–1130.

Ironside, R. (1956). Disorders of laughter due to brain lesions. *Brain*, *79*, 589–609.

Jorge, R.E., Robinson, R.G., Arndt, S.V., Forrester, A.W., Beisler, F., & Starkstein, S.E. (1993a). Comparison between acute and delayed onset depression following traumatic brain injury. *Journal of Neuropsychiatry*, *5*, 43–49.

Jorge, R.E., Robinson, R.G., Arndt, S.V., Starkstein, S.E., Forrester, A.W., & Geisler, F. (1993b). Depression following traumatic brain injury: A 1-year longitudinal study. *Journal of Affective Disorders*, *27*, 233–243.

Jorge, R.E., Robinson, R.G., Starkstein, S.E., Arndt, S.V., Forrester, A.W., & Geisler, F.H. (1993c). Secondary mania following traumatic brain injury. *American Journal of Psychiatry*, *150*, 916–921.

Katz, D.I. (1992). Neuropathology and neurobehavioral recovery from closed head injury. *Journal of Head and Trauma Rehabilitation*, *7*, 1–15.

Kinsella, G., Moran, C., & Ford, B. (1988). Emotional disorders and its assessment within the severe head injured population. *Psychological Medicine*, *18*, 57–63.

Kraepelin, E. (1921). *Manic Depressive Insanity and Paranoia*. Edinburgh: E & S Livingstone.

Kubos, K.L., Moran, T.H., & Robinson, R.G. (1987). Mania after brain injury: A controlled study of etiological factors. *Archives of Neurology*, *44*, 1069–1073.

Lewy, F.H. (1923). *Die Lehre von Tonus und der Bewegung*. Berlin: Springer.

Lipsey, J.R., Robinson, R.G., Pearlson, G.D., Rao, K., & Price, T.R. (1984). Nortriptyline treatment of post-stroke depression: A double-blind treatment trial. *Lancet*, *i*, 297–300.

Lishman, W.A. (1968). Brain damage in relation to psychiatric disability after head injury. *British Journal of Psychiatry*, *114*, 373–410.

Lishman, W.A. (1973). The psychiatric sequelae of head injury: A review. *Psychological Medicine, 3*, 304–318.

Lishman, W.A. (1988). Physiogenesis and psychogenesis in the post-concussional syndrome. *British Journal of Psychiatry, 153*, 460–469.

Mayberg, H.S., Starkstein, S.E., Sadzot, B., Preziosi, T., Andrezejewski, P.L., Dannals, R.F., Wagner, H.N., Jr., & Robinson, R.G. (1990). Selective inferior frontal lobe hypometabolism in depressed patients with Parkinson's disease. *Annals of Neurology, 28*, 57–64.

Mayeux, R., Stern, Y., & Rosen, J. (1981). Depression, intellectual impairment and Parkinson disease. *Neurology, 32*, 645–650.

Mayeux, R., Stern, Y., & Williams, J.B.W. (1986). Clinical and biochemical features of depression in Parkinson's disease. *American Journal of Psychiatry, 143*, 756–759.

Mayeux, R., Williams, J.B.W., & Stern, Y. (1984). Depression in Parkinson disease. *Advances in Neurology, 40*, 242–250.

Meyer, A. (1904). The anatomical facts and clinical varieties of traumatic insanity. *American Journal of Insanity, 60*, 373.

Mindham, R.H.S. (1970). Psychiatric symptoms in parkinsonism. *Journal of Neurology, Neurosurgery, and Psychiatry, 33*, 188–191.

Morris, P.L.P., Robinson, R.G., & Raphael, B. (1990). Prevalence and course of depressive disorders in hospitalized stroke patients. *International Journal of Psychiatry in Medicine, 20*, 349–364.

Morris, P.L.P., Robinson, R.G., & Raphael, B. (1992a). Lesion location and depression in hospitalized stroke patients: Evidence supporting a specific relationship in the left hemisphere. *Neuropsychiatry, Neuropsychology, and Behavioral Neurology, 3*, 75–82.

Morris, P.L.P., Robinson, R.G., Raphael, B., Samuels, J., & Molloy, P. (1992b). The relationship between risk factors for affective disorder and post-stroke depression in hospitalized stroke patients. *Australia and New Zeland Journal of Psychiatry, 26*, 208–217.

Morrison, J.H., Molliver, M.E., & Grzanna, R. (1979). Noradrenergic innervation of the cerebral cortex: Widespread effects of local cortical lesions. *Science, 205*, 313–316.

Nauta, W.J.H. (1971). The problem of the frontal lobe: A reinterpretation. *Journal of Psychological Research, 8*, 167–187.

Pappata, S., Dinh, S.T., Baron, J.C., Cambon, H., & Syrota, A. (1987). Remote metabolic effects of cerebrovascular lesions: Magnetic resonance and positron tomography imaging. *Neuroradiology, 29*, 1–6.

Parikh, R.M., Lipsey, J.R., Robinson, R.G., & Price, T.R. (1987). Two-year longitudinal study of post-stroke mood disorders: Dynamic changes in correlates of depression at one and two years. *Stroke, 18*, 579–584.

Parikh, R.M., Robinson, R.G., Lipsey, J.R., Starkstein, S.E., Fedoroff, J.P., & Price, T.R. (1990). The impact of post-stroke depression on recovery in activities of daily living over two-year follow-up. *Archives of Neurology, 47*, 785–789.

Perry, E.K., Curtis, M., & Dick, D.J. (1985). Cholinergic correlates of cognitive impairment in Parkinson disease: Comparisons with Alzheimer's disease. *Journal of Neurology, Neurosurgery, and Psychiatry, 48*, 413–421.

Prigatano, G.P. (1986). *Neuropsychological Rehabilitation after Brain Injury.* Baltimore: Johns Hopkins University Press.

Prigatano, G.P. (1987). Psychiatric aspects of head injury: Problem areas and suggested guidelines for research. In H.S. Levin, J. Grafman, & H.M. Eisenberg (Eds.), *Neurobehavioral Recovery from Head Injury* (pp. 215–232). Oxford, England: Oxford University Press.

Reding, J.J., Orto, L.A., Winter, S.W., Fortuna, I.M., DiPonte, P., & McDowell, F.H. (1986). Antidepressant therapy after stroke: A double-blind trial. *Archives of Neurology*, *43*, 763–765.

Robinson, R.G. (1979). Differential behavioral and biochemical effects of right and left hemispheric cerebral infarction in the rat. *Science*, *105*, 707–710.

Robinson, R.G., & Benson, D.F. (1981). Depression in aphasic patients: Frequency, severity and clinical–pathological correlations. *Brain and Language*, *14*, 282–291.

Robinson, R.G., Bolduc, P., & Price, T.R. (1987). A two year longitudinal study of post-stroke depression: Diagnosis and outcome at one and two year follow-up. *Stroke*, *18*, 837–843.

Robinson, R.G., Boston, J.D., Starkstein, S.E., & Price, T.R. (1988). Comparison of mania with depression following brain injury: Causal factors. *American Journal of Psychiatry*, *145*, 172–178.

Robinson, R.G., Kubos, K.L., Starr, L.B., Rao, K., & Price, T.R. (1983a). Mood changes in stroke patients: Relationship to lesion location. *Comprehensive Psychiatry*, *24*, 555–566.

Robinson, R.G., Lipsey, J.R., Bolla-Wilson, K., Bolduc, P.L., Pearlson, G.D., Rao, K., & Price, T.R. (1985). Mood disorders in left-handed stroke patients. *American Journal of Psychiatry*, *142*, 1424–1429.

Robinson, R.G., Lipsey, J.R., Rao, K., & Price, T.R. (1986). Two-year longitudinal study of post-stroke mood disorders: Comparison of acute-onset with delayed-onset depression. *American Journal of Psychiatry*, *143*, 1238–1244.

Robinson, R.G., Starr, L.B., Kubos, K.L., & Price, T.R. (1983b). A two year longitudinal study of post-stroke mood disorders: Findings during the initial evaluation. *Stroke*, *14*, 736–744.

Robinson, R.G., & Szetela, B. (1981). Mood change following left hemispheric brain injury. *Annals of Neurology*, *9*, 447–453.

Robinson, R.G., & Travella, J.I. (1996). Neuropsychiatry of mood disorders. In B.S. Fogel, R. Schiffer, & S.M. Rao (Eds.), *Neuropsychiatry* (pp. 287–305). Baltimore: Williams & Wilkins.

Ross, E.D., & Rush, A.J. (1981). Diagnosis and neuroanatomical correlates of depression in brain damaged patients. *Archives of General Psychiatry*, *38*, 1344–1354.

Sano, M., Stern, Y., & William, J. (1989). Coexisting dementia and depression in Parkinson's disease. *Archives of Neurology*, *46*, 1284–1286.

Shukla, S., Cook, B.L., Mukherjee, S., Godwin, C., & Miller, M.G. (1987). Mania following head trauma. *American Journal of Psychiatry*, *144*, 93–96.

Silver, J.M., Hales, R.E., & Yudofsky, S.C. (1990). Psychopharmacology of depression in neurologic disorders. *Journal of Clinical Psychiatry*, *51*, 33–39.

Sinyor, D., Jacques, P., Kaloupek, D.G., Becker, R., Goldenberg, M., & Coopersmith, H. (1986). Post-stroke depression and lesion location: An attempted replication. *Brain*, *109*, 539–546.

Starkstein, S.E., Bolduc, P.L., Mayberg, H.S., Preziosi, T.J., & Robinson, R.G. (1990a). Cognitive impairment and depression in Parkinson's disease: A follow-up study. *Journal of Neurology, Neurosurgery, and Psychiatry*, *53*, 597–602.

Starkstein, S.E., Bolduc, P.L., Preziosi, T.J., & Robinson, R.G. (1989a). Cognitive impairments in different states of Parkinson disease. *Journal of Neuropsychiatry and Clinical Neurosciences*, *1*, 243–248.

Starkstein, S.E., Fedoroff, J.P., Berthier, M.D., & Robinson, R.G. (1991). Manic depressive and pure manic states after brain lesions. *Biological Psychiatry*, *29*, 149–158.

Starkstein, S.E., Mayberg, H.S., Berthier, M.L., Fedoroff, P., Price, T.R., Dannals, R.F., Wagner, H.N., Leiguarda, R., & Robinson, R.G. (1990b). Mania after brain injury: neuroradiological and metabolic findings. *Annals of Neurology, 27,* 652–659.

Starkstein, S.E., Moran, T.H., Bowersox, J.A., & Robinson, R.G. (1988). Behavioral abnormalities induced by frontal cortical and nucleus accumbens lesions. *Brain Research, 473,* 74–80.

Starkstein, S.E., Pearlson, G.D., Boston, J., & Robinson, R.G. (1987a). Mania after brain injury: A controlled study of causative factors. *Archives of Neurology, 44,* 1069–1073.

Starkstein, S.E., Preziosi, T.J., Berthier, M.L., Bolduc, P.L., Mayberg, H.S., & Robinson, R.G. (1989b). Depression and cognitive impairments in Parkinson's disease. *Brain, 112,* 1141–1153.

Starkstein, S.E., & Robinson, R.G. (1988). Aphasia and depression. *Aphasiology, 2,* 1–20.

Starkstein, S.E., Robinson, R.G., Honig, M.A., Parikh, R.M., Joselyn, P., & Price, T.R. (1989c). Mood changes after right hemisphere lesion. *British Journal of Psychiatry, 155,* 79–85.

Starkstein, S.E., Robinson, R.G., & Preziosi, T.J. (1990c). Depression in Parkinson's disease. *Journal of Nervous and Mental Disease, 178,* 27–31.

Starkstein, S.E., Robinson, R.G., & Price, T.R. (1987b). Comparison of cortical and subcortical lesions in the production of post-stroke mood disorders. *Brain, 110,* 1045–1059.

Starr, L.B., Robinson, R.G., & Price, T.R. (1983). Reliability, validity, and clinical utility of the social functioning exam in the assessment of stroke patients. *Experimental Aging Research, 9,* 101.

Stevens, J.R. (1990). Psychiatric consequences of temporal lobectomy for intractable seizures. *Psychological Medicine, 20,* 529–545.

VanZomeren, A.H., & Saan, R.J. (1990). Psychological and social sequelae of severe head injury. In R. Braakman (Ed.), *Handbook of Clinical Neurology,* Vol. 13 (pp. 397–420). Amsterdam: Elsevier Science Publishers, B.V.

Wing, J.K., Cooper, J.E., & Sartorius, N. (1974). *The Measurement and Classification of Psychiatric Symptoms: An Instructional Manual for the PSE and CATEGO Programs.* New York: Cambridge University Press.

Regional Brain Function in Sadness and Depression

RICHARD J. DAVIDSON AND
JEFFREY HENRIQUES

Over the last 15, years there has been increased interest in the cerebral lateralization of emotion and emotion-related psychopathology (e.g., Davidson & Tomarken, 1989). Although numerous studies point to right-hemisphere specialization in the *perception* of emotional information (see Silberman & Weingartner, 1986), evidence suggests that the anterior regions of the right and left hemispheres play different roles with respect to the *production* of emotion. Following from Schneirla's argument (1959) that approach and withdrawal underlie all motivated behaviors across phylogeny, Davidson and others (i.e., Davidson, 1984, 1987, 1992, 1995; Davidson & Tomarken, 1989; Kinsbourne, 1978) have proposed that the anterior regions of the left and right hemispheres are specialized for approach and withdrawal behavior, respectively. For instance, the induction of a withdrawal-related emotion, such as disgust, has been shown to be associated with an increase in relative right-sided anterior activation, while increased relative left-sided activation accompanies approach-related emotions such as happiness (e.g., Davidson et al., 1990b; Fox & Davidson, 1986). Gray (1994) proposed similiar conceptual systems with a different functional anatomy and has labeled these systems the Behavioral Approach System (BAS) and the Behavioral Inhibition System (BIS).

At the same time, factor analytic studies of mood have identified two broad orthogonal factors: positive affect (PA) and negative affect (NA), (Tellegen,

1985; Watson & Tellegen, 1985). These two factors appear to tap behavior reflective of approach and withdrawal. NA is described generally as subjective distress and includes mood states such as fear, disgust, and anxiety (Watson, Clark, & Carey, 1988), prototypical withdrawal-related emotions (Davidson & Tomarken, 1989). PA does not reflect happiness per se, but rather "one's level of pleasurable engagement with the environment" (Watson, Clark, & Carey, 1988, p. 347). High PA is characterized by enthusiasm, mental alertness, and determination, while low PA is characterized by lethargy and fatigue. Studies using these affect dimensions have shown that it is the loss of PA that differentiates depression from other negative affect states such as anxiety (Bouman & Luteijn, 1986; MacLeod, Byrne, & Valentine, 1996; Watson, Clark, & Carey, 1988).

Although investigations of experimentally induced affect demonstrate consistent changes in frontal asymmetry across subjects between approach- and withdrawal-related emotion conditions (i.e., Davidson et al., 1990b), these changes in relative asymmetry are superimposed on considerable individual variation in absolute asymmetry. These asymmetries in absolute anterior activation are predicted to reflect affective style and to affect an individual's vulnerability to particular types of psychopathology (Davidson, 1998). In line with this, studies have shown that individuals with relative left-sided frontal activation are characterized by high levels of PA and self-reported activity in the BAS (e.g., Harmon-Jones & Allen, 1997; Jacobs & Snyder, 1996; Sutton & Davidson, 1997; Tomarken et al., 1992). Subjects with relative right-sided frontal activation are characterized by high levels of NA and self-reported activity in the BIS (Sutton & Davidson, 1997; Tomarken et al., 1992). Within this model, absolute anterior asymmetry by itself does not produce a particular pattern of emotional behavior or psychopathology; instead, anterior asymmetry is seen as a diathesis for the expression of emotional behavior, *given an appropriate affect elicitor*. For instance, individuals with increased relative right anterior activation report more NA in response to emotion-eliciting film clips than do subjects with relatively more left anterior activation (Tomarken, Davidson, & Henriques, 1990; Wheeler, Davidson, & Tomarken, 1993).

Within the context of this model, sadness and depression which are associated with decreased PA, should be associated with decreased left frontal activation, and individuals who are characterized by a relatively stable pattern of left anterior hypoactivation should be more susceptible to the elicitation of sad mood and at increased risk for depression. Note that this model is only proposing a relation between left anterior function and sad mood and depression, not one involving the relative pattern of activation between the two hemispheres. Variations in right anterior function should reflect variations in NA among individuals. Thus, depressed individuals who have increased right frontal activity would be expected to be at risk for withdrawal-related emotions as well and would typically present a clinical picture of a depressed and anxious mood. Individuals who have concurrent low right frontal activation should be less susceptible to withdrawal-related emotions, as well as to approach-related emotions, and would typically present a clinical picture of depressed flattened affect. This variability in predicted symptom profile mirrors the clinical literature (e.g., Baumeister, 1990; Roth et al., 1972).

The evidence for decreased left anterior activation in depression has grown slowly, and the results of studies that have examined patterns of cerebral activation during the elicitation of sadness seem to suggest different conclusions. One of the assumptions that appears to underlie work in this area is that sadness and depression are on the same continuum and that the differences are merely one of degree. That assumption may not, however, be correct. Sadness is only a part of depression, and it may be that the other symptoms, such as loss of interest, loss of pleasure, and social withdrawal, play a much larger role in the differences in regional brain activation that have been observed between depressed and nondepressed subjects.

STUDIES OF CEREBRAL INACTIVATION AND LESIONS

Investigators who have used sodium amytal to selectively anesthetize a cerebral hemisphere have found that inactivation of the left hemisphere produces a dysphoric reaction in some subjects, while inactivation of the right hemisphere is associated with euphoria or indifference (e.g., Alema & Rosadini, 1964; Christianson et al., 1993; Lee et al., 1990; Terzian, 1964). Although some authors (e.g., Flor-Henry, 1979) have interpreted these data in the context of a right-hemisphere role for sadness and depression, it should be noted that the dysphoric reaction described does not occur immediately after the left hemisphere has been anesthetized but emerges as the hemisphere resumes functioning and the language disturbances and hemiplegia resolve (Terzian, 1964). This suggests that the dysphoric reaction observed following left-hemisphere barbiturization is not necessarily the result of a disinhibited right hemisphere but rather could result from decreased activation in the left hemisphere. Additionally, lesion studies have shown that increased tearfulness and crying were associated with left-sided lesions (e.g., Gainotti, 1972; House et al., 1989; Sackeim et al., 1982). Thus, in these studies, sad mood is associated with left-sided inactivation.

A number of investigators who have studied mood disturbances in epileptics have found that patients with left-sided epileptogenic lesions report significantly higher levels of depression than do patients with right-sided lesions during the interictal period (e.g., Altshuler et al., 1990; Bear & Fedio, 1977; Black, 1975; Gasparrini et al., 1978; Mendez et al., 1994; Perini, 1986; Perini & Mendius, 1984). Given that the region of epileptic focus is usually characterized by hypometabolism during the interictal period (Engel, 1984), these studies are consistent with the idea of an association between left anterior hypoactivation and depression.

For the most part, these studies have not addressed the issue of the anterior/posterior dimension within the hemisphere, an important issue given the differential role these regions play in behavior (see Davidson, 1992). Robinson and coworkers have systematically and elegantly investigated the nature of post-stroke mood disturbance (e.g., Lipsey et al., 1983; Robinson et al., 1984, 1985; Robinson & Szetela, 1981; Starkstein, Robinson, & Price, 1987). They have used computerized tomography scans to precisely specify lesion location and have used standardized diagnostic interviews to characterize the nature of the emotional disturbance. They have found that the severity of post-stroke depression was positively related to the lesion's proximity to the frontal pole in the left hemisphere such that more anterior lesions were associated with increased depression (Lipsey et al., 1983; Robinson et al., 1984). Investigation of right-hemisphere damage and depression point to an inverse relation such that more posterior lesions were associated with increased severity of depression (Robinson et al., 1984).

The depression observed in these patients is phenomenologically similar to clinical depression (Lipsey et al., 1986), and comparisons of depressed patients with and without stroke-induced lesions reveal that both groups have similar levels of depression. The only difference between groups is the greater cognitive and physical impairment observed in post-stroke depressed patients relative to neurologically intact depressed patients (Lipsey et al., 1986). Given this difference in cognitive function, it should be noted that the severity of post-stroke depression has not been found to be related to the severity of the functional impairment produced by the stroke; rather, it is lesion location that appears to be the critical variable (Robinson & Price, 1982).

Although one study has replicated Robinson's work (Sinyor et al., 1986), a second study has not found an increased incidence of major depression among subjects with left-hemisphere lesions (House et al., 1990). Gainotti (1989) has argued that because not all subjects with left anterior lesions become depressed the hypothesis of a relation between left frontal inactivation and depression should be rejected. His view is predicated on the idea that left frontal lesions are sufficient to produce depression. Davidson (1993) has offered an alternative framework for understanding this corpus of evidence based on a diathesis–stress model. While subjects with left anterior lesions are presumed to be at increased risk for depression, the fact that not all of these subjects become depressed merely demonstrates that decreased left anterior activation is not *sufficient* for the occurrence of depression. It is quite possible that the House et al. (1990) subjects, while having the diathesis, simply had not had a sufficient level of stress to elicit a depressive episode. In fact, there were differences between the patient samples studied by House and Robinson: Fewer than half of the subjects in the House et al. (1990) study had been hospitalized as a result of their stroke, and less than one-third lived alone. In contrast, only one third of the subjects examined by Robinson and Price (1982) were married, and all had been hospitalized for their strokes.

The findings from this literature appear to be generally supportive of the idea that decreases in left-sided activation, specifically in the anterior cortical zones, are associated with sadness and depression. None of the studies reviewed thus far has, however, provided a concurrent assessment of cerebral function. Thus, these findings do not rule out the possibility that the observed changes in mood are the result of changes elsewhere in the brain. To that end, it is necessary to investigate cerebral functioning in an anatomically intact population. This question has been addressed with both electrophysiological and radioactive ligand studies.

ELECTROENCEPHALOGRAM STUDIES

Methodological Issues

Interpretation of the growing corpus of work utilizing electroencephalography (EEG) can be difficult for a number of reasons, including the use of different parameters, variability in the sites from which data were recorded, and variability in the frequency bands analyzed. Furthermore, there are some studies that cannot be interpreted because of methodological flaws, including failure to control for type I error, failure to transform raw EEG, and failure to remove muscle and eye movement artifact. Raw values of relative and absolute power are not normally distributed (Gasser, Bacher, & Mocks, 1982). In fact, "[t]hese deviations [from normality] are usually rather gross" (Gasser et al., 1982, p. 119), and this poses problems for the use of parametric statistics. Gasser, Bacher, and Mocks (1982) examined several different methods of data transformation and found that a log transformation of absolute power resulted in the best approximation of a normal distribution. Relative power more closely approximated a normal distribution before transformation, and using a $\log(x/1 - x)$ transform resulted in an almost perfect normal distribution. Some investigators do not remove epochs contaminated by muscle artifact either in the assumption that electromyographic (EMG) activity is symmetrical or in the belief that the filtering of all signals above 30 Hz removes EMG activity. Evidence suggests that EMG activity is not symmetrical (Volavka et al., 1981), and EMG power can be detected in bands as low as 10 Hz (see Davidson, 1988). This makes it difficult to interpret the results of studies that do not remove EMG artifact, especially those recording from the temporal regions, which are particularly susceptible to muscle artifact (e.g., Flor-Henry et al., 1979; Ulrich et al., 1984).

The EEG measures used by investigators fall into two broad categories: measures of amount (e.g., relative power) and measures of variability (e.g., coefficient of variation). Investigators use these measures to examine activity in broad frequency, bands (e.g., 0.5–30 Hz) or in specific frequency bands (e.g., delta [1–4 Hz], theta [4–8 Hz], alpha [8–13 Hz], beta 1 [13–20 Hz]). Although studies vary with regard to the specific frequency bands examined, almost all assess activity in the alpha band (e.g., Henriques & Davidson, 1990, 1991; Matousek, Capone, & Okawa, 1981; Perris et al., 1981). Power in the alpha band is inversely correlated with relative brain activation, with a *decrease* in alpha power indicative of an *increase* in brain activation (Lindsley & Wicke, 1974). Davidson et al. (1990a) examined patterns of activation during performance of spatial and verbal tasks and found that greater power suppression occurred in all bands, in the hemisphere putatively most activated. This suggests that increased activation is associated with decreases in power across bands. It is less clear what differences in variability reflect. For the most part, increases in variability have been interpreted as reflecting increases in activity, based on the assumption that cortical activation would be associated with neuronal desynchrony and thus increased variability in the EEG. Flor-Henry et al. (1979) examined both power and variability and reported decreases in variability coincident with increases in power.

Studies of Induced Sadness

In one of the earliest studies of induced sadness, Tucker et al. (1981) recorded the EEG activity from across the head during the induction of depression and euphoria. Differences between the two mood states were only observed in the frontal regions. Relative to the euphoric mood state, depressed mood was associated with more left and less right alpha power, indicating that depression was associated with relative right-sided activation. Ahern and Schwartz (1985) investigated EEG asymmetry in response to questions designed to elicit happy, excited, neutral, sad, or fearful responses. This study did not report data from the individual hemispheres and did not include any assessment of whether these differential moods had been induced. Their asymmetry data showed no difference in frontal alpha asymmetry between happiness and sadness. Both of these emotion conditions had relatively more left-sided activation than did the other three emotion conditions studied. Given the contradictory results found thus far, it is clear that more studies are needed to examine the relations between patterns of EEG activation and induced sad mood in normal individuals. One of the critical problems in this work is the need to verify that the intended emotion was indeed induced. Ideally, measures other than simple self-report should be used because there are strong expectancy effects in studies that use mood induction. Measures of spontaneous facial behavior can be fruitfully used as an unobtrusive index of the induced emotion (e.g., Davidson et al., 1990b).

Studies of Depression

Most EEG studies of depression have compared depressed and nondepressed subjects' resting patterns of brain electrical activity. Unfortunately, not all studies have included frontal measures (e.g., Cazard, 1989; Cazard, Ricard, & Facchetti, 1992; Ulrich et al., 1984). Henriques and Davidson (1991) examined the activity in four different frequency bands at six scalp sites in each hemisphere in a group of clinically depressed individuals. The one region where depressed subjects differed from normal controls was in the midfrontal region and involved the patterning of alpha power. Depressed subjects had relative right-sided frontal activation as a result of hypoactivation in the left hemisphere.

These findings mirror earlier work with subclinically depressed people (Schaffer, Davidson, & Saron, 1983). Because there is not a clear consensus in the literature regarding referencing strategies (see Davidson, 1988; Lehman, 1987; Nunez, 1981), data were derived with three different reference montages, and the pattern of left frontal hypoactivation was consistent across montages. We have also found this pattern of left frontal hypoactivation in remitted depressed patients (Henriques & Davidson, 1990). A recent study replicated these results, finding that both currently depressed and previously depressed subjects had less left frontal activation than never depressed controls (Gotlib, Ranganath, & Rosenfeld, 1998). Similar findings have been reported in a small group of bipolar subjects with seasonal affective disorder (Allen et al., 1993). Another study that examined the stability of frontal asymmetry in a group of 25 depressed subjects over an 8 week period found that changes in symptom severity were unrelated to frontal asymmetry (Hitt, Allen, & Duke, 1995). Furthermore, the intraclass correlations between the two testing occasions ranged from 0.51 to 0.81. All of these findings point to a trait-like role for decreased left frontal activation in depression, supporting the view that left hypoactivation serves as a diathesis for the experience of depression.

While studies have reported differences in posterior asymmetry, these findings have been mixed (e.g., Henriques & Davidson, 1990; von Knorring, 1983). d'Elia and Perris (1973, 1974) found decreases in left posterior variability among depressed subjects, and this variability increased on recovery. In contrast, von Knorring (1983) found that depressed subjects had more variability in the right hemisphere than did controls. Increased right posterior activation (decreased relative alpha power) has been reported by Pozzi et al. (1995) and Suzuki et al. (1996). Other studies suggest that depression is associated with decreased right posterior activation. Cazard (1989) recorded from the parietal regions and found that depressed subjects had less variability in the right than left hemisphere, while controls had similar variability in the two hemispheres. Recovery was associated with an increase in variability in both hemispheres and the loss of any asymmetry. A subsequent study found decreased right posterior variability in all depressed subjects, while only the most severe cases also had decreased left posterior variability (Cazard, Ricard, & Facchetti, 1992). We have found decreased right posterior activation in remitted depressed patients (Henriques & Davidson, 1990), but not in currently depressed subjects (Henriques & Davidson, 1991).

All of the aforementioned studies have examined subjects during resting conditions. A more consistent pattern of decreased right posterior activation in depression emerges when subjects are compared during cognitive task performance, and these results are consistent with those from behavioral studies that depressed subjects have a selective impairment in spatial task performance (e.g., Miller et al., 1995). We compared depressed and nondepressed subjects on psychometrically matched verbal and spatial tasks and found that depressed subjects performed worse than controls on the spatial task but performed similar to controls on the verbal task (Henriques & Davidson, 1997). EEGs recorded during these tasks showed that depressed subjects showed no increase in activation in the right posterior regions during spatial task performance. Control subjects, in contrast, had a pattern of relative right-sided activation during the spatial task and relative left-sided activation during the verbal task. Using the same tasks, Reid, Allen, and Duke (1995) had similar results. In a study examining patterns of EEG activation in response to lateralized facial stimuli, Davidson, Schaffer, and Saron (1985) found that depressed subjects had an inverse relationship between frontal and parietal asymmetries that was not seen in control subjects. Among depressed subjects, larger decreases in left frontal activation were associated with greater decreases in right parietal activation.

In work examining EEG patterns of activation in elderly depressed subjects, the pattern observed is one of a global decrease in activation compared with nondepressed subjects (Pollock & Schneider, 1990). This pattern of increased alpha power across the head also characterizes recovered elderly depressed people (Pollock & Schneider, 1989). Global decreases in activation have also been found by Roemer et al. (1992), who additionally found greater left-sided power in the theta, alpha, and beta bands among depressed subjects.

Although there has not been enough work done on EEG changes associated with sadness to draw any firm conclusions (Ahern & Schwartz, 1985; Tucker et al., 1981), depression appears to be associated with decreased left-sided anterior EEG activation (e.g., Allen et al., 1991; Gotlib, Ranganath, & Rosenfeld, 1998; Henriques & Davidson, 1990, 1991; Schaffer, Davidson, & Saron, 1983). The patterning of posterior asymmetry in depression is less clear. Findings include left-sided decreases in activation (e.g., d'Elia & Perris, 1973, 1974), right-sided increases (von Knorring, 1983), right-sided decreases (e.g., Allen et al., 1991; Cazard, 1989; Henriques & Davidson, 1990), and bilateral decreases (Pollock & Schneider, 1989, 1990). Heller and associates (1997) have suggested that differences in posterior asymmetry reflect differences in anxious arousal such that right-sided activation reflects the somatic arousal and tension associated with anxious arousal whereas left-sided activation is associated with the worry and verbal rumination of anxious apprehension. In fact, a recent study comparing anxious and nonanxious depressed subjects found that those who were nonanxious were characterized by decreased activation over the right parietotemporal sites and those who were anxious had increased right posterior activation (Bruder et al., 1997). Relations between increased right posterior activation and increased anxiety in depression has also been reported by Matousek (1991).

EVOKED POTENTIAL STUDIES

Methodological Issues

In evoked potential studies, when subjects are required to make a discrimination between a target and a nontarget stimulus, there is an identifiable positive peak occurring at about 300 msec post-stimulus (P300). The classic P300 waveform has a posterior distribution and has been hypothesized as reflecting an updating in memory of the stimulus representation (Coles, Gratton, & Fabiani, 1990). Its elicitation reflects, among other things, the psychological value or meaning of the stimulus and the relative probability of the stimulus' occurrence. The components of the evoked potential waveform that occur within the first 250 msec of stimulus onset are believed to be associated with early sensory and attentional processes (Naatanen & Picton, 1987). To the best of our knowledge, there are no studies that have examined event-related potentials (ERPs) during the elicitation of sadness.

Studies of Depression

There is a considerably larger corpus of work with ERP studies of depression than with EEG studies of depression (for reviews, see Henriques & Davidson, 1989; Zahn, 1986); however, relatively few have examined the issue of asymmetry and depression (e.g., Bruder et al., 1995; Tenke et al., 1993). In studies that have not examined asymmetry, some have not found differences between depressed and nondepressed subjects in P3 amplitude (e.g., Giedke, Thier, & Bolz, 1981) or in latency (e.g., Giedke, Thier, & Bolz, 1981; Kraiuhin et al., 1990; Pfefferbaum et al., 1984). Other investigators have reported that depressed subjects have decreased P3 amplitudes compared with controls (e.g., Diner, Holcomb, & Dykman, 1985; Pfefferbaum et al., 1984; Thier, Axmann, & Giedke, 1986). The results of examinations of other components of the evoked potential waveform are also mixed, with some investigators reporting increased amplitudes among depressed subjects (e.g., Elton, 1984; Khanna, Mukundan, & Channabasavanna, 1989; Vasile et al., 1989), others reporting no differences (e.g., Diner, Halcomb, & Dykman, 1985; Knott et al., 1991; Plooij-van Gorsel, 1984; Thier, Axmann, & Giedke, 1986), and still others reporting decreases (e.g., Giedke, Thier, Bolz, 1981; Roth et al., 1981).

Bruder (1992) has suggested that the use of overly simple tasks has resulted in the failure to find consistent differences between depressed and nondepressed subjects. Similar reasoning may explain why the EEG literature, reviewed above, reports variability in resting posterior differences yet consistent right posterior decreases during cognitive tasks. In addition to using more complex tasks, Bruder and his associates have examined the issue of asymmetry in the evoked potentials of depressed and nondepressed subjects (e.g., Bruder et al., 1995; Tenke et al., 1993). They have recorded evoked potentials during spatial and temporal discrimination tasks and have found that control subjects who had a strong left ear (right hemisphere) advantage during a complex tone task had right greater than left P3 amplitudes. This asymmetry was seen at different sites across the hemisphere. Depressed subjects, in addition to having lower P3 amplitudes than controls, did not show this normal right greater than left asymmetry (Bruder et al., 1995). In a study comparing typical and atypical depressed subjects, Bruder et al. (1991) found that typical depressed subjects had a longer P3 latency in an audiospatial task but not a temporal task than did normal controls and atypical depressed subjects. This investigation also found that the P3 latency in typical depressed subjects was longer for stimuli presented to the right hemifield (i.e., left hemisphere) than to the left hemifield. Atypical depressed subjects and normal controls did not show this asymmetry.

In summary, studies have failed to demonstrate consistent differences in P3 amplitudes between depressed and nondepressed subjects (e.g., Bruder et al., 1995; Diner, Holcomb, & Dykman, 1985; Giedke, Thier, & Bolz, 1981). The performance of a right hemisphere task, but not a left hemisphere task, however, is associated with increased P3 latency in typical depressed subjects (Bruder et al., 1995) and with a lack of the relative right-sided asymmetry in P3 amplitude seen in controls (Tenke et al., 1993), providing some evidence of impairment in right posterior function in depression, although the significance of latency differences in P3 is not entirely clear.

STUDIES OF CEREBRAL METABOLISM AND BLOOD FLOW

Methodological Issues

Studies of regional cerebral blood flow (rCBF) and glucose metabolism have the advantage over EEG and ERP studies of being able to provide better spatial resolution, and, furthermore, recent advances allow rCBF and glucose metabolism studies to assess the functions of subcortical structures, which measures of brain electrical activity cannot do. The increase in spatial resolution is, however, accompanied by a loss of temporal resolution and an increase in cost. Both metabolism and blood flow studies use a radioactive tracer to examine cerebral activation. The supposition underlying these studies is that increased neuronal activation is accompanied by an increase in metabolism and an associated increase in blood flow.

A particularly important methodological issue in the assessment of lateralized changes in neuroimaging studies is how putatively asymmetrical changes are measured. In most neuroimaging studies, if a focus of activation exceeds an arbitrary statistical threshold in one hemisphere but not in the other, a lateralized effect is reported. A formal test of the Hemisphere X Condition or Hemisphere X Group interaction must, however, be performed. This interaction test formally assesses whether the change in one hemisphere is significantly different from the change in the opposite hemisphere. Without such a test of the interaction term, it is simply not possible to know whether a reported lateralized effect is indeed truly asymmetrical. For example, if a focus exceeds threshold in one hemisphere and falls just below threshold in the other hemisphere, a lateralized effect would be claimed yet a formal test of the interaction would show that the interaction was clearly not significant. In addition, it is possible for there to be a significant interaction without any of the main effects being significant. Thus, we must exercise considerable caution in interpreting putatively lateralized changes that have been reported in the recent neuroimaging studies of emotion.

Blood Flow Studies of Induced Sadness

It was not until recently that investigators began to use rCBF technologies to study sadness, and, in contrast to studies of depression, most have found that sadness is associated with increased cerebral activation. In a study in which subjects were asked to recall or imagine a sad event, sadness was associated with increases in the inferior and orbitofrontal regions (Pardo, Pardo, & Raichle, 1993). Among women these increases were bilateral, whereas among men these increases were seen only in the left hemisphere. Because these investigators only compared the sad mood to a resting control condition, it is unclear how much of the observed increases were specific to sadness rather than to the processes involved in memory retrieval and imagery per se.

In a study that examined both happiness and sadness, sadness was associated with increased global blood flow relative to a neutral mood, whereas happiness was associated with decreased global blood flow (Schneider et al., 1994). Mood changes were induced by having the subjects view happy and sad facial expressions and asking the subjects to try and experience the mood being displayed. The efficacy of the mood induction was assessed with the Positive and Negative Affective Schedule scales, and the investigators found a significant correlation between the increase in negative mood reported and the increase in cerebral blood flow. The frontal poles were the only regions that showed lateralized differences between the emotions: Sadness was associated with left greater than right blood flow, whereas happiness was associated with right greater than left blood flow in this region. However, the three-way interaction of Region, Hemisphere, and Emotion condition was clearly not significant, casting some doubt on this specific finding.

A subsequent study by the same group did not find any global differences in blood flow between happy and sad induced moods (Schneider et al., 1995). They did report significant differences in subcortical blood flow such that sadness was associated with increased left and decreased right CBF in the amygdala, increases in the caudate, and decreases in the mamillary body and posterior cingulate. Although there were no cortical asymmetries, there was a trend for increased left frontotemporal blood flow to be associated with increased reports of both negative and positive affect. George et al. (1995) found that sadness relative to happiness was associated with bilateral increases in the prefrontal cortex, the thalamus, and the basal ganglia and with increases in the right anterior cingulate. Highlighting the importance of comparing sadness to another emotional state, when these investigators compared sadness to a neutral condition there was a different pattern of increased activation, including an increase in the left lateral prefrontal region and bilateral increases in the anterior cingulate.

Baker, Frith, and Dolan (1997) recently found that both elated and depressed mood states were associated with bilateral increases in orbitofrontal blood flow and with increased blood flow in the superior region of the left dorsolateral prefrontal cortex and in the right lateral premotor area. These investigators used a combination of the Velten technique (Velten, 1968) and music (portions of "Russia under the Mongolian Yoke" from Prokofiev's score for "Alexander Nevsky" played at half speed) to induce a depressed mood. Relative to the neutral condition, depressed mood was also associated with increases in the posterior cingulate cortex. Decreases in CBF were observed in the right caudate, the right dorsolateral prefrontal cortex, and the bilateral rostral medial prefrontal cortex. Unfortunately, these investigators did not directly compare the elated and depressed moods. Moreover, subjects were performing cognitive tasks during the time that the positron emission tomography (PET) data were acquired, and it is not clear whether the mood effects persisted throughout cognitive task performance. Additionally, a formal statistical assessment of the lateralized changes was not performed.

Another recent study examined film-induced and recalled happiness, sadness, and disgust and found that all three emotions were associated with increased activation in the prefrontal cortex, the thalamus, and bilateral regions within the anterior temporal cortex (Lane et al., 1997). In addition, sadness was associated with unique increases in activation in the caudate, putamen, lateral cerebellum, and the cerebellar vermis. There were no significant asymmetries observed.

Only Gemar et al. (1996) have reported on decreases in activation in response to induced sadness. These investigators found that, in contrast to a neutral recall condition, self-generated sadness was associated with decreases in blood flow in the left dorsolateral prefrontal cortex, the left medial prefrontal cortex, and the left temporal cortex. The investigators also included a resting control condition, and, when the self-generated sadness condition was compared with the resting control condition, a different pattern of findings emerged, thus underscoring the critical importance of the control condition in such neuroimaging studies.

Blood Flow Studies of Depression

A different pattern emerges from the literature on depression. One of the earliest studies found that depressed subjects had significantly lower gray matter flow in the left hemisphere than did controls (Mathew et al., 1980). The pattern of flow reduction in the right hemisphere was similar but not significant. Just as the initial investigations of stroke-induced mood changes did not consider the issue of location within the hemisphere (e.g., Black, 1975), this study examined activity only on the hemispheric level. Global decreases in both the right and left hemispheres of unipolar depressed subjects have been reported by a number of investigators (Bonne & Krauz, 1997; Gustafson, Risberg, & Silfverskiöld, 1981; Iidaka et al., 1997; Mayberg et al., 1994; Rush et al., 1982; Sackeim et al., 1990; Warren et al., 1984). Regions with the largest decrease in rCBF include selective frontal, superior temporal, central, and anterior parietal regions (Sackiem et al., 1990), as well as inferior frontal and cingulate cortex (Mayberg et al., 1994), and the severity of depression has been correlated with the magnitude of the bilateral decreases in frontal activity (Iidaka et al., 1997).

Using single photon emission computerized tomography (SPECT), Delvenne et al. (1990) examined a group of 38 depressed and 16 control subjects. Activity in a slice 5 cm above the orbitomeatal line revealed that subjects classified as bipolar and/or endogenous had significantly lower left than right activity, but the hemispheric differences between controls and unipolar subjects were not significant. This reduction in left hemisphere flow was most pronounced in the frontal region. Reischies, Hedde, and Drochenir (1989) found that depressed subjects in both the acute and remitted phases had a pattern of relative right-sided frontal activation compared with controls, who had relative left-sided asymmetry in this region. Investigators using [195m]Au in the measurement of CBF found that depressed subjects had significantly lower CBF in the left frontal and in all of the right hemisphere regions (frontal, temporal, parietal, and occipital) than did a group of normal control subjects (Schlegel et al., 1989). There was an age difference between the two groups, and this may have accounted for some of the observed differences. With the regional means provided by the authors, however, and computation of a frontal/hemisphere ratio, which eliminates the problem of differences in overall flow between the two groups, the data show that depressed subjects have lower frontal/hemisphere ratios than do controls, and this between-group difference is largest in the left hemisphere. Bilateral prefrontal decreases have also been reported by other authors (Chabrol et al., 1986; Ito et al., 1996; Schroeder et al., 1989).

A study of elderly depressed subjects found global decreases in rCBF compared with controls (Lesser et al., 1994). Using Tc-HMPAO as a tracer, the investigators found bilateral decreases in the orbital frontal, inferior temporal, and parietal regions in addition to global decreases in blood flow throughout the right hemisphere. Global flow decreases in elderly depressed subjects have also been found by other investigators (Hoyer, Oesterreich, & Wagner, 1984; Philpot et al., 1993).

Investigators at Hammersmith Hospital in London, England, have produced a large body of data on this topic over the last 5 years. Using PET measures of CBF, Bench et al. (1992) found that depressed subjects, in contrast to nondepressed controls, had decreased flow in a region consisting of the left anterior cingulate and the left dorsolateral prefrontal cortex. A subsequent study replicated these findings in another 40 depressed subjects (Bench et al., 1993). Ratings of patient symptomatology were subjected to a principal components analysis, and three factors were identified. The first factor was anxiety and psychomotor agitation, which was associated with an increase in blood flow in the right posterior cingulate and bilateral increases in the inferior parietal lobules. The second factor was depression and psychomotor retardation, and this was associated with decreases in the following regions in the left hemisphere: dorsolateral prefrontal cortex, inferior frontal, superior temporal, and inferior parietal. The final factor was cognitive impairment as identified by the Mini-Mental State Examination (MMSE), and this was associated with decreased flow in the left medial prefrontal cortex, the right anterior thalamus, the right superior temporal gyrus, and the right postcentral gyrus. More than half of these subjects were rescanned following treatment. Recovery was found to be associated with increased blood flow in the left dorsolateral prefrontal cortex, bilateral regions in the medial prefrontal cortex including the anterior cingulate, and in a region of the posterior parietal cortex (Bench, Frakowiak, & Dolan, 1995). Italian investigators found similar results: Depressed subjects had decreased left frontal blood flow, and, when they were rescanned after 6 months of tricyclic antidepressant therapy, these subjects had increases in these regions. Similar findings were obtained with the dopamine agonist amineptine (Passero, Nardini, & Battistini, 1995).

Somewhat contradictory results were reported by Drevets et al. (1992). Like the Hammersmith group, these investigators used ^{15}O, but they used a bolus injection instead of inhalation. The implications of these different methods is that an injection of ^{15}O results in a scan reflecting approximately 40 seconds of activity in comparison with about 10 minutes of data obtained with ^{15}O inhalation. Drevets et al. (1992) reported that depressed subjects with a family history of depression had increased activation in the left orbitofrontal region compared with controls. Interestingly, they did observe a significant correlation ($r = -0.62$) between depression and left frontal activation in the dorsolateral region such that increased severity of depression was associated with decreased activation in this left anterior region. Furthermore, a recently published study by this group reports decreased activation in a subgenual region of the left prefrontal cortex among a more heterogeneous group of depressed subjects relative to nondepressed controls (Drevets et al., 1997).

Other researchers who have not found decreases in left anterior blood flow include Silfverskiöld and Risberg (1989), who found no global or regional differences between depressed subjects and a group of age- and sex-matched controls. Gur et al. (1984) examined a group of medicated unipolar depressed subjects and found that they did not significantly differ from controls in the pattern and overall level of CBF. Nonsignificant group differences in rCBF were also reported by Maes et al. (1993). Uytdenhoef et al. (1983) found that depressed subjects had increased left frontal flows as well as decreased flows in the right posterior region, but it is unclear if there was any control for type I error in this study. Higher global flow values in depressed subjects than in controls were reported by Rosenberg et al. (1988). Surprisingly, the depressed subjects were older than the controls, which would lead us to expect overall decreases in activation (see above).

To summarize, studies of depression, in contrast to studies of induced sadness, have typically reported decreased left frontal blood flow (Bench et al., 1992, 1993; Delvenne et al., 1990; Passero, Nardini, & Battistini, 1995), and recovery has been found to be associated with increases in these regions (Bench et al., 1995; Passero, Nardini, & Battistini, 1995). Likewise, Drevets et al. (1992) found a negative relation between left dorsolateral prefrontal blood flow and symptom severity. A comparable number of investigators have found that depressed subjects are characterized by global decreases in blood flow (Bonne & Krausz, 1997; Gustafson, Risberg, & Silfverskiöld, 1981; Mathew et al., 1980; Mayberg et al., 1994; Rush et al., 1982; Sackeim et al., 1990; Warren et al., 1984). Global decreases in blood flow are also typical of elderly depressed subjects (Hoyer, Oesterreich, & Wagner, 1984; Lesser et al., 1994; Philpot et al., 1993).

Studies of Glucose Metabolism in Depression

Although no studies have yet been done examining patterns of glucose metabolism during the induction of sadness, the results of metabolism studies of depression are mostly consistent with results in the rCBF literature. An early study of glucose metabolism in a small group of unipolar and bipolar depressed subjects did not find any differences in left/right asymmetry for the frontal cortex (Baxter et al., 1985), but a subsequent study indicated that this failure to find a consistent decrease in left frontal activation among the depressed subjects was because of the concurrent decrease in right frontal activation (Baxter et al., 1989). In this study, the ratio of the metabolic rate for the left dorsal anterolateral prefrontal cortex to whole hemisphere was significantly lower in depression. Recovery from depression was associated with increases in this index. Among bipolar and unipolar depressed subjects this ratio was also decreased in the right hemisphere, but it was only the reduced left prefrontal to whole hemisphere ratio that distinguished all three types of depression studied: unipolar depression, bipolar depression, and obsessive-compulsive disorder with depression. Bilateral decreases in frontal metabolism have also been reported by other groups (Biver et al., 1994; Francois et al., 1995). Biver et al. (1994) also found bilateral decreases in parietal metabolism.

Austin et al. (1992) reported that depressed subjects had decreased overall metabolism compared with controls. After controlling for age, medication, and endogenous subtype, they found a significant negative correlation between anterior activation and Hamilton Rating Scale for Depression (HRSD) scores. As in the Baxter et al. (1989) study, this negative relation was seen bilaterally. Global decreases in metabolism were also found in a small sample of depressed subjects with seasonal affective disorder (SAD) (Cohen et al., 1992). In contrast with other studies, Cohen et al. (1992) also found frontal asymmetry differences between groups such that depressed subjects had left greater than right metabolic activity in an anterior frontal region in contrast to controls who had greater relative right-sided activation. This result, however, emerged from unprotected t-tests comparing the groups across 26 different regions of interest. The finding they report disappears following Bonferroni correction. Moreover, the data are based on a sample of seven patients with seasonal affective disorder.

In a small study of 10 bipolar and unipolar depressed subjects, Martinot et al. (1990) found that depressed subjects had a significantly higher right/left ratio in the prefrontal cortex than did controls. This asymmetry was the result of decreased left prefrontal metabolism in the depressed subjects. Depressed subjects also had a relative hypofrontal pattern of activation compared with controls, who had more anterior than posterior activation. Although recovery was associated with an increase in left prefrontal metabolism such that there was no asymmetry, euthymic depressed subjects still had a pattern of hypofrontal activation. In a study of bipolar subjects, Kato et al. (1995) found that depression was associated with a decrease in left frontal metabolism and that left frontal metabolism was correlated negatively with HRSD scores. Bipolar subjects scanned in manic and euthymic states had decreased right frontal metabolism compared with controls. Negative correlations between left frontal metabolism and HRSD scores have also been found in a sample of bulimic subjects (Andreason et al., 1992). Nonsignificant differences were reported by Buchsbaum et al. (1984). Their use of a series of shocks to the subjects' right forearm during FDG uptake may, however, have obscured group differences in asymmetry by increasing activity in the left hemisphere.

Like rCBF, global metabolic decreases in elderly depressed subjects have been reported (e.g., Kumar et al., 1993). Studies of elderly subjects with Parkinson's disease have found that it is bilateral decreases in the frontal region that distinguishes patients with and without depression (Mayberg et al., 1990; Ring et al., 1994).

In most of the metabolism and rCBF studies reviewed here, decreased left frontal activation was found during depression. The reports are mixed as to whether these decreases occur in only the left hemisphere (e.g., Bench et al., 1992, 1993; Delvenne et al., 1990; Martinot et al., 1990) or in both the left and right frontal regions (e.g., Baxter et al., 1989; Chabrol et al., 1986; Francois et al., 1995; Sackeim et al., 1990; Schroeder et al., 1989). In several studies, activation in the prefrontal regions of the left hemisphere was negatively correlated with severity of depression (Andreason et al., 1992; Baxter et al., 1989; Bench et al., 1993; Drevets et al., 1992; Kato et al., 1995), and a number of investigators have found that remission is associated with reversal of the observed left frontal hypoactivation (Baxter et al., 1989; Bench et al., 1995; Martinot et al., 1990; Passero, Nardini, & Battistini, 1995). When the depressed subjects are older, bilateral decreases appear to be more prevalent (e.g., Hoyer, Oesterreich, & Wagner, 1984; Kumar et al., 1993). Decreased activation in the posterior regions has been reported for the right side (e.g., Schlegel et al., 1989; Uytdenhoef et al., 1983) and for both sides (e.g., Biver et al., 1994; Lesser et al., 1994; Sackiem et al., 1990).

In a new study in our laboratory, Abercrombie et al. (1998) found that, among depressed patients, PET-derived measures of glucose metabolism in the amygdala predicted the severity of dispositional NA (see Figs. 11.1 and 11.2). These findings, along with a similar observation by Drevets et al. (1992), suggest that

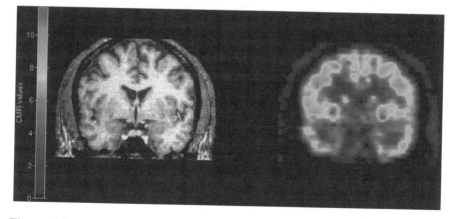

Figure 11.1. Illustration of PET–MRI coregistration and amygdalar region of interest delineation. Representative image planes in the coronal orientation for one participant are shown. The PET image plane is presented beside its corresponding coregistered MRI plane. Units of the PET color scale are in mg/100 g/min. Glucose metabolism extracted according to these MR-defined regions of interest was then used for the correlational analysis depicted in Figure 11.2. (Adapted from Abercrombie et al., 1998.)

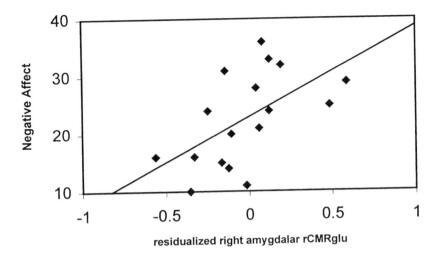

Figure 11.2. Scatter plot of correlation in depressed subjects ($N = 17$; $r(15) = 0.56$; $P < 0.02$) between dispositional negative affect (assessed with the PANAS Negative Affect Scale—Trait Version; Watson, Clark, & Tellegen, 1988) and glucose metabolism in the right amygdala (residualized for global metabolic rate). (Adapted from Abercrombie et al., 1998.)

variations in activation in the amygdala play an important role in determining the intensity of NA exhibited by depressed patients. In light of the role of the amygdala in a broad constellation of NA characteristics that include several different anxiety disorders (see Davidson & Irwin, 1998), it may well be that amygdala activation accounts for some of the comorbidity between anxiety and depression.

SUMMARY

It is clear from this review that there are a host of conceptual and methodological issues that still plague research on this topic. We believe that the most fruitful general approach has been and will continue to be the examination of relations between measures of emotional state and/or symptoms and specific patterns of regional brain activity. There appear to be fewer replicated findings in the literature on the effects of experimentally induced sadness on regional brain function than in the literature on depression. In part, this lack of consistency is a function of the failure of investigators to independently verify the presence of sadness. Another major contributor to the inconsistency among studies is the variability in control conditions that have been used. It is essential that investigators attempt to isolate specific features of sadness while controlling for sensory, perceptual, and memorial processes associated with the specific form of emotion elicitation. It is also important to include more than one emotion in these studies to ascertain whether the observed effects are indeed specific to sadness or are more general characteristics of emotion per se. Most of the neuroimaging studies of sadness have used injected O^{15} water as a tracer. This results in an uptake period of about 40 seconds. Such studies depend on very critical timing in the presentation of the activation condition in relation to tracer injection. Fluctuations in the intensity of elicited emotion during this critical period will affect the data obtained.

The literature on depression is somewhat more consistent, though many different patterns of regional brain abnormalities have been reported. Here it is important to emphasize the obvious point that considerable heterogeneity exists in the symptoms of depression, even among very carefully diagnosed patients meeting specific DSM-IV criteria. The strategy pioneered by Bench, Dolan, and their colleagues to examine relations between specific symptom clusters and patterns of regional brain function is particularly helpful. With such a strategy, the heterogeneity among patients can be harnessed to one's advantage in dissecting those circuits that appear to vary with changes in specific patterns of symptoms. A further refinement of this strategy would include testing patients on objective laboratory measures of emotional reactivity and emotion regulation and then examining the relations between specific patterns of performance on these laboratory tasks and measures of regional brain function (see Davidson, 1998). Another important strategy for future research is to examine regional brain function in patients who are performing tasks under different incentive and feedback conditions because extant evidence suggests that depressed patients may be underresponsive to reward (e.g., Henriques, Glowacki, & Davidson, 1994) as well as overresponsive to negative feedback (Elliott et al., 1997).

Finally, studies that combine neurochemical and functional neuroanatomical approaches to characterize regional neurochemical abnormalities are needed. For example, Mann and colleagues (1996) recently examined differences in regional glucose metabolism between depressed patients and healthy controls in response to fenfluramine, a serotonin agonist. Healthy controls showed significant increases in metabolism in left prefrontal and temporoparietal cortex and decreases in right prefrontal cortex, while depressed patients failed to show any significant change in response to the drug. These findings implicate abnormalities in lateralized prefrontal serotonergic function in depression. Although in need of replication, this finding helps to integrate the previously disparate reports on the neurochemistry and functional neuroanatomy of depression. The effects of treatment, particularly with medications that affect the serotonin system, on these lateralized abnormalities in serotonin function require study.

On the question of whether sadness in normal people is a good model system for clinical depression, the data are inconsistent. It is likely that cumulative exposure to depression will exert effects that are not going to emerge with brief mood inductions in normal people. On the other hand, there may be some features of the response that are similar, but any firm conclusions on this point must await more methodologically sophisticated studies that use appropriate control groups, statistical methods, and procedures to independently verify the presence of the intended emotion. We now have the tools to make rapid advances in the study of brain function and emotion in intact humans, and we expect much progress in the next decade.

REFERENCES

Abercrombie, H.C., Schaefer, S.M., Larson, C.L., Oakes, T.R., Lindgren, K.A., Holden, J.E., Perlman, S.E., Turski, P.A., Krahn, D.D., Benca, R.M., & Davidson, R.J. (1998). Metabolic rate in the right amygdala predicts negative affect in depressed patients. *NeuroReport, 9*, 3301–3307.

Ahern, G.L., & Schwartz, G.E. (1985). Differential lateralization for positive and negative emotion in the human brain: EEG spectral analysis. *Neuropsychologia, 23*, 745–755.

Alema, G., & Rosadini, G. (1964). Données cliniques et E.E.G. de l'introduction d'amytal sodium dans la circulation encéphalique, concernant l'état de conscience. *Acta Neurochirurgica, 12*, 241–257.

Allen, J.J., Iacono, W.G., Depue, R.A., & Arbisi, P. (1993). Regional electroencephalographic asymmetries in bipolar seasonal affective disorder before and after exposure to bright light. *Biological Psychiatry, 33*, 642–646.

Allen, K.M., Blascovich, J., Tomaka, J., & Kelsey, R.M. (1991). Presence of human friends and pet dogs as moderators of autonomic responses to stress in women. *Journal of Personality and Social Psychology, 61*, 582–589.

Altshuler, L.L., Devinsky, O., Post, R.M., & Theodore, W. (1990). Depression, anxiety, and temporal lobe epilepsy. *Archives of Neurology, 47*, 284–288.

Andreason, P.J., Altemus, M., Zametkin, A.J., King, A.C., Lucinio, J., & Cohen, R.M. (1992). Regional cerebral glucose metabolism in bulimia nervosa. *American Journal of Psychiatry, 149*, 1506–1513.

Austin, M.-P., Dougall, N., Ross, M., Murray, C., O'Carroll, R.E., Moffoot, A., Ebmeier, K.P., & Goodwin, G.M. (1992). Single photon emission tomography with ^{99m}Tc-exametazime in major depression and the pattern of brain activity underlying the psychotic/neurotic continuum. *Journal of Affective Disorders, 26*, 31–44.

Baker, S.C., Frith, C.D., & Dolan, R.J. (1997). The interaction between mood and cognitive function studied with PET. *Psychological Medicine, 27*, 565–578.

Baumeister, R.F. (1990). Suicide as escape from self. *Psychological Review, 97*, 90–113.

Baxter, L.R., Phelps, M.E., Mazziotta, J.C., Schwartz, J.M., Gerner, R.H., Selin, C.E., & Sumida, R.M. (1985). Cerebral metabolic rates for glucose in mood disorders. *Archives of General Psychiatry, 42*, 441–447.

Baxter, L.R., & Schwartz, J.M., Phelps, M.E., Mazziotta, J.C., Guze, B.H., Selin, C.E., Gerner, R.H., & Sumida, R.M. (1989). Reduction of prefrontal cortex glucose metabolism common to three types of depression. *Archives of General Psychiatry, 46*, 243–250.

Bear, D.M., & Fedio, P. (1977). Quantitative analysis of interictal behavior in temporal lobe epilepsy. *Archives of Neurology, 34*, 454–467.

Bench, C.J., Frackowiak, R.S., & Dolan, R.J. (1995). Changes in regional cerebral blood flow on recovery from depression. *Psychological Medicine, 25*, 247–261.

Bench, C.J., Friston, K.J., Brown, R.G., Frackowiak, R.S., & Dolan, R.J. (1993). Regional cerebral blood flow in depression measured by positron emission tomography the relationship with clinical dimensions. *Psychological Medicine, 23*, 579–590.

Bench, C.J., Friston, K.J., Brown, R.G., Scott, L.C., Frackowiak, R.S.J., & Dolan, R.J. (1992). The anatomy of melancholia—focal abnormalities of cerebral blood flow in major depression. *Psychological Medicine, 22*, 607–615.

Biver, R., Goldman, S., Delvenne, V., Luxen, A., De Maertelaer, V., Hubain, P., Mednlewicz, J., & Lotstra, F. (1994). Frontal and parietal metabolic disturbances in unipolar depression. *Biological Psychiatry, 36*, 381–388.

Black, F.W. (1975). Unilateral brain lesions and MMPI performance: A preliminary study. *Perceptual and Motor Skills, 40*, 87–93.

Bonne, O., & Krausz, Y. (1997). Pathophysiological significance of cerebral perfusion abnormalities in major depression—Trait or state marker? *European Neuropsychopharmacology, 7*, 225–233.

Bouman, T.K., & Luteijn, F. (1986). Relations between the pleasant events schedule, depression, and other aspects of psychopathology. *Journal of Abnormal Psychology, 95*, 373–377.

Bruder, G.E. (1992). P300 findings for depressives and anxiety disorders. *Annals of the New York Academy of Science, 658*, 205–222.

Bruder, G.E., Fong, R., Tenke, C.E., Liete, P., Towey, J.P., Stewart, J.E., McGrath, P.J., & Quitkin, F.M. (1997). Regional brain asymmetries in major depression with or without an anxiety disorder: A quantitative electroencephalographic study. *Biological Psychiatry, 41*, 939–948.

Bruder, G.E., Tenke, C.E., Stewart, J.W., Towey, J.P., Leite, P., Voglmaier, M., & Quitkin, F.M. (1995). Brain event-related potentials to complex tones in depressed patients: Relations to perceptual asymmetry and clinical features. *Psychophysiology, 32*, 373–381.

Bruder, G.E., Towey, J.P., Stewart, J.W., Friedman, D., Tenke, C., & Quitkin, F.M. (1991). Event-related potential in depression: Influence of task, stimulus hemifield, and clinical features on P3 latency. *Biological Psychiatry, 30*, 233–246.

Buchsbaum, M.S., Cappelletti, J., Ball, R., Hazlett, E., King, A.C., Johnson, J., Wu, J., & DeLisi, L.E. (1984). Positron emission tomographic image measurement in schizophrenia and affective disorders. *Annals of Neurology, 15* (suppl.), S157, 65.

Cazard, P. (1989). Hemisphere asymmetry of alpha burst frequency of occurrence variations in depression. *International Journal of Neuroscience, 47*, 181–191.

Cazard, P., Ricard, F., & Facchetti, L. (1992). [Depression and functional EEG asymmetry]. *Annales Medico-Psychologiques (Paris), 150*, 230–239 [From Medline, Unique Identifier No. 94136917].

Chabrol, H., Barrere, M., Guell, A., Bes, A., & Moron, P. (1986). Hypofrontality of cerebral blood flow in depressed adolescents [letter to the editor]. *American Journal of Psychiatry, 143*, 263–264.

Christianson, S.-A., Saisa, J., Garvill, J., & Silfvenius, H. (1993). Hemisphere inactivation and mood-state changes. *Brain and Cognition, 23*, 127–144.

Cohen, R.M., Gross, M., Nordahl, T.E., Semple, W.E., Oren, D.A., & Rosenthal, N. (1992). Preliminary data on the metabolic pattern of patients with winter seasonal affective disorder. *Archives of General Psychiatry, 49*, 545–552.

Coles, M.G.H., Gratton, G., & Fabiani, M. (1990). Event related potentials. In J.T. Cacioppo & L.G. Tassinary (Eds.), *Principles of Psychophysiology* (pp. 413–455). New
York: Cambridge University Press.

Davidson, R.J. (1984). Affect, cognition, and hemispheric specialization. In C.E. Izard, J.
Kagan, & R. Zajonc (Eds.), *Emotion, Cognition, and Behavior* (pp. 320–365). New
York: Cambridge University Press.

Davidson, R.J. (1987). Cerebral asymmetry and the nature of emotion: Implications for
the study of individual differences and psychopathology. In R. Takahashi, P. Flor-
Henry, J. Gruzelier, & S. Niwa (Eds.), *Cerebral Dynamics, Laterality, and Psychopathology* (pp. 71–83). New York: Elsevier Science Publishers.

Davidson, R.J. (1988). EEG measures of cerebral asymmetry: Conceptual and methodological issues. *International Journal of Neuroscience, 39,* 71–89.

Davidson, R.J. (1992). Emotion and affective style: Hemispheric substrates. *Psychological Science, 3,* 39–43.

Davidson, R.J. (1993). Cerebral asymmetry and emotion: Conceptual and methodological conundrums. *Cognition and Emotion, 7,* 115–138.

Davidson, R.J. (1995). Cerebral asymmetry, emotion, and affective style. In R.J. Davidson
and K. Hugdahl (Eds.), *Brain Asymmetry* (pp. 361–387). Cambridge, MA: MIT Press.

Davidson, R.J. (1998). Affective style and affective disorders: Perspectives from affective neuroscience. *Cognition and Emotion, 12,* 307–330.

Davidson, R.J., Chapman, J.P., Chapman, L.J., & Henriques, J.B. (1990a). Asymmetrical
brain electrical activity discriminate between psychometrically-matched verbal and
spatial cognitive tasks. *Psychophysiology, 27,* 528–543.

Davidson, R.J., Ekman, P., Saron, C.D., & Friesen, W.V. (1990b). Approach-withdrawal
and cerebral asymmetry: Emotional expression and brain physiology I. *Journal of Personality and Social Psychology, 58,* 330–341.

Davidson, R.J., & Irwin, W. (1999). The functional neuroanatomy of emotion and affective style. *Trends in Cognitive Science, 3,* 11–21.

Davidson, R.J., Schaffer, C.E., & Saron, C. (1985). Effects of lateralized presentations of
faces on self-reports of emotion and EEG asymmetry in depressed and non-depressed
subjects. *Psychophysiology, 22,* 353–364.

Davidson, R.J., & Tomarken, A.J. (1989) Laterality and emotion: An electrophysiological approach. In F. Boller & J. Grafman (Eds.), *Handbook of Neuropsychology*
(pp. 419–441). Amsterdam: Elsevier.

d'Elia, G., & Perris, C. (1973). Cerebral functional dominance and depression. *Acta Psychiatrica Scandinavica, 49,* 191–197.

d'Elia, G., & Perris, C. (1974). Cerebral functional dominance and memory functions.
Acta Psychiatrica Scandinavica, Suppl. 255, 143–157.

Delvenne, V., Delecluse, F., Hubain, P.P., Schoutens, A., De Maertelaer, V., &
Mendlewicz, J. (1990). Regional cerebral blood flow in patients with affective disorders. *British Journal of Psychiatry, 157,* 359–365.

Diner, B.C., Holcomb, P.J., & Dykman, R.A. (1985). P_{300} in major depressive disorder.
Psychiatry Research, 15, 175–184.

Drevets, W.C., Price, J.L., Simpson, J.R., Todd, R.D., Reich, T., Vannier, M., & Raichle,
M.E. (1997). Subgenual prefrontal cortex abnormalities in mood disorders. *Nature,
386,* 824–827.

Drevets, W.C., Videen, T.O., Price, J.L., Preskorn, S.H., Carmichael, T., & Raichle, M.E.
(1992). A functional anatomical study of unipolar depression. *The Journal of Neuroscience, 12,* 3628–3641.

Elliott, R., Sahakian, B.J., Herrod, J.J., Robbins, T.W., & Paykel, E.S. (1997). Abnormal response to negative feedback in unipolar depression: Evidence for a diagnosis specific impairment. *Journal of Neurology, Neurosurgery and Psychiatry, 63*, 74–82.

Elton, M. (1984). A longitudinal investigation of event-related potentials in depression. *Biological Psychiatry, 19*, 1635–1649.

Engel, J. (1984). The use of positron emission tomographic scanning in epilepsy. *Annals of Neurology, 15* (suppl.), S180–S191.

Flor-Henry, P. (1979). Laterality, shifts of cerebral dominance, sinistrality, and psychosis. In J. Gruzelier & P. Flor-Henry (Eds.), *Hemisphere Asymmetries of Function in Psychopathology* (pp. 3–19). New York: Elsevier/North-Holland Biomedical Press.

Flor-Henry, P., Koles, Z.J., Howarth, B.G., & Burton, L. (1979). Neurophysiological studies of schizophrenia, mania, and depression. In J. Gruzelier & P. Flor-Henry (Eds.), *Hemisphere Asymmetries of Function in Psychopathology* (pp. 189–222). New York: Elsevier/North-Holland Biomedical Press.

Fox, N.A., & Davidson, R.J. (1986). Taste-elicited changes in facial signs of emotion and the asymmetry of brain electrical activity in human newborns. *Neuropsychologia, 24*, 417–422.

Francois, A., Biver, F., Goldman, S., Luxen, A., Mendlewicz, J., & Lotstra, F. (1995). [Decrease in the frontal-superobasal metabolic ratio in unipolar depression] [in French]. *Acta Psychiatrica Belgica, 95*, 234–245.

Gainotti, G. (1972). Emotional behavior and hemispheric side of the lesion. *Cortex, 8*, 41–55.

Gainotti, G. (1989). Disorders of emotions and affect in patients with unilateral brain damage. In F. Boller & J. Grafman (Eds.), *Handbook of Neuropsychology* (pp. 345–361). Amsterdam: Elsevier.

Gasparrini, W.G., Satz, P., Heilman, K.M., & Coolidge, F.L. (1978). Hemispheric asymmetries of affective processing as determined by the Minnesota Multiphasic Personality Inventory. *Journal of Neurology, Neurosurgery, and Psychiatry, 41*, 470–473.

Gasser, T., Bacher, P., & Mocks, J. (1982). Transformation towards the normal distribution of broad band spectral parameters of the EEG. *Electroencephalography and Clinical Neurophysiology, 53*, 119–124.

Gemar, M.C., Kapur, S., Segal, Z.V., Brown, G.M., & Houle, S. (1996). Effects of self-generated sad mood on regional cerebral activity: A PET study in normal subjects. *Depression, 4*, 81–88.

George, M.S., Ketter, T.A., Parekh, P.I., Horwitz, B., Herscovitch, P., & Post, R.M. (1995). Brain activity during transient sadness and happiness in healthy women. *American Journal of Psychiatry, 152*, 341–351.

Giedke, H., Thier, P., & Bolz, J. (1981). The relationship between P_3-latency and reaction time in depression. *Biological Psychology, 13*, 31–49.

Gray, J.A. (1994). Three fundamental emotion systems. In P. Ekman & R.J. Davidson (Eds.), *The Nature of Emotion: Fundamental Questions* (pp. 243–247). New York: Oxford University Press.

Gotlib, I.H., Ranganath, C., & Rosenfeld, J.P. (1998). Frontal EEG alpha asymmetry, depression, and cognitive functioning. *Cognition and Emotion, 12*, 449–478.

Gur, R.E., Skolnick, B.E., Gur, R.C., Caroff, S., Rieger, W., Obrist, W.D., Younkin, D., & Reivich, M. (1984). Brain function in psychiatric disorders. *Archives of General Psychiatry, 41*, 695–699.

Gustafson, L., Risberg, J., & Silfverskiöld, P. (1981). Regional cerebral blood flow in organic dementia and affective disorders. *Advances in Biological Psychiatry, 6*, 109–116.

Harmon-Jones, E., & Allen, J.J.B. (1997). Behavioral activation sensitivity and resting frontal EEG asymmetry: Covariation of putative indicators related to risk for mood disorders. *Journal of Abnormal Psychology, 106,* 159–163.

Heller, W., Nitschke, J.B., Etienne, M.A., & Miller, G.A. (1997). Patterns of regional brain activity differentiate types of anxiety. *Journal of Abnormal Psychology, 106,* 376–385.

Henriques, J.B., & Davidson, R.J. (1989). Affective disorders. In G. Turpin (Ed.), *Handbook of Clinical Psychophysiology* (pp. 357–392). London: Wiley.

Henriques, J.B., & Davidson, R.J. (1990). Regional brain electrical asymmetries discriminate between previously depressed and healthy control subjects. *Journal of Abnormal Psychology, 99,* 22–31.

Henriques, J.B., & Davidson, R.J. (1991). Left frontal hypoactivation in depression. *Journal of Abnormal Psychology, 100,* 535–545.

Henriques, J.B., & Davidson, R.J. (1997). Brain electrical asymmetries during cognitive task performance in depressed and nondepressed subjects. *Biological Psychiatry, 42,* 1039–1050.

Henriques, J.B., Glowacki, J.M., & Davidson, R.J. (1994). Reward fails to alter response bias in depression. *Journal of Abnormal Psychology, 103,* 460–466.

Hitt, S.K., Allen, J.J.B., & Duke, L.M. (1995). Stability of resting frontal alpha asymmetry in major depression [abstract]. *Psychophysiology, 32,* S40.

House, A., Dennis, M., Molyneux, A., Warlow, C., & Hawton, K. (1989). Emotionalism after stroke. *British Medical Journal, 298,* 991–994.

House, A., Dennis, M., Warlow, C., Hawton, K., & Molyneux, A. (1990). Mood disorders after stroke and their relation to lesion location. *Brain, 113,* 1113–1129.

Hoyer, S., Oesterreich, K., & Wagner, O. (1984). Depression in old age and its relation to primary dementia: Variations in brain blood flow and oxidative metabolism. *Monographs of Neural Science, 11,* 187–192.

Iidaka, T., Nakajima, T., Suzuki, Y., Okazaki, A., Maehara, T., & Shiraishi, H. (1997). Quantitative regional cerebral blood flow measured by Tc-99m HMPAO SPECT in mood disorder. *Psychiatry Research: Neuroimaging, 68,* 143–154.

Ito, H., Kawashima, R., Awata, S., Ono, S., Sato, K., Goto, R., Koyama, M., Sato, M., & Fukuda, H. (1996). Hypoperfusion in the limbic system and prefrontal cortex in depression: SPECT with anatomic standardization technique. *Journal of Nuclear Medicine, 37,* 410–414.

Jacobs, G.D., & Snyder, D. (1996). Frontal brain asymmetry predicts affective style in men. *Behavioral Neuroscience, 110,* 3–6.

Kato, T., Shioiri, T., Murashita, J., Hamakawa, H., Takahashi, Y, Inubushi, T., & Takahashi, S. (1995). Lateralized abnormality of high energy phosphate metabolism in the frontal lobes of patients with bipolar disorder detected by phase-encoded 31P-MRS. *Psychological Medicine, 25,* 557–566.

Khanna, S., Mukundan, C.R., & Channabasavanna, S.M. (1989). Middle latency evoked potentials in melancholic depression. *Biological Psychiatry, 25,* 494–498.

Kinsbourne, M. (1978). Evolution of language in relation to lateral action. In M. Kinsbourne (Ed.), *Asymmetrical Function of the Brain* (pp. 553–556). New York: Cambridge University Press.

Knott, V., Lapierre, Y., Griffiths, L, de Lugt, D., & Bakish, D. (1991). Event related potentials and selective attention in major depressive illness. *Journal of Affective Disorders, 23,* 43–48.

Kraiuhin, C., Gordon, E., Coyle, S., Sara, G., Rennie, C., Howson, A., Landau, P., &

Meares, R. (1990). Normal latency of the P300 event-related potential in mild-to-moderate alzheimer's disease and depression. *Biological Psychiatry*, *28*, 372–386.

Kumar A., Newberg A., Alavi A., Berlin J., Smith R., & Reivich M. (1993). Regional cerebral glucose metabolism in late-life depression and Alzheimer disease a preliminary positron emission tomography study. *Proceedings of the National Academy of Sciences of the United States of America*, *90*, 7019–7023.

Lane, R.D., Reiman, E.M., Ahern, G.L., Schwartz, G.E., & Davidson, R.J. (1997). Neuroanatomical correlates of happiness, sadness, and disgust. *American Journal of Psychiatry*, *154*, 926–933.

Lee, G.P., Loring, D.W., Meader, K.J., & Brooks, B.B. (1990). Hemispheric specialization for emotion expression: A reexamination of results from intracarotid administration of sodium amobarbital. *Brain and Cognition*, *12*, 267–280.

Lehman, D. (1987). Principles of spatial analysis. In A.S. Gevins & A. Remond (Eds.), *Methods of Analysis of Brain Electrical and Magnetic Signals* (pp. 309–354). New York: Elsevier Science Publishing.

Lesser, I.M., Mena, I., Boone, K.B., Miller, B.L., Mehringer, C.M., & Wohl, M. (1994). Reduction of cerebral blood flow in older depressed patients. *Archives of General Psychiatry*, *51*, 677–686.

Lindsley, D.B., & Wicke, J.D. (1974). The electroencephalogram: Autonomous electrical activity in man and animals. In R. Thompson & M.N. Patterson (Eds.), *Biolelectric Recording Techniques* (pp. 3–83). New York: Academic Press.

Lipsey, J.R., Robinson, R.G., Pearlson, G.D., Rao, K., & Price, T.R. (1983). Mood change following bilateral hemisphere brain injury. *British Journal of Psychiatry*, *143*, 266–273.

Lipsey, J.R., Spencer, W.C., Rabins, P.V., & Robinson, R.G. (1986). Phenomenological comparison of poststroke depression and functional depression. *American Journal of Psychiatry*, *143*, 527–529.

MacLeod, A.K., Byrne, A., & Valentine, J.D. (1996). Affect, emotional disorder, and future-directed thinking. *Cognition and Emotion*, *10*, 69–86.

Maes, M., Dierckx, R., Meltzer, H.Y., Ingels, M., Schotte, C., Vandewoude, M., Calabrese, J., & Cosyns, P. (1993). Regional cerebral blood flow in unipolar depression measured with Tc-99m-HMPAO single photon emission computed tomography: Negative findings. *Psychiatry Research*, *50*, 77–88.

Mann, J.J., Malone, K.M., Diehl, D.J., Perel, J., Cooper, T.B., & Mintun, M.A. (1996). Demonstration in vivo of reduced serotonin responsivity in the brain of untreated depressed patients. *American Journal of Psychiatry*, *153*, 174–182.

Martinot, J.-L., Hardy, P., Feline, A., Huret, J.-D., Mazoyer, B., Attar-Levy, D., Pappata, S., & Syrota, A. (1990). Left prefrontal glucose hypometabolism in the depressed state: A confirmation. *American Journal of Psychiatry*, *147*, 1313–1317.

Mathew, R.J., Meyer, J.S., Francis, D.J., Semchuk, K.M., Mortel, K., & Claghorn, J.L. (1980). Cerebral blood flow in depression. *American Journal of Psychiatry*, *137*, 1449–1450.

Matousek, M. (1991). EEG patterns in various subgroups of endogenous depression. *International Journal of Psychophysiology*, *10*, 239–243.

Matousek, M., Capone, C., & Okawa, M. (1981). Measurement of the inter-hemispheral differences as a diagnostic tool in psychiatry. *Advances in Biological Psychiatry*, *6*, 76–80.

Mayberg, H.S., Lewis, P.L., Regenold, W., & Wagner, H.N. (1994). Paralimbic hypoperfusion in unipolar depression. *Journal of Nuclear Medicine*, *35*, 929–934.

Mayberg, H.S., Starkstein, S.E., Sadzot, B., Preziosi, T., Andrezejewski, P.I., Dannals, R.F., Wagner, H.N., & Robinson, R.G. (1990). Selective hypometabolism in the inferior frontal lobe in depressed patients with Parkinson's disease. *Annals of Neurology*, *28*, 57–64.

Mendez, M.F., Taylor, J.L., Doss, R.C., & Salguero, P. (1994). Depression in secondary epilepsy: Relation to lesion laterality. *Journal of Neurology, Neurosurgery, and Psychiatry*, *57*, 232–233.

Miller, E.N., Fujioka, T.A.T., Chapman, J.P., & Chapman, L.J. (1995). Hemispheric asymmetries of function in patients with major affective disorders. *Journal of Psychiatric Research*, *29*, 173–183.

Naatanen, R., & Picton, T. (1987). The N1 wave of the human electric and magnetic response to sound: A review and an analysis of the component structure. *Psychophysiology*, *24*, 375–425.

Nunez, P.L. (1981). *Electrical Fields of the Brain: The Neurophysics of EEG*. New York: Oxford University Press.

Pardo, J.V., Pardo, P.J., & Raichle, M.E. (1993). Neural correlates of self-induced dysphoria. *American Journal of Psychiatry*, *150*, 713–719.

Passero, S., Nardini, M., & Battistini, N. (1995). Regional cerebral blood flow changes following chronic administration of antidepressant drugs. *Progress in Neuro-Psychopharmacology and Biological Psychiatry*, *19*, 627–636.

Perini, G. (1986). Emotions and personality in complex partial seizures. *Psychotherapy Psychosomatic*, *45*, 141–148.

Perini, G., & Mendius, R. (1984). Depression and anxiety in complex partial seizures. *Journal of Nervous and Mental Disease*, *172*, 287–290.

Perris, C., von Knorring, L., Cumberbatch, J., & Marciano, F. (1981). Further studies of depressed patients by means of computerized EEG. *Advances in Biological Psychiatry*, *6*, 41–49.

Pfefferbaum, A., Wenegrat, B.G., Ford, J.M., Roth, W.T., & Kopel, B.S., (1984). Clinical application of the P3 component of event-related potentials. II. Dementia, depression and schizophrenia. *Electroencephalography and Clinical Neurophysiology*, *59*, 104–124.

Philpot, M.P., Banerjee, S., Needham-Bennett, H., Costa, D.C., & Ell, P.J. (1993). ^{99m}Tc-HMPAO single photon emission tomography in late life depression: A pilot study of regional cerebral blood flow at rest and during a verbal fluency task. *Journal of Affective Disorders*, *28*, 233–240.

Plooij-van Gorsel, E. (1984). Evoked potential correlates of information processing and habituation in depressive illness. *Annals of the New York Academy of Sciences*, *425*, 609–616.

Pollock, V.E., & Schneider, L.S. (1989). Topographic electroencephalographic alpha in recovered depressed elderly. *Journal of Abnormal Psychology*, *98*, 268–273.

Pollock, V.E., & Schneider, L.S. (1990). Topographic quantitative EEG in elderly subjects with major depression. *Psychophysiology*, *27*, 438–444.

Pozzi, D., Golimstock, A., Petracchi, M., Garcia, H., & Starkstein, S. (1995). Quantified electroencephalographic changes in depressed patients with and without dementia. *Biological Psychiatry*, *38*, 677–683.

Reid, S.A., Allen, J.J.B., & Duke, L.M. (1995). Differences in task-specific EEG activity of depressed and nondepressed subjects [abstract]. *Psychophysiology*, *32*, S61.

Reischies, F.M., Hedde, J.-P., & Drochenir, R. (1989). Clinical correlates of cerebral blood flow in depression. *Psychiatry Research*, *29*, 323–326.

Ring, H.A., Bench, C.J., Trimble, M.R., Brooks, D.J., Frackowiak, R.S., & Dolan R.J. (1994). Depression in Parkinson's disease. A positron emission study. *British Journal of Psychiatry*, *165*, 333–339.

Robinson, R.G., Kubos, K.L., Starr, L.B., Rao, K., & Price, T.R. (1984). Mood disorders in stroke patients. *Brain*, *107*, 81–93.

Robinson, R.G., Lipsey, J.R., Bolla-Wilson, K., Bolduc, P.L., Pearlson, G.D., Rao, K., & Price, T.R. (1985). Mood disorders in left-handed stroke patients. *American Journal of Psychiatry*, *142*, 1424–1429.

Robinson, R.G., & Price, T.R. (1982). Post-stroke depressive disorders: A follow-up of 103 patients. *Stroke*, *13*, 635–641.

Robinson, R.G., & Szetela, B. (1981). Mood change following left hemisphere brain injury. *Annals of Neurology*, *9*, 447–453.

Roemer, R.A., Shagass, C., Dubin, W., Jaffe, R., & Siegal, L. (1992). Quantitative EEG in elderly depressives. *Brain Topography*, *4*, 285–290.

Rosenberg, R., Vorstrop, S., Andersen, A., & Bolwig, T.G. (1988). Effect of ECT on cerebral blood flow in melancholia assessed with SPECT. *Convulsive Therapy*, *4*, 62–73.

Roth, M., Gurney, C., Garside, R.F., & Kerr, T.A. (1972). Studies in the classification of affective disorders. The relationship between anxiety states and depressive illness I. *British Journal of Psychiatry*, *121*, 147–161.

Roth, W.T., Pfefferbaum, A., Kelly, A.F., Berger, P.A., & Kopell, B.S. (1981). Auditory event-related potentials in schizophrenia and depression. *Psychiatry Research*, *4*, 199–212.

Rush, A.J., Schlesser, M.A., Stokely, E., Bonte, F.R., & Altshuller, K.Z. (1982). Cerebral blood flow in depression and mania. *Psychopharmacology Bulletin*, *18*, 6–8.

Sackeim, H.A., Greenberg, M.S., Weiman, A.L., Gur, R., Hungerbuhler, J.P., & Geschwind, N. (1982). Hemispheric asymmetry in the expression of positive and negative emotions. *Archives of Neurology*, *39*, 210–218.

Sackeim, H.A., Prohovnik, I., Moeller, J.R., Brown, R.P., Apter, S., Prudic, J., Devanand, D.P., & Mukherjee, S. (1990). Regional cerebral blood flow in mood disorders. I. Comparison of major depressives and normal controls at rest. *Archives of General Psychiatry*, *47*, 60–70.

Schaffer, C.E., Davidson, R.J., & Saron, C. (1983). Frontal and parietal electroencephalogram asymmetry in depressed and nondepressed subjects. *Biological Psychiatry*, *18*, 753–762.

Schlegel, S., Adenhoff, J.B., Eissner, D., Lindner, P., & Nickel, O. (1989). Regional cerebral blood flow in depression: Associations with psychopathology. *Journal of Affective Disorders*, *17*, 211–218.

Schneider, F., Gur, R.C., Jaggi, J.L., & Gur, R.E. (1994). Differential effects of mood on cortical cerebral blood flow: A [133]xenon clearance study. *Psychiatry Research*, *52*, 215–236.

Schneider, F., Gur, R.E., Mozley, L.H., Smith, R.J., Mozley, P.D., Censits, D.M., Alavi, A., & Gur, R.C. (1995). Mood effects on limbic blood flow correlate with emotional self-rating: A PET study with oxygen-15 labeled water. *Psychiatry Research: Neuroimaging*, *61*, 265–283.

Schneirla, T.C. (1959). An evolutionary and developmental theory of biphasic processes underlying approach and withdrawal. In M.R. Jones (Ed.), *Nebraska Symposium on Motivation* (pp. 1–42). Lincoln, NE: University of Nebraska Press.

Schroeder, J., Saver, H., Wilhelm, K.-R., Neidermeier, T., & Georgi, P. (1989). Regional cerebral blood flow in endogenous psychoses: A Tc-99m HMPAO-SPECT pilot study. *Psychiatry Research*, *29*, 331–333.

Silberman, E.K., & Weingartner, H. (1986). Hemispheric lateralization of functions related to emotion. *Brain and Cognition, 5,* 322–353.

Silfverskiöld, P., & Risberg, J. (1989). Regional cerebral blood flow in depression and mania. *Archives of General Psychiatry, 46,* 253–259.

Sinyor, D., Jacques, P., Kaloupek, D.G., Becker, R., Goldenberg, M., & Coopersmith, H. (1986). Poststroke depression and lesion location. An attempted replication. *Brain, 109,* 537–546.

Starkstein, S.E., Robinson, R.G., & Price, T.R. (1987). Comparison of cortical and subcortical lesions in the production of poststroke mood disorders. *Brain, 110,* 1045–1059.

Sutton, S.K., & Davidson, R.J. (1997). Prefrontal brain asymmetry: A biological substrate of the behavioral approach and inhibition systems. *Psychological Science, 8,* 204–210.

Suzuki, H., Mori, T., Kimura, M., & Endo, S. (1996). [Quantitative EEG characteristics of the state depressive phase and the state of remission in major depression]. *Seishin Shinkeigaku Zasshi, 98,* 363–367 [From Medline, Unique Identifier No. 96406773].

Tellegen, A. (1985). Structures of mood and personality and their relevance to assessing anxiety, with an emphasis on self-report. In A.H. Tuma & J. Maser (Eds.) *Anxiety and the Anxiety Disorders* (pp. 681–706). Hillsdale, NJ: Erlbaum.

Tenke, C.E., Bruder, G.E., Towey, J.P., Leite, P., & Sidtis, J.J. (1993). Correspondence between brain ERP and behavioral asymmetries in a dichotic complex tone test. *Psychophysiology, 30,* 62–70

Terzian, H. (1964). Behavioral and EEG effects of intracarotid sodium amytal injection. *Acta Neurochirurgica, 12,* 230–239.

Thier, P., Axmann, D., & Giedke, H. (1986). Slow brain potentials and psychomotor retardation in depression. *Electroencephalography and Clinical Neurophysiology, 63,* 570–581.

Tomarken, A.J., Davidson, R.J., & Henriques, J.B. (1990). Frontal brain asymmetry predicts affective responses to films. *Journal of Personality and Social Psychology, 59,* 791–801.

Tomarken, A.J., Davidson, R.J., Wheeler, R.E., & Doss, R.C. (1992). Individual differences in anterior brain asymmetry and fundamental dimensions of emotion. *Journal of Personality and Social Psychology, 62,* 676–687.

Tucker, D.M., Stenslie, C.E., Roth, R.S., & Shearer, S.L. (1981). Right frontal lobe activation and right hemisphere performance. *Archives of General Psychiatry, 38,* 169–174.

Ulrich, G., Renfordt, E., Zeller, G., & Frick, K. (1984). Interrelation between changes in the EEG and psychopathology under pharmacotherapy for endogenous depression. A contribution to the predictor question. *Pharmacopsychiatry, 17,* 178–183.

Uytdenhoef, P., Portelange, P., Jacquy, J., Charles, G., Linkowski, P., & Mendlewicz, J. (1983). Regional cerebral blood flow and lateralized hemispheric dysfunction in depression. *British Journal of Psychiatry, 143,* 128–132.

Vasile, R.G., Duffy, F.H., McAnulty, G., Bear, D., Mooney, J.J., Bloomingdale, K., Serchuck, L.K., & Schildkraut, J.J. (1989). Abnormal visual evoked response in melancholia. *Biological Psychiatry, 25,* 785–788.

Velten, E. (1968). A laboratory task for induction of mood states. *Behavior Research and Therapy, 6,* 473–482.

Volavka, J., Abrams, R., Taylor, M.A., & Reker, D. (1981). Hemispheric lateralization of fast EEG activity in schizophrenia and endogenous depression. *Advances in Biological Psychiatry, 6,* 72–75.

von Knorring, L. (1983). Interhemispheric EEG differences in affective disorders. In P.

Flor-Henry & J. Gruzelier (Eds.), *Laterality and Psychopathology* (pp. 315–326). New York: Elsevier Science Publishers B.V.

Warren, L.R., Butler, R.W., Katholi, C.R., McFarland, C.E., Crews, E.L., & Halsey, J.H. (1984). Focal changes in cerebral blood flow produced by monetary incentive during a mental mathematics task in normal and depressed subjects. *Brain and Cognition, 3,* 71–85.

Watson, D., Clark, L.A., & Carey, G. (1988). Positive and negative affectivity and their relation to anxiety and depressive disorders. *Journal of Abnormal Psychology, 97,* 346–353.

Watson, D., Clark, L.A., & Tellegen, A. (1988). Development and validation of brief measures of positive and negative affect: The PANAS scales. *Journal of Personality and Social Psychology, 54,* 1063–1070.

Watson, D., & Tellegen, A. (1985). Toward a consensual structure of mood. *Psychological Bulletin, 98,* 219–235.

Wheeler, R.E., Davidson, R.J., & Tomarken, A.J. (1993). Frontal brain asymmetry and emotional reactivity: A biological substrate of affective style. *Psychophysiology, 30,* 82–89.

Zahn, T.P. (1986). Psychophysiological approaches to psychopathology. In M.G.H. Coles, E. Donchin, & S.W. Porges (Eds.), *Psychophysiology: Systems, Processes, and Applications* (pp. 508–610). New York: The Guilford Press.

12

Anxiety, Stress, and Cortical Brain Function

JACK B. NITSCHKE, WENDY HELLER,
AND GREGORY A. MILLER

Much has been written about the survival value of panic and the benefits of anxiety for various aspects of human performance (e.g., Barlow, 1991; Lang, 1985; Miller & Kozak, 1993). Anxiety can be maladaptive, however, disrupting performance and interfering with both psychological and physical well-being. Consequently, the current, 4th edition of the *Diagnostic and Statistical Manual of Mental Disorders* (DSM-IV; American Psychiatric Association, 1994) distinguishes 11 different diagnoses it classifies as anxiety disorders.

The prevalence of anxiety disorders has led to an interest in the neural mechanisms that accompany them. The search for the brain circuitry of anxiety has benefitted from a large data base of animal research (e.g., Davis, 1992; Gray, 1982; LeDoux, 1993, 1995; Mineka, 1985), possible in part because of the ease of experimentally conditioning fear. Although research has greatly elucidated the subcortical circuits mediating fear in animals, the precise role of the cortex in human anxiety has eluded understanding.

The interpretation of neuropsychological studies based on electrophysiological, hemodynamic (blood flow), and behavioral methods has been hindered by inconsistencies in findings for particular cortical brain regions. Although many studies have reported or inferred asymmetries in regional cortical activity and function, the regions involved and the direction of the asymmetry have varied, as reviewed below. Methodological differences from study to study, albeit important, do not provide a cogent explanation for the conflicting patterns of brain activity reported in the literature.

Heterogeneity among the samples studied may explain the inconsistencies in the literature on brain function in anxiety. Research has been conducted on samples characterized by specific anxiety disorders as defined by the several DSM editions, by self-reports of anxiety on various questionnaires, and by experimentally induced anxiety. In recent work, we suggested that distinguishing between types of anxiety, which would be differentially represented in different subject samples, may help to resolve some of the discrepancies in the literature (Heller et al., 1997a; Heller & Nitschke, 1998; Nitschke et al., 1999).

In this chapter, we review the evidence connecting distinct types of anxiety with specific patterns of regional brain function and examine the implications of these associations for cognition. In addition, we consider the role of stress in anxiety and explore the relationships among stress, anxiety, and regional brain activity.

TWO TYPES OF ANXIETY

There is considerable disagreement as to the meaning of anxiety and its relationship to fear, panic, stress, and worry (e.g., Barlow, 1991; Borkovec et al., 1983; Eysenck, 1957; Heller & Nitschke, 1998; Heller et al., 1997a; Klein, 1981, 1987; Lang, 1968, 1978, 1985; Lazarus, 1993; Mathews, 1990; Miller & Kozak, 1993; Molina & Borkovec, 1994; Watson et al., 1995). Eysenck (1991) adheres to the traditional conditioning view that anxiety is a learned kind of fear. In contrast, Gray (1982, 1991) argues that anxiety encompasses both a fear state that is elicited by certain conditioned stimuli associated with punishment and anticipatory frustration elicited by other types of stimuli. Barlow (1991) distinguished fear from anxiety and argued instead that panic and fear are the same. In keeping with the categorization of anxiety disorders in the DSM-IV, we view anxiety as subsuming fear, panic, and worry.

In recent work, we have focused on two types (or dimensions) of anxiety that can be psychometrically distinguished (Nitschke et al., 2000) and that may account for the varied findings in research examining brain activity in anxiety (see Table 12.1). In accord with Barlow (1991), we defined one of these types as anxious apprehension, also referred to as worry (e.g., Borkovec et al., 1983), cognitive anxiety (e.g., Lehrer & Woolfolk, 1982; Schwartz, Davidson, & Goleman, 1978), anticipatory anxiety (e.g., Klein, 1981), and anticipatory frustration (e.g., Amsel, 1962). Anxious apprehension is characterized by a concern for the future and verbal rumination about negative expectations and fears. It is often accompanied by muscle tension, restlessness, and fatigue. Unlike Barlow, we do not equate anxiety with anxious apprehension.

Table 12.1. Characteristics of Anxious Apprehension and Anxious Arousal

	ANXIOUS APPREHENSION	ANXIOUS AROUSAL
Cardinal feature	Verbal rumination involving negative expectations or fears about future	Intense, immediate fear
Time scale	Ranging from immediate to distant future	Present or very immediate future
Related or synonymous constructs	Worry, cognitive anxiety, anticipatory anxiety	Panic, somatic anxiety
Somatic symptoms	Muscle tension	Increased heart rate, shortness of breath, dizziness, sweating, feeling of choking
General neuropsychological patterns*	Left-hemisphere engagement	Right-hemisphere engagement

*Neuropsychological inferences based on electrophysiological, hemodynamic, and behavioral findings in anxiety.

The second type of anxiety is anxious arousal, often referred to as somatic anxiety (e.g., Lehrer & Woolfolk, 1982; Schwartz, Davidson, & Goleman, 1978). Anxious arousal is the predominant type of anxiety present in panic. In addition to feelings of fear, anxious arousal is associated with such somatic symptoms as pounding heart and dizziness (Watson et al., 1995) but not with somatic features associated with anxious apprehension (e.g., muscle tension). Anxious arousal is more likely to be triggered by a threat perceived to represent an immediate danger, whereas anxious apprehension would be more salient for a threat that invokes fear and worry about the more distant future.

Of conceptual import, our distinction between anxious apprehension and anxious arousal does not correspond precisely to the distinction between trait anxiety and state anxiety. Trait anxiety is typically characterized by a disposition to worry, to be tense, and to interpret stressful situations as threatening (e.g., Eysenck, 1992; Spielberger, 1983). Most self-report measures of trait anxiety assess anxious apprehension and negative affect. A disposition toward anxious arousal could, however, be a trait characteristic.

On the other hand, state anxiety is generally associated with a more immediate fear response accompanied by those somatic symptoms characteristic of anxious arousal. A panic attack would be an extreme manifestation of state anxiety. Although not as common, state anxiety characterized by anxious apprehension could be induced by a specific stressor that elicits worry. Indeed, the presence of either type of anxiety in an individual is not static: Stressful events, social support, and coping skills can modulate one's level of each type of anxiety.

Available research suggests that anxious apprehension and anxious arousal are not mutually exclusive (e.g., Dien, 1999; Heller et al., 1997a). It follows that anxious apprehension and anxious arousal would be present to varying degrees in the different anxiety disorders. Anxious apprehension is particularly prominent in generalized anxiety disorder (GAD) and obsessive-compulsive disorder (OCD) in which worry and other cognitive symptoms predominate. In addition, GAD includes the subset of somatic features outlined above for anxious apprehension. Moreover, a cardinal feature of specific phobia, social phobia, and agoraphobia is persistent, excessive fear that usually reflects concern about the future. Panic disorder includes worry about having additional panic attacks and about the implications or consequences of an attack. In those disorders in which panic attacks may occur, such as panic disorder, specific phobia, and social phobia, DSM-IV criteria clearly indicate the presence of anxious arousal. Furthermore, there are likely to be individual differences and situational factors that influence the relative frequency and occurrence of each type of anxiety in a particular person.

The importance of taking into account the relative admixture of both types of anxiety becomes apparent when we consider the findings reviewed below showing that each type of anxiety is associated with distinct patterns of brain activity. In turn, our distinction between anxious apprehension and anxious arousal may help to explain the cognitive findings reported for anxiety.

STRESS AND ANXIETY

Stress is an important factor influencing the relationship between types of anxiety and brain function. In numerous neuropsychological and cognitive studies, researchers have employed stressful experimental conditions to elicit state anxiety, which, as noted above, is likely to involve anxious arousal as well as anxious apprehension.

The term *stress* has most often been used to refer to an external phenomenon (a stressor) that has an emotional impact on an individual. Many researchers have also, however, invoked the term *stress* to imply psychological stress, defined as the emotional response to an external event or stressor. Lazarus and colleagues have emphasized the interactive relationship between these two aspects of stress, arguing that potential stressors can be appraised as indicative of harm, threat, or challenge (for review, see Lazarus, 1993).

The distinction between potential sources of stress and the emotional sequelae that ensue is critical to an understanding of anxiety. Lazarus and others have shown that a one-to-one correspondence between a potential stressor and a subsequent emotional response does not exist (Lazarus, 1993). Rather, there are large individual differences in response to any particular event, and many factors (e.g., life history, coping style, trait anxiety) influence the degree to which an event is appraised as harmful or threatening. For example, anticipation of a public speech might not elicit anxiety in a college professor with years of experience but is likely to do so in a graduate student giving a talk at a conference for the first time. Thus, a thorough understanding of the relationship between stress and anxiety must take into account not only specific and contextual external conditions involved but also the role of individual differences in response to those conditions. The importance of this issue can perhaps be seen most clearly in the heightened vulnerability of trait-anxious people to exhibit cognitive abnormalities (e.g., attentional biases to threat) in response to various stressors (see discussion of cognitive studies of anxiety, below).

In a review of the neuropsychological and cognitive literatures on anxiety, it is important to consider the role of stressors, which often elicit anxious apprehension and anxious arousal, as well as the role of both types of anxiety as forms of psychological stress. Experimental manipulations of stressful situations, such as electrical shock, can be used to elicit anxious arousal. Similarly, researchers have often designed experiments to take advantage of stressful life circumstances, such as final examinations for medical students. In addition, a large literature about the effects of major life events and daily hassles has documented that life stress precipitates a variety of psychopathological states, including anxiety (e.g., Faravelli & Pallanti, 1989; Pollard, Pollard, & Corn, 1989; Rapee, Litwin, & Barlow, 1990; Roy-Byrne, Geraci, & Uhde, 1986). Electrical shock, final examinations, major life events, and daily hassles are examples of potential stressors that can result in psychological stress, such as anxious apprehension or anxious arousal. In the following sections, it will be apparent that stress is often a key variable in the association between anxiety and region-specific brain function.

NEUROPSYCHOLOGICAL STUDIES OF ANXIETY

We have proposed a neuropsychological framework for anxiety based on the two types of anxiety distinguished above (Heller et al., 1997a; Heller & Nitschke, 1998). Given the left-hemisphere dominance for language in most right-handed people, we have hypothesized that anxious apprehension would be associated with more left-hemisphere activity because of the strong verbal component inherent in worry and cognitive anxiety. Conversely, consistent with a neuropsychological model of emotion proposed by Heller (1990), the literature linking somatic arousal to posterior right-hemisphere regions of the brain (for review, see Heller, Nitschke, & Lindsay, 1997b) suggested to us that anxious arousal should be associated with more right posterior activity.

In addition, of relevance to both types of anxiety, unpleasant valence and negative affect have been shown to be associated with increased right anterior activity (for review, see Davidson, 1992, 1998; Heller, 1990; Heller & Nitschke, 1997). The effect of unpleasant valence on anterior brain activity in anxious apprehension is difficult to anticipate. The greater right than left anterior activity associated with unpleasant valence might serve to cancel the increase in left anterior activity expected for anxious apprehension. Alternatively, anxious apprehension might be associated with a bilateral increase in anterior activity. Due to the presence of unpleasant valence, anxious arousal should be associated with increased activity in right anterior as well as right posterior regions of the brain.

Electrophysiological and Hemodynamic Paradigms

The distinction between anxious apprehension and anxious arousal is well supported in the literature on regional brain activity. Increased left-hemisphere activity has been associated with anxiety in studies on populations better characterized by anxious apprehension than by anxious arousal. In a positron emission tomography (PET) study, Baxter et al. (1987) reported greater regional cerebral blood flow (rCBF) in the left orbital gyrus in OCD patients than in depressed and control participants. Similarly, Swedo et al. (1989) found that OCD patients showed more left orbital frontal and left anterior cingulate metabolism than nonpsychiatric controls. Wu et al. (1991) reported higher relative metabolism in the left inferior frontal gyrus for GAD patients than for nonpsychiatric controls. In another study, inpatients with GAD showed increases in left orbital frontal blood flow when asked to freely associate about threatening pictures presented before rCBF measurement (Johanson et al., 1992). Relative increases in activity for left subcortical regions (e.g., caudate, putamen, and thalamus) have also been reported in a number of studies (e.g., Fredrikson et al., 1993; Swedo et al., 1989).

Similar results have been obtained with electroencephalography (EEG). Using only left-hemisphere and midline leads, Buchsbaum et al. (1985) reported that GAD patients had more activity (less delta and alpha) than nonpsychiatric controls. Consistent findings were reported by Carter, Johnson, and Borkovec (1986) for beta activity in students classified as "worriers" or "nonworriers" when asked to "worry about a specific topic of personal concern."

Conversely, those authors reporting increased right-hemisphere activity in anxiety examined populations characterized by anxious arousal or employed experimental designs manipulating it. Using PET, Reiman et al. (1984) found that patients with panic disorder showed greater right-hemisphere than left-hemisphere blood flow, blood volume, and metabolic rate in the parahippocampal gyrus, whereas normal controls demonstrated no such asymmetry. In a single photon emission computerized axial tomography study, panic disorder patients who experienced a sodium-lactate-induced panic attack were found to have a significantly greater increase in right occipital blood flow than did patients who did not panic and controls (Stewart et al., 1988).

Consistent with this pattern, glucose metabolism changes indicative of increased right-hemisphere activity for GAD patients performing a Continuous Performance Task designed to induce anxious arousal were reported in two studies (Buchsbaum et al., 1987; Wu et al., 1991). In recent EEG work, Davidson et al. (2000) reported increased right anterior temporal, right lateral prefrontal, and right parietal activity in social phobics immediately before making a public speech, an experimental manipulation likely to elicit anxious arousal. Spider phobia has also been found to be associated with more right than left parietal activity (Merckelbach et al., 1999). In sum, across a number of different imaging technologies and experimental protocols, the increased right-hemisphere activity expected for anxious arousal emerges consistently in clinical populations.

Similar findings have emerged in nonclinical samples as well. When the state version of the State-Trait Anxiety Inventory (STAI; Spielberger, 1968, 1983) was administered immediately after arterial and venous catheterization and again after completion of the PET scans, high-anxious subjects had greater right than left blood flow, whereas low-anxious subjects showed no differences between the hemispheres (only frontal regions were measured; Reivich, Gur, & Alavi, 1983). In a population of nonpsychiatric volunteers, those administered diazepam intravenously showed decreases in rCBF across all cortical regions, particularly in the right frontal area, whereas those injected with a placebo showed no rCBF changes (Mathew, Wilson, & Daniel, 1985).

In an event-related potential (ERP) study, participants who scored high on both the trait and state versions of the STAI showed smaller N2 and P3 amplitudes over the right hemisphere than low-anxious participants (de Pascalis & Morelli, 1990). Because smaller amplitude in response to the probes of the lexical recognition task was assumed to reflect enhanced information processing, the high-anxious participants can be inferred to have demonstrated more right-hemisphere engagement on the task than did the low-anxious participants.

The fact that some studies have reported significant or near-significant increases in activity for regions in both right and left hemispheres could reflect the co-occurrence of both types of anxiety (e.g., Baxter et al., 1988; Fredrikson et al., 1993; Reiman et al., 1989). Alternatively, the bilateral orbital frontal findings reported by Baxter et al. for OCD patients might provide evidence for the hypothesis that increased right anterior activity in anxious apprehension reflects the presence of negative affect.

In two recent EEG studies, we directly tested the hypothesis of opposing patterns of asymmetry for anxious apprehension and anxious arousal. Heller et al. (1997a) selected participants on the basis of self-reported trait anxiety using the STAI. We then manipulated anxious arousal on a within-subject basis by contrasting brain activity (EEG alpha) during rest periods to brain activity during a

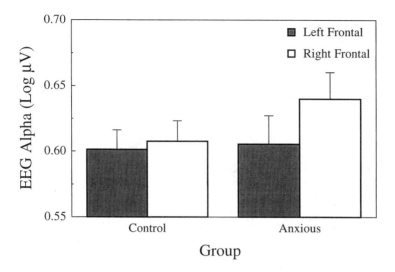

Figure 12.1. Mean log EEG alpha voltage (+SE) for left and right midfrontal regions for control ($N = 19$) and anxious ($N = 19$) groups averaged across the rest and listen periods of the fearful and sad narratives. Lower alpha values indicate greater brain activity. (From Heller et al., 1997a).

task in which participants listened to emotional narratives designed to elicit anxious arousal. As shown in Figure 12.1, anxious participants showed a larger frontal asymmetry in favor of the left hemisphere than did controls across both rest and listen periods. In contrast, when listening to the narratives, anxious participants showed a selective increase in right parietal activity that was not demonstrated by controls (Fig. 12.2).

The second study (Nitschke, 1998; Nitschke et al., 1999) employed a between-subjects design to compare participants scoring high on a questionnaire indexing anxious apprehension (Penn State Worry Questionnaire; Meyer et al., 1990) to others scoring high on the Anxious Arousal scale of the Mood and Anxiety Symptom Questionnaire (Watson et al., 1995). Figure 12.3 shows the patterns of hemispheric alpha asymmetry, with the anxious apprehension group showing more left-sided and the anxious arousal group showing more right-sided activity. Consistent with these findings, a recent ERP study also reported lateralized effects for the two types of anxiety in a between-subject design using different self-report measures (Dien, 1999). These studies provide further evidence for the utility of the distinction between anxious apprehension and anxious arousal in efforts to elucidate the neurophysiological mechanisms involved in anxiety and anxiety disorders.

An important consideration for any research on anxiety is the frequent comorbidity with depression. Despite this comorbidity, research has shown that brain function in anxiety differs substantially from brain function in depression

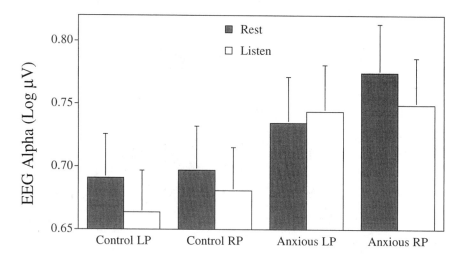

Figure 12.2. Mean log EEG alpha voltage (+SE) for left and right parietal regions for control (*N* = 19) and anxious (*N* = 19) groups during the rest and listen periods, averaged across fearful and sad narratives. Lower alpha values indicate greater brain activity. RP = right parietal; LP = left parietal. (From Heller et al., 1997a).

(for reviews, see Davidson et al., 1999; Heller & Nitschke, 1998). Although the finding of more right than left activity in anterior cortical regions for anxious arousal has also been reported for depression (e.g., Henriques & Davidson, 1991), the increased left-hemisphere activity reported for anxious apprehension and the increased right posterior activity associated with anxious arousal have not been found for depression. Indeed, other commonly reported findings for depression are in the opposite direction: decreased left anterior activity (e.g., George et al., 1994) and decreased right posterior activity (e.g., Post et al., 1987). In addition, several studies have reported bilateral decreases for anterior cortical regions in depression (e.g., Bench et al., 1992), a finding that has not emerged in the anxiety literature.[1] Although the differing patterns of brain activity reported for anxiety and for depression warrant the careful measurement of depression in studies examining anxiety, the EEG and hemodynamic findings distinguishing anxious apprehension from anxious arousal cannot be accounted for by comorbid depression.

Behavioral Paradigms

Complementing tests of our hypotheses using biological measures, regional brain activity can also be inferred from performance on tasks that depend on particu-

[1]Martinot et al. (1990) reported a bilateral decrease in prefrontal regions for OCD patients; however, despite not meeting criteria for DSM-III current major depressive episode, these patients may still have been characterized by significantly higher levels of depression than the nonpatient controls.

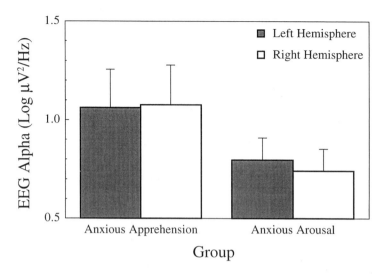

Figure 12.3. Mean log EEG alpha power (+SE) for left and right hemispheres (averaged across lateral frontal and parietal sites) for anxious apprehension ($N = 9$) and anxious arousal ($N = 19$) groups. Lower alpha values indicate greater brain activity. (From Nitschke et al., 1999).

lar brain regions. When samples of trait-anxious people are studied in the absence of experimental manipulations that might induce anxious arousal, results are typically consistent with the increased left-hemisphere activity hypothesized for anxious apprehension. Tucker et al. (1978) found that high-anxious subjects, as classified by the trait scale of the STAI, tended to report right-ear tones as louder and displayed a reduction in left lateral eye movements. Similarly, Tyler and Tucker (1982) found that high-anxious individuals tended to use a processing strategy characteristic of the left hemisphere, whereas low-anxious individuals were more likely to use a strategy characteristic of the right hemisphere.

In contrast, when experimental conditions involve an immediate anxiety-producing component, stimuli that can be interpreted as threatening, or stressful life circumstances, the data are consistent with the increased right-hemisphere activity predicted for anxious arousal. On a free-vision task of face processing (Chimeric Faces Task [CFT]; Levy et al., 1983) that typically elicits a left-hemispatial bias suggesting greater right posterior activity, Heller, Etienne, and Miller (1995) found that participants scoring high on the trait version of the STAI had larger left hemispatial (right-hemisphere) biases than those scoring low. This pattern was replicated in a population of major depressed subjects and in a non-clinical student population selected on the basis of recently developed anxiety and depression scales (Keller et al., 2000). Importantly, for the latter two samples, the relationship between anxiety and the CFT only emerged after the variance associated with depression was removed. This set of findings suggests that the strangeness and ambiguity of the CFT stimuli may lead to enhanced right-hemisphere processing in trait-anxious people (see discussion of lesion studies and anxiety below).

This interpretation is consistent with divided-visual-field studies demonstrating selective priming of the right hemisphere in response to threatening stimuli. In a series of studies, Van Strien and colleagues reported improved left-visual-field (right-hemisphere) performance on left-hemisphere tasks when threatening words were presented concurrently (see Van Strien & Heijt, 1995; Van Strien & Morpurgo, 1992).

Similar effects on right-hemisphere processing have been obtained under stress conditions. Gruzelier and Phelan (1991) tested medical students on a divided-visual-field lexical task under two conditions: 1 or 2 days before an examination and 4 weeks before or after the examination. They found that the left-hemisphere advantage in the nonstress condition gave way to a right-hemisphere advantage in the stress condition. Similarly, Asbjörnsen, Hugdahl, and Bryden (1992) found that the threat of electric shock eliminated the left-hemisphere advantage for a dichotic listening task.

Further support for our hypothesis of greater right-hemisphere activity in anxious arousal is provided by work conducted by Tucker and colleagues. In a study examining contralateral eye movements, Tucker et al. (1977) found significantly more left than right lateral eye movements during an anxiety-provoking task, suggesting greater right-hemisphere than left-hemisphere activation. These results were supported in a subsequent study in which an anxiety-producing experimental condition was associated with a reversal of the typical left-hemisphere superiority on a verbal task (Tucker et al., 1978). More recently, Johanson et al. (1998) found that spider phobics, a population primarily characterized by anxious arousal, performed significantly better on right-hemisphere than left-hemisphere tasks for a neuropsychological test battery. Taken together, the behavioral neuropsychology findings presented here are consistent with the hemodynamic and EEG studies reviewed above reporting greater left-hemisphere activity in anxious apprehension and greater right-hemisphere activity in anxious arousal.

LESION STUDIES AND ANXIETY

Complementing the EEG, hemodynamic, and behavioral paradigms often used in neuropsychological research, another common strategy for investigating the neuroanatomical bases of various functions is to examine the effects of brain damage on particular behaviors. This approach has been quite helpful in furthering our understanding of depression, which has been shown to be associated principally with lesions in the left frontal lobe (see Robinson & Manes, Chapter 10, this volume).

Unfortunately, lesion studies have not systematically examined anxiety, much less considered the distinction between anxious apprehension and anxious arousal. Furthermore, early stages of recovery from traumatic brain injury are often characterized by emotional disturbances, such as agitation, irritability, and emotional volatility, that make it difficult to assess the presence and region-specific impact of anxiety. Common sense would predict that anxiety would be a typical psychological response to the trauma of physical disability, illness, and accompanying life changes; however, in some cases, anxiety is notably absent. In fact, important inferences about the neuropsychology of anxiety can be drawn from those people in whom anxiety and emotional distress are not present.

Early descriptions of dramatically different emotional reactions after left versus right brain damage were systematically studied by Gainotti (1972) and later by Robinson and colleagues (e.g., Starkstein & Robinson, 1988). Left brain damage, particularly frontal, is associated with a "catastrophic" emotional propensity, marked by tearfulness, distress, and agitation. Right brain damage, in contrast, is more often accompanied by indifference, euphoria, or apathy, indicating a remarkable and inappropriate lack of anxiety. Research examining behavior after unilateral sodium amobarbital injection in populations without brain damage has provided almost identical findings (e.g., Ahern et al., 1994; Lee et al., 1990). In addition, attentional abnormalities (e.g., hemineglect, when patients ignore stimuli on the left side of space) and anosagnosia (when patients deny or minimize the existence of an illness or disability) are also often present in patients with right-hemisphere lesions. McGlynn and Schacter (1989) described a typical case of unawareness and indifference in a head-injured patient who had been a practicing physician before an automobile accident: "Shortly after regaining consciousness he insisted that he could soon return home and he began to make implausible plans for the future. . . . He confabulated about the cause of his illness . . . and exhibited no anxiety about his condition" (p. 170). The lack of anxiety in people with decreased right-hemisphere function due to a lesion parallels findings of increased right-hemisphere activity in anxious arousal.

Although the neuroanatomical damage is somewhat varied in the populations that have been studied, there is general agreement that the indifference reaction is most often reported after damage to right parietal regions (McGlynn & Schacter, 1989). This area has been shown to be differentially involved in processing emotional information, especially negative material (e.g., Borod et al., 1992; Heller & Levy, 1981), in spatial attention (e.g., Heilman, Watson, & Valenstein, 1985; Mesulam, 1981; see also Heller, 1993), and in monitoring responses to external sensory stimuli (e.g., Heilman & Van den Abell, 1979; Pardo, Fox, & Raichle, 1991). In addition, this and other right-hemisphere regions have been found to be uniquely involved in modulation and regulation of autonomic, cortical, and self-reported arousal (for reviews, see Heller, 1993; Heller et al., 1997b; Wittling, 1995), in the perception and integration of multimodal sensory integration (Goldberg & Costa, 1981), and in understanding the way in which objects and events are related to each other in a real-world context (Heller, 1994). Apropos of these observations, Bear (1986) referred to the right hemisphere as selectively engaged in "emotional surveillance."

Taken together, these results led Heller (1993) to describe a similar system confined to the right temporoparietal region "whose properties encompass the cognitive, attentional, and physiological attributes that would be useful for optimal efficiency in responding to environmental events" (pp. 480–481). This view is consistent with data described earlier suggesting that the right hemisphere is primed by material that could be interpreted as threatening (e.g., negative words, ambiguous stimuli) and with evidence that increased activity in this region accompanies anxious arousal. The absence of anxiety in patients with right parietal brain damage may be a manifestation of dysfunction in a broader network that not only governs withdrawal and avoidance behaviors (Davidson, 1992, 1998) but also attends to the external environment on an ongoing basis, monitors it for threat, orients toward potential threat, appraises the context for information regarding the possibility of threat, and exerts hierarchical control over the autonomic and somatic functions for responding to threat. That the cognitive biases typically found in anxiety appear to reflect the engagement of this right-hemisphere system is discussed in the next section.

COGNITIVE STUDIES OF ANXIETY

Cognitive Biases

As neuropsychological research on anxiety has matured during the 1980s and 1990s, an additional line of investigation has substantially advanced our knowledge about the cognitive concomitants of anxiety. There have been numerous reports of an attentional bias to threat in trait anxiety and the various anxiety disorders (for reviews, see Eysenck, 1992; Mathews & MacLeod, 1994; McNally, 1998), with some studies not finding effects unless state anxiety was induced (e.g., Broadbent & Broadbent, 1988; MacLeod, 1990; MacLeod & Mathews, 1988). This bias has emerged for subliminal as well as for supraliminal stimuli, suggesting that automatic, preattentive processing is involved (e.g., Bradley et al., 1995; MacLeod & Hagan, 1992; MacLeod & Rutherford, 1992; Mogg et al., 1993). Furthermore, attentional biases have been found to disappear in GAD patients, social phobics, spider phobics, and rape victims with post-traumatic stress disorder on remission (for review, see McNally, 1998), suggesting that such biases are state dependent.

Cognitive biases are also present in anxiety in the form of interpretation biases. Across a number of different paradigms involving ambiguous stimuli that can be interpreted as threatening or neutral, anxious people choose the threatening meaning. Similar to findings for attentional biases, the selective processing of ambiguous information in anxious individuals is most consistently observed in conditions eliciting state anxiety (e.g., MacLeod, 1990). Further evidence that these biases are state dependent is provided by research showing that recovered GAD patients do not exhibit the selective interpretation effect (Mathews, Richards, & Eysenck, 1989b; Eysenck et al., 1991).

Our neuropsychological framework for anxiety suggests that these attentional and interpretation biases are related to anxious arousal and to the emotion surveillance system of the right hemisphere. As reviewed above, this region of the brain has been shown to be primed by ambiguous and threatening stimuli and hypothesized to play a role in orienting to such stimuli. In addition, populations characterized by anxious arousal consistently show increased right-hemisphere activity at rest (e.g., Reiman et al., 1984), suggesting that anxious arousal is associated with the engagement of the emotional surveillance system, even in the absence of an emotional stimulus. This right-hemisphere system may correspond to the cortical processes that McNally (1998) postulated to accompany a subcortical circuit involved in attentional biases toward threat. Thus, anxious arousal can be hypothesized to produce a set of behaviors that include attentional and other cognitive responses designed to evaluate the presence of a threat.

In contrast to findings of attentional and interpretation biases in anxiety, results of studies examining explicit and implicit memory biases have been equivocal (for reviews, see Eysenck, 1992; Mathews & MacLeod, 1994; McNally, 1998). Previous work examining the neuropsychology of cognitive biases in depression may inform attempts to understand why some studies find memory biases in anxiety whereas others do not. Heller and Nitschke (1997) suggested that the negative memory bias reported so consistently in depression (for reviews, see Gotlib, Gilboa, & Kaplan, 2000; Mathews & MacLeod, 1994) is associated with more right than left cortical activity in anterior regions, the same pattern that emerges in studies examining negative affect. Similarly, the greater right than left anterior activity characterizing anxious arousal should be accompanied by a negative memory bias, as has been found in panic disorder patients (e.g., Amir et al., 1996a; Becker, Rinck, & Margraf, 1994; Cloitre et al., 1994) and post-traumatic stress disorder patients (Amir et al., 1996b; Vrana, Roodman, & Beckham, 1995). Conversely, many studies have found no memory biases in samples characterized better by anxious apprehension than by anxious arousal (e.g., MacLeod & McLaughlin, 1995; Mathews et al., 1989a; Mogg, Mathews, & Weinman, 1987; Nugent & Mineka, 1994; Rapee et al., 1994; Watts & Coyle, 1993). In sum, the neuropsychological perspective provided here can account for the dissociation among the different cognitive biases (cf. Eysenck, 1992; Williams et al., 1988).

Cognitive Impairments

An understanding of the neuropsychological mechanisms involved in anxiety may inform other cognitive research on anxiety as well. Unlike depression, which is accompanied by deficits in explicit memory, executive functions, and visuospatial skills (for review, see Heller & Nitschke, 1997), results for anxiety have been variable. Although numerous studies have reported impaired performance (particularly for trait-anxious people doing difficult tasks under stressful conditions that elicit state anxiety), others have found no effects of anxiety (for review, see Eysenck & Calvo, 1992). At times, high trait or state anxiety has even been associated with superior performance.

To explain these findings, Eysenck and Calvo (1992) argued that worry, or anxious apprehension, affects performance negatively by pre-empting processing and storage capacities of the working memory system. Working memory has been theorized to be comprised of three general systems: a central executive, an articulatory loop that involves verbal rehearsal and phonological storage, and a visuospatial processor (Baddeley, 1986). Eysenck and Calvo (1992) theorized that worry is particularly likely to disrupt the central processor and the articulatory loop.

This proposition is consistent with the neuropsychological data reviewed above that suggest a special role of the left hemisphere in anxious apprehension. Current research on the neural mechanisms associated with working memory suggests that dorsolateral prefrontal cortex is associated with the "central processor," that Broca's area in the left anterior region is associated with the rehearsal component of the articulatory loop, and that left posterior areas around the angular and supramarginal gyrus are associated with the phonological storage component of the articulatory loop (for review, see Gupta & MacWhinney, 1997). Cortical activity associated with apprehensive thoughts might thus interfere with information processing of other tasks in both anterior and posterior regions of the left hemisphere: the greater the level of worry, the greater the interference. Furthermore, it follows that performance would most likely be impaired on tasks that impose considerable demands on these components of the working memory system (Eysenck & Calvo, 1992).

Using our neuropsychological framework for anxious apprehension and anxious arousal as a guide, we have speculated about the brain regions involved in cognitive abnormalities accompanying anxiety. With the advancing sophistication of hemodynamic and electrophysiological imaging techniques, the time is ripe for research paradigms that can investigate simultaneously the specific cognitive characteristics and the patterns of regional brain activity associated with anxiety.

SUMMARY AND CONCLUSIONS

Considering a number of conceptualizations of anxiety, we argued for the utility of a distinction between anxious apprehension and anxious arousal. Like anxiety, stress is not a unitary construct, and understanding the relationships between external stressors and psychological stress is critical for research on anxiety. At the level of the cortex, we suspect a major role for left-hemisphere functions in anxious apprehension and for right-hemisphere functions in anxious arousal. Electrophysiological and hemodynamic studies have provided remarkably consistent evidence for our position that anxious apprehension is associated with more left-sided activity and anxious arousal with more right-sided activity. In addition, the utility of distinguishing the two types of anxiety is apparent when interpreting results for performance on left-hemisphere and right-hemisphere behavioral tasks. Corroborating evidence for the neuropsychological perspective espoused in this chapter has also been obtained from lesion studies and cognitive research.

In sum, the distinction between anxious apprehension and anxious arousal can resolve many of the inconsistencies that have emerged for the wide range of empirical approaches used in investigations of anxiety. Continued research is likely to provide greater specificity for the psychological and neurophysiological processes and anatomic regions involved in anxiety. To elucidate the mechanisms critical for each type of anxiety, the extensive animal research implicating various subcortical areas in fear and the increasing accuracy in hemodynamic imaging of the subcortex could contribute monumentally to the human work reviewed in this chapter primarily focused on cortical brain function.

REFERENCES

Ahern, G.L., Herring, A.M., Tackenburg, J.N., Schwartz, G.E., Seeger, J.F., Labiner, D.M., Weinand, M.E., & Oommen, K.J. (1994). Affective self-report during the intracarotid sodium amobarbital test. *Journal of Clinical and Experimental Neuropsychology, 16*, 372–376.

American Psychiatric Association (1994). *Diagnostic and Statistical Manual of Mental Disorders* (4th Ed.). Washington, DC: American Psychiatric Association.

Amir, N., McNally, R.J., Riemann, B.C., & Clements, C. (1996a). Implicit memory bias for threat in panic disorder: Application of the "white noise" paradigm. *Behaviour Research and Therapy, 34*, 157–162.

Amir, N., McNally, R.J., & Wiegartz, P.S. (1996b). Implicit memory bias for threat in posttraumatic stress disorder. *Cognitive Therapy and Research, 20,* 625–635.

Amsel, A. (1962). Frustrative nonreward in partial reinforcement and discrimination learning: Some recent history and a theoretical extension. *Psychological Review, 69,* 306–328.

Asbjörnsen, A., Hugdahl, K., & Bryden, M.P. (1992). Manipulations of subjects' level of arousal in dichotic listening. *Brain and Cognition, 19,* 183–194.

Baddeley, A.D. (1986). *Working Memory.* New York: Oxford University Press.

Barlow, D.H. (1991). Disorders of emotion. *Psychological Inquiry, 2,* 58–71.

Baxter, L.R., Phelps, M.E., Mazziotta, J.C., Guze, B.H., Schwartz, J.M., & Selin, C.E. (1987). Local cerebral glucose metabolic rates in obsessive-compulsive disorder. *Archives of General Psychiatry, 44,* 211–218.

Baxter, L.R., Schwartz, J.M., Mazziotta, J.C., Phelps, M.E., Pahl, J.J., Guze, B.H., & Fairbanks, L. (1988). Cerebral glucose metabolic rates in nondepressed patients with obsessive-compulsive disorder. *American Journal of Psychiatry, 145,* 1560–1563.

Bear, D.M. (1986). Hemispheric asymmetries in emotional function: A reflection of lateral specialization in cortical-limbic connections. In B.K. Doane & K.E. Livingston (Eds.), *The Limbic System: Functional Organization and Clinical Disorders* (pp. 29–42). New York: Raven Press.

Becker, E., Rinck, M., & Margraf, J. (1994). Memory bias in panic disorder. *Journal of Abnormal Psychology, 103,* 396–399.

Bench, C.J., Friston, K.J., Brown, R.G., Scott, L.C., Frackowiak, R.S.J., & Dolan, R.J. (1992). The anatomy of melancholia: Focal abnormalities of cerebral blood flow in major depression. *Psychological Medicine, 22,* 607–615.

Borkovec, T.D., Robinson, E., Pruzinsky, T., & DePree, J.A. (1983). Preliminary exploration of worry: Some characteristics and processes. *Behavior Research and Therapy, 21,* 9–16.

Borod, J.C., Andelman, F., Obler, L.K., Tweedy, J.R., & Welkowitz, J. (1992). Right hemisphere specialization for the identification of emotional words and sentences: Evidence from stroke patients. *Neuropsychologia, 30,* 827–844.

Bradley, B.P., Mogg, K., Millar, N., & White, J. (1995). Selective processing of negative information: Effects of clinical anxiety, concurrent depression, and awareness. *Journal of Abnormal Psychology, 104,* 532–536.

Broadbent, D.E., & Broadbent, M. (1988). Anxiety and attentional bias: State and trait. *Cognition and Emotion, 2,* 165–183.

Buchsbaum, M.S., Hazlett, E., Sicotte, N., Stein, M., Wu, J., & Zetin, M. (1985). Topographic EEG changes with benzodiazepine administration in generalized anxiety disorder. *Biological Psychiatry, 20,* 832–842.

Buchsbaum, M.S., Wu, J., Haier, R., Hazlett, E., Ball, R., Katz, M., Sokolski, K., Lagunas-Solar, M., & Langer, D. (1987). Positron emission tomography assessment of effects of benzodiazepines on regional glucose metabolic rate in patients with anxiety disorders. *Life Sciences, 40,* 2393–2400.

Carter, W.R., Johnson, M.C., & Borkovec, T.D. (1986). Worry: An electrocortical analysis. *Advances in Behavioral Research and Therapy, 8,* 193–204.

Cloitre, M., Shear, M.K., Cancienne, J., & Zeitlin, S.B. (1994). Implicit and explicit memory for catastrophic associations to bodily sensation words in panic disorder. *Cognitive Therapy and Research, 18,* 225–240.

Davidson, R.J. (1992). Anterior cerebral asymmetry and the nature of emotion. *Brain and Cognition, 20,* 125–151.

Davidson, R.J. (1998). Affective style and affective disorders: Perspectives from affective neuroscience. *Cognition and Emotion, 12*, 307–330.

Davidson, R.J., Abercrombie, H., Nitschke, J.B., & Putnam, K. (1999). Regional brain function, emotion, and disorders of emotion. *Current Opinion in Neurobiology, 9*, 228–234.

Davidson, R.J., Marshall, J.R., Tomarken, A.J., & Henriques, J.B. (2000). While a phobic waits: Regional brain electrical and autonomic activity in social phobics during anticipation of public speaking. *Biological Psychiatry* (in press).

Davis, M. (1992). The role of the amygdala in fear and anxiety. *Annual Review of Neuroscience, 15*, 353–375.

de Pascalis, V., & Morelli, A. (1990). Anxiety and individual differences in event-related potentials during the recognition of sense and nonsense words. *Personality and Individual Differences, 11*, 741–749.

Dien, J. (1999). Differential lateralization of trait anxiety and trait fearfulness: Evoked potential correlates. *Personality and Individual Differences, 26*, 333–356.

Eysenck, H.J. (1957). *The Dynamics of Anxiety and Hysteria.* New York: Praeger.

Eysenck, H.J. (1991). Neuroticism, anxiety, and depression. *Psychological Inquiry, 2*, 75–76.

Eysenck, M.W. (1992). *Anxiety: The Cognitive Perspective.* Hillsdale, NJ: Erlbaum.

Eysenck, M.W., & Calvo, M.G. (1992). Anxiety and performance: The processing efficiency theory. *Cognition and Emotion, 6*, 409–434.

Eysenck, M.W., Mogg, K., May, J., Richards, A., & Mathews, A. (1991). Bias in interpretation of ambiguous sentences related to threat in anxiety. *Journal of Abnormal Psychology, 100*, 144–150.

Faravelli, C., & Pallanti, S. (1989). Recent life events and panic disorder. *American Journal of Psychiatry, 146*, 622–626.

Fredrikson, M., Gustav, W., Greitz, T., Eriksson, L., Stonee-Elander, S., Ericson, K., & Sedvall, G. (1993). Regional cerebral blood flow during experimental phobic fear. *Psychophysiology, 30*, 126–130.

Gainotti, G. (1972). Emotional behavior and hemisphere side of lesion. *Cortex, 8,* 41–55.

George, M.S., Ketter, T.A., Perekh, P., Gill, D.S., Huggins, T., Marangell, L., Pazzaglia, P.J., & Post, R.M. (1994). Spatial ability in affective illness: Differences in regional brain activation during a spatial matching task. *Neuropsychiatry, Neuropsychology, and Behavioral Neurology, 7*, 143–153.

Goldberg, E., & Costa, L.D. (1981). Hemisphere differences in the acquisition and use of descriptive systems. *Brain and Language, 14*, 144–173.

Gotlib, I.H., Gilboa, E., & Kaplan, B.L. (2000). Cognitive functioning in depression: Nature and origins. In R.J. Davidson (Ed.), *Emotion and Psychopathology: The Wisconsin Symposium on Emotion.* New York: Oxford University Press (in press).

Gray, J.A. (1982). *The Neurophysiology of Anxiety.* New York: Oxford University Press.

Gray, J.A. (1991). Fear, panic, and anxiety: What's in a name? *Psychological Inquiry, 2*, 77–78.

Gruzelier, J., & Phelan, M. (1991). Stress induced reversal of a lexical divided visual-field asymmetry accompanied by retarded electrodermal habituation. *International Journal of Psychophysiology, 11*, 269–276.

Gupta, P., & MacWhinney, B. (1997). Vocabulary acquisition and verbal short-term memory: Computational and neural bases. *Brain and Language, 59*, 267–333.

Heilman, K.M., & Van den Abell, T. (1979). Right hemispheric dominance for mediating cerebral activation. *Neuropsychologia, 17*, 315–321.

Heilman, K.M., Watson, R.T., & Valenstein, E. (1985). Neglect and related disorders. In K.M. Heilman, & E. Valenstein (Eds.), *Clinical Neuropsychology* (pp. 243–293). New York: Oxford University Press.

Heller, W. (1990). The neuropsychology of emotion: Developmental patterns and implications for psychopathology. In N. Stein, B.L. Leventhal, & T. Trabasso (Eds.), *Psychological and Biological Approaches to Emotion* (pp. 167–211). Hillsdale, NJ: Lawrence Erlbaum.

Heller, W. (1993). Neuropsychological mechanisms of individual differences in emotion, personality, and arousal. *Neuropsychology, 7,* 476–489.

Heller, W. (1994). Cognitive and emotional organization of the brain: Influences on the creation and perception of art. In D. Zaidel (Ed.), *Neuropsychology* (pp. 271–292). San Diego, CA: Academic Press.

Heller, W., Etienne, M.A., & Miller, G.A. (1995). Patterns of perceptual asymmetry in depression and anxiety: Implications for neuropsychological models of emotion and psychopathology. *Journal of Abnormal Psychology, 104,* 327–333.

Heller, W., & Levy, J. (1981). Perception and expression of emotion in right-handers and left-handers. *Neuropsychologia, 19,* 263–272.

Heller, W., & Nitschke, J.B. (1997). Regional brain activity in emotion: A framework for understanding cognition in depression. *Cognition and Emotion, 11,* 637–661.

Heller, W., & Nitschke, J.B. (1998). The puzzle of regional brain activity in depression and anxiety: The importance of subtypes and comorbidity. *Cognition and Emotion, 12,* 421–447.

Heller, W., Nitschke, J.B., Etienne, M.A., & Miller, G.A. (1997a). Patterns of regional brain activity differentiate types of anxiety. *Journal of Abnormal Psychology, 106,* 376–385.

Heller, W., Nitschke, J.B., & Lindsay, D.L. (1997b). Neuropsychological correlates of arousal in self-reported emotion. *Cognition and Emotion, 11,* 383–402.

Henriques, J.B., & Davidson, R.J. (1991). Left frontal hypoactivation in depression. *Journal of Abnormal Psychology, 100,* 535–545.

Johanson, A.M., Gustafson, L., Passant, U., Risberg, J., Smith, G., Warkentin, S., & Tucker, D. (1998). Affective arousal and brain function in spider phobia. *Psychiatry Research: Neuroimaging, 84,* 101–110.

Johanson, A.M., Smith, G., Risberg, J., Silfverskiöld, P., & Tucker, D. (1992). Left orbital frontal activation in pathological anxiety. *Anxiety, Stress, and Coping: An International Journal, 5,* 313–328.

Keller, J., Nitschke, J.B., Bhargava, T., Deldin, P.J., Gergen, J.A., Miller, G.A., & Heller, W. (2000). Neuropsychological differentiation of depression and anxiety. *Journal of Abnormal Psychology* (in press).

Klein, D.F. (1981). Anxiety reconceptualized. In D.F. Klein, & J. Rabkin (Eds.), *Anxiety: New Research and Changing Concepts* (pp. 235–265). New York: Raven.

Klein, D.F. (1987). Anxiety reconceptualized. In D.F. Klein (Ed.), *Anxiety* (pp. 1–35). Basel: Karger.

Lang, P.J. (1968). Fear reduction and fear behavior: Problems in treating a construct. In J.M. Schlien (Ed.), *Research in Psychotherapy* (pp. 90–102). Washington, DC: American Psychological Association.

Lang, P.J. (1978). Anxiety: Toward a psychophysiological definition. In H.S. Akiskal & W.L. Webb (Eds.), *Psychiatric Diagnosis: Exploration of Biological Criteria* (pp. 365–389). New York: Spectrum.

Lang, P.J. (1985). The cognitive psychophysiology of emotion: Fear and anxiety. In A.H. Tuma & J.D. Maser (Eds.), *Anxiety and the Anxiety Disorders* (pp. 131–170). Hillsdale, NJ: Erlbaum.

Lazarus, R.S. (1993). From psychological stress to the emotions: A history of changing outlooks. *Annual Review of Psychology, 44,* 1–21.

LeDoux, J.E. (1993). Emotional networks in the brain. In M. Lewis & J.M. Haviland (Eds.), *Handbook of Emotions* (pp. 109–118). New York: Guilford.

LeDoux, J.E. (1995). Emotion: Clues from the brain. *Annual Review of Psychology, 46,* 209–235.

Lee, G.P., Loring, D.W., Meador, K.J., & Brooks, B.B. (1990). Hemispheric specialization for emotional expression: A reexamination of results from intracarotid administration of sodium amobarbital. *Brain and Cognition, 12,* 267–280.

Lehrer, P.M., & Woolfolk, R.L. (1982). Self-report assessment of anxiety: Somatic, cognitive, and behavioral modalities. *Behavioral Assessment, 4,* 167–177.

Levy, J., Heller, W., Banich, M.T., & Burton, L.A. (1983). Asymmetry of perception in free viewing of chimeric faces. *Brain and Cognition, 2,* 404–419.

MacLeod, C. (1990). Mood disorders and cognition. In M.W. Eysenck (Ed.), *Cognitive Psychology: An International Review* (pp. 9–56). Chichester, UK: Wiley.

MacLeod, C., & Hagan, R. (1992). Individual differences in the selective processing of threatening information, and emotional responses to a stressful life event. *Behaviour Research and Therapy, 30,* 151–161.

MacLeod, C., & Mathews, A.M. (1988). Anxiety and the allocation of attention to threat. *Quarterly Journal of Experimental Psychology: Human Experimental Psychology, 38,* 659–670.

MacLeod, C., & McLaughlin, K. (1995). Implicit and explicit memory bias in anxiety: A conceptual replication. *Behaviour Research and Therapy, 33,* 1–14.

MacLeod, C., & Rutherford, E.M. (1992). Anxiety and the selective processing of emotional information: Mediating roles of awareness, trait and state variables, and personal relevance of stimulus materials. *Behaviour Research and Therapy, 30,* 479–491.

Martinot, J.H., Allilaire, J.F., Mazolyer, B.M., Hantouche, E., Huret, J.D., Legaut-Demare, F., Deslauriers, A.G., Hardy, P., Pappata, S., Baron, J.C., & Syrota, A. (1990). Obsessive-compulsive disorder: A clinical neuropsychological and positron emission tomography study. *Acta Psychiatrica Scandinavica, 82,* 233–242.

Mathew, R.J., Wilson, W.H., & Daniel, D.G. (1985). The effect of nonsedative doses of diazepam on regional cerebral blood flow. *Biological Psychiatry, 20,* 1109–1116.

Mathews, A. (1990). Why worry? The cognitive function of anxiety. *Behaviour Research and Therapy, 28,* 455–468.

Mathews, A., & MacLeod, C. (1994). Cognitive approaches to emotion and emotional disorders. *Annual Review of Psychology, 45,* 25–50.

Mathews, A., Mogg, K., May, J., & Eysenck, M. (1989a). Implicit and explicit memory bias in anxiety. *Journal of Abnormal Psychology, 98,* 236–240.

Mathews, A., Richards, A., & Eysenck, M. (1989b). The interpretation of homophones related to threat in anxiety states. *Journal of Abnormal Psychology, 98,* 31–34.

McGlynn, S.M., & Schacter, D.L. (1989). Unawareness of deficits in neuropsychological syndromes. *Journal of Clinical and Experimental Neuropsychology, 11,* 143–205.

McNally, R.J. (1998). Information-processing abnormalities in anxiety disorders: Implications for cognitive neuroscience. *Cognition and Emotion, 12,* 479–495.

Merckelbach, H., Muris, P., Pool, K., & de John, P.J. (2000). Resting EEG asymmetry and spider phobia. *Anxiety, Stress, and Coping: An International Journal* (in press).

Mesulam, M.M. (1981). A cortical network for directed attention and unilateral neglect. *Annals of Neurology, 10,* 309–325.

Meyer, T.J., Miller, M.L., Metzger, R.L., & Borkovec, T.D. (1990). Development and validation of the Penn State Worry Questionnaire. *Behaviour Research and Therapy*, *28*, 487–495.

Miller, G.A., & Kozak, M.J. (1993). A philosophy for the study of emotion: Three-systems theory. In N. Birbaumer & A. Ohman (Eds.), *The Structure of Emotion: Physiological, Cognitive, and Clinical Aspects* (pp. 31–47). Seattle, WA: Hogrefe & Huber.

Mineka, S. (1985). Animal models of anxiety-based disorders: Their usefulness and limitations. In A.H. Tuma & J.D. Maser (Eds.), *Anxiety and the Anxiety Disorders* (pp. 199–244). Hillsdale, NJ: Erlbaum.

Mogg, K., Bradley, B.P., Williams, R., & Mathews, A. (1993). Subliminal processing of emotional information in anxiety and depression. *Journal of Abnormal Psychology*, *102*, 304–311.

Mogg, K., Mathews, A., & Weinman, J. (1987). Memory bias in clinical anxiety. *Journal of Abnormal Psychology*, *96*, 94–98.

Molina, S., & Borkovec, T.D. (1994). The Penn State Worry Questionnaire: Psychometric properties and associated characteristics. In G.C.L. Davey, & F. Tallis (Eds.), *Worrying: Perspectives on Theory, Assessment and Treatment* (pp. 265–283). Chichester, U.K.: John Wiley & Sons, Ltd.

Nitschke, J.B. (1998). *Differentiating Types of Anxiety, Depression, and Their Co-occurrence: Regional Brain Activity and Life Stress.* Unpublished doctoral dissertation, University of Illinois, Urbana-Champaign.

Nitschke, J.B., Heller, W., Imig, J.C., McDonald, R.P., & Miller, G.A. (2000). Distinguishing dimensions of anxiety and depression. *Cognitive Therapy and Research* (in press).

Nitschke, J.B., Heller, W., Palmieri, P.A., & Miller, G.A. (1999). Contrasting patterns of brain activity in anxious apprehension and anxious arousal. *Psychophysiology*, *36*, 628–637.

Nugent, K., & Mineka, S. (1994). The effect of high and low trait anxiety on implicit and explicit memory tasks. *Cognition and Emotion*, *8*, 147–163.

Pardo, J.V., Fox, P.T., & Raichle, M.E. (1991). Localization of a human system for sustained attention by positron emission tomography. *Nature*, *349*, 61–64.

Pollard, C.A., Pollard, H.J., & Corn, K.J. (1989). Panic onset and major events in the lives of agoraphobics: A test of contiguity. *Journal of Abnormal Psychology*, *98*, 318–321.

Post, R.M., DeLisi, L.E., Holcomb, H.H., Uhde, T.W., Cohen, R., & Buchsbaum, M. (1987). Glucose utilization in the temporal cortex of affectively ill patients: Positron emission tomography. *Biological Psychiatry*, *22*, 545–553.

Rapee, R.M., Litwin, E.M., & Barlow, D.H. (1990). Impact of life events on subjects with panic disorder and on comparison subjects. *American Journal of Psychiatry*, *147*, 640–644.

Rapee, R.M., McCallum, S.L., Melville, L.F., Ravenscroft, J., & Rodney, J.M. (1994). Memory bias in social phobia. *Behaviour Research and Therapy*, *32*, 89–99.

Reiman, E.M., Raichle, M.E., Butler, F.K., Herscovitch, P., & Robins, E. (1984). A focal brain abnormality in panic disorder, a severe form of anxiety. *Nature*, *310*, 683–685.

Reiman, E.M., Raichle, M.E., Robins, E., Mintum, M.A., Fusselman, M.J., Fox, P.T., Price, J.L., & Hackman, K.A. (1989). Neuroanatomical correlates of a lactate-induced anxiety attack. *Archives of General Psychiatry*, *46*, 493–500.

Reivich, M., Gur, R., & Alavi, A. (1983). Positron emission tomographic studies of sensory stimuli, cognitive process, and anxiety. *Human Neurobiology*, *2*, 25–33.

Roy-Byrne, P.P., Geraci, M., & Uhde, T.W. (1986). Life events and the onset of panic disorder. *American Journal of Psychiatry*, *143*, 1424–1427.

Schwartz, G.E., Davidson, R.J., & Goleman, D.J. (1978). Patterning of cognitive and so-
    matic processes in the self-regulation of anxiety: Effects of meditation versus exer-
    cise. *Psychosomatic Medicine, 40,* 321–328.

Spielberger, C.D. (1968). *Self-Evaluation Questionnaire. STAI Form X-2.* Palo Alto, CA:
    Consulting Psychologists Press.

Spielberger, C.D. (with Gorsuch, R.L., Lushene, R., Vagg, P.R., & Jacobs, G.A.). (1983).
    Manual for the State-Trait Anxiety Inventory (Form Y). Palo Alto, CA: Consulting
    Psychologists Press.

Starkstein, S.E., & Robinson, R.G. (1988). Lateralized emotional response following
    stroke. In M. Kinsbourne (Ed.), *Cerebral Hemisphere Function in Depression* (pp.
    23–47). Washington, DC: American Psychiatric Press.

Stewart, R.S., Devous, M.D., Rush, A.J., Lane, L., & Bonte, F.J. (1988). Cerebral blood
    flow changes during sodium-lactate-induced panic attacks. *American Journal of Psy-
    chiatry, 145,* 442–449.

Swedo, S.E., Schapiro, M.B., Grady, C.L., Cheslow, D.L., Leonard, H.L., Kumar, A.,
    Friedland, R., Rapoport, S.I., & Rapoport, J.L. (1989). Cerebral glucose metabolism
    in childhood-onset obsessive-compulsive disorder. *Archives of General Psychiatry,
    46,* 518–523.

Tucker, D.M., Antes, J.R., Stenslie, C.E., & Barnhardt T.M. (1978). Anxiety and lateral
    cerebral function. *Journal of Abnormal Psychology, 87,* 380–383.

Tucker, D.M., Roth, R.S., Arneson, B.A., & Buckingham, V. (1977). Right hemisphere
    activation during stress. *Neuropsychologia, 15,* 697–700.

Tyler, S.K., & Tucker, D.M. (1982). Anxiety and perceptual structure: Individual differ-
    ences in neuropsychological function. *Journal of Abnormal Psychology, 91,* 210–220.

Van Strien, J.W., & Heijt, R. (1995). Altered visual field asymmetries for letter naming
    and letter matching as a result of concurrent presentation of threatening and non-
    threatening words. *Brain and Cognition, 29,* 187–203.

Van Strien, J.W., & Morpurgo, M. (1992). Opposite hemispheric activations as a result
    of emotionally threatening and non-threatening words. *Neuropsychologia, 30,* 845–
    848.

Vrana, S.R., Roodman, A., & Beckham, J.C. (1995). Selective processing of trauma-rel-
    evant words in posttraumatic stress disorder. *Journal of Anxiety Disorders, 6,* 515–530.

Watson, D., Weber, K., Assenheimer, J.S., Clark, L.A., Strauss, M.E., & McCormick,
    R.A. (1995). Testing a tripartite model: I. Evaluating the convergent and discriminant
    validity of anxiety and depression symptom scales. *Journal of Abnormal Psychology,
    104,* 3–14.

Watts, F.N., & Coyle, K. (1993). Phobics show poor recall of anxiety words. *British Jour-
    nal of Medical Psychology, 66,* 373–382.

Williams, J.M.G., Watts, F.N., MacLeod, C., & Mathews, A. (1988). *Cognitive Psychol-
    ogy and Emotional Disorders.* Chichester, U.K.: Wiley.

Wittling, W. (1995). Brain asymmetry in the control of autonomic-physiologic activity.
    In R.J. Davidson, & K. Hugdahl (Ed.), *Brain Asymmetry* (pp. 305–357). Cambridge,
    MA: The MIT Press.

Wu, J.C., Buchsbaum, M.S., Hershey, T.G., Hazlett, E., Sicotte, N., & Johnson, J.C.
    (1991). PET in generalized anxiety disorder. *Biological Psychiatry, 29,* 1181–1199.

13

Violence Associated with Anger and Impulsivity

ANGELA SCARPA AND ADRIAN RAINE

According to the *Uniform Crime Report*, violent crime in the United States rose by 81% in the two decades between 1973 and 1992, and the largest increase was in aggravated assault (Stanton, Baldwin, & Rachuba, 1997). In view of the pervasiveness of violence and the tragic consequences it has on individuals and society, it is important to understand the factors that initiate and maintain the propensity to behave violently. In this context, anger and impulsivity become pivotal issues in the study of violence.

Paralleling the typologies of defensive and predatory aggression in the animal literature, human aggression has been primarily grouped into impulsive-emotional or controlled-instrumental subtypes (Vitiello & Stoff, 1997). *Impulsive-emotional violence* occurs suddenly, without forethought, and in response to some perceived threat, provocation, or insult, within the context of associated anger, high emotionality, and high impulsivity (Berkowitz, 1993). It may incorporate acts such as child physical abuse, assault, and murder/manslaughter, as well as less serious forms of physical and/or verbal aggression (e.g., biting, kicking, screaming). *Controlled-instrumental violence* involves a relatively nonemotional display of aggression directed at obtaining some goal, usually within the context of premeditation and manipulation. It may incorporate acts such as planned robberies, arsons, and serial murders, among others. These two forms of aggression have also been referred to in the literature as *reactive versus proactive* (Dodge & Coie, 1987) and *affective/defensive versus predatory* (Moyer, 1976).

The validity of these two types of aggressive behavior has been initially supported by several studies that show distinct differences among children and adolescents whose aggressive/violent behavior was classified as primarily impulsive-emotional or controlled-instrumental. According to these studies, youth with impulsive-emotional aggression (termed either *affective* or *reactive* aggression) tended to have an earlier age of onset of behavior problems, more stressful life events, a greater likelihood of comorbid psychiatric disorder or concurrent adjustment difficulties, and deficits in early stages of social information processing (Dodge & Coie, 1987; Dodge et al., 1997; Vitiello et al., 1990).

Along with these social, emotional, and cognitive differences, it is plausible that neurobiological variables also differentiate the two aggressive types. Impulsive-emotional aggression, in particular, may have biological correlates tied to its strong association with anger, impulsivity, or emotional disorders. Animal studies also have indicated distinct biological profiles between defensive and predatory aggression, as reviewed by Eichelman (1995), Reis (1974), and Vitiello and Stoff (1997). For example, defensive forms of animal aggression have been associated with intense autonomic activation, stimulation of the ventromedial hypothalamus, decreased serotonergic activity, and increased noradrenergic and dopaminergic activity. Predatory forms, on the other hand, have been associated with little autonomic activation, lesions of the frontomedial hypothalamus, lesions of the orbital prefrontal cortex, and increased cholinergic activity.

Few studies of biological bases of antisocial behavior in humans have categorized aggression or violence according to these subtypes. The purpose of this chapter is to review biological findings on crime and violence and then determine what can be concluded about the underpinnings of impulsive-emotional aggression based on these findings. The focus on biological findings does not preclude the clearly important role of social/environmental and psychological contributors to violence, but rather highlights one growing body of literature that may aid in a more complete understanding of emotionally violent behavior. This includes findings in neuropsychology (i.e., testing, brain lesions, and brain imaging studies) and related areas of neurochemistry, hormones, and psychophysiology.

FRAMEWORK

Previously, we have suggested that emotional aggression is related to "1) a predisposition to experience negative affect and arousal, 2) the inability to regulate or soothe negative affect or arousal, and 3) thought processes that will increase the likelihood of experiencing anger or making a decision to aggress" (Scarpa & Raine, 1997, p. 385). We further argued that biologic contributions could influence any of these risk factors and that the effect would be most pronounced when individuals were faced with stressful environments where emotional arousal and negative affect would be peaked. With these criteria, biological findings can be evaluated regarding their relationship to impulsive-emotional aggression.

The general theoretical framework of this chapter, then, is that a pattern of neurobiological influences is associated with each of the risk factors for impulsive-emotional aggression named above. Regarding the first two risks, negative affect (including depression, anxiety, and hostility), physiological arousal, and the inability to regulate affect and arousal have been ascribed to greater right cerebral activation, particularly in the frontotemporal regions (Cechetto & Saper, 1990; Demaree & Harrison, 1997; see also, Nitschke, Heller, & Miller, Chapter 12, this volume). Regarding the third risk, frontotemporal limbic dysfunction is related to impaired executive cognitive functioning, which encompasses abilities such as attention, planning, organization, abstract reasoning, self-monitoring, and the ability to use feedback to modulate behavior (Foster, Eskes, & Stuss, 1994; Wallace, Bachorowski, & Newman, 1991). This has been speculated to lead to cognitive biases that increase the chances of behaving aggressively in response to stressful and provocative situations (Giancola, 1995).

NEUROPSYCHOLOGY

Three areas of the brain have been most consistently described as related to the manifestation or inhibition of aggression: (*1*) the brain stem and hypothalamus, (*2*) the limbic system (including temporal cortex), and (*3*) the frontal cortex. Each of these three areas are interrelated in that components of the limbic system project to the hypothalamus, and the frontal cortex functions in modulating limbic and hypothalamic output. In general, neuropsychological findings about violence from studies using standardized tests, brain lesions in animals and humans, and brain imaging implicate frontal and temporal dysfunction.

Neuropsychological Tests

Anterior/frontal dysfunction in violent adult criminals has been implicated in neuropsychological studies with the Halstead-Reitan Neuropsychological Test Battery (Flor-Henry, 1973; Yeudall & Fromm-Auch, 1979) and the Luria-Nebraska Neuropsychological Battery (Bryant et al., 1984). Further support comes from a prospective study of 10–12-year-old boys with and without a paternal history of substance abuse. A composite score from five neuropsychological tests was used to measure impaired executive cognitive ability thought to reflect mild prefrontal dysfunction. Impaired executive cognitive functioning predicted reactive aggression 2 years later in the boys at high risk for substance abuse (Giancola et al., 1996). Reactive aggression was defined as an impulsive hostile reaction to frustration that is committed without forethought, closely resembling the impulsive-emotional form of aggression.

Others have suggested that brain dysfunction in criminals involves disruption to both frontal and temporal corticolimbic (i.e., hippocampal/amygdala) systems, localized to the left hemisphere (Flor-Henry, 1973; Yeudall & Fromm-Auch, 1979). Left hemisphere deficits in aggressive individuals are consistent with studies showing increased negative affect and arousal associated with relative activation of the right hemisphere (Nitschke, Heller, & Miller, Chapter 12, this volume).

Brain Lesion Studies

Multisite brain dysfunction, with particular focus on limbic system sites involving temporal and frontal projections, is also supported by lesion studies in animals and humans. Lesion studies in animals involve the ablation of localized brain sites and implicate the amygdala and prefrontal cortex in violence (Giancola, 1995; Siegel & Mirsky, 1990). Lesion studies in humans are generally less localized, as they involve brain trauma resulting from head injury, surgery, or epileptic seizures. Aggression is decreased, however, in patients with amygdalectomy (O'Callaghan & Carroll, 1982). Also, patients with known frontal lobe damage have shown a pattern of personality changes including impulsivity, argumentativeness, lack of concern for consequences of behavior, loss of social graces, distractibility, shallowness, lability, violence, and reduced ability to utilize symbols (termed *frontal lobe syndrome*) (Silver & Yudofsky, 1987).

The relationship between temporal lobe dysfunction and violence also has been studied in individuals with temporal lobe epilepsy (see Heilman et al., Chapter 15, this volume). Historically, it was believed that violent episodes may occur during (*ictal*), immediately after (*postictal*), or between (*interictal*) seizures, either as a direct result of brain stimulation or consequent to the confusion and disorganization following seizures. In a recent review of these studies, Volavka (1995) concluded that (*1*) seizure-related violence in epileptics is extremely rare; (*2*) although prisoners have a higher rate of seizure disorders relative to the general population, those without seizure disorders are equally as violent as those with seizure disorders; and (*3*) these studies have identified the same risk factors for violence that have been found in nonepileptic populations (i.e., young age, male gender, low IQ, low socioeconomic status, and adverse rearing environment). As such, effects of temporal lobe dysfunction secondary to seizure activity seem trivial, but these studies do not address whether nonseizure temporal lobe dysfunction increases violence.

Brain Imaging Studies

Recent reviews of brain imaging findings on violence support the neuropsychological findings of frontal and temporal deficits (Henry & Moffitt, 1997; Raine, 1993). Most of the structural studies with magnetic resonance imaging (MRI) and computerized tomography (CT) have implicated damage to the temporal lobe, whereas functional studies with single photon emission computerized tomography (SPECT) and positron emission tomography (PET) have found both temporal and frontal deficits.

Five of six recent analyses of antisocial/violent offendors not contained in the above reviews have also observed reduced frontal or temporal functioning in violent psychiatric patients (frontal and temporal deficits; Volkow et al., 1995), alcoholics with antisocial personality disorder (frontal deficits; Kuruoglu et al., 1996), violent offenders supsected of organic brain disease (temporal deficits; Seidenwurm et al., 1997), and murderers pleading not guilty by reason of insanity (frontal and temporal deficits; Raine, Buchsbaum, & La Casse, 1997; Raine et al., 1998a). Interestingly, one additional study showed *increased* functioning of the frontotemporal regions in drug-abusing psychopaths (Intrator et al., 1997). It is likely that discrepant findings may be a function of the different subject groups, types of violence, and experimental methods used in the various studies (Volkow et al., 1995).

The brain imaging studies by Raine et al. (1997, 1998a) are of special interest because they overcome some of the earlier methodological flaws in design. Frontal lobe glucose metabolism was assessed with PET in 41 murderers pleading not guilty by reason of insanity compared with 41 controls matched by age, sex, and presence/absence of schizophrenia. All participants with a history of seizure disorder, head trauma, or substance abuse were excluded. Murderers in this study failed to show the prefrontal activation observable in controls during a continuous performance task that is specifically designed to elicit such activation.

In addition to prefrontal deficits, significantly reduced glucose metabolism was also observed in the corpus callosum, superior parietal gyrus, and left angular gyrus, and left hemisphere deficits were found in the amygdala, thalamus, and medial temporal lobe. It was speculated by Raine, Buchsbaum, and La Casse (1997) that reduced functioning of the corpus callosum might result in a relative inability of the left hemisphere to control and regulate the more "emotional" right hemisphere.

In a recent reanalysis of the above data (Raine et al., 1998a), murderers were divided into those whose murders were planned, instrumental, and predatory in nature and those whose attacks were relatively impulsive, unplanned, and characterized by a high degree of emotional reactivity preceded by arguments. Results indicated that it was specifically the emotionally reactive murderers who were characterized by significant prefrontal dysfunction, whereas predatory murderers had levels of prefrontal glucose metabolism similar to controls. Raine (1993) speculated that, because the prefrontal cortex is involved in planning, regulating, and controlling behavior, those who plan their murders must have a reasonably functional prefrontal cortex. Conversely, those whose murders are impulsive and lacking in behavioral control are most likely to be lacking the regulatory influence of a functional prefrontal cortex.

Summary of Neuropsychological Findings

As is typical of most biological studies of violence, few studies examined separate effects for the form of violent behavior. There is some evidence to suggest, however, that frontal dysfunction is predominantly related to impulsive-emotional forms of aggression. First, a study with neuropsychological tests suggested that mild prefrontal dysfunction was predictive of reactive aggression in children (Giancola et al., 1996). Second, studies examining damage to the frontal cortex in noncriminal samples have shown a pattern of emotional and impulsive changes that has come to be called *frontal lobe syndrome* (Silver & Yudofsky, 1987). Third, the brain imaging findings suggest reduced prefrontal activation specifically in murderers whose crime was impulsive rather than instrumental (Raine et al., 1998a). Fourth, the frontal cortex has projections to the temporal lobe, limbic system, and hypothalamus, all of which are involved in the regulation and expression of emotion (Weiger & Bear, 1988).

Finally, if risk for impulsive-emotional aggression is highest when dysregulation of negative affect and arousal is peaked by environmental provocation, as suggested by Scarpa and Raine (1997), then aggression should increase when prefrontal dysfunction is combined with an adverse environment. In contrast to this suggestion, Raine et al. (1998b) found greater reductions in prefrontal functioning in murderers from benign home backgrounds relative to those from deprived backgrounds or to noncriminal controls. In a sample of juvenile delinquents, however, the highest rates of violence were found for those having a combination of neuropsychological impairment *and* a history of physical abuse or family violence (Lewis et al., 1989). This combination of emotional lability, impulsivity, and stressful experiences in violent individuals with frontal (or possibly frontotemporal limbic) dysfunction is consistent with impulsive-emotional aggression. The results of Raine et al. (1998b) need to be replicated, but they do suggest the intriguing possibility that frontal dysfunction itself can lead to disinhibited violent behavior in the absence of a "social push" for that behavior.

NEUROCHEMISTRY

A meta-analysis of 29 studies published before 1992, which examined neurotransmitter substances in antisocial children and adults, indicated overall effects for decreased metabolites of serotonin and norepinephrine in cerebrospinal fluid (CSF), and no effect for dopamine in antisocial individuals (Scerbo & Raine, 1993). These results were particularly moderated by the presence of alcohol abuse or affective instability. Indications of reduced CSF serotonin were found in all antisocial groups but were even more marked in suicide attempters and nonalcoholics. Indications of reduced CSF norepinephrine, however, were only found in antisocial samples who also had diagnoses of alcohol abuse, borderline personality disorder, depression, or dysthymia.

The relationship found between CSF noradrenergic activity and affective instability in violent samples is consistent with findings indicating increased likelihood of psychiatric disorder and emotion regulatory problems in individuals with impulsive-emotional aggression (Dodge et al., 1997; Vitiello et al., 1990). These findings suggest that reductions in serotonergic activity may underlie a general propensity to aggress, whereas the addition of a central norepinephrine disturbance may be related to impulsive-emotional aggression.

The idea that central norepinephrine mediates the affective instability associated with impulsive-emotional aggression is also consistent with frontotemporal limbic dysfunction. The primary source of central norepinephrine (i.e., the locus ceruleus) has projections to the hypothalamus through the median forebrain bundle. The hypothalamus, in turn, is densely interconnected with the limbic system and has both frontal and temporal cortical connections. These interconnections may comprise the neural substrate by which norepinephrine affects emotion and emotional expressivity. Together with a serotonergic-mediated propensity to aggress, such dysregulation of negative affect might increase the likelihood of impulsive-emotional aggression.

HORMONES

Although the release of hormones is also governed by the hypothalamus, the motivational and behavioral effects of different hormones seem to vary. The varying effects may serve to fine tune brain–behavior responses to emotions and to the environment. Studies on hormonal relationships to violence have generally examined testosterone, cortisol, and hypoglycemia. Testosterone production is regulated through the hypothalamic-pituitary-gonadal axis, cortisol production through the hypothalamic-pituitary-adrenal (HPA) axis, and hypoglycemia through the direct hypothalamic innervation of the sympathetic nervous system.

Testosterone

Overall, studies of testosterone and aggression have shown a positive association. Studies correlating testosterone with questionnaire measures of aggression in the general population have generally produced weak or nonsignificant findings, whereas studies of violent incarcerated inmates have more consistently produced results of moderate to large strength (for review, see Archer, 1991). Findings of increased testosterone in aggressive clinically referred children and young adults have been less consistent (Constantino et al., 1993; Dabbs, Jurkovic, & Frady, 1991; Scerbo & Kolko, 1994).

Most of these studies did not differentiate types of aggression or violence. Olweus et al. (1988), however, reported increased testosterone in male adolescents who self-reported high levels of both provoked (reactive) and unprovoked (proactive) aggressive behavior. One of the few studies of females also reported elevated testosterone levels in prisoners whose current offense was an *unprovoked* violent crime but not in those whose crime was defensive (i.e., violence in reaction to physical assault) (Dabbs et al., 1988). Others have found testosterone to be positively related to social dominance and status in prisoners (Ehrenkranz, Bliss, & Sheard, 1974) and competitive success (Mazur & Lamb, 1980). Altogether, these results suggest that the relationship of testosterone to violence may be primarily related to goal achievement found in controlled-instrumental aggression rather than to reactivity found in impulsive-emotional aggression.

Cortisol

Cortisol is a stress hormone released through HPA activation. Cortisol levels have been reported to be reduced in habitually violent offenders (Virkkunen, 1985), in aggressive schoolchildren (Tennes & Kreye, 1985), and in children and adolescents with conduct problems (Lahey & McBurnett, 1992; Susman, Dorn, & Chrousos, 1991), suggestive of possible low HPA activation or anxiety in these individuals. These results have not been consistently found, however, and cortisol effects may be moderated by other variables such as alcohol, comorbid anxiety, or environmental experiences. Buydens and Branchey (1992), for example, found that *increased* levels of cortisol characterized violent alcoholics. McBurnett et al. (1991) found *elevated* cortisol levels in conduct disordered children with comorbid anxiety disorder. Also, Scarpa (1997) reported that *increased* cortisol reactivity during a stressor interacted with physical abuse history to heighten the risk of aggression in clinically referred children with disruptive behavior disorders. Finally, in a study examining testosterone and cortisol in a group of disruptive children, resting levels of both hormones were positively associated with antisocial behavior problems, but cortisol was also positively related to internalizing (i.e., emotional) behavior problems and impulsivity (A. Scarpa & D.J. Kolko, unpublished data, 1996). These latter studies indicating a relationship between heightened cortisol level/reactivity in antisocial individuals with alcoholism, comorbid emotional problems, and impulsivity are consistent with impulsive-emotional aggression.

Hypoglycemia

Hypoglycemia is a blood sugar deficiency caused by an overproduction of insulin secreted by the pancreas. Hypoglycemia (or low blood sugar levels) may elicit irritability, aggression, confusion, amnesia, seizures, and eventually unconsciousness. A number of studies have linked hypoglycemia to violent and aggressive behavior, particularly in individuals with a history of alcohol abuse (Virkkunen, 1986; Virkkunen et al., 1989). These findings are qualified by the fact that, to date, there is no clear evidence indicating that violent offenders are hypoglycemic at the time of their violent offense (Kanarek, 1990).

Interestingly, hypoglycemia can occur as an indirect effect of cortisol overproduction. HPA-stimulated increases in cortisol lead to a rise in blood sugar, and, as part of a negative feedback loop, pancreatic glucogen is inhibited. Glucogen normally suppresses insulin, and so its reduction leads to insulin overproduction and a consequent drop in blood sugar level. In view of the relationship between hypoglycemia and negative affect and possibly with HPA arousal, hypoglycemia-related violence seems most closely linked to the impulsive-emotional form.

PSYCHOPHYSIOLOGY

The most commonly used psychophysiological measures recorded from antisocial populations have been skin conductance (SC), heart rate (HR), and cortical measures of electroencephalogram (EEG) and event-related potentials (ERP). Autonomic nervous system (ANS) activity produces SC through sympathetic mediation and HR through both sympathetic and parasympathetic mediation. Many of the ANS neurons exist in the brain and spinal cord and require input from the cortex, brain stem, hypothalamus, and spinal cord. In addition to brain stem influences, there is evidence to suggest that the frontal and temporal lobes are involved in the regulation of SC and HR (Heilman, Bowers, & Valenstein, 1993; Hugdahl et al., 1983; Nitschke, Heller, & Miller, Chapter 12, this volume; Raine, Reynolds, & Sheard, 1991). Reviews of psychophysiological studies and impulsive-emotional aggression have been recently published (Scarpa & Raine, 1997). These reviews are summarized here.

Skin Conductance

Reviews of SC studies indicate that (*1*) there is some evidence for SC underarousal in antisocial individuals, particularly with respect to nonviolent forms of crime; (*2*) SC-orienting deficits seem specific to antisocial individuals with concomitant schizotypal or schizoid features; (*3*) the findings up to 1978 of reduced SC responsivity to aversive stimuli in psychopaths generally have not been observed in more recent studies in either psychopathic or nonpsychopathic antisocial populations; and (*4*) the strongest findings support reduced SC classical conditioning and longer SC half-recovery times in antisocial populations. Reduced classical conditioning has been interpreted as reflecting a poorer ability to form conditioned emotional responses to potentially punitive situations, resulting in poor conscience development and antisocial behavior (Eysenck, 1977). Slower recovery rates imply slower dissipation of autonomic activation, possibly indicating slower recovery from an emotional fear state (Mednick, 1977).

In general, these results have been found in populations with primarily nonviolent forms of crime or in samples in which type of antisocial behavior was not distinguished (e.g., psychopathic populations). Only one of the reviewed SC arousal studies compared types of crime and found that underarousal characterized crimes of evasion (e.g., customs offenses) but not other forms of crime (Buikhuisen et al., 1985). Interestingly, the one SC responsivity study that specifically identified individuals characterized by affective violence showed *larger* SC responses to verbal stimuli in the violent group (Lakosina & Trunova, 1985). Finally, although not distinguished by type of antisocial behavior, several SC conditioning studies found poorer classical conditioning in only those antisocial individuals from high social class backgrounds (Raine & Venables, 1981) or good homes (Hemming, 1981). Thus, the overall SC findings of underarousal, response deficits, and poor conditioning do not seem to characterize impulsive-emotional aggression but rather relate to nonviolent forms of antisocial behavior.

Heart Rate

In terms of HR, studies of institutionalized adult offenders show no differences in resting HR. In contrast, all studies conducted to date on younger and predominantly noninstitutionalized or nonclinical populations show reduced resting HR levels in antisocial people (for review, see Raine, 1993). Reduced HR may reflect autonomic underarousal (Raine, Venables, & Williams, 1990a) or, alternatively, fearlessness to novel situations (Kagan, 1989; Venables, 1987).

Of two studies that examined violent behavior, both found the lowest resting HR levels in persons exhibiting violent behavior (Farrington, 1987; Wadsworth, 1976), but they did not specify types of violence. Only one known study distinguished form of aggression (Pitts, 1993). In that study, lower resting HR levels were exhibited in both proactive (i.e., controlled) and reactive (i.e., impulsive) aggressive schoolboys relative to nonaggressive controls. Interestingly, only the reactive subtype showed an increase in HR after a simulated provocation. These results are also consistent with a series of laboratory aggression studies by Zillmann and colleagues, which indicated that autonomic arousal facilitates aggressive behavior, particularly when participants were previously provoked and when the provocation was perceived as intentional or deliberate (for review, see Zillmann, 1983). With the exception of Farrington (1987) and Wadsworth (1976), these studies indicate HR underarousal in young, noninstitutionalized populations displaying mild levels of aggression or antisocial behavior and suggest that HR reactivity characterizes impulsive-emotional forms of aggression.

Electroencephalogram

Cortical EEG studies indicate that abnormalities exist in resting EEG in criminal populations, particularly violent recidivistic offending (Mednick et al., 1982), with the predominant deficit being excessive slow wave activity, particularly in the frontal cortex. Two out of three studies that examined premeditated versus impulsive/motiveless violent crime found diffusely abnormal EEG in the criminals whose offense was apparently without instrumental motive (Driver, West, & Faulk, 1974; Hill & Pond, 1952; Okasha, Sadek, Moneim, 1975). These abnormalities are thought to reflect either general underarousal (Raine, Venables, & Williams, 1990a) or cortical immaturity (Hare, 1970). In a review of EEG studies, however, Volavka (1995) suggested that the possibility of brain injury or cortical disinhibition, in addition to the hypotheses of underarousal and cortical immaturity, could not be ruled out. These studies indicate that abnormal EEG findings in antisocial populations may be related to impulsive-emotional forms of violence.

Event-Related Potentials

Cortical ERP studies generally indicate increased latencies in the early and middle components of ERP (i.e., brain stem auditory evoked potentials and N100) and enhanced late-component P300 amplitudes to stimuli of interest in antisocial samples. Raine (1993) has suggested that these processes may be conceptually and causally linked such that the early components relate to excessive filtering of stimuli and resulting underarousal that lead to sensation-seeking (related to the N100 findings), which may partly account for enhanced attention (i.e., increased P300) to events of interest. These ERP studies have primarily involved psychopathic populations.

Studies of violent individuals, however, have generally found *smaller* P300 amplitudes than nonviolent controls (Barratt et al., 1997; Branchey, Buydens-Branchey, & Lieber, 1988; Braverman, 1993; Gerstle, Mathias, & Stanford, 1988). Two of these studies included subjects who specifically displayed impulsive aggression (Barratt et al., 1997; Gerstle, Mathias, & Stanford, 1988). A recent study has replicated these results comparing three groups characterized by a history of impulsive aggression, aggression secondary to paranoid schizophrenia, or premeditated aggression (Stanford et al., 1998). Results from this study indicated reduced P300 amplitude in both the impulsive and schizophrenia-related aggression groups relative to the premeditated aggression group.

Prospective Psychophysiological Research

Findings of electrodermal (e.g., SC), cardiovascular (e.g., HR), and cortical (e.g., EEG and ERP) underarousal as a predisposition for the development of criminal behavior have been supported in prospective longitudinal studies (Loeb & Mednick, 1977; Mednick et al., 1982; Petersen et al., 1982; Raine, Venables, & Williams, 1990a). In addition, Raine, Venables, and Williams (1990b,c) found a reduced number of SC and HR orienting responses and larger N100 ERPs in 15-year-old criminals to be. The most common form of criminal offenses included burglary and theft, which suggests that these findings may be particularly relevant to the development of serious, but less violent, forms of crime.

Summary of Psychophysiological Findings

In sum, studies of SC, HR, and EEG, including prospective studies, implicate underarousal in the development of antisocial behavior. These studies, however, have consisted of individuals primarily committing nonviolent forms of crime or having less serious aggression. Autonomic reactivity of SC and HR, on the other hand, seems to characterize impulsive-emotional forms of aggression (Scarpa & Raine, 1997), especially when the aggressor is exposed to a provocation and perceives the provocation as intentional (Pitts, 1993; Zillmann, 1983). As such, consistent with the idea of impulsive-emotional aggression, these findings suggest that psychophysiological reactivity is related to aggression in the context of increased negative affect and thought processes that would increase the likelihood of negative affect.

Studies of ERP implicate reduced P300 amplitudes in impulsive-emotional aggressors. It has been suggested that such reduced amplitude is the result of problems with higher order cognitive processing and attention (Barratt et al., 1997) or more general low arousal (Gerstle, Mathias, & Stanford, 1998). Because underarousal in other systems seems related to nonviolent or mild aggressive behavior, deficits in cognitive processing may be the more likely explanation of reduced P300 in impulsively violent individuals. This would be consistent with executive cognitive dysfunction and affect dysregulation associated with frontotemporal deficits.

SUMMARY

Previous work has indicated the existence of several types of aggressive behavior in animals that primarily fall into two categories: defensive and predatory aggression. In humans, it has been suggested that two parallel forms of aggression or violence exist (i.e., impulsive-emotional and controlled-instrumental) with distinct biopsychosocial pathways (Vitiello & Stoff, 1997). The work of Dodge et al. (1997) indicates specific cognitive biases, emotional regulatory difficulties, and stressful life events in children with impulsive-emotional forms of aggression. Based on previous findings on the biological bases of antisocial behavior, this chapter was designed as an initial attempt to delineate neurobiological variables that may contribute to impulsive-emotional forms of violence. Few such studies specifically distinguish types of violence. Taken together, however, the research reviewed on neuropsychological, neurochemical, hormonal, and psychophysiological relationships to antisocial behavior suggest that there indeed may be specific biological underpinnings to impulsive-emotional aggression. The relationships are currently speculative, but point to the importance of distinguishing forms of violence in future research. An overall summary of these findings is presented in Table 13.1.

Neuropsychological testing, brain lesion, brain imaging, EEG, and ERP studies implicate multisite brain dysfunction, particularly affecting frontotemporal limbic sites, in relationship to violence. These findings must be qualified by the fact that many violent offenders have no substantial brain damage, lesions, or dysfunction, but this does not rule out the possibility of subtle neuropsychological effects on decision-making and impulse control. Giancola (1995), for example, suggests that frontal cortex impairments in executive cognitive functions involving planning, abstract reasoning, attention, and behavior regulation in response to environmental feedback may increase the risk for aggression by leading to (*1*) misattributions of threat and hostility in conflict sutuations, (*2*) inability to generate socially acceptable solutions in response to anger situations, (*3*) inability to execute actions that will avoid an argument or aggressive interaction, or (*4*) poor behavioral control over hostile cognitions and negative affect.

Table 13.1. Summary of Findings Relating Neuropsychology, Neurochemistry, Hormones, and Psychophysiology to Impulsive-Emotional Aggression in Humans

---

Neuropsychology
  Decreased frontotemporal functioning, possibly disrupting limbic functioning
    and activating the amygdala
  May be particularly localized to left hemisphere deficits and relative activation of the
    right temporal lobe
Neurochemistry
  Decreased central serotonin in combination with
  Decreased central norepinephrine
  No relationship with central dopamine
Hormones
  No relationship with testosterone
  Increased cortisol levels and reactivity
  Decreased blood sugar levels (i.e., hypoglycemia)
Psychophysiology
  EEG abnormalities, particularly increased alpha activity in frontal lobes
  Reduced P300 amplitude
  Increased heart rate reactivity
  Possibly larger skin conductance responses

Newman and colleagues (see Wallace, Bachorowski, & Newman, 1991) have suggested that frontal cortex impairments of executive functioning leads to the impulsivity found in many individuals with disinhibitory psychopathology (including antisocial people) by activating their responsivity in the face of competing reward and punishment. Thus, if frontal dysfunction (or multisite limbic dysfunction) exists in an aggressive individual, it seems most likely to relate to impulsive-emotional forms of aggression.

This conclusion is further supported by findings in related physiological systems, which include a combination of decreased serotonergic activity and noradrenergic dysregulation, cortisol reactivity indicative of HPA axis dysregulation, hypoglycemia, and autonomic HR reactivity. These biological systems seem to increase the propensity for negative affect and arousal, impair the ability to regulate that affect/arousal, and lead to biased thought processes, thus increasing risk for impulsive-emotional aggression (Scarpa & Raine, 1997).

CONCLUSION

Neurobiological effects on aggression are by no means simple or straightforward, and they reflect the complexity of the manifestation of violent behavior. First, as evidence of this complexity, the biological findings reviewed here are not an exhaustive list. Other biological factors that may contribute to crime and violence, but are not covered here, include those influenced by other types of brain injury or dysfunction, genetics, pregnancy and birth complications, physical appearance, diet, and exposure to toxins such as lead (for review, see Raine, 1993). Second, none of these factors has been found to individually and accurately predict violent behavior. Rather, they are to be viewed as risk factors that singly, or in combination, increase the likelihood that someone may react defensively and impulsively with aggression. Third, most of these studies were conducted with exclusively male samples. The generalization of such findings to female violence is thus extremely limited. Fourth, social and psychological factors have also been found to predispose to crime and violence, and such contributions need to be integrated into biological research to form a more comprehensive understanding of the manifestation of emotional aggression.

This last point is particularly relevant to individuals displaying impulsive-emotional aggression given their increased likelihood of stressful life events and physical abuse (Dodge et al., 1997). There are several examples of such complex interactions in biological research of antisociality. For example, the finding of lower resting HR in antisocial samples is particularly strong in those from higher social classes (Raine & Venables, 1984) and in intact families (Wadsworth, 1976). To explain such findings, it has been suggested that in relatively benign environments where the "social push" for antisocial behavior is lower, biological determinants of such behavior assume greater importance (Raine & Venables, 1981). Others have found that the risk for violent offending, on the other hand, is heightened when *both* biological and social risk factors are present. Mednick and Kandel (1988), for example, found the greatest degree of violence in individuals who had both minor physical anomalies (thought to reflect a disruption to fetal neural development in the first trimester of pregnancy) and came from unstable nonintact home environments. In a group of children with disruptive behavior disorders, Scarpa (1997) and Scerbo and Kolko (1995) found the greatest degree of aggression in those who had a history of physical abuse coupled with physiological or emotional dysregulation. Taken together, these latter studies demonstrate the sensitivity of individuals to adverse social environments, especially if they have predispositions that can influence their emotionality and emotion regulatory abilities.

Finally, the distinction between factors that are biological versus psychological or environmental is necessarily artificial. That is, any factor may directly or indirectly affect another. Some biological correlates of violence, for example, may be environmentally caused (e.g., brain damage resulting from blows to the head). Furthermore, the biological correlates reviewed herein are likely to have psychological effects (e.g., brain damage may impair intellectual and other cognitive functioning). This highlights again the complexity of human antisocial behavior and the mistake of conducting such research under the assumption of a false environmental versus biological dichotomy.

In conclusion, evidence is provided that suggests that impulsive-emotional forms of aggression (accompanied by anger and impulsivity) may indeed be partly mediated through neurobiological mechanisms. Because much of the violence occurring today involves interpersonal situations within familiar social circles, such as domestic violence and abuse, the examination of such reactive emotional aggression becomes crucial. As a more complete understanding is gained of the complex interplay of biological, cognitive, social, and emotional forces involved in such violence, we are afforded optimism that it can be minimized in the future.

REFERENCES

Archer, J. (1991). The influence of testosterone on human aggression. *British Journal of Psychology, 82*, 1–28.

Barratt, E.S., Stanford, M.S., Kent, T.A., & Felthous, A.R. (1997). Neuropsychological and cognitive psychophysiological substrates of impulsive aggression. *Biological Psychiatry, 41*, 1045–1061.

Berkowitz, L. (1993). *Aggression: Its Causes, Consequences, and Control.* New York: McGraw-Hill.

Branchey, M.H., Buydens-Branchey, L., & Lieber, C.S. (1988). P3 in alcoholics with disordered regulation of aggression. *Psychiatry Research, 25*, 49–58.

Braverman, E.R. (1993). Brain electrical activity mapping (BEAM) in patients who commit violent crimes: Are bitemporal abnormalities a characteristic? *Journal of Orthomolecular Medicine*, *8*, 154–156.

Bryant, E.T., Scott, M.L., Golden, C.J., & Tori, C.D. (1984). Neuropsychological deficits, learning disability, and violent behavior. *Journal of Consulting and Clinical Psychology*, *53*, 323–324.

Buikhuisen, W., Bontekoe, E.H.M., Plas-Korenhoff, C.D., & Buuren, S. (1985). Characteristics of criminals: The privileged offender. *International Journal of Law and Psychiatry*, *7*, 301–313.

Buydens, B.L., & Branchey, M.H. (1992). Cortisol in alcoholics with a disordered aggression control. *Psychoneuroendocrinology*, *17*, 45–54.

Cechetto, D., & Saper, C. (1990). In A. Loewy & K. Spyer (Eds.), *Central Regulation of Autonomic Functions* (pp. 208–223). New York: Oxford University Press.

Constantino, J.N., Grosz, D., Saenger, P., Chandler, D.W., Nandi, R., & Earls, F.J. (1993). Testosterone and aggression in children. *Journal of the American Academy of Child and Adolescent Psychiatry*, *32*, 1217–1222.

Dabbs, J.M., Jurkovic, G.J., & Frady, R.L. (1991). Salivary testosterone and cortisol among late adolescent male offenders. *Journal of Abnormal Child Psychology*, *19*, 469–478.

Dabbs, J.M., Ruback, R.B., Frady, R.L., et al. (1988). Saliva testosterone and criminal violence among women. *Personality and Individual Differences*, *9*, 269–275.

Demaree, H.A., & Harrison, D.W. (1997). Physiological and neuropsychological correlates of hostility. *Neuropsychology*, *35*, 1405–1411.

Dodge, K.A., & Coie, J.D. (1987). Social-information-processing factors in reactive and proactive aggression in children's peer groups. *Journal of Personality and Social Psychology*, *53*, 1146–1158.

Dodge, K.A., Lochman, J.E., Harnish, J.D., Bates, J.E., & Pettit, G.S. (1997). Reactive and proactive aggression in school children and psychiatrically impaired chronically assaultive youth. *Journal of Abnormal Psychology*, *106*, 37–51.

Driver, M.V., West, L.R., & Faulk, M. (1974). Clinical and EEG studies of prisoners charged with murder. *British Journal of Psychiatry*, *125*, 583–587.

Ehrenkranz, J., Bliss, E., & Sheard, M.H. (1974). Plasma testosterone: Correlation with aggressive behavior and social dominance in man. *Psychosomatic Medicine*, *36*, 469–475.

Eichelman, B. (1995). Animal and evolutionary models of impulsive aggression. In E. Hollander & D.J. Stein (Eds.), *Impulsivity and Aggression* (pp. 59–90). Chichester, U.K.: Wiley.

Eysenck, H.J. (1977). *Crime and Personality*, 3rd ed. St. Albans, England: Paladin.

Farrington, D.P. (1987). Implications of biological findings for criminological research (pp. 42–64). In S.A. Mednick, T.E. Moffitt, & S.A. Stack (Eds.), *The Causes of Crime: New Biological Approaches*. New York: Cambridge University Press.

Flor-Henry, P. (1973). Psychiatric syndromes considered a manifestation of lateralized-temporal-limbic dysfunction. In L. Laitiner & K. Livingston (Eds.), *Surgical Approaches in Psychiatry*. Lancaster, England: Medical and Technical Publishing.

Foster, J., Eskes, G., & Stuss, D. (1994). The cognitive psychology of attention: A frontal lobe perspective. *Cognitive Neuropsychology*, *11*, 133–147.

Gerstle, J.E., Mathias, C.W., & Stanford, M.S. (1998). Auditory P300 and self-reported impulsive aggression. *Progress in Neuropsychopharmacology and Biological Psychiatry*, *22*, 575–583.

Giancola, P.R. (1995). Evidence for dorsolateral and orbitofrontal prefrontal cortical involvement in the expression of aggressive behavior. *Aggressive Behavior*, *21*, 431–450.

Giancola, P.R., Moss, H.B., Martin, C.S., Krisci, L., & Tarter, R.E. (1996). Executive cognitive functioning predicts reactive aggression in boys at high risk for substance abuse: A prospective study. *Alcoholism: Clinical and Experimental Research, 20,* 740–744.

Hare, R.D. (1970). *Psychopathy: Theory and Practice.* New York: Wiley.

Heilman, K.M., Bowers, D., & Valenstein, E. (1993). In K.M. Heilman and E. Valenstein (Eds.), *Clinical Neuropsychology* (pp. 461–498). New York: Oxford University Press.

Hemming, J.H. (1981). Electrodermal indices in a selected prison sample and students. *Personality and Individual Differences, 2,* 37–46.

Henry, B., & Moffitt, T.E. (1997). Neuropsychological and neuroimaging studies of juvenile delinquency and adult criminal behavior. In D.M. Stoff, J. Breiling, & J.D. Maser (Eds)., *Handbook of Antisocial Behavior* (pp. 280–288). New York: Wiley.

Hill, D., & Pond, D.A. (1952). Reflections on one hundred capital cases submitted to electroencephalography. *Journal of Mental Science, 98,* 23–43.

Hugdahl, K., Franzen, M., Andersson, B., & Walldebo, G. (1983). Hear rate responses (HRR) to lateralized visual stimuli. *Pavlovian Journal of Biological Science, 18,* 186–198.

Intrator, J., Hare, R., Stritzke, P., Brichtswein, K., Dorfman, D., Harpur, T., Bernstein, D., Handelsman, L., Schaefer, C., Keilp, J., Rosen, J., & Machac, J. (1997). A brain imaging (single photon emission computerized tomography) study of semantic and affective processing in psychopaths. *Biological Psychiatry, 42,* 96–103.

Kagan, J. (1989). Temperamental contributions to social behavior. *American Psychologist, 44,* 668–674.

Kanarek, R.B. (1990). *Nutrition and Violent Behavior.* Report for the National Academy of Sciences Panel on the Understanding and Control of Violent Behavior.

Kuruoglu, A.C., Arikan, Z., Karatas, M., Arac, M., & Isik, E. (1996). Single photon emission computerized tomography in chronic alcoholism: Antisocial Personality Disorder may be associated with decreased frontal perfusion. *British Journal of Psychiatry, 169,* 348–354.

Lahey, B.B., & McBurnett, K. (1992). *Behavioral and Biological Correlates of Aggressive Conduct Disorder: Temporal Stability.* Paper presented to the annual meeting of the Society for Research in Child and Adolescent Psychopathology, Sarasota, FL.

Lakosina, N.D., & Trunova, M.M. (1985). The characteristics of emotional disorders on psychopathic personalities. *Soviet Neurology and Psychiatry, 18,* 35–45.

Lewis, D.O., Lovely, R., Yaeger, C., et al. (1989). Toward a theory of the genesis of violence: A follow-up study of delinquents. *Journal of the American Academy of Child and Adolescent Psychiatry, 28,* 431–436.

Loeb, J., & Mednick, S.A. (1977). A prospective study of predictors of criminality (pp. 245–254). In S.A. Mednick & K.O. Christiansen (Eds.), *Biosocial Bases of Criminal Behavior.* New York: Gardner Press.

Mazur, A., & Lamb, T.A. (1980). Testosterone, status, and mood in human males. *Hormones and Behavior, 14,* 236–246.

McBurnett, K., Lahey, B.B., Frick, P.J., et al. (1991). Anxiety, inhibition, and conduct disorder in children: II. Relation to salivary cortisol. *Journal of the American Academy of Child and Adolescent Psychiatry, 30,* 192–196.

Mednick, S.A. (1977). A bio-social theory of the learning of law-abiding behavior. In S.A. Mednick & K.O. Christiansen (Eds.), *Biosocial Bases of Criminal Behavior.* New York: Gardner Press.

Mednick, S.A., Volavka, J., Gabrielli, W.F., & Itil, T. (1982). EEG as a predictor of antisocial behavior. *Criminology, 19,* 219–231.

Moyer, K. (1976). *The Psychobiology of Aggression*. New York: Harper & Row.

O'Callaghan, M.A.J., & Carroll, D. (1982). *Psychosurgery: A Scientific Analysis*. Lancaster, England: Medical and Technical Publishing.

Okasha, A., Sadek, A.O., & Moneim, S.A. (1975). Psychosocial and electroencephalographic studies of Egyptian murderers. *British Journal of Psychiatry, 126*, 34–40.

Olweus, D., Mattson, A., Schalling, D., et al. (1988). Circulating testosterone levels and aggression in adolescent males: A causal analysis. *Psychosomatic Medicine, 50*, 261–272.

Petersen, I., Matousek, M., Mednick, S.A., Volavka, J., & Pollock, V. (1982). EEG antecedents of thievery. *Criminology, 19*, 219–229.

Pitts, T. (1993). *Cognitive and Psychophysiological Differences in Proactive and Reactive Aggressive Boys*. Doctoral dissertation, Department of Psychology, University of Southern California.

Raine, A. (1993). *The Psychopathology of Crime: Criminal Behavior as a Clinical Disorder*. San Diego: Academic Press.

Raine, A., Buchsbaum, M.S., & La Casse, L. (1997). Brain abnormalities in murderers indicated by positron emission tomography. *Biological Psychiatry, 42*, 495–508.

Raine, A., Meloy, J.R., Bihrle, S., Stoddard, J., LaCasse, L., & Buchsbaum, M.S. (1998a). Reduced prefrontal and increased subcortical brain functioning assessed using positron emission tomography in predatory and affective murderers. *Behavioral Sciences and the Law, 16*, 319–332.

Raine, A., Reynolds, G.P., & Sheard, C. (1991). Neuroanatomical mediators of electrodermal activity in normal human subjects: A magnetic resonance imaging study. *Psychophysiology, 28,* 548–558.

Raine, A., Stoddard, J., Bihrle, S., & Buchsbaum, M. (1998b). Prefrontal glucose deficits in muderers lacking psychosocial deprivation. *Neuropsychiatry, Neuropsychology, and Behavioral Neurology, 11*, 1–7.

Raine, A., & Venables, P.H. (1981). Classical conditioning and socialization—A biosocial interaction? *Personality and Individual Differences, 2*, 273–283.

Raine, A., & Venables, P.H. (1984). Tonic heart rate level, social class, and antisocial behavior. *Biological Psychology, 18*, 123–132.

Raine, A., & Venables, P.H. (1992). Antisocial behavior: Evolution, genetics, neuropsychology, and psychophysiology. In A. Gale & M. Eysenck (Eds.), *Handbook of Individual Differences: Biological Perspectives*. London: Wiley.

Raine, A., Venables, P.H., & Williams, M. (1990a). Relationships between CNS and ANS measures of arousal at age 15 and criminality at age 24. *Archives of General Psychiatry, 47*, 1003–1007.

Raine, A., Venables, P.H., & Williams, M. (1990b). Orienting and criminality: A prospective study. *American Journal of Psychiatry, 147*, 933–937.

Raine, A., Venables, P.H., & Williams, M. (1990c). Relationships between N1, P300, and CNV recorded at age 15 and criminal behavior at age 24. *Psychophysiology, 27*, 567–575.

Reis, D.J. (1974). Central neurotransmitters in aggression. In S.H. Frazier (Ed.), *Aggression*, Vol. 52 (pp. 119–148). Baltimore: Williams & Wilkins.

Scarpa, A. (1997). Aggression in physically abused children: The interactive role of emotion regulation. In A. Raine et al. (Eds.), *Biosocial Bases of Violence* (pp. 341–344). New York: Plenum Publishing.

Scarpa, A., & Raine, A. (1997). Psychophysiology of anger and violent behavior. *The Psychiatric Clinics of North America* [Special issue on anger, aggression, and violence], *20,* 375–394.

Scerbo, A.S., & Kolko, D.J. (1994). Salivary testosterone and cortisol in disruptive children: Relationship to aggressive, hyperactive, and internalizing behaviors. *Journal of the American Academy of Child and Adolescent Psychiatry, 33*, 1174–1184.

Scerbo, A.S., & Kolko, D.J. (1995). Child physical abuse and aggression: Preliminary findings on the role of internalizing problems. *Journal of the American Academy of Child and Adolescent Psychiatry, 8*, 1060–1066.

Scerbo, A.S., & Raine, A. (1993). Neurotransmitters and antisocial behavior: A meta-analysis. Cited in A. Raine (Ed.), *The Psychopathology of Crime: Criminal Behavior as a Clinical Disorder* (pp. 86–92). San Diego: Academic Press.

Seidenwurm, D., Pounds, T.R., Globus, A., & Valk, P.E. (1997). Temporal lobe metabolism in violent subjects: Correlation of imaging and neuropsychiatric findings. *American Journal of Neuroradiology, 18*, 625–631.

Siegel, A., & Mirsky, A.F. (1990). *The Neurobiology of Violence and Aggression*. National Academy of Sciences Conference on the Understanding and Control of Violent Behavior, San Destin, FL.

Silver, J.M., & Yudofsky, S.C. (1987). Aggressive behavior in patients with neuropsychiatric disorders. *Psychiatric Annals, 17*, 367–370.

Stanford, M.S., Greve, K.W., Mathias, C.W., & Houston, R.J. (1998). *Murderers not Guilty by Reason of Insanity and Impulsive Aggressive Psychiatric Outpatients: An EEG/ERP Comparison*. Paper presented at the meeting of the Scoiety for Psychophysiological Research. Denver, CO.

Stanton, B., Baldwin, R.M., & Rachuba, L. (1997). A quarter century of violence in the United States: An epidemiologic assessment. *The Psychiatric Clinics of North America* [Special issue on anger, aggression, and violence], *20*, 269–282.

Susman, E.J., Dorn, L.D., & Chrousos, G.P. (1991). Negative affect and hormone levels in young adolescents: Concurrent and predictive perspectives. *Journal of Youth and Adolescence, 20*, 167–190.

Tennes, K., & Kreye, M. (1985). Children's adrenocortical response to classroom activities in elementary school. *Psychosomatic Medicine, 47*, 451–460.

Venables, P.H. (1987). Autonomic and central nervous system factors in criminal behavior. In S.A. Mednick, T.E. Moffitt, & S.A. Stack (Eds.), *The Causes of Crime: New Biological Approaches* (pp. 110–136). Cambridge: Cambridge University Press.

Virkkunen, M. (1985). Urinary free cortisol secretion in habitually violent offenders. *Acta Psychiatrica Scandinavica, 72*, 40–44.

Virkkunen, M. (1986). Reactive hypoglycemia tendency among habitually violent offenders. *Nutrition Reviews, 44*, 94–103.

Virkkunen, M., De Jong, J., Bartko, J., et al. (1989). Relationship of psychobiological variables to recidivism in violent offenders and impulsive fire setters. *Archives of General Psychiatry, 46*, 600–603.

Vitiello, B., Behar, D., Hunt, J., Stoff, D., & Ricciuti, A. (1990). Subtyping aggression in children and adolescents. *Journal of Neuropsychiatry and Clinical Neuroscience, 2*, 189–192.

Vitiello, B., & Stoff, D.M. (1997). Subtypes of aggression and their relevance to child psychiatry. *Journal of the American Academy of Child and Adolescent Psychiatry, 36*, 307–315.

Volavka, J. (1995). *Neurobiology of Violence*. Washington, D.C.: American Psychiatric Press.

Volkow, N.D., Tancredi, L.R., Grant, C., Gillespie, H., Valentine, A., Mullani, N., Wang, G.J., & Hollister, L. (1995). Brain glucose metabolism in violent psychiatric patients: A preliminary study. *Psychiatry Research Neuroimaging, 61*, 243–253.

Wadsworth, M.E.J. (1976). Delinquency, pulse rate, and early emotional deprivation. *British Journal of Criminology, 16,* 245–256.

Wallace, J.F., Bachorowski, J., & Newman, J.P. (1991). Failures of response modulation: Impulsive behavior in anxious and impulsive individuals. *Journal of Research in Personality and Individual Differences, 25,* 23–44.

Weiger, W.A., & Bear, D.M. (1988). An approach to the neurology of aggression. *Journal of Psychiatric Research, 22,* 85–98.

Yeudall, L.T., & Fromm-Auch, D. (1979). Neuropsychological impairments in various psychopathological populations. In J. Gruzelier & P. Flor-Henry (Eds.), *Hemisphere Asymmetries of Function and Psychopathology* (pp. 5–13). New York: Elsevier/North Holland.

Zillmann, D. (1983). Arousal and aggression. In R.G. Geen & E.I. Donnerstein (Eds.), *Aggression: Theoretical and Empirical Reviews,* Vol. 1 (pp. 75–101). New York: Academic Press.

14

Differentiation of States and Causes of Apathy

DONALD T. STUSS, ROBERT VAN REEKUM,
AND KELLY J. MURPHY

Apathy is best characterized in behavioral terms as an absence of responsiveness to stimuli as demonstrated by a lack of self-initiated action. The main thesis of this chapter is that there are different kinds of apathy. Each is separable on the basis of both the anatomical regions and the psychological mechanisms involved. The chapter is organized into four main sections written with the aim of establishing support for this thesis. In the first section, definitions of apathy are reviewed, and we introduce our approach to defining apathy states. The second section describes common causes of apathy and outlines the neuroanatomical regions involved. In the third section, we present our proposed conceptualization of the different kinds of apathy. The fourth section contains a review of what is known about treatment interventions for apathy.

THE DEFINITIONS OF APATHY

We use *apathy* as our general label. The word apathy consists of the prefix *a*, meaning without, and *pathos*, the Greek word for *passion*. Apathy is therefore most commonly defined as a lack of interest or emotion. In this sense, synonyms such as *indifference* and *flat affect* are commonly used in the neurological and neuropsychiatric literature. However, *pathos* can also indicate suffering. Dictionary synonyms and adjectival phrases provided for apathy include *destitute of feeling, insensible, indifferent, impassive, lethargic, stoic,* and *unconcerned.* Although there is a clear communal theme among these phrases and words, there is also a range of connotations and thus the potential for a lack of precision in the clinical definition of apathy.

One reason concepts of apathy lack precision is the fact that apathy is often secondary to different neurological and psychiatric disorders and as such is often considered to incorporate some of the features of the related disorder or syndrome into its definition. For example, Fisher (1983) described the disorder abulia as impaired spontaneity in action and speech against a background of normal intellectual content, reduced range of movement, mental slowness, decreased attention in the presence of increased distractibility, and apathy. Clearly, abulia and apathy overlap or are coexistent in Fisher's conceptualization. Marin (1990, p. 22), in an admirable attempt to refine and limit the range of the term apathy, suggested the following definition: "diminished motivation not attributable to diminished level of consciousness, cognitive impairment, or emotional distress," excluding not only states such as depression, demoralization, delirium, and dementia but also abulia, akinesia, and akinetic mutism. Hence, Marin's view of apathy appears to differ from that of Fisher. Marin views apathy and abulia as being mutually exclusive, whereas Fisher (1983) views apathy as being a characteristic of abulia. Distinct definitions of strongly related states are clearly very difficult to achieve.

Marin (1991, 1996) differentiated between apathy as a symptom of other problems (such as depression or altered level of consciousness) and apathy as a syndrome. In the description of apathy as a syndrome by Marin, Biedrzycki, and Firinciogullari (1991), the key feature remains a lack of motivation (amotivational state). In his more recent reformulation, Marin (1996) adopted a diagnostic-based approach to propose criteria for the diagnosis of apathy. The inclusion criterion is the presence of amotivation in any of the realms of affect, behavior, and cognition, and exclusion criteria include the presence of disordered arousal, depression, or causative cognitive impairment.

Recently, Berrios and Gili (1995) proposed a more philosophical conceptualization of disorders involving pathology of action, stating that such disorders were best described as an "absence of will." Although it is not clear whether all manifestations of apathy reflect a disturbance of will, there is a sense of the importance of the concept of an absence of self-initiated behavior in the definition of apathy.

We argue for a formulation of apathy that differs in several ways from the concepts of apathy reviewed above. Apathy cannot be clinically defined as simply a lack of motivation. First, there are difficulties inherent in the assessment of motivation. To be amotivated is to be lacking in the inner urge that moves or prompts one to action. The assessment of inner urges is problematic and usually necessitates inference based on observations of affect or behavior. Second, when one considers all of the pathological and clinical states that may produce apathy (see below and Marin, 1990, 1991, 1996; Marin, Biedrzycki, & Firinciogullari, 1991), almost all of these "states" contain features in addition to the narrow "lack of motivation" definition. Employing syndromal criteria, like that suggested by Marin, is also potentially limiting. Recent accumulation of knowledge in neuroanatomy and neuropsychology provides support for the specification of different kinds of apathy. Consider, for example, frontal lobe injury, a major cause of apathy. There is now empirical data demonstrating the specificity of attention and memory functions within the frontal lobes (Shallice & Burgess, 1991; Stuss et al., 1994a,b; Stuss, Picton, & Alexander, 1999). Stuss and Benson (1986) have indeed distinguished between two kinds of apathetic behavior: disorders of drive primarily related to the medial frontal regions and disorders of arousal primarily related to lower neural axes such as the brain stem reticular formation, specific brain stem nuclei, and the thalamus. It is thus likely that behavioral disorders fitting under the umbrella of apathy might also demonstrate greater anatomical and functional specificity in the frontal lobes of the brain and related brain structures.

Our definition of apathy, "an absence of responsiveness to stimuli as demonstrated by a lack of self-initiated action," allows for objective behavioral measurements. We contend that apathy is not a singly definable state, nor is it a single syndrome. Apathy can be divided into separable types or states that differ in both the functional disturbances underlying the clinical presentation and the neural substrates of involvement. Using an adjectival phrase with the term *apathy* provides us with the necessary increases in scope and specificity of definition. Furthermore, the use of adjectival modifiers promotes greater consistency across studies in terms of identifying the type of apathetic behavior being investigated and how this behavior is measured.

CAUSES OF APATHY

An overview of the reported causes of apathetic behavior (Table 14.1) is essential for clinical purposes and for providing the background context against which our proposed conceptualization of apathy is introduced. To provide a background for our neurological dissociations, the examples presented below selectively review three major central nervous system (CNS) causes of apathy: localized brain dysfunction, dementias, and psychiatric disorders. Other causes of apathy, which are not easily related to CNS disturbances, are noted in Table 14.1 but not discussed.

Localized Brain Dysfunction

The most commonly described focal neurologic cause of apathetic behavior is damage to the frontal lobes. Early clinical case studies frequently reported a

Table 14.1. Common Causes of Apathy States*

Localized brain dysfunction
    Dorsolateral prefrontal cortical damage
    Medial frontal (cingulate gyrus/supplementary motor area) damage
    Frontal systems damage involving subcortical connections to basal ganglia and
        thalamus
    Dopaminergic hypoactivity affecting mesolimbic areas
    Brain stem lesions affecting catecholamine function (ventral tegmental nucleus of the
        thalamus)
    Limbic drive dysfunction (bilateral lesions of the amygdala and anterior temporal
        poles, as in human Klüver-Bucy syndrome)
Dementia
    Frontal/subcortical dementias
    Later stages of all progressive dementias
Psychiatric disorders
    Major depressive episodes
    Schizophrenia (the negative symptoms)
    Grief and adjustment disorders
Other causes
    Lack of environmental incentive or reward (institutionalization, role loss,
        dissatisfaction)
    Loss of primary sensory function (deafness, blindness)
    Metabolic disturbances
    Sleep disorders
    Chronic pain

---

*Based on both Marin (1996) and our clinical experience.

diminution in initiated behavior (for reviews, see Stuss & Benson, 1986; Stuss et al., 1992). This apathy was observed behaviorally but was also demonstrated on neuropsychological tests such as verbal fluency (Belyi, 1979; Masdeu & Shewmon, 1980). In fact, a key observation that led to the use of frontal lobotomies for psychiatric disturbances was that frontal lobe lesions in monkeys made the animals more placid (Jacobsen, 1936; Moniz, 1937). Both left dorsolateral and superior medial frontal regions demonstrate the most decreased verbal fluency (Stuss et al., 1998).

    Another commonly reported acquired neurological cause of apathetic behavior is damage to the basal ganglia, particularly if the damage is bilateral. A review of 240 patients with lesions in the caudate nucleus, putamen, or globus pallidus revealed that apathy was the most common behavioral disorder after basal ganglia stroke, occurring in approximately 13% of cases (Bhatia & Marsden, 1994). The apathetic behavior was most common after caudate lesions (26%), and was never found in the 20 patients with putamen lesions. The behavioral consequence of basal ganglia damage was called *psychic akinesia*, a disturbance of psychic autoactivation (Ali-Cherif et al., 1984; Habib & Poncet, 1988; Laplane et al., 1984; Percheron et al., 1994) linked to an impaired dopaminergic mesolimbic system (Poncet & Habib, 1994). There is a dramatic decrease in spontaneous behavior of any kind, including thought, and verbal fluency (Alexander, Naeser, & Palumbo, 1987). The observed behavioral aspontaneity contrasts with the relatively normal reaction to external stimuli and commands. In other words, such individuals respond appropriately to external stimulation from the people and general environment around them, but they do not demonstrate self-initiated behavior.

Another common focal neurologic cause of apathy is damage to the dorsomedial thalamic nucleus. This is also most striking and persistent with bilateral lesions (Bogousslavsky et al., 1988; Guberman & Stuss, 1983; McGilchrist et al., 1993). Patients with dorsomedial thalamic damage often exhibit apathetic behaviors consistent with those described above.

The extreme form of apathetic behavior is akinetic mutism wherein the patient exhibits normal sleep–wake cycles but rarely, if at all, initiates behavior in any modality (Plum & Posner, 1980). The proposed causes are variable. Some researchers have suggested that akinetic mutism is related to disruption in the ascending input from the reticular activating system, perhaps due to medial forebrain bundle lesions (e.g., Cairns et al., 1941; Ross & Stewart, 1981). Still others have proposed that the etiology for akinetic mutism is a loss of limbic drive and activation secondary to bilateral anterior cingulate lesions, which is believed to play a role in limbic motivation (e.g., Devinsky, Morrell, & Vogt, 1995; Laplane et al., 1984; Mega & Cummings, 1994). Akinetic mutism has also been reported secondary to bilateral globus pallidus/internal capsule lesions. This is particularly true for lesions with ventral extension because these may disconnect the anterior cingulate from involvement in limbic motivational activity (Mega & Cohenour, 1997).

In most of the focal neurologic etiologies of apathy noted above and in Table 14.1, there is a direct or indirect anatomical involvement of the frontal lobes and/or limbic drive. Each of the nonfrontal areas mentioned above has extensive reciprocal connections with the frontal lobes and are component parts of frontal systems (Fuster, 1989; Pandya & Barnes, 1987; Stuss & Benson, 1986). Moreover, similar apathetic behaviors have been shown after pathology in deep frontal white matter (Poncet & Habib, 1994). Descriptions of apathetic behavior after capsular genu infarct note behavioral sequelae that are consistent with the interruption of the inferior and anterior thalamic peduncles, resulting in functional deactivation of the ipsilateral frontal cortex (Tatemichi et al., 1992; Yasuda et al., 1990). Bilateral lesions of the amygdala and anterior temporal poles, as in human Klüver-Bucy syndrome, often results in apathy that is likely due to limbic drive damage (Marin, 1996). Evidence from neuroimaging research also demonstrates a link between the frontal lobes and apathy even in the absence of focal frontal brain damage. For example, McGilchrist et al. (1993), using single photon emission computed tomography (SPECT) to measure regional cerebral blood flow, found hypometabolism in the frontal brain regions of a patient presenting with apathetic behavior following bilateral dorsomedial thalamic lesions. It appears that frontal lobe involvement, involvement of structures supportive of frontal system function, and/or dysfunction in limbic motivational regions are a necessary requirement for apathy secondary to most focal neurologic disorders.

Dementia

Patients with frontotemporal lobar dysfunction (frontal lobe dementia) often exhibit apathy as an important symptom (Snowden, Neany, & Mann, 1996). Similar to patients with acquired basal ganglia lesions, individuals who have progressive disorders involving the basal ganglia, such as Parkinson's disease and Huntington's disease, have impaired initiation of behavior (Mayberg, 1994). Such patients often reveal varying degrees of apathy, bradyphrenia (slowness in thinking), and psychomotor slowing. Huntington's and Parkinson's disease patients may also be depressed, however, and the influence of depression on behavior must be dissociated from the influence of apathy. A large percentage of patients with Alzheimer's disease have also been reported to have apathy and diminished initiative (Bozzola, Gorelick, & Freels, 1992; Reichman et al., 1996). Such lack of interest of some Alzheimer's disease patients in self-care and other personal activities may exist in some patients independent of depression or other symptoms (Reichman et al., 1996). In a SPECT study of 40 Alzheimer patients, the degree of apathy was correlated with decreased right temporoparietal perfusion (Ott, Noto, & Fogel, 1996). For aging individuals, there is some suggestion that the degree of apathy is related to the severity of the cognitive disorder (Forsell et al., 1993). These findings suggest that apathy secondary to Alzheimer's disease may be qualitatively different from apathy due to some focal lesions in which intellectual functioning as measured by IQ tests may be intact (even though specific cognitive disorders may be revealed).

Psychiatric Disorders

Apathy related to psychiatric diagnoses has primarily been recognized in patients with depression and schizophrenia. In depression, the emphasis has been on differentiation of apathy and depression in various neurological populations (Starkstein et al., 1992). Starkstein and colleagues (1992) studied depression and apathy in idiopathic Parkinson's disease patients. Approximately 12% showed apathy as their primary psychiatric problem, while 30% were both apathetic and depressed. Apathy was related more to slowness of speed on Trail Making Test Part B than to accuracy of performance, and depression was associated with increased errors but not significant slowness of response time, suggesting that apathy and depression were dissociable. Such a dissociation between apathy and depression has also been reported in other patient groups. Marin et al. (1993) found that apathy in the absence of depression was seen most frequently in patients with Alzheimer's disease and right hemisphere stroke, and less frequently in patients with left hemisphere stroke or in normal subjects. In the subjects with major depression, apathy scores were positively associated with depression scores, although apathy was occasionally absent in some of these subjects. Forsell et al. (1993) studied elderly depressed subjects with and without dementia and found that the mood symptoms of this population clustered into two groups: mood disturbance and motivational disturbance. Mood symptoms were most frequent in those subjects with mild dementia, and motivational disturbances were most frequent in those with more advanced disease. Thus, although apathy may be seen in depression, it is also dissociable from depression.

Research on schizophrenia has had a significant impact on the understanding of apathy since the distinction between positive and negative symptoms was first made (Andreasen, 1982; Crow, 1985). The negative symptoms clearly include the concept of apathy. Frith (1987) argued that negative symptoms reflect a subjective internal failure of willed intention, in other words, a deficit in initiation. Crow (1995) argued that the negative symptoms could reflect a failure in brain development. This hypothesis would be compatible with the correlation between negative symptoms with cognitive impairment and the presence of personality change in these patients before the actual onset of the diagnosed illness. Strauss (1993), following Frith and Done (1989), suggested that positive and negative symptoms could be related to two separate anatomical systems: positive symptoms to dysfunction in the interaction of frontal/septohippocampal systems and negative symptoms to abnormalities in frontostriatal interconnections.

In summary, our selective review of causes of apathetic behavior leads to two conclusions. First, the term *apathy* has been used quite differently by different authors, and there appears to be a range of behavioral and affective changes that are inadequately described under single definitional or syndromal descriptions of apathy. For example, disorders of "willed" intention are very different from the difficulty in initiation found in patients with degrees of akinetic mutism. It is difficult to ascribe this entire range of apathetic behaviors simply to a lack of motivation. Second, there appears to be increasing evidence of frontal/subcortical or frontolimbic circuitry involved in most types of neurologically based apathy.

A CONCEPTUALIZATION OF APATHY STATES

In this section we outline different types of apathy. The kinds of apathy are differentiated by inclusion of an adjective modifier that denotes the major qualities of the kind of apathetic behavior referred to. The different forms of apathy are related to damage to different regions in frontal anatomical functional systems. To some degree, our proposed conceptualization of apathy states derives from the model of frontal lobe function developed over the years by Stuss and colleagues (e.g., Alexander, Benson, & Stuss, 1989; Stuss, 1991b; Stuss et al., 1995, 1998; Stuss & Benson, 1986, 1987).

Apathy Related to Disturbed Arousal

Frequently apathy is described as a symptom associated with many disorders of arousal. In considering apathy related to disturbed arousal, the distinct aspects of disturbed arousal should be differentiated. Fernandez-Duque and Posner (1997) suggest, for example, that alerting and orienting are dissociable, with separate mechanisms and different biochemical bases. This is similar to the concept of phasic and tonic attention (Benson & Geshwind, 1975) or the different types of delirium (Lipowsky, 1990). Others (Plum & Posner, 1980) describe a continuum of arousal, from coma through stupor to obtundation. In all of these disorders of arousal related to brain stem reticular activity system dysfunction, there is a lack of self-initiated activity. The apathy is usually not the most obvious problem in these patients, however, and as such the clinical value of the apathy label is likely to be limited. In our conceptualization, we exclude all disorders of arousal in which there is an impaired sleep–wake cycle. Similarly, if the cortex is so profoundly damaged that there is no content of consciousness despite normal arousal—the persistent vegetative state—it would be inappropriate to label a patient as simply apathetic.

One particular disorder, akinetic mutism, deserves to be labeled apathy associated with disturbed arousal. Damage limited to the dopaminergic ventral tegmental brain stem nucleus or its projections to frontal cortex via the medial forebrain bundle will result in diminished general responsiveness against a background of normal sleep–wake cycles and intact cortical functions. Although the patient is cognitively capable, self-initiated and purposeful cortical functioning does not normally occur. Occasionally, however, under conditions of emotionally potent stimuli or when requests are not cognitively demanding, responsiveness may be observed. Considering this type of apathy as arousal apathy may be appropriate as the medial forebrain bundle conveys ascending reticular activating system information to modulate the effects of arousal in the cortex.

Apathy Associated with Frontal System Dysfunction

This apathy is related not just to the frontal lobes themselves but also to frontal/subcortical connectivity (for an overview of frontal/subcortical connections, see Alexander, DeLong, & Strick, 1986; Cummings, 1993; Mega & Cummings, 1994). Five frontal/subcortical circuits have been described. Each circuit includes the same general brain regions: frontal lobe, striatum, globus pallidus, substantia nigra, and thalamus. The five circuits are divisible into two major functional categories, motor and behavioral. Although damage to any of the five could be considered within the general term *executive apathy*, we propose that damage to any one of the five circuits results in distinctly different forms of executive apathy.

The two motor circuits are the oculomotor and the general motor circuits. The relation of each to the frontal lobes is to the frontal eye fields and the supplementary motor area (SMA), respectively. For the two motor circuits, two different types of apathetic behavior have been described. For the oculomotor circuit, there is a tendency not to initiate responses to the contralateral side. This occurs for both vision (Hécaen & Albert, 1978) and motor (Spiers et al., 1990) responses. This is frequently evidenced in neglect. Damage to the SMA circuit results in two types of reported apathetic behavior. There is a decrease in verbal output as evidenced by a decrease in verbal fluency (Alexander, Benson, & Stuss, 1989; Stuss & Benson, 1986). While diminished verbal fluency is frequently observed after left dorsolateral frontal lesions, it is also common after damage to either the right or left SMA (Stuss et al., 1998). The second type of apathetic behavior associated with SMA pathology is the alien hand disorder. Although most commonly described as a type of impulsive behavior (i.e., a positive but unwilled activity of the contralateral [usually left] hand), there have also been descriptions of occasional apathy, an inability to move the left hand at will (Baynes et al., 1997; Feinberg et al., 1992; Tanaka et al., 1996).

The three behavioral circuits are related to the dorsolateral prefrontal, lateral orbital, and anterior cingulate regions, respectively. The dorsolateral prefrontal circuit has been proposed as originating in the convexity of the lateral surface of the anterior frontal lobe. The lateral orbital circuit initiates in Brodmann area 10. The anterior cingulate is the site of origin for the final behavioral circuit. Different types of apathetic behavior have been associated with damage to these three behavioral circuits (Bhatia & Marsden, 1994). Apathy, because it is a disorder of self-initiated behavior, is particularly susceptible to damage to these frontal/subcortical circuits because each is an effector circuit enabling action in the environment (Cummings, 1993).

The dorsolateral prefrontal circuit is characterized by a decrease in verbal fluency as well as by disturbance in active selection of behaviors. This lack of behavioral response after dorsolateral frontal damage can be considered as apathetic behavior. Arousal is normal, and general cognitive functions are intact. The specific type of executive apathy can be explained by a simple model of responsiveness (Stuss, 1991a,b; Stuss, Picton, & Alexander, 1999). In any behavior, there is an input and a response-output pathway. Incoming information is compared with stored information—a constructed model or template. This normally leads to a response of some type, including the potential generation of a new, adapted model. At the level of executive functions, the responses are those that require flexibility, selection, novel responsiveness, and so on, controlling the more automatic functions of posterior areas. If there is damage to the template (the specific type of executive process) or to the comparator, then the outcome is impaired behavior or the absence of behavior. Thus, in the above examples, the absence of behavior could be considered as executive apathy (i.e., the absence of initiated behavior secondary to a disorder of executive cognitive functioning.

Damage to the lateral orbitofrontal cortex results in personality blunting and change. Again, this can be viewed as a type of apathetic behavior due perhaps to the absence of limbic affective input. As noted earlier, orbitofrontal lobotomies were often performed to make patients easier to get along with. A current example related to the ventral medial frontal region but perhaps appropriate here involves the demonstrated inability to anticipate selection of response in a gambling task. Despite normal arousal, the absence of responses would reflect a disorder of self-initiated behavior, or apathy (Bechara et al., 1996).

The most obvious frontal type of apathy results from damage to the anterior cingulate. Damage to this region, particularly if bilateral, results in apathy and lack of initiation. The classification of anterior cingulate executive apathy is itself too broad, and even more specific subtyping may be required. Devinsky, Morrell, and Vogt (1995) point to the considerable anatomical and connective specificity of the anterior cingulate. The association to the rostral limbic system suggests that a major role of the cingulate is to assess the motivational information from internal and external stimuli. Because of the connectivity, however, subtypes of apathetic behavior might result from cingulate pathology. For example, chronic pain patients treated with cingulomotomy continue to feel pain, but they are no longer bothered by it (Foltz & White, 1968). Damage to the anterior cingulate results in affective placidity, lack of emotional response, and altered social interactions—all of which are reflective of apathy. Anterior cingulate damage can also result in impaired response selection and decision to respond (symptoms representative of apathetic behavior), as well as impaired movement execution itself. Devinsky and colleagues suggest very specific anatomical localization for the different subtypes of apathy: affective placidity (connection of Brodmann areas 24/25 with the amygdala), impaired response selection (gyral surface of anterior cingulate, areas 24a' and 24b'), and impaired movement execution (interconnection of 24c' with the SMA). In other words, the types of apathy revealed are related to the cingulate itself and to the connections of the cingulate with other regions.

The five frontal sites of origin result in different types of apathy, and this distinction is paralleled in the subcortical regions of each circuit. That is, damage to different parts of the same circuit can result in similar impairments. Thus, damage to the frontal lobes of the dorsolateral prefrontal circuit will lead to similar results as damage to the connected subcortical areas such as the caudate, globus pallidus, and thalamus. Because of the compressed nature of these subcortical regions, however, differentiation of forms of apathy specific to one circuit is almost impossible to determine. Nevertheless, some dissociation at this level has been suggested. Studies of the basal ganglia indicate that different types of apathy may occur (Schultz et al., 1993; Williams et al., 1993). Similar suggestions of dissociation have been reported after thalamic lesions. McAlonan, Robbins, and Everitt (1993) suggested that the dorsal medial nucleus, through its interconnections with the ventral striatal pallidal and prefrontal cortex, might be involved in response selection. A flat affect (unconcern), and physical withdrawal and akinesia, may differentiate dorsomedial and anterior thalamic lesions (Graff-Radford et al., 1984; Stuss et al., 1988).

The above types of apathy associated with frontal system dysfunction are related more to the direct effector responsiveness in which the frontal lobes play an important role. A more abstract form of apathy also likely exists, related to the frontal lobes and primarily their limbic connections. Evidence is accumulating for the role of the anterior frontal lobes (the right frontal, ventral medial, and possibly polar regions have been particularly implicated) in awareness of self and social awareness (Damasio et al., 1994; Stuss, 1991a,b; Stuss, Picton, & Alexander, 1999; Wheeler, Stuss, & Tulving, 1997). Self and social awareness is a metacognitive ability that is necessary to mediate information from a personal, social past and current history with projections to the future. The key feature of this apathy appears to be intact knowledge of behavior, even of intention, but a lack of action in one's own self-interest—a type of "social apathy" (Stuss, Picton, & Alexander, 1999). The patient appears not to have a mental model of his or her own self that serves to organize perceptions and actions. This type of social apathy is evident in the clinical descriptions of patients such as Phineas Gage, those with the Capgras syndrome, and even in disorders of humour (Alexander, Stuss, & Benson, 1979; Damasio et al., 1994; Shammi & Stuss, 1999; Stuss & Benson, 1986).

Comparisons Between our Conceptualization of Apathy States and Other Views

Our approach to understanding apathy shares some commonalties with other conceptualizations of apathy. The idea of apathy being associated with frontal/subcortical circuits has been discussed by others (e.g., Bhatia & Marsden, 1994; Cummings, 1993; Mega & Cummings, 1994). The separation of positive and negative symptoms in schizophrenia has led to the proposal of distinct frontal system dysfunctions underlying the two symptom groupings (Frith, 1987; Frith & Done, 1989; Strauss, 1993). Mega and Cohenour (1997), in their review of akinetic mutism, proposed that there may be three different kinds of disturbed activation of behavior: motor, cognitive, and limbic. Our idea of comparison and generation processes in the construction of models of the world is somewhat similar to that of Godefroy and Rousseaux's "relative judgment theory" (1997). Turkstra and Bayles (1992), in their model of mutism, suggested that speech production depended on five interrelated processes: arousal; cognitive processes; affect and drive; motor initiation; planning; programming and coordination; and execution of movement. If verbal output is considered as a measure of apathy, as has been done, then it is clear that disturbances in very different mechanisms and brain areas could lead to the same decreases in output. Our research on verbal fluency has shown that impairments in different processes can affect self-initiated behavior such as word generation (Stuss et al., 1998; Troyer et al., 1998).

In summary, our conceptualization of apathy states is based on the known clinical presentations and separable neuroanatomical substrates of apathetic behaviors. This conceptualization will of necessity be modified as we continue to learn more about the various types of apathy and their neural correlates. For example, as our knowledge of the specificity of functioning within the frontal lobes increases, and our mapping of the interconnections of frontal, cognitive, and limbic regions is completed, our understanding of the exact nature of the circuits may alter. We are arguing more for an approach than for absolute distinction among these frontal system types of apathy. We do not have experimental data, and in reality it may be difficult to dissociate unique causes. The major point is this: If the causes of observable apathy are distinguishable to some degree, then treatment and rehabilitation can be more specific. At present, we believe that the presented view of apathy states is a useful framework within which to view apathy disorders, as well as a guide for targeting specific treatment interventions.

TREATMENT INTERVENTIONS

In this section, we summarize the evidence gathered to date on the treatment of apathy. Past research and clinical efforts have typically used the concept of apathy as a syndrome. We attempt to relate, as much as possible, the available treatment information to our proposed conceptualization of apathy states.

Pharmacotherapy

Two broad introductory comments need to be made. First, little research into the efficacy of medication therapy for apathy states has been completed to date. This in part probably reflects the view of many that apathy is not a significant problem, if it is a "problem" at all. The clinical relevance of apathy is likely to vary depending on the clinical setting and/or the philosophical viewpoint of the assessor of its relevance. For example, in a busy nursing home, with severe problems for staff posed by the disinhibited and aggressive behavior of some residents, apathetic residents are likely to be largely viewed as somewhat ideal behaviorally. On the other hand, apathy in a rehabilitation setting may become a very significant deterrent to progress. The risks associated with treating apathy in chronic care settings need to be offset by compelling reasons to treat the apathy (e.g., residents who are so apathetic that they no longer eat).

The second comment relates to the potential temptation to infer neurotransmitter bases for apathy states based on response to treatment. This approach, while ultimately somewhat validated by other types of data for the dopamine hypothesis of schizophrenia (which of course has its origins in the observed response to dopamine-blocking drugs), has been less successful in other domains. Clearly additional evidence related to neurotransmitter dysfunction over and above observations of treatment response are required before the neurotransmitter bases of apathy states can be fully understood.

In some case studies akinetic mutism has been treated with bromocriptine (Crismon et al., 1988; Echiverri et al., 1988; Ross & Stewart, 1981) or methylphenidate (Daly & Love, 1958; Weinberg, Auerbach, & Moore, 1987). Although we have excluded apathetic behavior that is coexistent with fluctuating arousal from our precise definition of apathy, it is of relevance that this type of apathy is common in states such as post-traumatic amnesia, and some success has been reported with pharmacological treatment (Jackson, Corrigan, & Arnett, 1985; Mysiw, Jackson, & Corrigan, 1988).

Medications used for this "executive" kind of apathy fall broadly into the three categories of dopaminergic drugs, amphetamines, and atypical neuroleptics. Gualtieri et al. (1989) have suggested that apathy in traumatic brain injured (TBI) patients may have its origins in the axonal shearing of brain stem structures, with secondary lowering of monoamine transmission, including dopamine, to striatum and cortex. If the suggestion of Gualtieri et al. (1989) is correct, then medications dependent on an intact presynaptic neuron may be less effective in TBI-related apathy. This very hypothesis led Gualtieri et al. (1989) to study the efficacy of amantadine, a drug that increases dopaminergic activity. Benefit in the treatment of apathy in TBI patients was reported with amantadine; however, the results were limited by methodological problems. Van Reekum et al. (1995) performed an N of 1 randomized double-blind, placebo-controlled study that showed effectiveness of amantadine in improving initiation/participation in a subject with a profound apathy beginning after a TBI. Rehabilitation was facilitated by amantadine in this subject.

Although not directly assessing apathy, other studies have used amantadine for indications that may have formed part of an apathy state. Improvement in appetite, talkativeness, and activity level were noted in long-term geriatric care patients treated with amantadine (Roca et al., 1990). Andersson et al. (1992) reported cognitive improvement (i.e., increases in visual attention, speed of information processing, attention span, learning capacity, and alertness) in two severe TBI cases treated with amantadine. Reversal of "mute, immobile states" were noted with amantadine when used for the end-stage of Alzheimer's disease (Erkulwater & Pillai, 1989). Amantadine may also play a role in reducing fatigue and frontal system cognitive impairments associated with multiple sclerosis (Cohen & Fisher, 1989). Although the mechanism of action of amantadine is likely to be related to increased dopaminergic activity, additional changes in the brain (e.g., improved frontal system cognitive functioning) in response to amantadine are being identified. For example, Semlitsch, Anderson, and Saletu (1992) found that the P300 amplitude of targets in an auditory odd-ball paradigm was significantly augmented (by 30% over baseline) in subjects with mild dementia who received amantadine.

Bromocriptine is a dopamine agonist that has also been studied in apathy states. Powell et al. (1996) performed an open study of 11 apathetic subjects (after TBI or subarachnoid hemorrhage) and showed improvements in motivation and frontal cognitive functioning, but an absence of change in mood, with bromocriptine. Parks et al. (1992) showed improved range of affect, less social withdrawal, and increased assertiveness with bromocriptine in a single male subject after subarchnoid haemorrhage (related to an anterior communicating artery aneurysm on the right side), who also had evidence of a lacunar infarct in the head of the left caudate. Some "marginal" improvement in right superior frontoparietal lobe perfusion was seen in serial HMPAO SPECT scanning with bromocriptine, and there was also improvement in frontal system, but not visuospatial, cognitive functioning. Muller and von Cramon (1994) also noted improvement in motivational behavior with bromocriptine in 4 of 15 subjects treated with bromocriptine; in this series of subjects cognition was not improved with bromocriptine.

Methylphenidate is a frequently used amphetamine, particularly for children with attention deficit hyperactivity disorder. Several case reports of improvement in motivational behavior with methylphenidate exist (Marin et al., 1995). An open study of 88 elderly subjects in a rehabilitation center (for cerebrovascular accidents and so forth) using amphetamine showed that half of the subjects improved significantly, one-fourth did not change, and one-fourth dropped out because of the side effects (Clark & Mankikar, 1979). Branconnier and Cole (1980) performed a randomized clinical trial of methylphenidate in elderly apathetic subjects and found improved "vigour." Kaplitz (1975) also completed a randomized clinical trial with methylphenidate. They studied subjects with "senile apathy"; nurses and physicians noted improvements in interest, involvement, activity level, and self-esteem.

Much of the methylphenidate evidence reviewed above is limited by diagnostic and assessment issues. More recently, Maletta and Winegarden (1993) reported on three severely demented residents of long-term institutions who showed gradual onset of apathy "eventually resulting in severe anorexia . . . with consideration of permanent feeding tube placement." Methylphenidate led to significant and almost immediate improvement in appetite with weight increase. Galynker et al. (1997) studied 27 subjects with dementia (Alzheimer's disease and vascular) and found that negative symptoms and cognition both improved with methylphenidate, while mood symptoms did not. Watanabe et al. (1995) reported on a 38-year-old apathetic male. Neuropsychological testing showed frontal system deficits, and magnetic resonance imaging showed infarcts in the subcortical white matter, basal ganglia, cerebellum, and left thalamus. Methylphenidate led to increased interest, social behavior, and hygiene. The pre-methylphenidate SPECT scan showed bilateral frontal hypoperfusion, and the post-methylphenidate SPECT scan showed significantly increased perfusion frontally.

Finally, Volkow et al. (1997) found that methylphenidate's effects on brain function were to some extent dependent on the levels of dopamine D_2 receptors throughout the brain and between individuals. Methylphenidate consistently decreased relative (to whole brain) metabolism in the basal ganglia and increased it in the cerebellum. Frontotemporal metabolism was increased in subjects with high D_2 receptors and was decreased in subjects with low D_2 receptors.

Although the traditional neuroleptics have done little to improve negative symptoms in schizophrenia, and might even have worsened negative symptoms, the newer "atypical" neuroleptics generally have been shown to have treatment efficacy for negative symptoms (Arvanitis & Miller, 1997; Tran et al., 1997). These atypical neuroleptics have effects on multiple neurotransmitter subsystems, and it is as yet unknown which effect is most important in terms of the impact on negative symptoms. A leading candidate, however, appears to be the antagonistic binding to $5\text{-}HT_2$ receptors.

There is little research investigating the concepts of self and social awareness in pharmacologic studies. Close review of some of the studies discussed above, however, suggests that subjects did improve in terms of social skills and awareness and acted to preserve their "self" to a greater degree in response to pharmacologic interventions.

In summary, there is preliminary support for the use of amantadine and other dopaminergic agents, as well as methylphenidate, for the pharmacologic treatment of some types of apathy. Much of this literature seems to point to the need to increase dopaminergic activity in the brain as a necessary requirement of successful treatment of apathy with medications, although dopaminergic receptor subtype specificity and interactions with other neurotransmitter systems may also be important. Because a dopaminergic strategy has been used successfully in so many different patient groups, it should be evaluated in patients with focal lesions resulting in apathy. This approach may be a necessary initial step upon which specific behavioral treatments are applied. The type of lesion may determine treatment response, with, for example, presynaptic neuronal damage dictating the need for medications that exert direct postsynaptic effects. Finally, this literature has been somewhat illustrative in terms of identifying changes within the brain, particularly involving frontal/subcortical functioning, in response to successful pharmacologic treatment of apathy, and as such this is broadly supportive of the systems we suggest are involved in some apathy states.

Rehabilitation Interventions—Behavioral Therapy

Although rare, there have been reports of successful behavioral therapy treatment of apathetic states. For example, Rosenthal and Meyer (1971) used a behavior modification technique with a young woman diagnosed with clinical abulia. These researchers used a combination of therapy techniques to increase the opportunity for reward (environmental reinforcers); to reframe the cause of problem behaviors using cognitive restructuring; and to set goals, identify goal obstacles, and establish problem-solving techniques for overcoming these obstacles. The therapy intervention they employed had considerable success. It is important to note, however, that their client's abulia was not due to central nervous system (CNS) damage but rather had its origin in non-CNS causes related to lack of environmental incentive or reward and grief and adjustment disorders (see Table 14.1).

Kopelowicz et al. (1997) performed a pilot study with six subjects with schizophrenia, three of whom had "deficit" syndrome (i.e., cognitive impairment and increased neurological signs) and three of whom did not (i.e., negative symptoms without cognitive impairment). All received 12 weeks of social skills training. Improvements in social skills and negative symptoms in the nondeficit group were more impressive than in the deficit group, suggesting that comorbid cognitive impairments may limit rehabilitation efficacy.

Other potentially useful approaches to rehabilitation of apathetic individuals are based on behavioral rehabilitation of frontal lobe deficits (Prigatano, 1999; Sohlberg, Mateer, & Stuss, 1993; Stuss et al., 1994c). The authors suggested using one or more aspects of the following protocol of behavior therapy with frontal lobe patients: teaching clients compensatory strategies; providing practice on executive tasks (e.g., self-initiation and monitoring); and facilitating self-awareness and generalization to other behavioral situations. For example, a frontal lobe patient exhibiting problems initiating and maintaining social interactions might be taught initiation strategies specific to social situations and provided with an opportunity for supervised practice of these learned strategies along with therapy interventions (e.g., didactic training) designed to increase self and social awareness. All three of these steps would be reciprocally connected, thereby reinforcing each other. The relationship between frontal systems pathology and apathy indicates that investigation of rehabilitation strategies for frontal lobe injury may also have utility with patients presenting with apathy.

In summary, behavioral rehabilitation of apathetic behaviors is an area requiring considerable future study. The kind of apathy state and the nature of its cause (e.g., CNS or non-CNS) are factors that must be considered in the development and evaluation of behavioral therapy interventions for individuals presenting with apathetic disorders. We cannot rehabilitate what we do not know (Stuss, 1987).

CONCLUSION

Our review of apathetic behavior and our apathy model lead us to conclude that there is no single definition or syndrome of apathy. Although having a single definition or syndrome may be appealing, it inherently limits experimental and clinical approaches, as was the idea of the frontal syndrome. Not all symptoms of apathy co-occur. Indeed, there is now considerable evidence in the literature for clinical presentations of separable forms of apathetic behavior.

There are different kinds of apathy, related to different pathophysiological bases and psychological mechanisms. Although the term *apathy* is still useful as a very general description of behavior, it is more parsimonious to describe the types of apathetic behavior in the context of their pathophysiological and/or psychological mechanisms. For example, when discussing apathy associated with disturbed arousal, it is likely worthwhile to distinguish between conditions of altered arousal from the apathy of akinetic mutism that may occur in the presence of normal sleep–wake cycles. Moreover, there are different types of executive apathetic disorders, resulting from disturbances in cognitive/affective processes due to damage to specific frontal/subcortical circuits. The major value in differentiating these executive apathys is to differentiate the specific cause of the behavior. In many regards it may be best to refer to the different kinds of executive apathy behaviors according to their cognitive dysfunction rather than as apathy. Finally, social apathy may be the most devastating and the most important type to recognize. The absence of an abstract model of one's self in society may require the motivation of external environmental support. One avenue for research is the pursuit of pharmacological interventions in conjunction with social awareness and social behavior training.

Treatment of apathetic behaviors by pharmacotherapy, behavioral therapy, or both will be most efficacious when the underlying pathophysiological basis and/or disturbance in psychological mechanisms is clearly understood. In this chapter, we have attempted to further approaches to treatment by pointing out potentially different causes of apathetic states and their associated underlying etiologies. The recognition of the types of apathy is a call for the initiation of rehabilitative efforts.

ACKNOWLEDGMENTS

Our ongoing research funding, which provided assistance in preparation of this chapter, is gratefully acknowledged: Medical Research Council of Canada and the Ontario Mental Health Foundation (D.T.S.); Alzheimer Society of Canada and the Kunin-Lunenfeld Applied Research Unit (R.V.R.); and Rotman Research Institute postdoctoral fellowship (K.J.M.).

DEDICATION

This chapter is dedicated to the memory of D. Frank Benson, M.D., who was originally to be our co-author.

REFERENCES

Alexander, G.E., DeLong, M.R., & Strick, P.L. (1986). Parallel organization of functionally segregated circuits linking basal ganglia and cortex. *Annual Review of Neuroscience, 9,* 357–381.

Alexander, M.P., Benson, D.F., & Stuss, D.T. (1989). Frontal lobes and language. *Brain and Language, 37(4),* 656–691.

Alexander, M.P., Naeser, M.A., & Palumbo, C.L. (1987). Correlations of subcortical CT lesion sites and aphasia profiles. *Brain, 110(4),* 961–991.

Alexander, M.P., Stuss, D.T., & Benson, D.F. (1979). Capgras syndrome: A reduplicative phenomenon. *Neurology, 29(3),* 334–339.

Ali-Cherif, A., Royere, M.L., Gosset, A., Poncet, M., Salamon, G., & Khalil, R. (1984). Behavioral and mental activity disorders after carbon monoxide poisoning. Bilateral pallidal lesions. *Revue Neurologique (Paris), 140(6–7),* 401–405.

Andersson, S., Berstad, J., Finset, A., & Grimsmo, J. (1992). Amantadine in cognitive failure in patients with traumatic brain injuries. *Tidsskrift for den Norske Laegeforening, 112(16),* 2070–2072.

Andreasen, N.C. (1982). Negative symptoms in schizophrenia: Definition and reliability. *Archives of General Psychiatry, 39(7),* 784–788.

Arvanitis, L.A., & Miller, B.G. (1997). Multiple fixed doses of "Seroquel" (Quetiapine) in patients with acute exacerbation of schizophrenia: A comparison of haloperidol and placebo. The Seroquel trial 13 study group. *Biological Psychiatry, 42(4),* 233–246.

Baynes, K., Tramo, M.J., Reeves, A.G., & Gazzaniga, M.S. (1997). Isolation of a right hemisphere cognitive system in a patient with anarchic (alien) hand sign. *Neuropsychologia, 35(8),* 1159–1173.

Bechara, A., Tranel, D., Damasio, H., & Damasio, A.R. (1996). Failure to respond autonomically to anticipated future outcomes following damage to prefrontal cortex. *Cerebral Cortex, 6(2),* 215–225.

Belyi, B. (1979). On the syndrome of lack of spontaneity in tumors of the frontal lobes. *Journal of Neurology and Psychiatry, 7,* 901–907.

Benson, D.F., & Geshwind, N. (1975). Psychiatric conditions associated with focal lesions of the central nervous system. In S. Arieti & M. Reiser (Eds.), *American Handbook of Psychiatry, Vol. 4: Organic Disorders and Psychosomatic Medicine* (pp. 208–243). New York: Basic Books.

Berrios, G.E., & Gili, M. (1995). Abulia and impulsiveness revisited: A conceptual history. *Acta Psychiatrica Scandinavica, 92(3),* 161–167.

Bhatia, K.P., & Marsden, C.D. (1994). The behavioral and motor consequences of focal lesions of the basal ganglia in man. *Brain, 117(4)*, 859–876.

Bogousslavsky, J., Ferrazzini, M., Regli, F., Assal, G., Tanabe, H., & Delaloye-Bischof, A. (1988). Manic delirium and frontal-like syndrome with paramedian infarction of the right thalamus. *Journal of Neurology, Neurosurgery, and Psychiatry, 51(1)*, 116–119.

Bozzola, F.G., Gorelick, P.B., & Freels, S. (1992). Personality changes in Alzheimer's disease. *Archives of Neurology, 49(3)*, 297–300.

Branconnier, R., & Cole, J.O. (1980). The therapeutic role of methylphenidate in senile organic brain syndrome. *Proceedings of the Annual Meeting of the American Psychopathological Association, 69*, 183–196.

Cairns, H., Oldfield, R.C., Pennybacker, J.B., & Whitteridge, D. (1941). Akinetic mutism with an epidermoid cyst of the third ventricle. *Brain, 64*, 273–290.

Clark, A.N., & Mankikar, G.D. (1979). *d*-Amphetamine in elderly patients refractory to rehabilitation procedures. *Journal of the American Geriatrics Society, 27(4)*, 174–177.

Cohen, R.A., & Fisher, M. (1989). Amantadine treatment of fatigue associated with multiple sclerosis. *Archives of Neurology, 46(6)*, 676–680.

Crismon, M.L., Childs, A., Wilcox, R.E., & Barrow, N. (1988). The effect of bromocriptine in speech dysfunction in patients with diffuse brain injury (akinetic mutism). *Clinical Neuropharmacology, 11(5)*, 462–466.

Crow, T. (1985). The two-syndrome concept: Origins and current status. *Schizophrenia Bulletin, 11(3)*, 471–486.

Crow, T. (1995). Brain changes and negative symptoms in schizophrenia. *Psychopathology, 28(1)*, 18–21.

Cummings, J.L. (1993). Frontal-subcortical circuits and human behavior. *Archives of Neurology, 50(8)*, 873–880.

Daly, D.D., & Love, J.G. (1958). Akinetic mutism. *Neurology (Minneapolis), 8*, 238–242.

Damasio, H., Grabowski, T., Frank, R., Galaburda, A. M., & Damasio, A. (1994). The return of Phineas Gage: Clues about the brain from the skull of a famous patient. *Science, 264(5162)*, 1102–1105.

Devinsky, O., Morrell, M., & Vogt, B.A. (1995). Contributions of anterior cingulate cortex to behavior. *Brain, 118(1)*, 279–306.

Echiverri, H.C., Tatum, W.O., Merens, T.A., & Coker, S.B. (1988). Akinetic mutism: Pharmacologic probe of the dopaminergic mesencephalofrontal activating system. *Pediatric Neurology, 4(4)*, 228–230.

Erkulwater, S., & Pillai, R. (1989). Amantadine and the end-stage dementia of Alzheimer's type. *Southern Medical Journal, 82(5)*, 550–554.

Feinberg, T.E., Schindler, R.J., Flanagan, N.G., & Haber, L.D. (1992). Two alien hand syndromes. *Neurology, 42(1)*, 19–24.

Fernadez-Duque, D., & Posner, M.I. (1997). Relating the mechanisms of orienting and alerting. *Neuropsychologia, 35(4)*, 477–486.

Fisher, C.M. (1983). Honoured guest presentation: Abulia minor vs. agitated behavior. *Clinical Neurosurgery, 31*, 9–31.

Foltz, E.L., & White, L.E. (1968). The role of rostral cingulumotomy in "pain" relief. *International Journal of Neurology, 6(3–4)*, 353–373.

Forsell, Y., Jorm, A.F., Fratiglioni, L., Grut, M., & Winblad, B. (1993). Application of DSM-III-R criteria for major depressive episode to elderly subjects with and without dementia. *American Journal of Psychiatry, 150(8)*, 1199–1202.

Frith, C.D. (1987). The positive and negative symptoms of schizophrenia reflect impairments in the perception and initiation of action. *Psychological Medicine, 17(3)*, 631–648.

Frith, C., & Done, J. (1989). Positive symptoms of schizophrenia. *British Journal of Psychiatry, 154*, 569–570.

Fuster, J.M. (1989). *The Prefrontal Cortex: Anatomy, Physiology, and Neuropsychology of the Frontal Lobe*, 2nd Ed. New York: Raven Press.

Galynker, I., Ieronimo, C., Rosenblum, J., Vilkas, N., & Rosenthal, R. (1997). Methylphenidate treatment of negative symptoms in patients with dementia. *Journal of Neuropsychiatry and Clinical Neurosciences, 9(2)*, 231–239.

Godefroy, O., & Rousseaux, M. (1997). Novel decision making in patients with prefrontal or posterior brain damage. *Neurology, 49(3)*, 695–701.

Graff-Radford, N.R., Eslinger, P.J., Damasio, A.R., & Yamada, T. (1984). Nonhemorrhagic infarction of the thalamus: Behavioral, anatomic, and physiologic correlates. *Neurology, 34(1)*, 14–23.

Gualtieri, T., Chandler, M., Coons, T.B., & Brown, L.T. (1989). Amantadine—A new clinical profile for traumatic brain injury. *Clinical Neuropharmacology, 12(4)*, 258–270.

Guberman, A., & Stuss, D.T. (1983). The syndrome of bilateral paramedian thalamic infarction. *Neurology, 33(5)*, 540–546.

Habib, M., & Poncet, M. (1988). Loss of vitality, of interest, and of the affect (athymhormia syndrome) in lacunar lesions of the corpus striatum. *Revue Neurologique (Paris), 144(10)*, 571–577.

Hécaen, H., & Albert, M.L. (1978). *Human Neuropsychology*. New York: Wiley, 1978.

Jackson, R.D., Corrigan, J.D., & Arnett, J.A. (1985). Amitriptyline for agitation in head injury. *Archives of Physical Medicine and Rehabilitation, 66(3)*, 180–181.

Jacobsen, C.F. (1936). Studies of cerebral function in primates. *Comparative Psychological Monographs, 13*, 1–60.

Kaplitz, S.E. (1975). Withdrawn, apathetic geriatric patients responsive to methylphenidate. *Journal of the American Geriatrics Society, 23(6)*, 271–276.

Kopelowicz, A., Liberman, R.P., Mintz, J., & Zarate, R. (1997). Comparison of efficacy of social skills training for deficit and nondeficit negative symptoms in schizophrenia. *American Journal of Psychiatry, 154(3)*, 424–425.

Laplane, D., Baulac, M., Widlocher, D., & Dubois, B. (1984). Pure psychic akinesia with bilateral lesions of basal ganglia. *Journal of Neurology, Neurosurgery, and Psychiatry, 47(4)*, 377–385.

Lipowski, Z.J. (1990). *Delirium: Acute Confusional States*. New York: Oxford University Press.

Maletta, G.J., & Winegarden, T. (1993). Reversal of anorexia by methylphenidate in apathetic, severely demented nursing home patients. *American Journal of Geriatric Psychiatry, 1*, 234–243.

Marin, R.S. (1990). Differential diagnosis and classification of apathy. *American Journal of Psychiatry, 147(1)*, 22–29.

Marin, R.S. (1991). Apathy: A neuropsychiatric syndrome. *Journal of Neuropsychiatry and Clinical Neurosciences, 3(3)*, 243–254.

Marin, R.S. (1996). Apathy and related disorders of diminished motivation. In L.J. Dickstein, M.B. Riba, & J.M. Oldham (Eds.), *Review of Psychiatry*, Vol. 15. Washington, DC: American Psychiatric Press.

Marin, R.S., Biedrzycki, R.C., & Firinciogullari, S. (1991). Reliability and validity of the apathy evaluation scale. *Psychiatry Research, 38(2)*, 143–162.

Marin, R.S., Firinciogullari, S., & Biedrzycki, R.C. (1993). The sources of convergence between measures of apathy and depression. *Journal of Affective Disorders*, *28(2)*, 117–124.

Marin, R.S., Firinciogullari, S., & Biedrzycki, R.C. (1994). Group differences in the relationship between apathy and depression. *Journal of Nervous and Mental Disease*, *182*, 235–239.

Marin, R.S., Fogel, B.S., Hawkins, J., et al. (1995). Apathy: A treatable syndrome. *Journal of Neuropsychiatry and Clinical Neurosciences*, *7(1)*, 23–30.

Masdeu, J.C., & Shewmon, D.A. (1980). Left medial parietal lobe and receptive language functions. *Neurology*, *30(10)*, 1137–1138.

Mayberg, H.S. (1994). Frontal lobe dysfunction in secondary depression. *Journal of Neuropsychiatry and Clinical Neurosciences*, *6(4)*, 428–442.

McAlonan, G.M., Robbins, T.W., & Everitt, B.J. (1993). Effects of medial dorsal thalamic and ventral pallidal lesions on the acquisition of a conditioned place preference: Further evidence for the involvement of the ventral striatopallidal system in reward-related processes. *Neuroscience*, *52(3)*, 605–620.

McGilchrist, I., Goldstein, L.H., Jadresic, D., & Fenwick, P. (1993). Thalamo-frontal psychosis. *British Journal of Psychiatry*, *163*, 113–115.

Mega, M.S., & Cohenour, R.C. (1997). Akinetic mutism: Disconnection of frontal-subcortical circuits. *Neuropsychiatry, Neuropsychology, and Behavioral Neurology*, *10(4)*, 254–259.

Mega, M.S., & Cummings, J.L. (1994). Frontal-subcortical circuits and neuropsychiatric disorders. *Journal of Neuropsychiatry and Clinical Neurosciences*, *6(4)*, 358–370.

Moniz, E. (1937). Prefrontal leucotomy in treatment of mental disorders. *American Journal of Psychiatry*, *93*, 1379–1385.

Muller, U., & von Cramon, D.Y. (1994). The therapeutic potential of bromocriptine in neuropsychological rehabilitation of patients with acquired brain damage. *Progress in Neuro-Psychopharmacology and Biological Psychiatry*, *18(7)*, 1103–1120.

Mysiw, W.J., Jackson, R.D., & Corrigan, J.D. (1988). Amitryptiline for post-traumatic aggression. *American Journal of Physical Medicine and Rehabilitation*, *67(1)*, 29–33.

Ott, B.R., Noto, R.B., & Fogel, B.S. (1996). Apathy and loss of insight in Alzheimer's disease: A SPECT imaging study. *Journal of Neuropsychiatry and Clinical Neurosciences*, *8(1)*, 41–46.

Pandya, D.N., & Barnes, C.L. (1987). Architecture and connections of the frontal lobe. In E. Perecman (Ed.), *The Frontal Lobes Revisited* (pp. 41–72). New York: IRBN Press.

Parks, R.W., Crockett, D.J., Manji, H.K., & Ammann, W. (1992). Assessment of bromocriptine intervention for the treatment of frontal lobe syndrome: A case study. *Journal of Neuropsychiatry and Clinical Neurosciences*, *4(1)*, 109–111.

Percheron, G., Fenelon, G., Leroux-Hugon, V., & Feve, A. (1994). History of the basal ganglia system. Slow development of a major cerebral system. *Revue Neurologique (Paris)*, *150(8–9)*, 543–554.

Plum, F., & Posner, J.B. (1980). The pathologic physiology of signs and symptoms of coma. *The Diagnosis of Stupor and Coma*, 3rd Ed. Philadelphia: Davis.

Poncet, M., & Habib, M. (1994). Isolated involvement of motivated behavior and basal ganglia diseases. *Revue Neurologique (Paris)*, *150(8–9)*, 588–593.

Powell, J.H., al-Adawi, S., Morgan, J., & Greenwood, R.J. (1996). Motivational deficits after brain injury: Effects of bromocriptine in 11 patients. *Journal of Neurology, Neurosurgery, and Psychiatry*, *60(4)*, 416–421.

Prigatano, G.P. (1999). Motivation and awareness in cognitive neurorehabilitation. In D.T. Stuss, G. Winocur, & I.H. Robertson (Eds.), *Cognitive Neurorehabilitation* (pp. 240–251). Cambridge: Cambridge University Press.

Reichman, W.E., Coyne, A.C., Amirneni, S., Molino, B., & Egan, S. (1996). Negative symptoms in Alzheimer's disease. *American Journal of Psychiatry, 153(3)*, 424–426.

Roca, R.P., Santmyer, K., Gloth, F.M., & Denman, S.J. (1990). Improvements in activity and appetite among long-term care patients treated with amantadine. A clinical report. *Journal of the American Geriatrics Society, 38(6)*, 675–677.

Rosenthal, T.L., & Meyer, V. (1971). Case report: Behavioral treatment of clinical abulia. *Conditional Reflex, 6(1)*, 22–29.

Ross, E.D., & Stewart, R.M. (1981). Akinetic mutism from hypothalamic damage: Successful treatment with dopamine antagonists. *Neurology, 31(11)*, 1435–1439.

Schultz, W., Apicella, P., Ljungberg, T., Romo, R., & Scarnati, E. (1993). Reward-related activity in the monkey striatum and substantia nigra. *Progress in Brain Research, 99*, 227–235.

Semlitsch, H.V., Anderer, P., & Saletu, B. (1992). Topographic mapping of long latency "cognitive" event-related potentials (P300): A double blind, placebo-controlled study with amantadine in mild dementia. *Journal of Neural Transmission. Parkinson's Disease and Dementia Section, 4*, 319–336.

Shallice, T., & Burgess, P.W. (1991). Deficits in strategy application following frontal lobe damage in man. *Brain, 114(2)*, 727–741.

Shammi, P., & Stuss, D.T. (1999). Humour in the right frontal lobe. *Brain, 122*, 657–666.

Snowden, J.S., Neary, D., & Mann, D.M.A. (1996). *Fronto-temporal Lobar Degeneration: Fronto-temporal Dementia, Progressive Aphasia, and Semantic Dementia.* New York: Churchill Livingstone.

Sohlberg, M.M., Mateer, C.A., & Stuss, D.T. (1993). Contemporary approaches to the management of executive control dysfunction. *Journal of Head Trauma Rehabilitation, 8*, 45–58.

Spiers, P.A., Schomer, D.L., Blume, H.W., Kleefield, J., O'Reilly, G., Weintraub, S., Osborne-Shaefer, P., & Mesulam, M.M. (1990). Visual neglect during intracarotid amobarbital testing. *Neurology, 40(10)*, 1600–1606.

Starkstein, S.E., Fedoroff, J.P., Price, T.R., Leiguarda, R., & Robinson, R.G. (1992). Anosognosia in patients with cerebrovascular lesions: A study of causative factors. *Stroke, 23(10)*, 1446–1453.

Strauss, M.E. (1993). Relation of symptoms to cognitive deficits in schizophrenia. *Schizophrenia Bulletin, 19(2)*, 215–231.

Stuss, D.T. (1987). Contribution of frontal lobe injury to cognitive impairment after closed head injury—Methods of assessment and recent findings. In H.S. Levin, J. Grafman, & H.M. Eisenberg (Eds.), *Neurobehavioral Recovery After Head Injury* (pp. 166–177). New York: Oxford University Press.

Stuss, D.T. (1991a). Disturbance of self-awareness after frontal system damage. In G. Prigatano & D. Schacter (Eds.), *Awareness of Deficit after Brain Injury: Clinical and Theoretical Issues* (pp. 63–83). New York: Oxford University Press.

Stuss, D.T. (1991b). Self, awareness, and the frontal lobes: A neuropsychological perspective. In J. Strauss & G.R. Goethals (Eds.), *The Self: Interdisciplinary Approaches* (pp. 255–278). New York: Springer-Verlag.

Stuss, D.T., Alexander, M.P., Hamer, L., Palumbo, C., Dempster, R., Binns, M., Levine, B., & Izukawa, D. (1998). The effects of focal anterior and posterior brain lesions on verbal fluency. *Journal of the International Neuropsychological Society, 4*, 265–278.

Stuss, D.T., Alexander, M.P., Palumbo, C.L., Buckle, L., et al. (1994a). Organizational strategies of patients with unilateral or bilateral frontal lobe injury in word list learning tasks. *Neuropsychology*, *8(3)*, 355–373.

Stuss, D.T., & Benson, D.F. (1986). *The Frontal Lobes*. New York: Raven Press.

Stuss, D.T., & Benson, D.F. (1987). The frontal lobes and control of cognition and memory. In E. Perecman (Ed.), *The Frontal Lobes Revisited* (pp. 141–158). New York: IRBN Press.

Stuss, D.T., Eskes, G.A., & Foster, J.K. (1994b). Experimental neuropsychological studies of frontal lobe functions. In F. Boller & J. Grafman, (Eds.), *Handbook of Neuropsychology*, Vol. 9 (pp. 149–185). Amsterdam: Elsevier.

Stuss, D.T., Gow, C.A., & Hetherington, C.R. (1992). "No longer Gage": Frontal lobe dysfunction and emotional changes. *Journal of Consulting and Clinical Psychology*, *60*, 349–359.

Stuss, D.T., Guberman, A., Nelson, R., & LaRochelle, S. (1988). The neuropsychology of paramedian thalamic infarction. *Brain and Cognition*, *8*, 348–378.

Stuss, D.T., Mateer, C., & Sohlberg, M.M. (1994c). Innovative approaches to frontal lobe deficits. In M.A.J. Finlayson & S.H. Garner (Eds.), *Brain Injury Rehabilitation*: *Clinical Considerations* (pp. 212–237). Baltimore: Williams & Wilkins.

Stuss, D.T., Picton, T.W., & Alexander, M.P. (1999). Consciousness, self awareness, and the frontal lobes. In S. Salloway, P. Malloy, & J. Duffy (Eds.), *The Frontal Lobes and Neuropsychiatric Illness*. Washington, DC: American Psychiatric Press.

Stuss, D.T., Shallice, T., Alexander, M.P., & Picton, T.W. (1995). A multidisciplinary approach to anterior attentional functions. *Annals of the New York Academy of Sciences*, *769*, 191–211.

Tanaka, Y., Yoshida, A., Kawahata, N., Hashimoto, R., & Obayashi, T. (1996). Diagnostic dyspraxia. Clinical characteristics, responsible lesion, and possible underlying mechanism. *Brain*, *119(3)*, 859–873.

Tatemichi, T.K., Desmond, D.W., Prohovnik, I., Cross, D.T., Gropen, T.I., Mohr, J.P., & Stern,Y. (1992). Confusion and memory loss from capsular genu infarctions: A thalamocortical disconnection syndrome? *Neurology*, *42(10)*, 1966–1979.

Tran, P.V., Hamilton, S.H., Kuntz, A.J., Potvin, J.H., Andersen, S.W., Beasley, C., Jr., & Tollefson, G.D. (1997). Double-blind comparison of olanzapine versus risperidone in the treatment of schizophrenia and other psychotic disorders. *Journal of Clinical Psychopharmacology*, *17(5)*, 407–418.

Troyer, A.K., Moscovitch, M., Winocur, G., Alexander, M.P., & Stuss, D.T. (1998). Clustering and switching on verbal fluency: The effects of focal frontal- and temporal-lobe lesions. *Neuropsychology*, *4*, 137–143.

Turkstra, L.S., & Bayles, K.A. (1992). Acquired mutism: Physiopathy and assessment. *Archives of Physical and Medical Rehabilitation*, *73(2)*, 138–144.

Van Reekum, R., Bayley, M., Garner, S., Burke, I.M., Fawcett, S., Hart, A., & Thompson, W. (1995). N of 1 study: Amantadine for the amotivational syndrome in a patient with traumatic brain injury. *Brain Injury*, *9(1)*, 49–53.

Volkow, N.D., Wang, G.J., Fowler, J.S., Logan, J., Angrist, B., Hitzemann, R., Lieberman, J., & Pappas, N. (1997). Effects of methylphenidate on regional brain glucose metabolism in humans: Relationship to dopamine D2 receptors. *American Journal of Psychiatry*, *154(1)*, 50–55.

Watanabe, M.D., Martin, E.M., DeLeon, O.A., Gaviria, M., Pavel, D.G., & Trepashko, D.W. (1995). Successful methylphenidate treatment of apathy after subcortical infarcts. *Journal of Neuropsychiatry and Clinical Neurosciences*, *7(4)*, 502–504.

Weinberg, R.M., Auerbach, S.H., & Moore, S. (1987). Pharmacologic treatment of cognitive deficits: A case study. *Brain Injury, 1(1)*, 57–59.

Wheeler, M.A., Stuss, D.T., & Tulving, E. (1997). Toward a theory of episodic memory: The frontal lobes and autonoetic consciousness. *Psychological Bulletin, 121(3)*, 331–354.

Williams, G.V., Rolls, E.T., Leonard, C.M., & Stern, C. (1993). Neuronal responses in the ventral striatum of the behaving macaque. *Behavioural Brain Research, 55*, 243–252.

Yasuda, Y., Akiguchi, I., Ino, M., Nabatabe, H., & Kameyama, M. (1990). Paramedian thalamic and midbrain infarcts associated with palilalia. *Journal of Neurology, Neurosurgery, and Psychiatry, 53(9)*, 797–799.

V

CLINICAL IMPLICATIONS

15

Neurological Disorders and Emotional Dysfunction

KENNETH M. HEILMAN, LEE X. BLONDER,
DAWN BOWERS, AND GREGORY P. CRUCIAN

The domain of emotion, as it has been conceptualized in behavioral neurology and neuropsychology, includes two major divisions: emotional experience and emotional behaviors. Whereas emotional experiences can be transient (happy, sad, angry, frightened, or surprised), emotional moods have a longer duration. Moods include depression, elation, agitation, and anxiety. Affective disorders can be considered emotional states that are chronic and pathological. Emotions can also be described in terms of their valence (positive or negative) and their level of arousal (low to high). Some have also drawn a distinction between primary emotions (e.g., happy, sad, angry, frightened) and social emotions (see Ross, Homan, & Buck, 1994), or those that derive from attachment (e.g., love, shame). There are several types of emotional behaviors including, autonomic–endocrine–visceral and communicative (verbal–semantic, facial, prosodic, and gestural–postural) with receptive and expressive components. Other dimensions of emotion include emotional imagery and emotional memory.

The brain is critical for mediating emotional experiences and behavior. Therefore, diseases that injure the brain may change both emotional experience and behavior. In this chapter, we discuss how diseases of the brain may affect emotional experience and emotional behavior. Diseases of the brain, like diseases in other parts of the body, may induce an emotional response. In addition, there are many diseases and conditions that can be induced or enhanced by emotional responses. Emotional response to diseases and emotionally induced diseases are not, however, unique to neurological disorders and are not discussed in this chapter.

The ideal chapter on how diseases of the brain affect emotional processes would first discuss how the brain mediates emotions in normal subjects. Unfortunately, the means by which the brain normally mediates emotion is not entirely known, and much of what we know comes from studies of patients with neurological disorders. Recently, functional imaging has added to our understanding of the role of the brain in emotions. There is also a rich literature on animal studies of emotional mediation. Unfortunately, it is unclear how much of this literature is relevant to the understanding of human emotion. Therefore, this chapter focuses primarily on observations of humans, but occasionally we refer to animal studies.

Based on the work of Papez (1937), it has been thought that the limbic circuits play a very important role in the mediation of emotional experience. Although subsequently many portions of the Papez circuit (e.g., hippocampus) have been demonstrated to be important for processes such as memory, recent work has demonstrated that other portions of the limbic system such as the amygdala are important for emotions in humans. The cerebral cortex and basal ganglia also play important roles. Many disorders of the basal ganglia, such as Parkinson's disease, are associated with neurotransmitter defects. Neurotransmitters are critical for the activation and modulation of cortical and limbic systems. The frontal lobes have strong connections not only with the limbic system and basal ganglia but also with other areas of the cortex that may be important in mediating emotions. Therefore, in addition to the posterior neocortex, the basal ganglia, portions of the limbic system, and the frontal lobes play critical roles in emotions. In this chapter, we discuss both the frontal and posterior neocortical, limbic, and basal ganglia disorders that are associated with changes of emotional experience or behavior, and based on these disorders, we discuss how the brain may mediate emotional communication and experience.

CORTICAL DYSFUNCTION

Left Hemisphere Damage

Communication deficits

Comprehension. Developing an appropriate emotion depends, in part, on communication with other people. Perhaps the two most important types of communication are speech and gestures, including facial expressions. Speech carries at least two types of messages, propositional and prosodic. Emotion can be conveyed by either words or prosody. The propositional or linguistic content is conveyed by a complex code that requires an auditory or visual process, phonemic or orthographic decoding, and lexical semantic analysis.

In most people, including left-handed people, the left hemisphere mediates propositional language. Therefore, injury particularly to the posterior portions of the left hemisphere may impair the comprehension of propositional speech. Patients with Wernicke's, transcortical sensory, global, or mixed transcortical aphasia may have difficulties in comprehending propositional speech. Patients with pure word deafness may also have problems understanding emotion that is based on verbal–propositional speech. Often these aphasic syndromes are associated with reading disorders or alexia. Alexia with or without aphasia may also impair the comprehension of written material that can induce or communicate emotion. Therefore, if the development of an appropriate emotional state depends on the comprehension of either spoken or written propositional language, patients with aphasia or alexia may be unable to develop the appropriate emotional state.

Although patients with comprehension disturbances may be unable to understand propositional messages, many are still able to understand emotional intonations (prosody) and emotional facies (Barrett et al., 1997; Kanter et al., 1986). When the propositional and prosodic messages are congruent, the addition of emotional prosody may help aphasic patients understand the propositional message (Bowers et al., 1987; Heilman, Scholes, & Watson, 1975).

Expression. Almost all patients with aphasia have problems expressing verbal–propositional messages. Many patients with aphasia also have difficulty writing their messages (agraphia). Agraphia, however, even in the absence of aphasia, may also impair written expression of language. Therefore, if the communication of emotion depends on propositional language, individuals with aphasia and agraphia may be impaired.

Hughlings Jackson (1932) noted that even severely, nonfluent aphasic patients with left hemisphere lesions could express their emotion by intoning simple recurrent utterances with prosodic emotional intonations. In addition, when nonfluent aphasic patients become angry or frustrated, it is not unusual for them to express their emotional feelings by using explicatives. Hughlings Jackson (1932) posited that perhaps it was the right hemisphere that was mediating these activities, and the role of the right hemisphere in expressing emotional intonations is discussed later. Roeltgen, Sevush, and Heilman (1983) demonstrated that patients with aphasia and agraphia could write emotional words better than nonemotional words. Although it appears that the left hemisphere is dominant in propositional speech, emotional words may be mediated by the right hemisphere and this will also be discussed in a later section.

Emotional experience and mood

Goldstein (1948) noted that patients with left hemisphere lesions often demonstrated an agitated or anxious depression. Goldstein called this emotional mood the "catastrophic reaction." Gainotti (1972) replicated Goldstein's observations. The catastrophic reaction is more likely to be seen with anterior than posterior left hemisphere lesions (Benson, 1979; Robinson & Sztela, 1981). We discuss the possible mechanisms of this mood change in a subsequent section.

Right Hemisphere Damage

Communication defects

Perceptual and comprehension disorders. As discussed, it appears that in most right-handed and left-handed people it is the left hemisphere that mediates the lexical–semantic processes important for speech. However, Borod and colleagues (1992) presented emotional and nonemotional tasks that included word identification, sentence identification, and word discrimination to right hemisphere–damaged (RHD) patients, left hemisphere–damaged (LHD) patients, and controls. They found that the RHD subjects were more impaired in the emotional condition than the LHD patients or the controls.

Speech, however, can convey another message that, unlike the message conveyed by words, is conveyed by changes in prosody, including the amplitude, pitch, timbre, and tonal contours of speech. During the last two to three decades there have been multiple studies that suggest patients with right temporal parietal damage have difficulty comprehending emotional prosody (Heilman, Scholes, & Watson, 1975; Heilman et al., 1984; Ross, 1981). In addition, as previously discussed, there have also been reports of patients with severe word comprehension deficits associated with disorders such as pure word deafness (Kanter et al., 1986) and global aphasia (Barrett et al., 1997), who, despite being unable to understand words, have been able to understand emotional prosody, thereby giving further support to the postulate that the right hemisphere has a dominant role in the comprehension of emotional prosody.

The mechanism underlying this prosodic hemispheric asymmetry is not entirely known. Patients with right hemisphere lesions, especially in the temporal parietal regions, may be unable to discriminate (same or different) between various emotional prosodies, suggesting that the deficit is not one of denotation or verbal–lexical labeling (Tucker, Watson, & Heilman, 1977). These findings suggest that the right hemisphere contains emotional prosodic representations and that these representations are stored in the right temporal parietal region. Therefore, injury to these representations may impair the comprehension of emotional prosody.

When involved in an emotional discussion with a significant other, we may have been told, "It's not what you said, but how you said it." In such cases, the propositional word message and the emotional prosodic message may be incongruent. When emotionally intoned sentences were presented to RHD and LHD patients, comprehension of emotional prosody was more disrupted by incongruent propositional content for RHD patients, whereas comprehension of the propositional content was more disrupted by the incongruent emotional prosody in LHD subjects (Bowers et al., 1987).

Gestures such as facial expressions are also important in emotional communication and appropriate development of the emotional state. Repeated studies have demonstrated that RHD patients are impaired in comprehending emotional facial expressions (Borod et al., 1986; Bowers et al., 1985; Cicone, Wapner, & Gardner, 1980; DeKosky et al., 1980; Schmitt, Hartje, Wilmes, 1997; Peper & Irle, 1997). It has also been demonstrated that this deficit cannot be accounted for by a purely lower level perceptual disorder (Blonder et al., 1993; Borod et al., 1998; Bowers et al., 1987) or a higher order semantic–conceptual deficit (Blonder et al., 1993). It is also not directly related to a face-processing deficit, and perhaps the best explanation of the deficit seen with these patients is that they have degraded emotional facial representations.

Support for this postulate comes from the observation that RHD subjects have a defect in imagery for emotional faces but not objects. In contrast, subjects with left-hemisphere disease have impaired imagery for objects but not emotional faces (Bowers et al., 1991). Stimulation studies of epileptic patients suggest that these emotional facial representations are stored in the posterior portion of the temporal lobe (Fried et al., 1982).

Expressive deficits. Bloom et al. (1990, 1993) and Borod et al. (2000) studied emotional and nonemotional discourse production, including the ability to use words to convey emotion, in patients with right-hemisphere and left-hemisphere lesions as well as normal controls. In the nonemotional condition, LHD subjects were particularly impaired, whereas in the emotional condition, RHD patients demonstrated deficits. Emotional content facilitated the pragmatic performance of LHD subjects.

The speech of patients with right-hemisphere disease often lacks emotional prosody (Ross, 1981; Tucker, Watson, & Heilman, 1977). This prosodic expressive deficit can be formally tested by asking patients to express neutral sentences with different emotional prosodies. Expressive deficits can exist with and without prosodic comprehension deficits (Ross & Mesulam, 1979). The patients who appear to have expressive but not comprehension deficits often have lesions in the anterior portions of the right hemisphere. Ross (1981) has suggested that an expressive–receptive dichotomy of emotional prosody associated with right-hemisphere lesions may parallel the manner in which the left-hemisphere lesions disrupt the comprehension and expression of propositional speech.

Patients with right-hemisphere dysfunction may have problems not only comprehending facial expressions but also expressing emotions using facial gestures. This has been demonstrated both in the laboratory (Buck & Duffy, 1980) and in natural situations (Blonder et al., 1993).

Emotional experience and mood

Patients with right cortical dysfunction may appear indifferent or even euphoric (Babinski, 1914; Gainotti, 1972). There are several mechanisms that may account for this profound indifference associated with right-hemisphere dysfunction. Although communicative defects may partially account for the indifference associated with right-hemisphere dysfunction, the changes in the mood associated with right-hemisphere dysfunction are included in the later discussion of mechanisms.

Emotional memory

To learn if patients with hemispheric dysfunction have specific problems with the acquisition of emotional memories or anterograde emotional memory deficits, Wechsler (1973) presented two stories to patients with right-hemisphere and left-hemisphere strokes. One story was designed to elicit an emotional response, and the other story contained little or no emotion. Whereas the patients with left-hemisphere lesions recalled more from the emotion-charged story than from the emotion-neutral story, the patients with right-hemisphere disease did not detect any difference between the stories, thereby suggesting that the emotional aspects of the story did not benefit their memory.

To study retrograde emotional memory deficits, Cimino and coworkers (1988) asked patients to tell stories about events that happened to them in the past. These stories were then given to judges who assessed the emotional content. These judges found that RHD patients' stories had less emotional content than did those of LHD patients. Borod et al. (1996) also studied recall of subjects' positive and negative emotional experiences and nonemotional experiences. Judges thought that the experiences described by the RHD subjects had less emotional intensity than those described by the LHD or normal subjects.

Somewhat different findings have been described by Bowers et al. (1998) who also examined the emotionality of autobiographical memories recalled by patients with focal hemispheric strokes. In that study, there was no explicit demand that subjects describe emotional memories per se. Rather, subjects were instructed merely to recall personal memories associated with specific cues words (i.e., the Crovitz paradigm). Content ratings by blinded judges revealed no overall differences in the types of emotional topics (e.g., weddings, death, and illness) covered by the stroke groups. The memories of the LHD group were, however, less intensely positive than were those of the RHD or control groups. There were no group differences in the intensity of negative memories. Because there was no evidence of depression according to various mood scales, it is difficult to attribute these valence asymmetries to the presence of depression per se. To account for these findings, one could posit that left-hemisphere lesions may alter the retrieval of information from semantic networks that are uniquely concerned with pleasant events. Lesions of the left hemisphere either directly hamper this process or create a mood bias whereby such networks are not readily primed.

The neuropsychological mechanisms accounting for the emotional anterograde and retrograde deficits described above remain unknown. One possibility is that the subjects with right-hemisphere disease have an expressive deficit. Although recall in these studies depended on propositional speech, as discussed above, patients with right-hemisphere disease may be impaired at expressing emotions even when using words. A second possibility is related to mood. When testing memory, subjects generally perform better with recognition than recall. Recognition paradigms provide subjects with cues that help activate the neural nets that store these memories. Depressed subjects will better recall sad than happy events (Yang & Rehm, 1993). This phenomenon has been termed *mood congruence*. Mood congruence may be a special form of cuing. Subjects with right-hemisphere lesions may perform poorer with emotional memory tests because they have a flattened affect, and emotional memories would be incongruent with their mood.

Bilateral Frontal Cortical Dysfunction

Neurological disorders can induce injuries to both sides of the brain. For example, trauma and tumors can injure both frontal lobes. Vascular diseases, especially of the anterior cerebral artery, may also induce bilateral lesions of the frontal lobes. Bilateral frontal lobe dysfunction may have profound effects on emotional behavior and experience. There have been many important case reports of patients who had bilateral frontal lobe lesions and had profound changes of emotional behavior and responses. These cases include the famous Gage described by Harlow (1868), Patient A described by Brickner (1934, 1936), and Ackerly and Benton's case along with the cases reported by Damasio and Anderson (1993). In general, these patients suffered with emotional indifference and apathy unless frustrated, when they would often become inappropriately aggressive.

There have been several studies with positron emission tomography (PET) of subjects with a history of aggressive behavior and violence (e.g., murderers). The studies revealed reduced activity in the frontal lobes (Raine et al., 1994; Volkow et al., 1995).

Normal people avoid stimuli or situations that have been know to produce emotions with negative valence (e.g., fear, anger, sadness, disgust) and to approach stimuli or situations that induce emotions of positive valence. Bilateral disorders of the frontal lobe may interfere with this process. Damasio and Anderson (1993) suggest that the response selection impairment is due to a "defect in the activation of somatic markers . . . that mark the ultimate consequences of the response option with a negative or positive somatic state." They also indicate that the frontal lobes are critical for this process and suggest that the orbital and lower mesial frontal regions may be the most important portion of the frontal lobes.

Corticobulbar Dysfunction

Bilateral dysfunction of the corticobulbar pathways may induce a pseudobulbar palsy. Associated with this pseudobulbar palsy may be involuntary emotional expressions. These abnormal emotional expressions are stereotypical and do not show degrees of intensity or a spectrum of emotional expressions. Usually, patients with pseudobulbar palsy either laugh, cry, or both. The latter is very similar to the cry of an infant who, even in the absence of neocortex, may cry. When patients express these emotions, however, they often are not experiencing the emotion that they are expressing.

It has been posited that bilateral interruption of the corticobulbar pathways release or disinhibit subcortical centers that mediate these emotional behaviors. Wilson (1924) suggested that this subcortical center was in the region of the pons, and Poeck (1969) suggested that these expressions are programmed in the diencephalon (hypothalamus and thalamus). Sackeim et al. (1982) noted that, although patients with pseudobulbar emotional expressions had bilateral lesions, those with larger left-hemisphere lesions were more likely to cry and those with right-sided lesions were more likely to laugh.

LIMBIC SYSTEM DYSFUNCTION

Emotional Communication

Unlike dysfunction of the cerebral cortex, emotional communication disorders are not frequently encountered with limbic dysfunction. Adolphs et al. (1994), however, described a woman who had bilateral damage to the amygdala and a concomitant disturbance in the processing of faces expressing fear. Although Young et al. (1995) found that identification of facial emotion was disturbed in their patient D.R. after partial bilateral amygdala ablation, other aspects of face processing were also impaired, including recognition of familiar faces and detection of direction of gaze on faces. Adolphs et al. (1994) also demonstrated that unilateral amygdala damage did not interfere with the processing of fearful faces and that bilateral lesions were necessary. In line with this observation, Bowers and colleagues (1999) examined 26 patients after anterior temporal resections involving approximately 45%–55% of the volume of the right or left amygdala. Relative to controls, these patients had no difficulty processing emotional faces, fearful or otherwise. These findings reinforce the view that unilateral amygdala lesions are not sufficient to disrupt the networks involved in the detection of fear/threat from nonverbal social signals.

Functional imaging studies in normal subjects have also provided converging evidence that the amygdala is important in the processing of fearful faces (Breiter et al., 1996; Irwin et al., 1996; Phillips et al., 1997). Amygdala activation has even been demonstrated with functional magnetic resonance imaging (fMRI) under conditions in which subjects are unaware that fearful faces have been briefly shown (Whalen et al., 1998). In this study, faces depicting fear or happiness were presented for 33 msec and were then immediately followed by masking stimuli consisting of neutral faces. Although the masking procedure inhibited subject's overt awareness of having viewed an emotional face, it nevertheless did not interfere with a process via which fearful, but not happy, faces differentially activated the amygdala.

Some evidence suggests that the amygdala's role in processing affective displays of fear or anger is not modality specific (Scott et al., 1997). Scott and coworkers (1997) examined their patient (D.R.) who had partial bilateral amygdala damage. Not only was this patient impaired at recognizing facial expressions of fear and anger (see Young et al., 1995), she was also impaired at recognizing vocal intonation patterns (prosody) associated with fear and anger. No hearing deficits existed to account for this prosody perception defect. Other investigators have reported disturbances in the recognition of nonverbal fear signals that may be modality specific. Ghika-Schmid et al. (1997) described a patient with bihippocampal damage (left more than right) whose recognition of vocal expressions of fear was selectively disrupted relative to other types of emotional prosody. The perception of fear faces was intact, although perception of other facial expressions was severely impaired (e.g., contempt, surprise).

Before final conclusions can be made about modality or category specificity of emotional processing, it is crucial to verify that comparable levels of difficulty existed among various facial and/or intonational emotion stimuli, both within and across modalities. Regarding prosody, it is equally important to examine a full range of auditory processing abilities, from basic acoustic to linguistic prosody tasks.

Emotional Experience

Paul Broca (1878) called a group of anatomically related structures on the medial wall of the cerebral hemispheres "le grand lobe limbique." Papez (1937) thought that a circuit in this limbic lobe that included the cingulate gyrus, hippocampus, fornix, mammillary bodies, and anterior thalamus was a core component of the central mechanisms subserving emotional feeling and expression. In part, Papez's postulate about the limbic system came from the knowledge that the hypothalamus was important in mediating rage responses (Bard, 1934). Subsequent studies have, however, revealed that lesions in several areas of the Papez circuit are associated with memory rather than emotional deficits.

Yakovlev (1948) posited that another brain circuit may be an important element of the limbic system. This basal lateral circuit includes the orbital frontal and insular cortex, the uncinate fasciculus, the anterior temporal cortex, the amygdala, and the dorsomedial nucleus of the thalamus. Kluver and Bucy (1937) demonstrated that bilateral ablation of the anterior temporal lobe, which interrupts this basal lateral limbic circuit of Yakovlev, changed aggressive rhesus monkeys into tame and placid animals. Akert et al. (1961) demonstrated that it was not the removal of temporal lobe cortex but rather of the amygdala that induced this tameness. Subsequent studies revealed that amygdala stimulation induced rage and that specific ablation induced placidity (Ursin, 1960; Woods, 1956). Investigators also demonstrated that the amygdala was important for fear, and a series of studies performed by Davis (1989) and LeDoux (1993) demonstrated that the amygdala was critical for fear conditioning.

Animal studies revealed that whereas septal lesions can cause a rage-like state (Brady & Nauta, 1955), septal stimulation can induce an extremely positive emotion (Olds, 1958). Some of the emotional changes described in animals with septal and amygdala lesions and stimulation have also been observed in humans. Tumors of the septal region in humans have been reported to cause rage-like attacks with increased irritability and agitation (Poeck & Pilleri, 1961; Zeman & King, 1958). In contrast, stimulation of the septal region has been reported to be pleasant and even sexually arousing (Heath, 1964). Bilateral temporal lesions in humans that included the amygdala have been reported to reduce rage and to induce placidity (Poeck, 1969). Morris and coworkers (1991) demonstrated that removal of the right amygdala reduces the experience and autonomic nervous system–visceral response to stimuli that before ablation induced emotions of negative valence. The experience and response to stimuli that induced emotions with positive valence was unchanged.

Viral and inflammatory diseases, such as herpes simplex, rabies, and limbic encephalitis may destroy portions of the limbic system and thus may be associated with many abnormal emotional behaviors, including depression, agitation, and anxiety. It is difficult to ascertain exactly how these diseases induce emotional changes.

Partial seizures with complex symptoms, also called *temporal lobe epilepsy* or *psychomotor seizures*, often start in limbic structures. These seizures may be associated with emotional symptoms. Emotional changes may be seen during a seizure. Mood changes may also be seen in epileptics even between seizures (the so-called interictal phenomenon). Gascon and Lombrosco (1971) described patients with temporal lobe seizures who laughed as part of their epileptic phenomena (gelastic seizures). All of Gascon and Lombrosco's patients had right-sided seizures. Chen and Forster (1973) described 10 patients who had gelastic seizures, but seven of the ten had left-sided seizures. Alternatively, some patients may cry during seizures. This is called *dacrystic epilepsy*. Unfortunately, these cases are so rare that clear lateralization has not been demonstrated. Offen et al. (1976) reviewed six patients with dacrystic epilepsy; four had right temporal dysfunction, one had left-sided dysfunction, and in one the locus was unknown.

The relationship between epilepsy and aggression remains unclear. Mark and Erwin (1970) and Pincus (1980) think that there is a relationship between temporal lobe epilepsy and aggression, but Stevens and Hermann (1981) note that there are no well-controlled studies to support this relationship. Of all the emotions reported with seizures, fear is the emotion most frequently reported (Williams, 1956). Ictal fear has been reported with both right and left temporal seizure foci (Strauss, Risser, & Jones, 1982). Within the temporal lobe, when fear is associated with a seizure, the amygdala appears to be the critical structure (Glore, 1972). Interictal abnormalities of mood appear to be frequently associated with patients who have temporal lobe epilepsy. The most common abnormalities appear to be anxiety and depression. Men with left-sided foci appear to have more fear than those with right-sided foci (Strauss, Risser, & Jones, 1982). In addition, patients with temporal lobe epilepsy seem to have a higher incidence of attempted or successful suicide than control subjects (Hawton, Fagg, & Marsack, 1980). Flor-Henry (1969) and Bear and Fedio (1977) demonstrated that interictally, patients with right hemisphere foci are more likely to show emotional changes such as sadness or elation.

Interictal aggressiveness, like aggressiveness during a seizure, remains controversial and continues to be a source of many medicolegal arguments. Although Taylor (1959) reported that temporal epileptics had a higher incidence of interictal aggression, Stevens and Hermann (1981), as previously discussed, noted that these observations have not been validated by detailed, controlled studies

BASAL GANGLIA DISEASES

Disorders of the basal ganglia are commonly thought to primarily induce defects in motor performance. Basal ganglia disorders are, however, known to affect both emotional experience and emotional communication. In some cases, the emotional changes associated with basal ganglia diseases can even precede the motor symptoms (e.g., Huntington's disease). In this section we review some of the emotional experiences and communicative changes associated with diseases of the basal ganglia and discuss the possible pathophysiologies of these changes.

Parkinson's Disease

Emotional communication

Facial expressions. One of the core symptoms of Parkinson's disease (PD) is the expressionless or "masked" face. Neurologists have long distinguished between disorders of volitional facial expression that result from lesions to the motor strip or corticobulbar projections and those of spontaneous facial expression that result from subcortical lesions, particularly those involving the basal ganglia. Thus, it has been observed that PD patients are able to make facial expressions to command but that spontaneous facial expression tends to be "flat" (Rinn, 1984). Two recent studies have, however, found diminished emotional facial expressivity even during posed conditions, suggesting that both systems are affected by PD (Borod et al., 1990; Jacobs et al., 1995a). Lack of facial expressivity is not thought to reflect depressed mood, as lack of expressivity is more prevalent than dysphoria among PD patients (Rinn, 1984). Furthermore, in two studies of spontaneous facial expressions, there was no correlation between depression scores and facial expressivity scores, again suggesting that diminished facial expressivity is not simply a function of depressed mood (Katsikitis & Pilowsky, 1991; Smith, Smith, & Ellgring, 1996).

Clinical observations of masked facies in PD patients have been confirmed by experimental studies. Buck and Duffy (1980) videotaped PD, LHD, and RHD patients and normal controls while each participant viewed a set of emotionally evocative slides. Raters then watched the videotapes and rated the subjects' emotional expressivity on a seven point scale. Results showed that RHD and PD patients were rated as significantly less expressive than LHD aphasics and normal controls.

Scott, Caird, and Williams (1984) found deficits in PD patients' ability to produce facial expressions of anger. Brozgold et al. (1998) found that PD patients showed significantly greater negative affect than controls while relating an unpleasant experience, yet were deficient in expressing positive affect while conveying a pleasant experience. Katsikitis and Pilowski (1988, 1991) used a microcomputer program to quantify facial expressions of PD patients who had observed a series of amusing slides. They found that PD patients smiled less frequently than did controls. Pitcairn et al. (1990) showed that PD patients produced a greater proportion of false smiles (smiles lacking a cheek raise) than did controls.

Smith, Smith, and Ellgring (1996) used the Facial Action Coding system developed by Ekman and Friesen (1978) to analyze both spontaneous and posed facial expressions. They found that PD patients displayed less emotional reactivity to emotionally laden film clips than did the normal control group.

Furthermore, in moderately affected PD patients, the intensity of spontaneous smiles was lower than the intensity of posed smiles. The findings of Smith, Smith, and Ellgring (1996) corroborate those of Pitcairn and collaborators (1990) in that the PD group produced fewer true or "felt" smiles than did the controls during the spontaneous condition. This loss of facial expressivity was not associated with diminished capacity to experience emotion, as Smith and colleagues found that patient ratings of subjective emotion experienced in response to the video clips were comparable, if not more intense, than ratings by controls.

Studies have also shown that PD patients are impaired in the perception of emotional facial expressions, although these results are less consistent. Blonder, Gur, and Gur (1989) found that PD patients could name or match facial emotions as well as the control group. When facial identity recognition versus facial emotion recognition were compared within the PD group, however, the investigators found that PD patients made significantly more errors in the emotional than in the nonemotional task. Within the controls, the two face tasks were performed comparably. Scott, Caird, and Williams (1984) found deficits in the ability of PD patients to recognize angry facial expressions. Jacobs et al. (1995b) discovered impairments in the ability to discriminate facial emotion among nondemented PD patients.

Prosody. A second channel of nonverbal communication of emotion that has received considerable attention over the last few decades is prosody, mainly intonation, stress, and timing. Disorders of prosody, particularly monopitch and loss of volume in the voice, are characteristic of parkinsonian speech. These findings have been observed both clinically and experimentally. For example, Darley, Aronson, and Brown (1969) performed a judgment study of speech characteristics in PD and found that monopitch, monoloudness, and increased rate were among the most pronounced prosodic abnormalities. Acoustic analyses of parkinsonian speech have also found evidence of monotone production (Canter, 1963; Kent & Rosenbek, 1982).

Many consider that speech disorders in PD are related to defects of motor programing. Prosodic disturbances in PD may, however, have an emotional dimension. Scott, Caird, and Williams (1984) found that PD patients had difficulty producing anger through prosody. Blonder, Gur, and Gur (1989) found that PD patients' ability to convey different emotions through prosody was judged to be impaired, and the intensity of their emotional prosody was also rated as less expressive than that of normal controls. Similar results were found by Borod et al. (1990). This evidence supports the idea that parkinsonian prosody compromises patients' ability to express emotion through the voice. Scott, Caird, and Williams (1984), Blonder, Gur, and Gur (1989), and Borod et al. (1990) found that PD patients were also impaired in their ability to comprehend emotion conveyed through prosodic intonations.

Emotional experience

Although PD is characterized by akinesia, a resting tremor, and rigidity, Parkinson (1817) noted that his patients were often unhappy. There are now many reports in the literature documenting depression in patients with PD (Brown et al., 1988; Gotham, Brown, & Marsden, 1986; Liu et al., 1997; Mayeux et al., 1981, 1984; Vogel, 1982; for review, see Cummings, 1992). Cummings (1992) estimates that depression occurs in approximately 40% of PD patients. Of those, about half have major depression.

Some studies suggest that depression in PD patients may have a reactive component. As discussed by Lindgren (1996), PD is associated with continual loss of function during the illness that can affect not only patients but also their spouses, producing states of "chronic sorrow." Gotham, Brown, and Marsden (1986) compared PD patients, arthritis sufferers, and normal controls on measures of depression and found that both the PD patients and the arthritis sufferers were depressed. In addition, depression in both patient groups was similar in that it was characterized by pessimism, hopelessness, decreased motivation, and increased concerns regarding health. Despite these data, the bulk of the evidence indicates that depression in PD is most likely due to depletion of brain catecholamines and serotonin, dysregulation of frontal subcortical connections involved in emotion regulation, or a combination these processes.

The depression associated with PD is atypical. Schiffer et al. (1988) applied Research Diagnostic Criteria to 16 depressed PD patients and 20 depressed patients with multiple sclerosis and found that the depression in the PD patients was often accompanied by anxiety and panic. Stein et al. (1990) found that 38% of the PD patients in their sample of 24 met *Diagnostic and Statistical Manual of Mental Disorders*, third edition, revised (DSM-III-R), criteria for a diagnosis of a concurrent anxiety disorder. This rate exceeds that found in the general population as well as in individuals with chronic medical conditions. These authors also note that there were no differences in disease severity between the anxious PD patients and those who lacked anxiety disorders, suggesting that anxiety is not simply a reaction to disability.

As discussed earlier with regard to cortical dysfunction, whereas patients with left hemisphere disease are often depressed, those with right hemisphere dysfunction are often indifferent or even euphoric. Several studies have examined the relationship between mood and laterality of parkinsonian motor symptoms. Neither Barber et al. (1985), Blonder, Gur, and Gur (1989), nor St. Clair et al. (1998) found differences in self-reported depression between right and left hemiparkinson patients. Fleminger (1991), however, showed that symptoms of atypical depression (i.e., depression with relatively little anhedonia and prominent anxiety) were increased fivefold in patients with left hemiparkinsonism, suggesting right basal ganglia dysfunction. Fleminger's finding is contradicted in a study by Starkstein et al. (1988), who found depression following left but not right basal ganglia infarcts. This finding is also inconsistent with the reports of emotional changes associated with cortical dysfunction that we previously discussed.

One problem associated with the diagnosis of depression in patients with PD is that many instruments used to measure depression confound the symptoms of physical illness and normal aging with those of dysphoria. For example, the Beck Depression Inventory, reported by Cummings (1992) to be the instrument most widely used to measure depression in PD patients, includes both somatic and ideational items. When Direnfield et al. (1984) excluded items associated with neurologic symptomatology from the Beck Depression Inventory, they found that PD patients, those suffering from Alzheimer's disease, and hospitalized controls exhibited no differences in dysphoria. In a study by Blonder, Gur, and Gur (1989), PD patients' scores on the Zung Depression Inventory were significantly higher (more depressed) than those of age-matched controls when somatic indicators were included. When these items were excluded, there were no statistically significant between-group differences. In contrast, Levin, Llabre, and Weiner (1988) performed internal consistency reliability analyses of the Beck Depression Inventory in 119 PD patients and 76 controls and found that the instrument was a valid measure of dysphoric mood in the PD patients.

From a neuropharmacological perspective, it is not surprising that PD patients show symptoms of dysphoria. It is well documented that these patients have depletion of brain norepinephrine and serotonin (Scatton et al., 1983). Norepinephrine and serotonin were initially implicated as etiological agents in depressive mood when hypertensive patients receiving reserpine therapy developed dysphoria (Lemieux, Davignon, & Genest, 1956). Reserpine acts by depleting central and peripheral norepinephrine and serotonin. Chan-Palay and Assan (1989) found extensive cell loss in the rostral and caudal portions of the locus coeruleus of depressed PD patients while those who had not been depressed showed relative sparing of caudal neurons. These findings implicate noradrenergic systems in the etiology of parkinsonian depression. The involvement of these neurotransmitters in mood is further substantiated by the therapeutic efficacy of monoamine oxidase inhibitors, tricyclic compounds, and selective serotonin reuptake inhibitors (SSRIs) in the treatment of depression associated with PD.

Several studies have evaluated the effects of levodopa on patients' mood and yielded somewhat inconsistent findings (see Mayeux, 1983). Spigset and von Scheele (1997) reported two patients who increased their own dosage of levodopa to 1500–2000 mg/day to induce feelings of euphoria. Maricle et al. (1995) found that mood elevation, anxiety reduction, and a corresponding increase in tapping speed were related to levodopa but not to placebo infusion in a sample of PD patients.

Price, Farley, and Hornykiewicz (1978) showed that PD patients have significantly reduced levels of dopamine in the limbic paraolfactory gyrus and the nucleus accumbens. These levels correlate with the amount of dopamine reduction in the neostriatum. There is also evidence that the dopaminergic innervation of these limbic structures may be anatomically related to the nigrostriatal fiber system. Investigators have proposed that degeneration of dopaminergic terminals in the ventral tegmental region underlies parkinsonian mood disorders, and interindividual differences in the extent to which this system is involved may explain variability in the incidence of depression in PD (Cantello et al., 1989). How changes in neurotransmitter systems induce changes in mood, however, remains to be determined.

Huntington's Disease

Emotional communication

Published studies of facial processing in patients with Huntington's disease (HD) are limited to perception. Jacobs et al. (1995b) administered tests of emotional and nonemotional facial perception to five patients with HD and found impaired performance. They suggest that these deficits may be related to degeneration of the tail of the caudate in HD. Sprengelmeyer et al. (1996) found that HD patients were impaired in the recognition of surprised, fearful, sad, angry, and disgusted facial expressions, with severe deficits in the recognition of disgust. They attribute this profound impairment in disgust recognition to HD-associated atrophy in paleocortical regions, including the periamygdalar and pyriform cortex. More recently, Phillips et al. (1997) showed fMRI activation of the anterior insula during the perception of disgusted faces by normal individuals. This region is connected to a limbic–striatal–thalamic circuit. This finding may explain the loss of recognition of disgust by HD patients. The amygdala is known to atrophy in HD and, as discussed with regard to the limbic system, this region has been associated with the processing of emotional facial expressions. Emotional prosody has not been fully studied in patients with HD. Speedie et al. (1990), however, reported that patients with HD were also impaired in the comprehension of prosodic signals.

Emotional experience

Huntington's disease or Huntington's chorea is characterized by involuntary dance-like movements and intellectual decline. Huntington (1872) reported that many patients with this disease have emotional disorders and that there was a high rate of suicide associated with the disorder. Emotional dysfunction is highly prevalent in HD. Mayeux (1983) estimates that most if not all patients with HD manifest some type of emotional disorder, including apathy or irritability, depression, manic-depression, agitation, hostility, aggression, promiscuity, and suicidal behavior (see also Brothers, 1964; Folstein, Folstein, & McHugh, 1979; Mayberg et al., 1992; Mayeux et al., 1981). Emotional changes may precede the motor or cognitive symptoms, suggesting that cerebral dysfunction and not reactive disorders is responsible

(Heathfield, 1967; Kosky, 1981). In addition, different emotional symptoms may be seen during different stages of the disease. Apathy usually occurs late in the disease when there are intellectual deterioration and signs of frontal lobe dysfunction.

When Mayberg et al. (1992) measured regional cerebral glucose metabolism in depressed and nondepressed HD patients and normal controls, they found that both groups of HD patients had reductions in caudate, putamen, and cingulate metabolism. The depressed HD patients were distinguished from their nondepressed counterparts by orbital–frontal–inferior prefrontal hypometabolism, implicating paralimbic frontal regions in mood disturbance. This pattern has also been observed in depressed PD patients (Mayberg et al., 1990).

Ranen et al. (1996) noted complete cessation of severe irritability and aggression in two HD patients after treatment with an SSRI. SSRIs, as well as tricyclic antidepressants, have been used to treat depression in HD. Bipolar disorders and apathy have also been treated with lithium and butyrophenone. Although neurotransmitters such as gamma-aminobutyric acid and acetylcholine are reduced in the basal ganglia, the mechanisms underlying the mood changes associated with this disease remain unknown.

Progressive Supranuclear Palsy

Patients with progressive supranuclear palsey (PSP) have akinesia and axial rigidity similar to that seen with PD. These patients do not, however, have a resting tremor, but do have supranuclear palsies of their cranial nerves. For example, PSP, patients may be impaired in looking up or down to command. When the head is rapidly flexed and extended, however, the eye may then move up and down (ocular cephalic reflex).

When Steele, Richardson, and Olszewski (1964) first reported this disorder, they noted that their patients were often irritable. Like other patients with diseases that involve the basal ganglia, however, patients with PSP may also have apathy and depression. Litvan et al. (1996) examined emotional disorders in 22 patients with PSP, and found that 91% exhibited apathy, 18% dysphoria, and 18% anxiety. Menza, Cocchiola, and Golbe (1995) found that 42% of the PSP patients suffered from mild depression or anxiety and that these rates were comparable to those found in the PD group. Both cognitive and functional imaging studies of PSP patients show evidence of frontal lobe dysfunction (Blin et al., 1990; Grafman et al., 1990). Litvan et al. (1996) attribute the high incidence of apathy in their sample of PSP patients to dysfunction in the medial frontal/subcortical system.

Wilson's Disease

Wilson's disease (WD) is principally characterized by neuropathological changes in the putamen and globus pallidus, although other structures are also affected. Patients with WD may exhibit tremors, athetoid movements, and dysarthria. A significant proportion of patients with WD are reported to have emotional disturbances, including depression, anxiety, aggression, and personality changes (Dening & Berrios 1989; Rathbun, 1996; Sternleib & Scheinberg, 1964). In Rathbun's series (1996), 50% of the WD patients had been hospitalized for psychiatric disorders before they were diagnosed with WD, reaffirming the importance of thorough neurological and medical examinations of patients with psychiatric disorders. Dening and Berrios (1989) found a correlation between psychiatric and neurological symptoms but not between psychiatric and hepatic symptoms, suggesting that the emotional changes accompanying WD are primarily related to brain dysfunction and not a psychological reaction to their disease.

Striatonigral Degeneration

Garcia-Campayo and Sanz-Carrillo (1994) reviewed the scant literature on psychiatric disorders accompanying striatonigral degeneration (SND), a syndrome that resembles PD but usually is not associated with tremor and responds less well to the dopaminergic medication than do patients with PD. Neuropathologically, SND is characterized by neuronal loss in the putamen, globus pallidus, and substantia nigra. Previous published reports of mood changes associated with this disorder include depression (Bannister & Oppenheimer, 1972; Fearnley & Lees, 1990; Feve et al., 1977), anxiety (Scully, Mark, & McNeely, 1983), and emotional lability (Fearnley & Lees, 1990).

Garcia-Campayo and Sanz-Carrillo (1994) reported a patient who initially presented with major depression with no neurologic symptoms or signs. The depression was successfully treated with imipramine. Several months later, the patient developed an unsteady gait and suffered repeated falls and a recurrence of depression. Neurological examination revealed extrapyramidal motor symptoms, and an MRI scan showed putamenal atrophy. The diagnosis of SND was confirmed 2 years later when the patient came to autopsy. Garcia-Campayo and Sanz-Carrillo (1994) suggest that, as in PD, dysfunction in neurotransmitter systems involved in mood regulation may lead to emotional disturbance in SND.

Other Basal Ganglia Disorders

Emotional communication

Cancelliere and Kertesz (1990) mapped cerebral infarcts on CT scans and found that most individuals with deficits in the comprehension of facial affect had sustained damage to the basal ganglia and the anterior temporal lobe, suggesting basal ganglia involvement in facial affect perception.

Emotional experience

Sydenham's chorea, which may be seen with diseases such as rheumatic fever and systemic lupus, may also be associated with irritability and apathy. Trautner et al. (1988) report affective disorders in five patients with idiopathic basal ganglia calcification. Four of the five patients had unipolar depression, whereas the fifth was described as hypomanic. They also review previous reports of mood disorders in patients with calcification of the basal ganglia.

Starkstein et al. (1988) compared mood in stroke patients whose infarcts were confined to either the left or right basal ganglia or to the left or right thalamus and found that the patients with left-sided lesions of the basal ganglia had a higher frequency and severity of depression than did any of the other groups. Seven of eight patients with left-sided basal ganglia lesions showed major depression, whereas only one of seven patients with right-sided basal ganglia lesions had major depression. Furthermore, none of the patients with restricted thalamic lesions showed major depression.

Affective Disorders and Basal Ganglia Dysfunction

There have been several studies of basal ganglia function in patients with primary affective disorders. For example, some investigators have shown reductions in putamenal or caudate volumes in patients who suffer from major depression (Husain et al., 1991; Krishnan et al., 1992). Figiel et al. (1991) found a higher number of caudate hyperintensities in patients with late onset unipolar depression than in patients with early onset unipolar depression. These subjects had no past history of any disease associated with subcortical structural changes on MRI.

Results from studies of basal ganglia dysfunction in patients with bipolar disorder are inconsistent. Swayze et al. (1992) did not find differences in caudate or putamenal volumes between bipolar subjects and normal controls. Aylward et al. (1994) found that males with bipolar disorder had larger caudate volumes than did normal control males. Sharma et al. (1992) examined patients with bipolar disorder who were being treated with lithium. Proton magnetic resonance spectroscopy showed changes in the metabolite ratios in the basal ganglia spectra. These findings may have been due to either the action of lithium or the relationship of bipolar disorder itself and basal ganglia dysfunction.

POSSIBLE MECHANISMS OF EMOTIONAL COMMUNICATION DISORDERS

Studies of patients with left-hemisphere dysfunction have demonstrated that their verbal lexicon (auditory word images) and semantics (meaning) are dissociable. Whereas the left hemisphere contains a verbal lexicon and verbal semantics, perhaps the right hemisphere contains prototypic facial iconic and prosodic echoic emotional representations, as well as emotional semantics. To test this postulate, Blonder, Bowers, and Heilman (1991) examined subjects with right-hemisphere and left-hemisphere damage by presenting them with sentences, generated by a computer, that described either an emotional gesture (e.g., emotional face) or a scene that may induce an emotion (e.g., the children tracked mud all over new white carpet). Compared with both left-hemisphere damage and control subjects, the subjects with right-hemisphere damage did well noting the emotion associated with the description of scenes that was designed to test their emotional semantics. In contrast, the subjects with right-hemisphere damage performed poorly in recognizing the description of emotional gestures. These results cannot be explained by a visuospatial defect because the stimuli were verbal. These results suggest an iconic representational defect.

Further evidence that RHD subjects have an emotional facial iconic defect comes from a study by Bowers et al. (1991). If patients have lost their representations of prototypic emotional facial expressions, they should not only fail to recognize emotional faces and be unable to recognize descriptions of emotional faces but they also should not be able to image emotional faces. Bowers et al. (1991) demonstrated that RHD subjects could image objects, but they could not image emotional faces. In contrast, LHD subjects could image emotional faces but not objects.

Although we presented evidence that the representations of emotional faces may be stored in a sensory–iconic form, there is an alternative possibility. When subjects are asked that when they use a screw driver to remove a screw, do they rotate their arm in a clockwise or a counterclockwise direction, most subjects report that when they attempted to answer this question they had to covertly move their arm. Functional imaging studies have also demonstrated that when subjects are asked to think about making a movement without actually making the movement, their premotor cortex demonstrates activation.

Patients with PD often have mask-like faces and often do not spontaneously express facial emotions. To test this motor representational hypothesis, we studied PD patients' ability to image and comprehend emotional faces. Compared with control subjects, patients with PD were impaired (Jacobs et al., 1995a). These observations suggest that to comprehend or image an emotional face, one may have to activate motor representations.

Patients with emotional face discrimination and comprehension defects often have coexisting problems in discriminating and comprehending emotional prosody. It has been estimated that approximately 40%–45% of RHD patients are impaired on both face and prosody affect tasks versus 22% of LHD patients (Bowers et al., 1996). Dissociations between the ability to perceive facial affect versus the ability to perceive emotional prosody have been clinically described (Ross, 1981). To determine the frequency of modality-specific disturbances in a large population, Bowers et al. (1996) examined 105 patients with MRI-verified ischemic hemispheric lesions using the Florida Affect Battery. This battery consists of facial, prosodic, and cross-modal tasks designed to identify general and specific subtypes of affect disturbance (modality-specific, anomic, and agnosic variants). Approximately 22% of the RHD patients were uniquely impaired on face perception tasks versus 2% of the left hemisphere group. Of note, relatively few patients were found to have an "isolated" prosody perception defect, and the lesions in these "pure cases" included ones in the insula and temporal region. Taken together, these observations suggest that prosodic and facial emotional representations are, in part, independent.

Darwin believed that the means by which we express emotions are innate. If the facial expression of emotion is innate, there should be little or no difference in emotional expression across cultures. To learn if the expression of emotion is innate, Izard (1977) and Ekman, Sorenson, and Freisen (1969) performed cross-cultural studies of facial emotional expression and found that the same seven to nine emotional facial expressions appeared to be universal, thereby providing support for Darwin's hypothesis that emotional expressions are innate. Therefore, unlike the left hemisphere's phonological or orthographic lexicon, which is culturally specific and therefore learned, the right hemisphere's emotional representations may be primarily inborn rather than learned.

POSSIBLE MECHANISMS OF EMOTIONAL EXPERIENCE

As discussed earlier, dysfunction of the cortex, limbic system, and basal ganglia induces changes in emotional experience and mood. In this section we explore the possible mechanisms. We briefly review the classic feedback and central theories and the more recent revisions of these theories. Then, based on the changes in emotional experience and mood associated with neurological disorders, we attempt to develop a model of how the brain mediates emotional experience.

Feedback Theories

Facial feedback hypothesis

Darwin (1872) noted that, "He who gives violent gesture increases his rage." Tomkins (1962, 1963) posited that it was the feedback of these facial emotions to the brain that induced emotional feeling. Many of the patients we discussed who have right-hemisphere dysfunction have a reduced ability to express facial emotions and also are emotionally indifferent, thereby providing some support to the facial feedback hypothesis. Laird (1974) experimentally manipulated facial expressions and found that subjects felt emotions, providing support for the facial feedback hypothesis. There are, however, many unresolved problems with the facial feedback theory of emotional experience.

One of the major problems is that it is, at least in part, circular. If facial feedback induces emotional experience, what induces facial emotion? Second, we recently had the opportunity to examine and test a young woman who had Guillian-Barré syndrome. This is a neuropathy that can affect the cranial nerves. During her disease, the patient had total facial paralysis. When presented with a set of standardized slides that have been shown to evoke emotional experience and responses in normal subjects (Greenwald, Cook, & Lang, 1989), this woman's emotional responses were the same as those of the controls. After she recovered full facial mobility she was tested again, and her emotional experiences to these slides were unchanged from her previous test results (Keillor et al., 1999). Also unsupportive of the facial feedback hypothesis of emotional experience is the observation that patients with pseudobulbar palsy may express strong facial emotions that they are not feeling (Poeck, 1969). It is possible, however, that these patients' brain lesions also interrupt facial feedback to the brain. As we discussed, patients with PD and parkinsonian symptoms may have a mask-like face but feel sad and depressed.

Visceral feedback hypotheses

William James (1890) proposed that stimuli that provoke emotion induce changes in the viscera and autonomic nervous system and that it is the self-perception of these visceral changes that produces emotional experience. To have visceral feedback, one needs efferent and afferent systems. The autonomic nervous system has two components, the sympathetic and parasympathetic. The descending sympathetic neurons receive projections from the hypothalamus, and the hypothalamus receives projections from many limbic and paralimbic areas, including the amygdala. The most important parasympathetic nerve is the vagus. The vagus originates in the dorsal motor nucleus situated in the brain stem and projects to the viscera such as the heart. The amygdala not only projects to the hypothalamus but also sends direct projections to the nucleus of the solitary tract and the dorsal motor nucleus of the vagus. In this manner, the amygdala may directly influence the parasympathetic system. The amygdala receives neocortical input. Although the amygdala may be the most important part of the limbic system to influence autonomic nervous system and viscera, stimulation of other areas, including the insula and orbitofrontal cortex, can also induce autonomic and visceral changes, and these structures also receive input from the neocortex.

With regard to feedback, the major nerve that carries visceral afferent information back to the brain is the vagus. These afferents terminate in the nucleus of the solitary tract, which projects to the central nucleus of the amygdala. The central nucleus of the amygdala projects to other amygdala nuclei and the insula. The amygdala and insula, in turn, project to the temporal, parietal, and frontal lobes.

As we discussed above, in humans the neocortex and limbic cortex plays a critical role in the analysis and interpretation of various stimuli. Luria and Simernitskaya (1977) thought that the right hemisphere may be more important than the left in perceiving visceral changes. James' feedback theory was challenged by Cannon (1927), who thought that the viscera have insufficient afferent input to the brain to be important in inducing emotional experience. Using a heartbeat detection paradigm, Katkin et al. (1982) found that normal subjects can accurately detect their heartbeat. They also reported that the subjects who had the strongest emotional responses to negative slides were the subjects who were best able to detect their own heartbeat (Hantas, Katkin, & Blasovich, 1982).

Cannon (1927) also argued that the separation of the viscera from the brain that occurs with cervical spinal cord injuries does not eliminate emotional experience. Hohmann (1966), however, studied patients with spinal cord injuries at different levels and found that patients with either high or low spinal cord transection did experience emotions, but patients with lower lesions reported stronger emotions than those with higher lesions. Higher cervical lesions would be more likely to affect efferent control of the viscera and injure the autonomic nervous system's afferent output. Therefore, Hohmann's observations provide partial support for the visceral feedback theory. Cannon (1927) thought that because the same visceral responses occur with different emotions, feedback of these visceral responses could not account for the variety of emotions that humans experience. Ax (1953) and others have, however, demonstrated that different visceral–autonomic reactions are associated with different emotions.

Although many of Cannon's objections (1927) to the visceral feedback theory could be refuted, there are still observations that are inconsistent with this theory. Marañon (1924) injected epinephrine into normal subjects. Epinephrine does not cross the blood–brain barrier but does affect the autonomic nervous system and viscera, inducing increased activity of the heart. After the injection with visceral–autonomic activation, Marañon inquired as to the nature of the emotion felt by these subjects and found that injections of epinephrine were not associated with emotional experience but rather with "as if" feelings.

Because visceral–autonomic activation, by itself, did not induce an emotional experience, Schacter and Singer (1962) posited that another element is needed to induce emotions. Schachter and Singer (1962) also injected epinephrine into experimental subjects and reported that pharmacologically induced autonomic and visceral activation did not, by itself, produce an emotion. When this injection with visceral–autonomic activation was accompanied with an appropriate cognitive set, however, an emotion could be induced. Some cognitive sets may, by themselves, produce an emotion. Schacter and Singer (1962), however, found that the emotion induced by a cognitive set was stronger in the subjects who received epinephrine than in those who did not receive epinephrine.

Although Schachter and Singer's study (1962) suggested that visceral feedback together with centrally mediated cognition are important for emotional experience, observations in our laboratory do not entirely support these findings. Recently, we attempted to further test the autonomic–visceral feedback theory and to learn if, as suggested by Luria and Simernitskaya (1977), the right hemisphere plays a dominant role in perceiving visceral changes. Using a shock anticipation paradigm in brain-lesioned subjects, we found that, compared with normal control subjects, patients with right-hemisphere lesions had a reduced autonomic response. Although their autonomic response was reduced, they showed no differences in the experience of anticipatory anxiety (Slomine, 1995). In addition, in the clinic one can see patients who have strong emotions (e.g., fear) associated with medial temporal lobe or amygdala seizures. Sometimes patients become aware that they are beginning to have a seizure, and the fear of having a seizure may lead to a fearful cognitive set. Autonomic and visceral changes may be associated with these partial seizures, and the patients may be aware of these changes and therefore experience fear. In many epileptic patients, however, the emotional experience is often the first symptom or aura. Therefore, in these patients, cognitive set comes after the experience rather than before the experience. Schachter and Singer's attribution theory (1962) cannot account for these observations.

The studies we have discussed do not preclude the possibility that visceral and facial feedback play some role in emotional experience. Although feedback may influence emotional experience, the evidence we reviewed suggests that feedback does not play a critical role in emotional experience. In addition, the feedback theories cannot explain the mood changes induced by neurological diseases.

Central Theories

Subcortical (diencephalic) theories

To account for emotional experience, Walter Cannon (1927) proposed that afferent stimuli enter the brain and are transmitted from the thalamus to the hypothalamus. The hypothalamus activates the endocrine and autonomic nervous system, and it is these systems that induce the physiological changes in the viscera. These autonomic and visceral changes are primarily adaptive and aid in the survival of the organism. Emotional experience is induced by the hypothalamus feeding back to the cortex.

LeDoux and coworkers (1990) have modified Cannon's (1927) thalamic–hypothalamic emotion circuit to include the amygdala in fear conditioning. These investigators conditioned animals by associating a nociceptive stimulus with an auditory stimulus. Although ablation of the auditory thalamus and amygdala interrupted the behavioral emotional response to the conditioned stimulus, ablation of the auditory cortex did not. Therefore, LeDoux et al. (1990), like Cannon (1927), do not propose a critical role for the cortex in the interpretation of stimuli in the mediation of emotional experience. Whereas conditioned stimuli similar to those used by LeDoux et al. (1990) may induce emotion without cortical interpretation, as we discussed, there is overwhelming evidence that in humans the neocortex is critical for interpreting the meaning of many stimuli that induce an emotional experience. The diencephalic–hypothalamic theory of Cannon (1927) and the diencephalic–limbic (amygdala) theory of LeDoux et al. (1990) also fail to explain how humans can experience a variety of emotions.

Modular theory

There are at least two ways in which the brain may mediate a variety of emotional experiences. One possibility is that the brain may contain specialized or devoted emotional systems for each emotional experience such that each emotion is uniquely mediated. Therefore, there would be a special system for fear, anger, happiness, and so forth. A second possibility is that each emotion is not uniquely mediated but that the neural apparatus that mediates one emotion may not only play a role in other emotions but also mediate nonemotional functions.

The second or nondevoted systems postulate is consistent with the "dimensional" view of emotion. Wundt (1903) proposed that emotional experiences vary in three dimensions, quality, activity, and excitement (arousal). Osgood, Suci, and Tannenbaum (1957) performed factor analyses on verbal assessments of emotional judgements and found that the variance could be accounted for by three major dimensions: valence (positive/negative, pleasant/unpleasant), arousal (calm/excited), and control or dominance (in control/out of control). Using this type of multidimensional view, one can define the different emotional experiences by using one or more of these three dimensions. For example, fear would be unpleasant; high arousal, out of control; and sadness could be unpleasant and low arousal. Psychophysiological studies with normal subjects have supported this dimensional view (Greenwald, Cook, & Lang, 1989). Frijda (1987) also explored the cognitive structure of emotion and found that "action readiness" was an important component or dimension.

Heilman (1994, 1997) posited that conscious experience of emotion may be mediated by anatomically distributed modular networks. This distributed network has three major modules: one that helps determine the valence, a second that controls arousal, and a third that mediates motor activation with either approach or avoidance behaviors.

Valence. In prior sections we discussed the studies that demonstrated that whereas people with left-hemisphere lesions are often sad and anxious, those with right-hemisphere lesions often appear indifferent or euphoric. Gainotti (1972) proposed that patients' psychological response to their own illness may account for some of the emotional asymmetries observed between patients with right-hemisphere and left-hemisphere lesions. Whereas patients with left-hemisphere disease are often aphasic and have a hemiparesis of their preferred hand, those with right-hemisphere damage often are unaware of their disabilities (anosognosia). Other observations are not, however, consistent with this reaction postulate.

Terzian (1964) and Rossi and Rosadini (1967) studied the emotional reactions of patients recovering from selective hemispheric barbiturate-induced anesthesia (the Wada test). These investigators noted that whereas barbiturate injections into the left carotid artery were often associated with catastrophic reactions, injections into the right hemisphere were associated with indifference or euphoria. Because the Wada test is a diagnostic study that only causes transient hemiparesis and aphasia, it is unlikely that it would cause a reactive depression. In addition, we have seen RHD stroke patients who are emotionally indifferent but who are aware of their deficits and do not demonstrate anosognosia or verbally explicit denial of illness.

The catastrophic–depressive reaction associated with left-hemisphere lesions is seen most commonly in patients who have anterior (frontal) perisylvian lesions (Benson, 1979; Robinson & Sztela 1981). It is possible that the hemispheric emotional asymmetries reported by Gainotti (1972) and others are related to emotional communication disorders associated with frontal lesions, as discussed earlier, rather than differences in emotional experience. Although defects in emotional expression may account for some of the behavioral observations by Goldstein (1948), Babinski (1914), and Gainotti (1972), they cannot explain the results of Gasparrini et al. (1978), who administered the Minnesota Multiphasic Inventory to a group of LHD and RHD patients. The LHD patients were not severely aphasic, and the RHD and LHD patients were balanced for cognitive and motor defects. The Minnesota Multiphasic Inventory does not require emotionally intoned speech or facial expressions. Gasparrini et al. (1978) found that whereas patients with left-hemisphere disease showed a marked elevation of the depression scale, patients with right-hemisphere disease did not. Therefore, the right–left differences in emotional behavior observed by Gainotti (1972) and others cannot be attributed to emotional expressive disorders or to severity of the motor or cognitive deficit.

Starkstein, Robinson, and Price (1987) also studied emotional changes associated with stroke and found that about one third of stroke patients had depression. They found that depression was associated with both left frontal and left caudate lesions and also that the closer to the frontal pole the lesion was located, the more severe the depression. Many of the patients with left-hemisphere lesions and depression were also anxious. In contrast, patients with right frontal lesions were often indifferent or even euphoric. Not all investigators agree, however, that after stroke there is more depression with left-hemisphere than with right-hemisphere lesions. House et al. (1990) and Milner (1974) could not replicate the emotional symmetries found in other reports.

To learn if there are discrete physiological changes of the brain associated with depression, several groups of investigators studied patients with primary depression using functional imaging. Several of these investigators noted a decrease in activation in the left frontal lobe as well as in the left cingulate gyrus (Bench et al., 1992; Phelps et al., 1984). Drevets and Raichle (1992), however, found increased activity in the left prefrontal cortex, amygdala, basal ganglia, and thalamus.

Davidson et al. (1979) and Tucker (1981) investigated the hemispheric valence hypothesis by studying normal subjects using electrophysiological techniques and confirmed the results of the ablation studies. Unfortunately, it is not known how the right and left hemisphere may influence emotional valence. Fox and Davidson (1984) suggest that left hemisphere–mediated positive emotions are related to approach behaviors and that right hemisphere–mediated negative emotions are related to avoidance behaviors. In our laboratory, we studied emotions and approach-avoidance behavior. We found that negative emotions can be associated with both approach and avoidance behaviors (Crucian et al., 1997). For example, fear and anger both have a negative valence, but fear is associated with avoidance and anger approach. In addition, this approach–avoidance model does not explain how the two hemispheres are differently organized such that they make opposite contributions to mood or how other emotions are mediated, nor does it explain the role of other areas in the brain such as the basal ganglia and limbic system.

With regard to the limbic system, the amygdala, which is critical for negative emotions such as fear and anger, when bilaterally ablated, induces a reduction in the experience of these emotions. To learn if the right amygdala may be more important than the left in mediating emotions with negative valence, Morris and coworkers (1991) showed slides with positive and negative valence to a subject before and after temporal lobectomy. This study demonstrated that ablation of the right anterior temporal lobe, which included the amygdala, reduced the patient's experience of negative emotions.

Tucker and Williamson (1984) think that hemispheric valence asymmetries may be related to asymmetrical control of neuropharmacological systems, with the left hemisphere being more cholinergic and dopaminergic than the right hemisphere, and the right hemisphere being more noradrenergic than the left hemisphere. Robinson and Starkstein (1989) reported that pharmacological changes in the two hemispheres may be different after stroke. They reported that strokes in the right hemisphere appear on PET images to increase serotonergic receptor binding and that left-hemisphere strokes lower serotonergic binding. The lower the serotonergic binding, the more severe the depression. Although it is well known from clinical psychiatry that neurotransmitter systems may have a profound influence on mood, the mechanism by which the pharmacological changes induce mood remain unknown. In addition, as we discussed above, moods and emotions may not be synonymous and may be mediated differently.

Arousal. Arousal has both behavioral and physiological components. Behaviorally, an aroused organism is awake, alert, and prepared to process stimuli. An unaroused organism is lethargic to comatose and not prepared to process stimuli. Physiologically, arousal has several definitions. In the central nervous system, arousal usually refers to the excitatory state of neurons or to the propensity of neurons to discharge when appropriately activated. In functional imaging, arousal is usually measured by increases of blood flow, and electrophysiologically, it is measured by desynchronization of the EEG or by the amplitude and latency of evoked potentials. Outside the central nervous system, arousal usually refers to activation of the sympathetic nervous system and the viscera such as the heart.

Arousal and attention are intimately linked and appear to be mediated by a modular cortical limbic reticular network (Heilman, 1979; Mesulam, 1981; Watson, Valenstein, & Heilman, 1981). An overview of this network is presented here, but for details one should refer to the original articles or, for a review, see Heilman, Watson, and Valenstein (1993b).

Much of what we know about the anatomical basis of this network initially came from studies of monkeys and patients with discrete brain lesions. More recently, functional imaging has confirmed much of the ablation research. In humans, lesions of the inferior parietal lobe are most often associated with disorders of attention and arousal (Critchley, 1966; Heilman, Valenstein, & Watson, 1983). In monkeys, temporoparietal ablations are also associated with attentional disorders (Heilman, Pandya, & Geschwind, 1970; Lynch, 1980). Physiological recordings from neurons in the parietal lobes of monkeys appear to support the postulate that the parietal lobe is important in attention. Unlike neurons in primary sensory cortex, the rate of firing of these "attentional" neurons in the parietal lobe appears to be associated with the significance of the stimulus to the monkey such that relevant stimuli are associated with higher firing rates than are unimportant stimuli (see Bushnell, Goldberg, & Robinson, 1981; Lynch, 1980).

Sensory information projects to the thalamic relay nuclei. From the thalamus, these modality-specific sensory systems project to the primary sensory cortices. Each of these primary sensory cortices (e.g., visual, tactile, auditory) projects only to its associated cortex. For example, Brodmann's area 17, the primary visual cortex, projects to Brodmann's area 18. Subsequently, each of these modality-specific association areas converges on polymodal areas such as the frontal cortex (periarcuate, prearcuate, and orbitofrontal), and both banks of the superior temporal sulcus (Pandya & Kuypers, 1969). Both of these latter sensory polymodal convergence areas project to the supramodal inferior parietal lobe (Mesulam et al., 1977).

Whereas the determination of stimulus novelty may be mediated by modality-specific sensory association cortex, stimulus significance requires knowledge as to both the meaning of the stimulus and the motivational state of the organism. The motivational state depends on at least two factors: immediate biological needs and long-term goals. It has been demonstrated that portions of the limbic system together with the hypothalamus monitor the internal milieu and develop drive states. Therefore, limbic input into regions important in determining stimulus significance may provide information about immediate biological needs. Portions of the limbic system such as the cingulate gyrus, project to both the inferior parietal lobe and the frontal lobe. Regarding long-term goals, the frontal lobe has been demonstrated to play a major role in goal-oriented behavior and set development (Damasio & Anderson, 1993; Stuss & Benson, 1986). Frontal input into the attentional–arousal systems may provide information about goals that are not motivated by immediate biological needs. Studies of cortical connectivity in monkeys have demonstrated that the temporoparietal region has strong connections not only with portions of the limbic system (i.e., cingulate gyrus) but also with the frontal cortex.

Stimulation of the mesencephalic reticular formation (MRF) in animals induces behavioral and physiological arousal (Moruzzi & Magoun, 1949). In contrast, bilateral lesions of the MRF induce coma, and unilateral lesions cause the ipsilateral hemisphere to be both behaviorally and physiologically hypoaroused (Watson et al., 1974). The polymodal and supramodal cortical areas we discussed above not only determine stimulus significance but also modulate arousal by influencing the MRF (Segundo, Naguet, & Buser, 1955). The exact means by which these cortical areas influence the MRF and the MRF influences the cortex remain unknown.

There are, however, at least three possible mechanisms by which the MRF may influence cortical processing. Shute and Lewis (1967) describe an ascending cholinergic reticular formation. The nucleus basalis, which is in the basal forebrain, receives input from the reticular formation and has cholinergic projections to the entire cortex. These cholinergic projections appear to be important for increasing neuronal sensitivity (Sato et al., 1987). The MRF may also influence the cortical activity through thalamic projections. Steriade and Glenn (1982) demonstrated that nonspecific thalamic nuclei, such as centralis lateralis and paracentralis, project to widespread cortical regions and that these thalamic nuclei can be activated by stimulation of the mesencephalic reticular formation. The third mechanism that may help account for cortical arousal involves the thalamic nucleus reticularis. This thin nucleus envelops the thalamus and projects to all the sensory thalamic relay nuclei. Physiologically, the nucleus reticularis inhibits the thalamic relay of sensory information (Scheibel & Scheibel, 1966). When cortical limbic networks determine that a stimulus is significant or novel, however, corticofugal projections may inhibit the inhibitory nucleus reticularis, thereby allowing the thalamic sensory nuclei to relay sensory information to the cortex.

The level of activity of the peripheral autonomic nervous system usually mirrors the level of arousal in the central nervous system. One means of measuring peripheral autonomic arousal is by assessing hand sweating. When the hand sweats, there is a change in resistance. To learn if there were differences in the hemispheric control of sweating, Heilman, Schwartz, and Watson (1978) studied RHD and LHD patients and normal controls. These subjects received nociceptive stimuli (electric shock) that was uncomfortable but not painful. The RHD patients had a reduced arousal response compared with controls and LHD patients. Subsequently, other investigators also reported similar findings.

For example, Morrow et al. (1981) and Schrandt, Tranel, and Damasio (1989) also found that RHD patients had a reduced skin response to emotional stimuli. There was, however, another interesting finding. Compared with normal subjects, LHD patients appeared to have a greater autonomic response (Heilman, Schwartz, & Watson, 1978). Using changes in heart rate as a measure of arousal, Yokoyama et al. (1987) obtained results similar to those with galvanic skin response. Using functional imaging, Perani et al. (1993) also found that, in patients with right hemisphere stroke, there is also a metabolic depression of the left hemisphere. Unfortunately, LHD control patients were not included.

The mechanisms underlying the asymmetrical hemispheric control of arousal remain unknown. Because lesions restricted to the right hemisphere were not found to directly interfere with the left hemisphere's corticofugal projections to the reticular system or the reticular system's corticopetal influence on the left hemisphere, one could propose that the right hemisphere's control of arousal may be related to privileged communication that the right hemisphere has with the reticular activating system. Alternatively, portions of the right hemisphere may play a dominant role in computing stimulus significance. The increased arousal associated with left-hemisphere lesions also remains unexplained. Perhaps the left hemisphere maintains some type of inhibitory control over the right hemisphere or the reticular activating system.

Motor activation and approach–avoidance. Some emotions do not call for action (e.g., sadness, satisfaction), but others do (e.g., anger, fear, joy, surprise). When emotions are associated with action, this action may be toward the stimulus (approach) or away from the stimulus (avoidance) that induced the emotion. People want to avoid emotions that are unpleasant and approach situations that induce pleasant emotions, but this is not what we are addressing when we discuss approach and avoidance. Rather, we are addressing the behavior associated with the emotion and not the plans for structuring the behavior in relation to the stimuli that induce the emotions. For example, whereas one would like to avoid situations that induce anger, when one does become angry, one has a propensity to approach the stimulus that is inducing this emotion. Joy, a positive emotion, is also associated with approach behaviors.

Primbram and McGuiness (1975) use the term *activation* to denote the physiological readiness to respond to stimuli. We have posited that motor activation or motor intention is mediated by a modular network that includes portions of the cerebral cortex, basal ganglia, and limbic system (for a detailed review, see Heilman, Bowers, & Valenstein, 1993a; Heilman & Watson, 1989). The dorsolateral frontal lobe appears to be a critical portion of this motor preparatory network (Heilman, 1978; Watson, Miller, & Watson, Valenstein, & Heilman, 1981). Physiological recordings from cells in the dorsolateral frontal lobe reveal neurons that have enhanced activity when the animal is presented with a stimulus that is meaningful and predicts movement (Goldberg & Bushnell, 1981).

The dorsolateral frontal lobe receives input from the cingulate gyrus and from posterior cortical association areas that are modality specific, polymodal, and supramodal. Input from these posterior neocortical areas may provide the frontal lobe information about the stimulus, including its meaning and its spatial location. The limbic system (e.g., the cingulate gyrus, which is not only part of the Papez circuit but also receives input from Yakolov's basal lateral circuit) may provide information as to the organism's motivational state. The dorsolateral frontal lobe has nonreciprocal connections with the basal ganglia (e.g., caudate), which in turn projects to the globus pallidus, and the globus pallidus projects to the thalamus, which projects back to the frontal cortex (Alexander, DeLong, & Strick, 1986).

The dorsolateral frontal lobe also has extensive connections with the nonspecific intralaminar nuclei of the thalamus (centromedian and parafasicularis). These intralaminar nuclei, which can be activated by the mesencephalic reticular system, may gate motor activation by their influence on the basal ganglia, especially the putamen, or by influencing the thalamic portion of motor circuits (ventralis lateralis pars oralis). Finally, the dorsolateral frontal lobe has strong input into the premotor areas. The observation that lesions of the dorsolateral frontal lobe, the cingulate gyrus, the basal ganglia, the intralaminar nuclei, and the ventrolateral thalamus may all cause akinesia supports the postulate that this system mediates motor activation.

The right hemisphere appears to play a special role in motor activation or intention. Coslett and Heilman (1989) demonstrated that right-hemisphere lesions are more likely to be associated with contralateral akinesia than are those of the left hemisphere. Howes and Boller (1975) measured reaction times (a measure of the time taken to initiate a response) of the hand ipsilateral to a hemispheric lesion and demonstrated that right-hemisphere lesions were associated with slower reaction times than were left-hemisphere lesions. As previously discussed, however, this finding may be related to the important role of the right hemisphere in mediating attention and arousal. Heilman and Van Den Abell (1979) measured the reduction in reaction times of normal subjects who received warning stimuli directed to either their right or left hemisphere. They found that, independent of the hand used, the warning stimuli delivered to the right hemisphere reduced reaction times to midline stimuli more than warning stimuli delivered to the left hemisphere.

Whereas some emotions (e.g., anger and joy) are associated with approach behaviors, other emotions (e.g., fear and disgust) are associated with avoidance behaviors. Unfortunately, the portions of the brain that mediate approach and avoidance behaviors have not been entirely elucidated. Denny-Brown and Chambers (1958) suggested that the frontal lobes mediate avoidance behaviors and the parietal lobes mediate approach behaviors. Denny-Brown and Chambers (1958) also suggested that approach and avoidance behaviors may be reciprocal such that a loss of one behavior may release the other behavior. Therefore, because the frontal lobes mediate avoidance behavior, frontal lobe lesions would cause inappropriate approach behaviors, and because the parietal lobes mediate approach behaviors, parietal lesions would induce avoidance. In support of this postulate are those patients with frontal lesions who demonstrate a variety of approach behaviors, including manual grasp reflexes, visual grasp reflexes, rooting and sucking responses, magnetic apraxia, utilization behaviors, and defective response inhibition. Unfortunately, the specific area or areas within the frontal lobes that when damaged cause approach behaviors have not been entirely elucidated. Animals with frontal lesions show an increase in aggressive behavior. Patients with left dorsolateral frontal lesions (which should induce an emotion of negative valence, increased arousal, and approach behaviors) are also prone to hostility and anger (Grafman et al., 1986).

Denny-Brown and Chambers (1958) demonstrated that, in contrast to the manual grasp response associated with frontal lesions, patients with parietal lesions may demonstrate a palmar avoiding response. Patients with parietal lesions, especially of the right side, may not only fail to move or have a delay in moving their arms, head, and eyes toward a part of space that is opposite the parietal lesion, but may also deviate their eyes, head, and arms toward ipsilateral hemispace. In addition, unlike patients with frontal lesions who cannot withhold their response to stimuli, patients with parietal lesions may not be able to respond to stimuli (neglect). These avoidance responses are more severe with right-hemisphere than with left-hemisphere lesions.

SUMMARY

Emotions may be divided into two major divisions, experience and behavior. Because the brain is critical for mediating emotional experience and behavior, diseases of the brain may induce changes in emotional behavior and experience.

Disorders of almost all portions of the cerebral hemisphere, including the cortex, limbic system, and basal ganglia, have been associated with changes in emotional experience and behavior. Dysfunction of the cerebral cortex may be associated with disorders of emotional communication. Whereas deficits of the left hemisphere appear to impair the comprehension and expression of propositional language, deficits of the right hemisphere may be associated with an impaired ability to comprehend and express emotional gestures, such as facial expressions and emotional prosody. Some patients have either prosodic or facial emotional deficits. Some have only expressive or receptive deficits. Others, however, may be globally impaired either within or across modalities. The posterior portions of the neocortex appear to be important for comprehension, and the anterior portions seem to be important for expression of both emotional prosody and facial gestures.

Injury and dysfunction of the limbic system may also alter emotional communication and experience. For example, amygdala damage may be associated with an impaired ability to recognize emotional faces and with a reduction of affect, especially anger, rage, and fear. In contrast, lesions of the septal region may be associated with increased rage-like behaviors. Seizures frequently emanate from the limbic system, and seizures that start in the amygdala can induce fear and perhaps even rage.

Disorders of the basal ganglia may also be associated with defects of emotional communication and, experience. Patients with PD may not only be impaired in communicating emotions, showing both expressive and receptive deficits, but also are often depressed and anxious. Patients with HD may have emotional comprehension deficits with an impaired ability to recognize emotional faces and prosody. Patients with HD may also have mood changes even before their motor dysfunction becomes manifest.

Many of the defects in emotional experience may be related to the associated changes in neurotransmitter systems. Unfortunately, how alteration of neurotransmitters induces mood changes remains unknown.

In this chapter, we review the feedback and central theories of emotional experience. Although we argue against the postulate that feedback is critical to the experience of emotions, we do suspect that feedback may influence emotions. Emotions may be conditioned and may use thalamic–limbic circuits. Most emotional behaviors and experiences are, however, induced by complex stimuli that an isolated thalamus could not interpret.

The cerebral cortex of humans has complex modular systems that analyze stimuli, develop percepts, and interpret meaning. We discuss the proposal that the experience of emotions is dimensional. Almost all primary emotions can be described with two or three factors, including valence, arousal, and motor activation. The determination of valence is based on whether the stimulus is beneficial (positive) or detrimental (negative) to a person's well being. Whereas the right frontal lobe and its subcortical connections appear to be important in the mediation of emotions with negative valence, the left frontal lobe and its subcortical connections may be important in the mediation of emotions with positive valence. Depending on the nature of the stimulus, some positive and some negative emotions are associated with high arousal (e.g., joy and fear) and others with low arousal (e.g., satisfaction and sadness). Whereas the right parietal lobe appears to be important in mediating the arousal response, the left hemisphere appears to inhibit the arousal response. Some positive and negative emotions (e.g., anger, fear, and joy) are associated with motor activation and others (e.g., sadness) are not. The right frontal lobe appears to be important in motor activation. The motor activation associated with emotions may be either approach or avoidance behaviors. Whereas approach behaviors may be mediated by the parietal lobes, avoidance behaviors may be mediated by the frontal lobes.

The cortical areas we have discussed have rich connections. In addition, these neocortical areas also contain rich connections with the limbic system, basal ganglia, thalamus, and reticular system. Therefore, the anatomic modules that mediate valence, arousal, and activation systems are richly interconnected and form a modular network. Emotional experience depends on the patterns of neural activation of this modular network, and the neurotransmitter systems that are altered in many neurological diseases may play a critical role in altering the patterns of activation.

REFERENCES

Akert, K., Greusen, R.A., Woolsey, C.N., & Meyer, D.R. (1961). Kluver-Bucy syndrome in monkeys with neocortical ablations of temporal lobe. *Brain, 84*, 480–498.

Adolphs, R., Tranel, D., Damasio, H., & Damasio, A. (1994). Impaired recognition of emotion in facial expressions following bilateral damage to the human amygdala. *Nature, 372*, 669–672.

Alexander, G.E., DeLong, M.R., & Strick, P.L. (1986). Parallel organization of functionally segregated circuits linking basal ganglia and cortex. *Annual Review in Neuroscience, 9*, 357–381.

Ax, A.F. (1953). The physiological differentiation between fear and anger in humans. *Psychosomatic Medicine, 15*, 433–442.

Aylward, E.H., Roberts-Twillie, J.V., Barta, P.E., Kumar, A.J., Harris, G.J., Geer, M., Peyser, C.E., & Pearlson, G.D. (1994). Basal ganglia volumes and white matter hyperintensities in patients with bipolar disorder. *American Journal of Psychiatry, 151*, 687–693.

Babinski, J. (1914). Contribution à l'étude des troubles mentaux dans l'hémiplégie organique cérébrale (anosognosie). *Revue Neurologique, 27*, 845–848.

Bannister, R., & Openheimer, D.R. (1972). Degenerative diseases of the nervous system associated with autonomic failure. *Brain, 95*, 457–474.

Barber, J., Tomer, R., Sroka, H., & Myslobodsky, M.S. (1985). Does unilateral dopamine deficit contribute to depression? *Psychiatry Research, 15*, 17–24.

Bard, P. (1934). Emotion. I: The neuro-hormonal basis of emotional reactions. In C. Murchison (Eds.), *Handbook of General Experimental Psychology*. Worchester, MA: Clark University Press.

Barrett, A.M., Crucian, G.P., Raymer, A.M., & Heilman, K.M. (1997). Spared comprehension of emotional prosody in a patient with global aphasia [abstract]. *Journal of the International Neuropsychological Society, 3(1),* 57.

Bear, D.M., & Fedio, P. (1977). Quantitative analysis of interictal behavior in temporal lobe epilepsy. *Archives of Neurology, 34,* 454–467.

Bench, C.J., Friston, K.J., Brown, R.G., Scott, L.C., Frackowiak, R.S., & Dolan, R.J. (1992) The anatomy of melancholia; focal abnormalities of blood flow in major depression. *Psychological Medicine, 22,* 607–615.

Benson, D.F. (1979). Psychiatric aspects of aphasia. In D.F. Benson (Ed.), *Aphasia, Alexia, and Agraphia* (pp. 174–180). New York: Churchill-Livingstone.

Blin, J., Baron, J.C., Dubois, B., Pillon, B., Cambon, H., Cambier, J., & Agid, Y. (1990). Positron emission tomography study in progressive supranuclear palsy. Brain hypometabolic pattern and clinicometabolic correlations. *Archives of Neurology, 47,* 747–752.

Blonder, L.X., Bowers, D., & Heilman, K.M. (1991). The role of the right hemisphere in emotional communication. *Brain, 114,* 1115–1127.

Blonder, L.X., Burns, A.F., Bowers, D., Moore, R., & Heilman, K.M. (1993). Right hemisphere facial expressivity during natural conversation. *Brain and Cognition, 21(1),* 44–56.

Blonder, L.X., Gur, R.E., & Gur, R.C. (1989). The effects of right and left hemiparkinsonism on prosody. *Brain and Language, 36,* 193–207.

Bloom, R.L., Borod, J.C., Obler, L.K., & Gerstman, L.J. (1993). Suppression and facilitation of pragmatic performance: Effects of emotional content on discourse following right and left brain damage. *Journal of Speech and Hearing Research, 36(6),* 1127–1135.

Bloom, R.L., Borod, J.C., Obler, L.K., & Koff, E. (1990). A preliminary characterization of lexical emotional expression in right and left brain-damaged patients. *International Journal of Neuroscience, 55(2–4),* 71–80.

Borod, J.C., Andelman, F., Obler, L.K., Tweedy, J.R., & Welkowitz, J. (1992). Right hemisphere specialization for the identification of emotional words and sentences: Evidence from stroke patients. *Neuropsychologia, 30(9),* 827–844.

Borod, J.C., Cicero, B., Obler, L.K., Welkowitz, J., Erhan, H., Santschi, C., Grunwald, I., Agosti, R., & Whalen, J. (1998). Right hemisphere emotional perception: Evidence across multiple channels. *Neuropsychology, 12,* 446–458.

Borod, J.C., Koff, E., Perlman Lorch, M., & Nicholas, M. (1986). The expression and perception of facial emotion in brain-damaged patients. *Neuropsychologia, 24(2),* 169–180.

Borod, J.C., Rorie, K.D., Haywood, C.S., Andelman, F., Obler, L.K., Welkowitz, J., Bloom, R.L., & Tweedy, J.R. (1996). Hemispheric specialization for discourse reports of emotional experiences: Relationships to demographic, neurological, and perceptual variables. *Neuropsychologia, 34(5),* 351–359.

Borod, J.C., Rorie, K.D., Pick, L., Bloom, R.L., Andelman, F., Campbell, A., Obler, L.K., Tweedy, J.R., Welkowitz, J., & Sliwinski, M. (2000) Verbal pragmatics following unilateral stroke: Emotional content and valence. *Neuropsychology, 14,* 112–124.

Borod, J.C., Welkowitz, J., Alpert, M., Brozgold, A.Z., Martin, C., Peselow, E., & Diller, L. (1990). Parameters of emotional processing in neuropsychiatric disorders: Conceptual issues and a battery of tests. *Journal of Communicative Disorders, 23,* 247–271.

Bowers, D., Bauer, R.M., Coslett, H.B., & Heilman, K.M. (1985). Processing of faces by patients with unilateral hemispheric lesions. I. Dissociation between judgments of facial affect and facial identity. *Brain and Cognition, 4*, 258–272.

Bowers, D., Blonder, L., Feinberg, T., & Heilman, K. (1991). Differential impact of right and left hemisphere lesions on facial emotion versus object imagery. *Brain, 114*, 2593–2609.

Bowers, D., Blonder, L., Slomine, B., & Heilman, K. (1996). Nonverbal affect signals: Patterns of impairment following hemispheric strokes using the Florida affect battery. [abstract] *Neurology, 46(2)*, S28.003.

Bowers, D., Coslett, H.B., Bauer, R.M., Speedie, L.J., & Heilman, K.M. (1987). Comprehension of emotional prosody following unilateral hemispheric lesions: Processing defect versus distraction defect. *Neuropsychologia, 25*, 317–328.

Bowers, D., Glantz, M., Heilman, K., Morris, K., Blonder, L., Cimino, C., & Kortenkamp, S. (1998). *Valence effects in the recall of autobiographical memories: Findings from patients with hemispheric strokes.* Submitted for publication.

Bowers, D., Rogish, M., Eckert, M., Kortemkamp, S., Gilmore, R., & Roper, S. (1999). *Decoding nonverbal social signals of fear and threat by patients with unilateral temporal ablations involving the amygdala.* Paper presented at the International Neuropsychology Society, Boston, MA.

Brady, J.V., & Nauta, W.J. (1955). Subcortical mechanisms in control of behavior. *Journal of Comparative and Physiological Psychology, 48*, 412–420.

Breiter, H., Etcoff, N., Whalen, P.J., Kennedy, W., Rauch, S., Buckner, R., Strauss, M., Hyman, S., & Rosen, B. (1996). Response and habituation of the human amygdala during visual processing of facial expression. *Neuron, 17(5)*, 875–887.

Brickner, R.M. (1934). An interpretation of frontal lobe function based upon the study of a case of partial bilateral frontal lobectomy. *Research Publication of the Association for Research in Nervous and Mental Disease, 13*, 259–351.

Brickner, R.M. (1936). *The Intellectual Functions of the Frontal Lobes: Study Based Upon Observation of a Man After Partial Bilateral Frontal Lobectomy.* New York: Macmillan.

Broca, P. (1878). Anatomie comparée des circonvolutions cérébrales: Le grand lobe limbique et al scissure limbique dans la série des mammifères. *Revue Anthropologique, 1*, 385–498.

Brothers, C. (1964). Huntington's chorea in Victoria and Tasmania. *Neurological Science, 1*, 405–420.

Brown, R.G., MacCarthy, B., Gotham, A.M., Der, G.J., & Marsden, C.D. (1988). Depression and disability in Parkinson's disease: A follow-up of 132 cases. *Psychological Medicine, 18*, 49–55.

Brozgold, A.Z., Borod, J.C., Martin, C.C., Pick, L.H., Alpert, M., & Welkowitz, J. (1998). Social functioning and facial emotional expression in neurological and psychiatric disorders. *Applied Neuropsychology, 5(1)*, 15–23.

Buck, R., & Duffy, R. (1980). Nonverbal communication of affect in brain-damaged patients. *Cortex, 16*, 351–362.

Bushnell, M.C., Goldberg, M.E., & Robinson, D.L. (1981). Behavioral enhancement of visual responses in monkey cerebral cortex. I. Modulation of posterior parietal cortex related to selected visual attention. *Journal of Neurophysiology, 46*, 755–772.

Cancelliere, A.E., & Kertesz, A. (1990). Lesion localization in acquired deficits of emotional expression and comprehension. *Brain and Cognition, 13*, 133–147.

Cannon, W.B. (1927). The James-Lange theory of emotion: A critical examination and an alternative theory. *American Journal of Psychology, 39,* 106–124.

Cantello, R., Aguggia, M., Gilli, M., Delsedime, M., Chiardo, C.I., Riccio, A., & Mutani, R. (1989). Major depression in Parkinson's disease and the mood response to intravenous methylphenidate: Possible role of the "hedonic" dopamine synapse. *Journal of Neurology, Neurosurgery, and Psychiatry, 52,* 724–731.

Canter, G. (1963). Speech characteristics of patients with Parkinson's disease. Intensity, pitch, and duration. *Journal of Speech and Hearing Disorders, 29,* 221–229.

Chan-Palay, V., & Assan, E. (1989). Alterations in catecholamine neurons of the locus coeruleus in senile dementia of the Alzheimer type and Parkinson's disease with and without dementia and depression. *Journal of Comparative Neurology, 287,* 373–392.

Chen, R.C., & Forster, F.M. (1973). Cursive epilepsy and gelastic epilepsy. *Neurology, 23,* 1019–1029.

Cicone, M., Waper, W., & Gardner, H. (1980). Sensitivity to emotional expressions and situations in organic patients. *Cortex, 16,* 145–158.

Cimino, C.R., Verfaellie, M., Bowers, D., & Heilman, K.M. (1988). Emotional autobiographical memory in right-hemisphere-damaged patients [abstract]. *Journal of Clinical and Experimental Neuropsychology, 10(1),* 86.

Coslett, H.B., & Heilman, K.M. (1989). Hemihypokinesia after right hemisphere strokes. *Brain and Cognition, 9,* 267–278.

Critchley, M. (1966). *The Parietal Lobes.* New York: Hafner.

Crucian, G.P., Preston, L.M., Raymer, A.M., & Heilman, K.M. (1997). Dissociation of behavioral action and emotional valence in the expression of affect [abstract]. *Neurology, 48(Suppl. 3),* S50.004.

Cummings, J.L. (1992). Depression and Parkinson's disease: A review. *American Journal of Psychiatry, 149,* 443–454.

Damasio, A.R., & Anderson, S.W. (1993). The frontal lobes. In K.M. Heilman & E. Valenstein (Eds.), *Clinical Neuropsychology,* 3rd ed. (pp. 409–460). New York: Oxford University Press.

Darley, F., Aronson, A., & Brown, J. (1969). Differential diagnostic patterns of dysarthria. *Journal of Speech and Hearing Research, 12,* 246–269.

Darwin, C. (1872). *The Expression of Emotion in Man and Animals.* London: Murray.

Davidson, R.J., Schwartz, G.E., Saron, C., Bennett, J., & Goleman, D.J. (1979). Frontal versus parietal EEG asymmetry during positive and negative affect. *Psychophysiology, 16,* 202–203.

Davis, M. (1989). Neural systems involved in fear conditioning. *Annals of the New York Academy of Sciences, 563,* 165–183.

DeKosky, S., Heilman, K.M., Bowers, D., & Valenstein, E. (1980). Recognition and discrimination of emotional faces. *Brain and Language, 9,* 206–214.

Dening, T.R., & Berrios, G.E. (1989). Wilson's disease. Psychiatric symptoms in 195 cases. *Archives of General Psychiatry, 46,* 1126–1134.

Denny-Brown, D., & Chambers, R.A. (1958). The parietal lobe and behavior. *Research Publications Associations for Research in Nervous and Mental Disease, 36,* 35–117.

Direnfeld, L.K., Albert, M.L., Volicer, L., Langlais, P.J., Marquis, J., & Kaplan, E. (1984). The possible relationship of laterality to dementia and neurochemical findings. *Archives of Neurology, 41,* 935–941.

Drevets, W.C., & Raichle, M.E. (1992). Neuroanatomic circuits in depression. *Psychopharmacology Bulletin, 28,* 261–274.

Ekman, P., & Friesen, W. (1978). *Facial Action Coding System.* Palo Alto, CA: Consulting Psychologists Press.

Ekman, P., Sorenson, E.R., & Freisen, W.V. (1969). Pancultural elements in facial displays of emotions. *Science, 164,* 86–88.

Fearnley, J.M., & Lees, A.J. (1990). Striatonigral degeneration. A clinicopathological study. *Brain, 113,* 1823–1842.

Feve, J.R., Mussini, J.M., Mathe, J.F., et al. (1977). Dégénérescence striatonigirique: Etude clinique et anatomique d'un cas ayant réagi très favorablement à la L-DOPA. *Revue Neurologique, 133,* 271–278.

Figiel, G.S., Krishnan, K.R.R., Doraiswamy, P.M., Rao, V.P., Nemeroff, C.B., & Boyko, O.B. (1991). Subcortical hyperintensities on brain magnetic resonance imaging: A comparison between late age onset and early onset elderly depressed subjects. *Neurobiology of Aging, 26,* 245–247.

Fleminger, S. (1991). Left-sided Parkinson's disease is associated with greater anxiety and depression. *Psychological Medicine, 21,* 629–638.

Flor-Henry, P. (1969). Psychosis and temporal lobe epilepsy: A controlled investigation. *Epilepsia, 10,* 363–395.

Folstein, S.E., Folstein, M.F., & McHugh, P.R. (1979). Psychiatric syndromes in Huntington's disease. *Advances in Neurology, 23,* 281–289.

Fox, N.A., & Davidson, R.J. (1984). Hemispheric substrates for affect: A developmental model. In N.A. Fox & R.J. Davidson (Eds.), *The Psychobiology of Affective Development* (pp. 353–381). Hillsdale, NJ: Erlbaum.

Fried, I., Mateer, C., Ojemann, G., Wohns, R., & Fedio, P. (1982). Organization of visuospatial functions in human cortex. *Brain, 105,* 349–371.

Frijda, N.H. (1987). Emotion, cognitive structure, and action tendency. *Cognition and Emotion, 1,* 115–143.

Gainotti, G. (1972). Emotional behavior and hemispheric side of lesion. *Cortex, 8,* 41–55.

Garcia-Campayo, J.J., & Sanz-Carrillo, C. (1994). Psychiatric onset in striatonigral degeneration. *European Journal of Psychiatry, 8,* 84–88.

Gascon, G.C., & Lombrosco, C.T. (1971). Epileptic (gelastic) laughter. *Epilepsia, 12,* 63–76.

Gasparrini, W.G., Satz, P., Heilman, K.M., & Coolidge, F.L. (1978). Hemispheric asymmetries of affective processing as determined by the Minnesota Multiphasic Personality Inventory. *Journal of Neurology, Neurosurgery, and Psychiatry, 41,* 470–473.

Ghika-Schmid, F., Chika, J., Vuilleumier, P., Assal, G.L., Vuadens, P., Scherer, K., Maeder, P., Uske, A., & Bogousslavsky, J. (1997). Bihippocampal damage with emotional dysfunction: Impaired auditory recognition of fear. *European Neurology, 38,* 276–283.

Gloor, P. (1972). Temporal lobe epilepsy. In B. Eleftheriou (Ed.), *Advances in Behavioral Biology: The Neurobiology of the Amygdala,* Vol. 2 (pp. 423–427). New York: Plenum Press.

Goldberg, M.E., & Bushnell, B.C. (1981). Behavioral enhancement of visual responses in monkey cerebral cortex: II. Modulation in frontal eye fields specifically to related saccades. *Journal of Neurophysiology, 46,* 773–787.

Goldstein, K. (1948). *Language and Language Disturbances.* New York: Grune & Stratton.

Gotham, A.M., Brown, R.G., & Marsden, C.D. (1986). Depression in Parkinson's disease: A quantitative and qualitative analysis. *Journal of Neurology, Neurosurgery, and Psychiatry, 49,* 381–389.

Grafman, J., Litvan, I., Gomez, C., & Chast, T.N. (1990). Frontal lobe function in progressive supranuclear palsy. *Archives of Neurology, 47*, 553–558.

Grafman, J., Vance, S.C., Weingartner, H., Salazarm A.M., & Amin, D. (1986). The effects of lateralized frontal lesions on mood regulation. *Brain, 109*, 1127–1140.

Greenwald, M.K., Cook, E.W., & Lang, P.J. (1989). Affective judgment and psychophysiological response: Dimensional co-variation in the evolution of pictorial stimuli. *Journal of Psychophysiology, 3*, 51–64.

Hantas, M., Katkin, E.S., & Blasovich, J. (1982). Relationship between heartbeat discrimination and subjective experience of affective state. *Psychophysiology, 19*, 563.

Harlow, J.M. (1868). Recovery after severe injury to the head. *Publication of the Massachusetts Medical Society (Boston), 2*, 327–346.

Hawton, K., Fagg, J., & Marsack, P. (1980). Association between epilepsy and attempted suicide. *Journal of Neurology, Neurosurgery, and Psychiatry, 43*, 168–170.

Heath, R.G. (1964). Pleasure response of human subjects to direct stimulation of the brain: Physiologic and psychodynamic considerations. In R.G. Heath (Ed.), *The Role of Pleasure in Behavior*. New York: Harper & Row.

Heathfield, K.W.G. (1967). Huntington's chorea. *Brain, 90*, 203–232.

Hécaen, H., Ajuriagerra, J., & de Massonet, J. (1951). Les troubles visuoconstuctifs par lésion parieto-occipitale droit. *Encéphale, 40*, 122–179.

Heilman, K.M. (1979). Neglect and related disorders. In K.M. Heilman & E. Valenstein (Eds.), *Clinical Neuropsychology* (pp. 268–307). New York: Oxford University Press.

Heilman, K.M. (1994). Emotion and the brain: A distributed modular network mediating emotional experience. In D.W. Zaidel (Ed.), *Neuropsychology* (pp. 139–158). San Diego: Academic Press.

Heilman, K.M. (1997). The neurobiology of emotional experience. *Journal of Neuropsychiatry and Clinical Neurosciences, 9*, 439–448.

Heilman, K.M., Bowers, D., Speedie, L., & Coslett, B. (1984). Comprehension of affective and nonaffective speech. *Neurology, 34*, 917–921.

Heilman, K.M., Bowers, D., & Valenstein, E. (1993a). Emotional disorders associated with neurological disease. In K.M. Heilman & E. Valenstein (Eds.), *Clinical Neuropsychology*, 3rd Ed., (pp. 461–497). New York: Oxford University Press.

Heilman, K.M., Pandya, D.N., & Geschwind, N. (1970). Trimodal inattention following parietal lobe ablations. *Transactions of the American Neurology Association, 95*, 259–261.

Heilman, K.M., Scholes, R., & Watson, R.T. (1975). Auditory affective agnosia: Disturbed comprehension of affective speech. *Journal of Neurology, Neurosurgery, and Psychiatry, 38*, 69–72.

Heilman, K.M., Schwartz, H., & Watson, R.T. (1978). Hypoarousal in patients with the neglect syndrome and emotional indifference. *Neurology, 28*, 229–232.

Heilman, K.M., Valenstein, E., & Watson, R.T. (1983). Localization of neglect. In A. Kertesz (Ed.), *Localization in Neurology* (pp. 471–549). New York: Academic Press.

Heilman, K.M., & Van Den Abell, T. (1979). Right hemispheric dominance for mediating cerebral activation. *Neuropsychologia, 17*, 315–321.

Heilman, K.M., & Watson, R.T. (1989). Intentional motor disorders. In H.S Levin, H. M. Eisenberg, & A. Benton (Eds.), *Frontal Lobe Function* (pp. 199–213). New York: Oxford University Press.

Heilman, K.M., Watson, R.T., & Valenstein, E. (1993b). Neglect and related disorders. In K.M. Heilman & E. Valenstein (Eds.), *Clinical Neuropsychology*, 3rd ed. (pp. 279–336), New York: Oxford University Press.

Hohmann, G. (1966). Some effects of spinal cord lesions on experimental emotional feelings. *Psychophysiology, 3,* 143–156.

House, A., Dennis, M., Warlow, C., Hawton, K., & Molyneux, A. (1990). Mood disorders after stroke and their relation to lesion location. *Brain, 113,* 1113–1129.

Howes, D., & Boller, F. (1975). Evidence for focal impairment from lesions of the right hemisphere. *Brain, 98,* 317–332.

Hughlings Jackson, J. (1932). *Selected Writings of John Hughlings Jackson.* J. Taylor (Ed). London: Hodder and Stoughton.

Huntington, G.W. (1872). On chorea. *Medicine and Surgical Reports, 26,* 317–321.

Husain, M.M., McDonald, W.M., Doraiswamy, P.M., Figiel, G.S., Na, C., Escalona, P.R., Boyko, O.B., Nemeroff, C.B., & Krishnan, K.R.R. (1991). A magnetic resonance imaging study of putamen nuclei in major depression. *Psychiatry Research, 40(2),* 95–99.

Irwin, W., Davidson, R., Lowe, M., Mock, B., Sorenson, J., & Turski, P. (1996). Human amygdala activation detected with echo-planar functional magnetic resonance imaging. *Neuroreport, 7(11),* 1765–1769.

Izard, C.E. (1977). *Human Emotions.* New York: Plenum.

Jacobs, D.H., Shuren, J., Bowers, D., & Heilman, K.M. (1995a). Emotional facial imagery, perception, and expression in Parkinson's disease. *Neurology, 45,* 1696–1702.

Jacobs, D.H., Shuren, J., & Heilman, K.M. (1995b). Impaired perception of facial identity and facial affect in Huntington's disease. *Neurology, 45,* 1217–1218.

James, W. (1890). *The Principles of Psychology,* Vol. 2. New York: Dover Publications. Reprinted 1950.

Kanter, S.L., Day, A.L., Heilman, K.M., & Gonzalez-Rothi, L.J. (1986). Pure word deafness: A possible explanation of transient deterioration following EC-IC bypass. *Neurosurgery, 18,* 186–189.

Katkin, E.S., Morrell, M.A., Goldband, S., Bernstein, G.L., & Wise, J.A. (1982). Individual differences in heartbeat discrimination. *Psychophysiology, 19,* 160–166.

Katsikitis, M., & Pilowsky, I. (1988). A study of facial expression in Parkinson's disease using a novel microcomputer-based method. *Journal of Neurology, Neurosurgery, and Psychiatry, 51,* 362–366.

Katsikitis, M., & Pilowsky, I. (1991). A controlled study of facial expression in Parkinson's disease and depression. *Journal of Nervous and Mental Disease, 179,* 683–688.

Keillor, J.M., Barrett, A.M., Crucian, G.P., Kortenkamp, S., & Heilman, K.M. (1999). *Emotional experience and perception in a case of facial paralysis: A test of the facial feedback hypothesis.* Manuscript in preparation.

Kent, R., & Rosenbek, J. (1982). Prosodic disturbance and neurologic lesion. *Brain and Language, 15,* 259–291.

Kluver, H., & Bucy, P.C. (1937). "Psychic bindness" and other symptoms following bilateral temporal lobectomy in rhesus monkeys. *American Journal of Physiology, 119,* 352–353.

Kosky, R. (1981). Children and Huntington's disease: Some clinical observations of children-at-risk. *Medical Journal of Australia (Sydney), 1,* 405–407.

Krishnan, K.R.R., McDonald, W.M., Escalona, P.R., Doraiswamy, P.M., Na, C., Husain, M.M., Figiel, G.S., Boyko, O.B., Ellinwood, E.H., & Nemeroff, C.F. (1992). Magnetic resonance imaging of the caudate nuclei in depression. *Archives of General Psychiatry, 49,* 553–557.

Laird, J.E. (1974). Self-attribution of emotion: The effects of expressive behavior on the quality of emotional experience. *Journal of Personality and Social Psychology, 29,* 475–486.

LeDoux, J.E. (1993). Emotional memory systems in the brain. *Behavioral Brain Research*, *58*, 69–70.

LeDoux, J.E., Cicchetti, P., Xagoraris, A., & Romanski, L.M. (1990). The lateral amygdaloid nucleus: Sensory interface of the amygdala in fear conditioning. *Journal of Neuroscience*, *10*, 1062–1069.

Lemieux, G., Davignon, A., & Genest, J. (1956). Depressive states during rauwolfia therapy for arteriol hypertension. *Canadian Medical Association*, *74*, 522–526.

Levin, B.E., Llabre, M.M., & Weiner, W.J. (1988). Parkinson's disease and depression: Psychometric properties of the Beck Depression Inventory. *Journal of Neurology, Neurosurgery, and Psychiatry*, *51*, 1401–1404.

Lindgren, C.L. (1996). Chronic sorrow in persons with Parkinson's and their spouses. *Scholarly Inquiry for Nursing Practice*, *10*, 351–366.

Litvan, I., Mega, M.S., Cummings, J.L., & Fairbanks, L. (1996). Neuropsychiatric aspects of progressive supranuclear palsy. *Neurology*, *47*, 1184–1189.

Liu, C.Y., Wang, S.J., Fuh, J.L., Lin, C.H., Yang, Y.Y., & Liu, H.C. (1997). The correlation of depression with functional activity in Parkinson's disease. *Journal of Neurology*, *244*, 493–498.

Luria, A.R., & Simernitskaya, E.G. (1977). Interhemispheric relations and the functions of the minor hemisphere. *Neuropsychologia*, *15*, 175–178.

Lynch, J.C. (1980). The functional organization of posterior parietal association cortex. *Behavioral Brain Science*, *3*, 485–534.

Marañon, G. (1924). Contribution à l'étude de l'action émotive de l'adrénaline. *Revue Française d'Endocrinologie*, *2*, 301–325.

Maricle, R.A., Nutt, J.G., Valentine, R.J., & Carter, J.H. (1995). Dose–response relationship of levodopa with mood and anxiety in fluctuating Parkinson's disease: A double-blind, placebo-controlled study. *Neurology*, *45*, 1757–1760.

Mark, V.H., & Erwin, F.R. (1970). *Violence and the Brain*. New York: Harper & Row.

Mayberg, H.S., Robinson, R.G., Wong, D.F., Parikh, R., Bolduc, P., Price, T., Dannals, R.F., Links, J.M., Wilson, A.A., Ravert, H.T., & Wagner, H.N. Jr. (1988). PET imaging of cortical S2-serotonin receptors following stroke: Lateralized changes and relationship to depression. *American Journal of Psychiatry*, *145*(8), 937–943.

Mayberg, H.S., Starkstein, S.E., Peyser, C.E., Brandt, J., Dannals, R.F., & Folstein, S.E. (1992). Paralimbic frontal lobe hypometabolism in depression associated with Huntington's disease. *Neurology*, *42*, 1791–1797.

Mayberg, H.S., Starkstein, S.E., Sadzot, B., Preziosi, T., Andrezejewski, P.L., Dannals, R.F., Wagner, H.N., Jr., & Robinson, R.G. (1990). Selective hypometabolism in the inferior frontal lobe in depressed patients with Parkinson's disease. *Annals of Neurology*, *28*, 57–64.

Mayeux, R. (1983). Emotional changes associated with basal ganglia disorders. In K.M. Heilman & P. Satz (Eds.), *Neuropsychology of Human Emotion* (pp. 141–164). New York: Guilford Press.

Mayeux, R., Stern, Y., Cote, L., & Williams, J.B. (1984). Altered serotonin metabolism in depressed patients with Parkinson's disease. *Neurology*, *34*, 642–646.

Mayeux, R., Stern, Y., Rosen, J., & Leventhal, J. (1981). Depression, intellectual impairment, and Parkinson's disease. *Neurology*, *31*, 645–650.

Menza, M.A., Cocchiola, J., & Golbe, L.I. (1995). Psychiatric symptoms in progressive supranuclear palsy. *Psychosomatics*, *36*, 550–554.

Mesulam, M.-M. (1981). A cortical network for directed attention and unilateral neglect. *Annals of Neurology*, *10*, 309–325.

Mesulam, M.-M., Van Hoesen, G.W., Pandya, D.N., & Geschwind, N. (1977). Limbic and sensory connections of the inferior parietal lobule (area PG) in the rhesus monkey: A study with a new method for horseradish peroxidase histochemistry. *Brain Research*, *136*, 393–414.

Milner, B. (1974). Hemispheric specialization: Scope and limits. In F.O. Schmitt & F.G. Worden (Eds.), *The Neurosciences: Third Study Program* (pp. 75–89). Cambridge, MA: MIT Press.

Morris, M.K., Bradley, M., Bowers, D., Lang, P.J., & Heilman, K.M. (1991). Valence-specific hypoarousal following right temporal lobectomy. *Journal of Clinical and Experimental Neuropsychology*, *13(1)*, 42–43.

Morrow, L., Vrtunski, P.B., Kim, Y., & Boller, F. (1981). Arousal responses to emotional stimuli and laterality of lesions. *Neuropsychologia*, *19*, 65–71.

Moruzzi, G., & Magoun, H.W. (1949). Brainstem reticular formation and activation of the EEG. *Electroencephalogram and Clinical Neurophysiology*, *1*, 455–473.

Offen, M.L., Davidoff, R.A., Troost, B.T., & Richey, E.T. (1976). Dacrystic epilepsy. *Journal of Neurology, Neurosurgery, and Psychiatry*, *39*, 829–834.

Olds, J. (1958). Self-stimulation of the brain. *Science*, *127*, 315–324.

Osgood, C., Suci, G., & Tannenbaum, P. (1957). *The Measure of Meaning*. Urbana, IL: University of Illinois.

Pandya, D.M., & Kuypers, H.G.J.M. (1969). Cortico-cortical connections in the rhesus monkey. *Brain Research*, *13*, 13–36.

Papez, J.W. (1937). A proposed mechanism of emotion. *Archives of Neurology and Psychiatry*, *38*, 725–743.

Parkinson, J. (1817). *An Essay on the Shaking Palsy*. London: Sherwood, Neely, & Jones.

Peper, M., & Irle, E. (1997). The decoding of emotional concepts in patients with focal cerebral lesions. *Brain and Language*, *34*, 360–387.

Perani, D., Vallar, G., Paulesu, E., Alberoni, M., & Fasio, F. (1993). Left and right hemisphere contributions to recovery from neglect after right hemisphere damage. *Neuropsychologia*, *31*, 115–125.

Phelps, M.E., Mazziotta, J.C., Baxter, L., & Geiner, R. (1984). Positron emission tomographic study of affective disorders: Problems and strategies. *Annals of Neurology*, *15* (*Suppl.*), S149–S156.

Phillips, M.L., Young, A.W., Senior, C., Brammer, M., Andrew, C., Calder, A.J., Bullmore, E.T., Perrett, D.I., Rowland, D., Williams, S.C.R., Gray, J.A., & David, A.S. (1997). A specific neural substrate for perceiving facial expressions of disgust. *Nature*, *389*, 495–498.

Pincus, J.H. (1980). Can violence be a manifestation of epilepsy? *Neurology*, *30*, 304–307.

Pitcairn, T., Clemie, S., Gray, J., & Pentland, B. (1990). Non-verbal cues in the self-presentation of parkinsonian patients. *British Journal of Clinical Psychology*, *29*, 177–184.

Poeck, K. (1969). Pathophysiology of emotional disorders associated with brain damage. In P.J. Vinken & G.W Bruyn (Eds.), *Handbook of Clinical Neurology*, Vol. 3 (pp. 343–367). New York: Elsevier.

Poeck, K., & Pilleri, G. (1961). Wutverhalten und pathologischer Schlaf bei Tumor der vorderen Mitellinie. *Archiv für Psychiatrie und Nervenkrankheiten*, *201*, 593–604.

Pribram, K.H., & McGuiness, D. (1975). Arousal, activation, and effort in the control of attention. *Psychology Review*, *182*, 116–149.

Price, K., Farley, I., & Hornykiewicz, O. (1978). Neurochemistry of Parkinson's disease: Relation between striatal and limbic dopamine. In P. Roberts (Ed.), *Advances in Biochemical Psychopharmacology* (pp. 293–300). New York: Raven Press.

Raine, A., Buchsbaum, M.S., Stanley, J., Lottenberg, S., Abel, L., & Stoddard. J. (1994). Selective reductions in prefrontal glucose metabolism in murderers. *Biological Psychiatry, 36(6)*, 365–373.

Ramon y Cajal, S. (1955). *Studies on the Cerebral Cortex (Limbic Structures)* [L.M Kraft, Translator]. London: Lloyd-Luke.

Ranen, N.G., Lipsey, J.R., Treisman, G., & Ross, C.A. (1996). Sertraline in the treatment of severe aggressiveness in Huntington's disease. *Journal of Neuropsychiatry and Clinical Neurosciences, 8*, 338–340.

Rathbun, J.K. (1996). Neuropsychological aspects of Wilson's disease. *International Journal of Neuroscience, 85*, 221–229.

Rinn, W. (1984). The neuropsychology of facial expression: A review of the neurological and psychological mechanisms for producing facial expressions. *Psychological Bulletin, 95*, 52–77.

Robinson, R.G., Kubos, K.L., Starr, L.B., Rao, K., & Price, T.R. (1984). Mood disorders in stroke patients: Importance of location of lesion. *Brain, 107*, 81–93.

Robinson, R.G., & Starkstein, S. (1989). Mood disorders following stroke: New findings and future directions. *Journal of Geriatric Psychiatry, 22*, 1–15.

Robinson, R.G., & Sztela, B. (1981). Mood change following left hemisphere brain injury. *Annals of Neurology, 9*, 447–453.

Roeltgen, D.P., Sevush, S., & Heilman, K.M. (1983). Ponological agraphia: Writing by the lexical semantic route. *Neurology, 33*, 755–765.

Ross, E.D. (1981). The aprosodias: Functional–anatomic organization of the affective components of language in the right hemisphere. *Annals of Neurology, 38*, 561–589.

Ross, E.D., Homan, R., & Buck, R. (1994). Differential hemispheric lateralization of primary and social emotions. *Neuropsychiatry, Neuropsychology, and Behavioral Neurology, 7*, 1–19.

Ross, E.D., & Mesulam, M.M. (1979). Dominant language functions of the right hemisphere? Prosody and emotional gesturing. *Archives of Neurology, 36*, 144–148.

Rossi, G.S., & Rosadini, G. (1967). Experimental analysis of cerebral dominance in man. In C. Millikan & F.L. Darley (Eds.), *Brain Mechanisms Underlying Speech and Language* (pp. 167–175). New York: Grune & Stratton.

Roy-Byrne, P.P., Uhde, T.W., Sack, D.A., Linnoila, M., & Post, R.M. (1986). Plasma HVA and anxiety in patients with panic disorder. *Biological Psychiatry, 21*, 849–853.

Sackeim, H.A., Greenberg, M.S., Weiman, A.L., Gur, R.C., Hungerbuhler, I.P., & Geschwind, N. (1982). Hemispheric asymmetry in the expression of positive and negative emotions: Neurologic evidence. *Archives of Neurology, 39*, 210–218.

Sato, H., Hata, Y., Hagihara, K., & Tsumoto, T. (1987). Effects of cholinergic depletion on neuron activities in the cat visual cortex. *Journal of Neurophysiology, 58*, 781–794.

Scatton, B., Javoy-Agid, F., Rouquier, L., Dubois, B., & Agid, Y. (1983). Reduction of cortical dopamine, noradrenaline, serotonin and their metabolites in Parkinson's disease. *Brain Research, 275*, 321–328.

Schacter, S., & Singer, J.E. (1962). Cognitive, social, and physiological determinants of emotional state. *Psychological Review, 69*, 379–399.

Scheibel, M.E., & Scheibel, A.B. (1966). The organization of the nucleus reticularis thalami: A Golgi study. *Brain Research, 1*, 43–62.

Schiffer, R.B., Kurlan, R., Rubin, A., & Boer, S. (1988). Evidence for atypical depression in Parkinson's disease. *American Journal of Psychiatry, 145*, 1020–1022.

Schmitt, J., Hartje, W., & Wilmes, K. (1997). Hemispheric asymmetry in the recognition of emotional attitide conveyed by facial expression, prosody, and propositional speech. *Cortex, 33*, 65–81.

Schrandt, N.J., Tranel, D., & Damasio, H. (1989). The effects of total cerebral lesions on skin conductance response to signal stimuli. *Neurology, 39(Suppl. 1)*, 223.

Scott, S., Caird, F., & Williams, B. (1984). Evidence for an apparent sensory speech disorder in Parkinson's disease. *Journal of Neurology, Neurosurgery, and Psychiatry, 47*, 840–843.

Scott, S., Young, A., Calder, A., Hellawell, D., Aggleton, J., & Johnson, M. (1997). Impaired auditory recognition of fear and anger following bilateral amygdala lesions. *Nature, 385(16)*, 254–257.

Scully, R.E., Mark, E.J., & McNeely, B.U. (1983). Case records of the Massachusetts General Hospital. *New England Journal of Medicine, 23*, 1406–1414.

Segundo, J.P., Naguet, R., & Buser, P. (1955). Effects of cortical stimulation on electrocortical activity in monkeys. *Neurophysiology, 1B*, 236–245.

Sharma, R., Palamadai, N., Venkatasubramanian, M.B., & Davis, J.M. (1992). Proton magnetic resonance spectroscopy of the brain in schizophrenic and affective patients. *Schizophrenia Research, 8*, 43–49.

Shute, C.C.D., & Lewis, P.R. (1967). The ascending cholinergic reticular system, neocortical olfactory and subcortical projections. *Brain, 90*, 497–520.

Slomine, B.S. (1995). *Hemispheric Differences in Emotional Psychophysiology*. Unpublished doctoral dissertation, University of Florida, Gainesville.

Smith, M.A., Smith, M.K., & Ellgring, H. (1996). Spontaneous and posed facial expression in Parkinson's disease. *Journal of the International Neuropsychological Society, 2*, 383–391.

Speedie, L.J., Brake, N., Folstein, S.E., Bowers, D., & Heilman, K.M. (1990). Comprehension of prosody in Huntington's disease. *Journal of Neurology, Neurosurgery, and Psychiatry, 53*, 607–610.

Spigset, O., & von Scheele, C. (1997). Levodopa dependence and abuse in Parkinson's disease. *Pharmacotherapy, 17*, 1027–1030.

Sprengelmeyer, R., Young, A.W., Calder, A.J., Karnat, A., Lange, H., Homberg, V., Perrett, D.I., & Rowland, D. (1996). Loss of disgust. Perception of faces and emotions in Huntington's disease. *Brain, 119*, 1647–1665.

Starkstein, S.E., Robinson, R.G., Berthier, M.L., Parikh, R.M., & Price, T.R. (1988). Differential mood changes following basal ganglia versus thalamic lesions. *Archives of Neurology, 45*, 725–730.

Starkstein, S.E., Robinson, R.G., & Price, T.R. (1987). Comparison of cortical and subcortical lesions in the production of poststroke mood disorders. *Brain, 110*, 1045–1059.

St. Clair, J., Borod, J.C., Sliwinski, M., Cole, L.J., & Stern, Y. (1998). Cognitive and affective functioning in Parkinson's disease patients with lateralized motor signs. *Journal of Clinical and Experimental Neuropsychology, 20(3)*, 320–327.

Steele, J.C., Richardson, J.C., & Olszewski, J. (1964). Progressive supranuclear palsy: A heterogenous degeneration involving the brainstem, basal ganglia, and cerebellum with vertical gaze and pseudobulbar palsy, nuchal dystonia, and dementia. *Archives of Neurology, 10*, 333–359.

Stein, M.B., Heuser, I.J., Juncos, J.L., & Uhde, T.W. (1990). Anxiety disorders in patients with Parkinson's disease. *American Journal of Psychiatry, 147*, 217–220.

Steriade, M., & Glenn, L. (1982). Neocortical and caudate projections of intralaminar thalamic neurons and their synaptic excitation from the midbrain reticular core. *Journal of Neurophysiology, 48*, 352–370.

Sternlieb, L., & Scheinbeg, I.H. (1964). Penicillamine therapy for hepatolenticular degeneration. *Journal of the American Medical Association, 189,* 748–754.

Stevens, J.R., & Hermann, B.P. (1981). Temporal lobe epilepsy, psychopathology, and violence: The state of the evidence. *Neurology, 31,* 1127–1132.

Strauss, E., Risser, A., & Jones, M.W. (1982). Fear responses in patients with epilepsy. *Neurology, 39,* 626–630.

Stuss, D.T., & Benson, D.F. (1986). *The Frontal Lobes.* New York: Raven Press.

Swayze, V.W. II, Andreasen, N.C., Alliger, R.J., Yuh, W.T., & Ehrhardt, J.C. (1992). Subcortical and temporal structures in affective disorder and schizophrenia: A magnetic resonance imaging study. *Biological Psychiatry, 31,* 221–240.

Taylor, D.C. (1959). Aggression and epilepsy. *Journal of Psychiatric Research, 13,* 229–236.

Terzian, H. (1964). Behavioral and EEG effects of intracarotid sodium amytal injections. *Acta Neurochirugica, 12,* 230–240.

Tomkins, S.S. (1962). *Affect, Imagery, Consciousness, Vol. 1, The Positive Affects.* New York: Springer.

Tomkins, S.S. (1963). *Affect, Imagery, Consciousness, Vol. 2, The Negative Affects.* New York: Springer.

Trautner, R.J., Cummings, J.L., Read, S.L., & Benson, D.F. (1988). Idiopathic basal ganglia calcification and organic mood disorder. *American Journal of Psychiatry, 145,* 350–353.

Tucker, D.M. (1981). Lateral brain function, emotion, and conceptualization. *Psychological Bulletin, 89,* 19–46.

Tucker, D.M., Watson, R.T., & Heilman, K.M. (1977). Affective discrimination and evocation in patients with right parietal disease. *Neurology, 17,* 947–950.

Tucker, D.M., & Williamson, P.A. (1984). Asymmetric neural control in human self-regulation. *Psychological Review, 91,* 185–215.

Ursin, H. (1960). The temporal lobe substrate of fear and anger. *Acta Psychiatrica Scandinavica, 35,* 378–396.

Volkow, N.D., Tancredi, L.R., Grant, C., Gillespie, H., Valentine, A., Mullani, N., Wang, G.J., & Hollister, L. (1995). Brain glucose metabolism in violent psychiatric patients: A preliminary study. *Psychiatry Research, 61(4),* 243–253.

Vogel, H.P. (1982). Symptoms of depression in Parkinson's disease. *Pharmacopsychiatrica, 15,* 192–196.

Watson, R.T., Heilman, K.M., Miller, B.D., & King, F.A. (1974). Neglect after mesencephalic reticular formation lesions. *Neurology, 24,* 294–298.

Watson, R.T., Miller, B.D., & Heilman, K.M. (1978). Nonsensory neglect. *Annals of Neurology, 3,* 505–508.

Watson, R.T., Valenstein, E., & Heilman, K.M. (1981). Thalamic neglect: The possible role of the medial thalamus and nucleus reticularis thalami in behavior. *Archives of Neurology, 38,* 501–507.

Wechsler, A.F. (1973). The effect of organic brain disease on recall of emotionally charged versus neutral narrative texts. *Neurology, 23,* 130–135.

Whalen, P.J., Rauch, S., Etcoff, N., McInerney, S., Lee, M., & Jenike, M. (1998). Masked presentations of emotional facial expressions modulate amygdala activity without explicit knowledge. *Journal of Neuroscience, 18,* 411–418.

Williams, D. (1956). The structure of emotions reflected in epileptic experiences. *Brain, 79,* 29–67.

Williams, D. (1969). Neural factors related to habitual aggression. *Brain, 92,* 503–520.

Wilson, S.A.K. (1924). Some problems in neurology. II Pathological laughing and crying. *Journal of Neurology and Psychopathology, 16*, 299–333.

Woods, J.W. (1956). Taming of the wild Norway rat by rhinocephalic lesions. *Nature, 170*, 869.

Wundt, W. (1903). *Grundriss der Psychologie*. Stuttgart: Engelmann.

Yakovlev, P.I. (1948). Motility, behavior, and the brain: Stereodynamic organization and neural coordinates of behavior. *Journal of Nervous and Mental Disease, 107*, 313–335.

Yang, J.A., & Rehm, L.P. (1993). A study of autobiographical memories in depressed and nondepressed elderly individuals. *International Journal of Aging and Human Development, 36(1)*, 39–55.

Yokoyama, K., Jennings, R., Ackles, P., Hood, P., & Boller, F. (1987). Lack of heart rate changes during an attention-demanding task after right hemisphere lesions. *Neurology, 37*, 624–630.

Young, A.W., Aggleton, J.P., Hellawell, D.J., Johnson, M., Broks, P., & Hanley, J.R. (1995). Face processing impairments after amygdalotomy. *Brain, 118*, 15–24.

Zeman, W., & King, F.A. (1958). Tumors of the septum pellucidum and adjacent structures with abnormal affective behavior: An anterior midline structure syndrome. *Journal of Nervous and Mental Disease, 127*, 490–502.

16

Rehabilitation of Emotional Deficits in Neurological Populations: A Multidisciplinary Perspective

SARAH A. RASKIN, RONALD L. BLOOM, AND JOAN C. BOROD

Traditionally, pharmacological intervention and psychotherapy have been the predominant approaches for the treatment of emotional disorders. This chapter focuses on the treatment of affect rather than on therapy designed to adjust or alter mood. Techniques from a variety of disciplines are discussed to provide a framework for the treatment of emotional deficits in patients with neurological disorders.

The chapter begins by exploring different approaches to clinical management, including cognitive rehabilitation, speech–language rehabilitation, and numerous psychotherapeutic strategies. Techniques from these various approaches are applied to the assessment and treatment of emotional processing deficits. Next, a brief overview of the emotional deficits associated with selected neurological disorders (i.e., traumatic brain injury, stroke, Parkinson's disease, senile dementia of the Alzheimer's type, and multiple sclerosis) is provided. For an in-depth discussion, see Heilman et al. (Chapter 15, this volume).

Based on the model of fundamental emotional responses conceptualized in Part II of this volume, specific treatment strategies are proposed for depression, anxiety/stress, anger/irritability, apathy/indifference, and impaired affect. Detailed descriptions of these emotional disorders are given elsewhere in this volume. In this chapter, processes that underlie cognition, language, and speech, and their relationships to emotional processing, are discussed, and the need for a multidisciplinary approach to rehabilitation is emphasized.

CONTEMPORARY REHABILITATION

Approaches to Rehabilitation

We begin with a review of cognitive and speech–language rehabilitation techniques. These techniques provide a basis for the treatment of emotional disorders.

Cognitive rehabilitation and speech–language therapy

Cognitive rehabilitation or remediation is a form of intervention in which a series of procedures are applied by a trained practitioner to retrain or alleviate problems in a person's daily life due to deficits in cognitive functions (e.g., Sohlberg & Mateer, 1989). There are many theoretical models that support different types of cognitive rehabilitation currently in practice (e.g., Diller & Gordon, 1981; Sohlberg & Mateer, 1989). Similarly, speech–language therapy is a systematic approach to rehabilitation that emphasizes restoration of an individual's communication abilities. There are numerous theories that attempt to explain the relationships among brain, language, and behavior (Goodglass & Kaplan, 1983) and theoretical models that support a host of techniques designed to assist recovery of speech (Duffy, 1995) and language (Chapey, 1986).

Clinical models are still needed to form the basis of emotional rehabilitation, but models of emotional processing (e.g., Borod, 1993b) can provide a basis for intervention. In general, models of rehabilitation can be divided into two basic approaches: functional skills training and process-oriented rehabilitation. Both approaches have implications for the rehabilitation of emotional deficits in neurological populations.

Functional skills training. Functional skills training involves retraining specific skills of daily life, most often in a particular living or work environment. The skill to be retrained is broken down into component parts; the underlying cognitive requirements of the skill or task are not examined (Mayer, Keating, & Rapp, 1986). Generalization to other contexts is not a goal of treatment (Kirsch, Levine, & Fallon-Krueger, 1987). Although the targeting of specific tasks encountered in the individual's daily life can appear to have considerable ecological validity, the narrow focus and restricted generalizability may limit the potential for recovery. Practical limitations on the number of skills that can be targeted and trained make this approach less relevant for many patients. For example, in terms of emotional processing, one could train specific skills such as smiling when given a cue. The generalizability to a real life situation would, however, be limited.

The process approach. The process approach involves remediation of deficits in specific cognitive areas (e.g., memory). These areas are related to specific brain systems and can be analyzed into component parts. With regard to emotional processing, remediation could be conducted whether the problem occurred in a specific processing mode (e.g., perception), communication channel (e.g., facial), emotional dimension (e.g., pleasantness), or discrete emotion (e.g., happiness).

The process approach proceeds through one or more of these areas in a progression from less difficult to more difficult tasks. Many of these techniques are derived from the cognitive (e.g., Anderson, 1996), experimental (e.g., Raichle et al., 1994), and rehabilitation psychology (e.g., Wilson et al., 1994) literature. Individualized training programs are generally based on the specific patient's pattern of cognitive and communicative impairment and are oriented toward their vocational goals and ability to live independently. Within the process approach, three general methods have been utilized. The first, retraining, involves improvement or restoration of specific cognitive functions. The second involves training in the use of specific compensatory strategies that help the person adapt to his or her limitations. The third involves increasing the individual's awareness by training the capacity to regulate one's behavior. Each of these methods might be applied to emotional deficits.

Retraining was conceptualized by Luria (1963) as facilitating recovery of cognitive functions after brain injury through newly established connections within the central nervous system. Luria (1963) speculated that the underlying mechanism of recovery involves reorganization within the damaged brain region, as well as transfer of function to the opposite cerebral hemisphere. When one neural system breaks down, a second system may become operational and take over for the damaged system (Stein, Brailowsky, & Will, 1995).

Several approaches in speech–language pathology utilize the idea of transfer of function to the opposite side of the brain. For example, Melodic Intonation Therapy (Helm-Estabrooks, Nicholas, & Morgan, 1989) exploits right-hemisphere prosodic abilities to promote language use in patients with damage to language centers in the left hemisphere. Perhaps the opposite could be done for individuals with aprosodia (Ross, 1997).

Compensation training, on the other hand, is based on the idea that some processes cannot be regained following brain damage. Rather, the individual is shown how to work around the lost function. Examples include using a different sensory modality (e.g., tactile input for visuospatial deficits [Luria, 1963]) or employing an external aid (e.g., a notebook for memory loss [Sohlberg & Mateer, 1989]) or an alternative communication system, such as a computerized lapboard to help patients discuss family issues or state how they feel (Silverman, 1995). Persons with flat facial affect could, for example, be taught to exaggerate prosody.

The noetic approach focuses on increasing awareness of deficits and on the capacity to recognize and regulate behavior. This approach has been used primarily in individuals with frontal-system pathology. The individual learns through practice to internalize specific skills or behaviors and to apply them to a variety of situations (e.g., Cicerone & Wood, 1987; Sohlberg, Sprunk, & Metzelaar, 1988). Related to the noetic approach are metalinguistic forms of speech–language therapy (e.g., Myers, 1994).

Multidisciplinary treatment

Although it is essential that treatment be individualized, many programs have stressed the benefits of the milieu approach (Ben-Yishay et al., 1985). Depending on the nature of the deficits, this approach can include a neuropsychologist, speech–language pathologist, psychotherapist, social worker, vocational counselor, physiatrist, psychiatrist, occupational therapist, physical therapist, and/or recreational therapist. See Table 16.1 for a brief description of the typical functions of each member of the rehabilitation team.

In many settings, each professional operates independently, and the patient is scheduled for separate appointments with several services. In other settings, the team meets regularly to discuss each case but appointments remain separate. In milieu settings, issues are dealt with daily in as natural an environment as possible. In addition to individual sessions, there are frequent group sessions and community-based activities.

Caregiver participation

The patient's significant other is considered a critical member of the rehabilitation process. Most caregiver programs focus on education about the nature of the problem and its psychological, communicative, and neurological consequences. The second avenue focuses on altering the patient's environment and examining communication roles between partners. For example, Lubinski (1981) noted that certain environments may contain removable obstacles to communication (e.g., noise elimination). Lyons (1992) underscored the importance of working directly with a patient's significant others. People in the patient's environment are taught to establish and practice alternative modes of functioning and to accept patients' limitations.

Assessment Techniques for Rehabilitation

The evaluation of individuals who participate in rehabilitation requires some variation from the usual neuropsychological assessment techniques. An additional goal of this assessment is to determine the relative contributions of the individual's neurological disorder and his or her reaction to it. Diagnostic accuracy is extremely important so that treatment can be appropriately tailored. For example, in the case of depression, it is critical that standard self-report scales of depression not be the only measures employed. Standard scales typically contain

Table 16.1 Role of Rehabilitation Professionals

TITLE	DEGREE	CLINICAL FUNCTION
Neuropsychologist	Ph.D.	Perform cognitive, personality, and mood assessment
		May do rehabilitation
Speech Language Pathologist	M.A. CCC-SLP	Provide speech and language assessment and treatment
		Provide swallowing assessment and treatment
		May do rehabilitation
Psychotherapist	Ph.D. or M.A.	Perform psychotherapy
		May do personality and mood assessment
		May do relaxation training
Social Worker	M.S.W.	Provide discharge planning
		Mediate family meetings
		May do psychotherapy
Vocational Counselor	M.A.	Perform vocational assessment
		Provide vocational counseling
Physiatrist	M.D.	Perform physical examination
		Provide rehabilitation planning
		Prescribe medication (including pain relief)
Psychiatrist	M.D.	Perform personality and mood assessment
		Prescribe psychotropic medication
Occupational Therapist	M.A. O.T.R.	Evaluate hand functions
		Provide splints, braces
		Evaluate cognitive skills required for daily living
		Rehabilitate activities of daily living
Physical Therapist	M.A. R.P.T.	Evaluate motor functions
		Provide braces, cane
		Rehabilitate motor functions
		Provide pain management
Recreational Therapist	M.A. or B.A.	Evaluate recreational interests
		Train compensations needed to participate in recreational activities

vegetative items (e.g., lack of energy and trouble initiating activities) that could easily be due to neurological dysfunction rather than to depression per se. Testing of language, including pragmatics, should be augmented with informal observations of communication abilities in naturally occurring situations. It is critical that the speech–language examination also evaluate resonance, phonation, prosody, and respiration, as these processes may interfere with affective expression. Because it is likely that individuals will be tested both before and after treatment, objective and reliable clinical measures should be utilized. Finally, it is essential that measures of generalization be employed from the time of initial assessment. Measures of generalization should include those that are specific to processes being rehabilitated and those that assess everyday functioning.

Generalization of Treatment

The importance of generalizing treatment to daily life is ingrained in clinical practice (Raskin & Gordon, 1992). An understanding of generalization and how to facilitate it, however, are still, for the most part, lacking in the field of rehabilitation. Generalization of cognitive rehabilitation, for example, has been described by Gordon (1987) at three levels: (*1*) gains from remediation are observed on the same materials on separate occasions, (*2*) improvement on training tasks is also observed on similar but not identical sets of tasks, and (*3*) functions gained in training transfer to functions in day-to-day living.

Recently, Sohlberg and Raskin (1996) proposed generalization strategies (adapted from Anderson, 1996; Stokes & Baer, 1977) that could be broadly implemented in both research and clinical practice in emotional rehabilitation. These principles include actively planning for and programming generalization from the beginning of the treatment process, identifying reinforcements in the natural environment, programming stimuli common to training and real-world environments, and using sufficient examples when conducting treatment.

The most difficult of these principles is the selection of measures of generalization. Three approaches have been suggested (Sohlberg & Raskin, 1996). The first applies to the treatment targeted and might include a rating form targeting behaviors specifically trained, such as a questionnaire to be completed by a significant other regarding the patient's ability to verbally express sadness. The second includes measures of everyday functioning specific to the area of treatment, such as emotional expression. The final approach applies to the individual's daily life in more general terms. Measures of generalization should examine social interaction, productive activities, and independence. Examples of such measures include the Community Integration Questionnaire (Willer & Corrigan, 1994) and the Craig Handicap Assessment and Reporting Technique (Whiteneck et al., 1992).

Finally, generalization may be enhanced by having a spouse or significant other administer practice exercises that teach the patient to use compensatory strategies. Generalization may also be enhanced by having the patient practice using the system in a natural environment (e.g., school, workplace, or home).

TREATMENT OF EMOTION

The emotional deficits that follow neurological disorders and acquired brain injury have typically been treated with medication, cognitive therapy, and behavior therapy. Recent work suggests that affective difficulties are amenable to direct remediation techniques (Myers, 1998; Tompkins, 1995). For example, Hornak, Rolls, and Wade (1996) suggest that individuals who have deficits in the prosodic expression of emotion could be encouraged to take advantage of intact facial emotional expressions when talking to others (i.e., a compensation technique). In a similar vein, Borod, Bloom, and Haywood (1998) recommend that patients with right-brain damage who demonstrate deficits in the verbal expression of emotion be systematically exposed to a hierarchy of situations that gradually increase in emotional intensity.

Certain neurological etiologies have yielded predictable patterns of emotional disorders. For example, patients with left-brain damage and aphasia have shown relatively preserved emotional expression (Blonder et al., 1993) or have demonstrated increased emotional intensity while producing affective expressions (Kent et al., 1988; Montreys & Borod, 1998). In contrast, patients with right-brain damage have demonstrated reduced accuracy and intensity in producing emotional expression (Borod, 1993a). Cognitive and communication abilities can interact with emotional deficits and thereby influence treatment approaches. For example, auditory or attention deficits can impair the interpretation of emotional prosody or facial expression, and limitations in speech movement can reduce the production of verbal emotional expression.

Emotional Deficits Associated with Common Neurological Disorders

Traumatic brain injury

Traumatic brain injury produces a wide range of emotional changes, depending on the mechanism of injury and premorbid factors. Because of the susceptibility of the prefrontal cortex to damage in acceleration/deceleration injuries, common emotional changes with such injuries include apathy, impulsivity, poor emotional control, and poor social judgement. Individuals frequently experience depression, anxiety, and post-traumatic stress disorder. Depending on the consequences of the injury on daily living, individuals can experience a "shaken sense of self" (Kay, 1992) in which poor cognitive performance leads to poor social or occupational functioning, which in turn leads to lowered self-esteem, increased depression, and increased anxiety. Rehabilitation efforts must include attempts to interrupt this cycle and deal with the interacting cognitive and emotional symptoms together.

Stroke

Stroke has been the focus of cognitive rehabilitation, speech–language therapy, and a large number of studies aimed at treating depression. There is some controversy regarding lesion location and incidence of depression (Starkstein & Robinson, 1992). Treatment in the acute phase post-stroke must be different than that after more recovery has occurred. There is some evidence that depression following stroke becomes worse over time (Robinson & Price, 1982). In addition to depression, survivors of stroke may experience apathy and indifference (see Robinson & Manes, Chapter 10, this volume).

Parkinson's disease

Depression is the emotional disorder most frequently associated with Parkinson's disease (PD) (Cummings, 1986). The depression does not appear to be merely a reaction to the cognitive and motoric deficits because the symptoms do not covary (e.g., Mayeux et al., 1984). As would follow, treatment of the motor symptoms alone does not generally improve the depression. As in other neurological disorders, the diagnosis of depression must be made without reference to the masked face, reduced motor activity, speech disorder (i.e., dysarthria), and slow information processing commonly seen in PD. As PD is a progressive disorder, treatment of cognition and communication must be aimed at slowing progression rather than at amelioration. In addition to depression, a number of studies have shown deficits in PD patients relative to neurologically healthy normal adults for the perception and expression of facial and prosodic emotion (e.g., Borod et al., 1990; Brozgold et al., 1998; Buck & Duffy, 1980; Scott, Caird, & Williams, 1984).

Alzheimer's disease

Personality and psychiatric disturbances in senile dementia of the Alzheimer's type (SDAT) vary greatly according to premorbid personality and stage of the disease. The disease can lead to a wide range of behavioral and emotional difficulties and are often the earliest symptoms. Apathy is common, as are agitation and rage (Haley, Brown, & Levine, 1987). There is evidence of an increased incidence of depression, but this decreases as the disease progresses. Approximately 30% of SDAT patients meet criteria for clinical depression (Borod, 1996).

SDAT is a progressive disorder and thus must be treated with goals that are similar to those in PD. These include, for example, putting systems in place in anticipation of later deterioration. Frequently, these systems involve environmental modification. Behavioral symptoms appear to change somewhat predictably as the disease progresses. In early stages, individuals have mood swings and increased dependence. This is often followed by apathy, agitation, and/or restlessness; increased violence or anger; and frequent suspiciousness.

Multiple sclerosis

Multiple sclerosis is a demyelinating disease of the central nervous system that results in lesions of the myelin sheath. These lesions begin with inflammation and edema and later become plaque formations (Adams, 1993). In some individuals, the disorder is progressive, while in others there may be remission, possibly due to remyelination (Poser et al., 1983). There may also be diffuse effects, including cerebral atrophy (Adams, 1993). The most common symptoms are fatigue, motor weakness, motor incoordination, spasticity, visual disturbance, paresthesia, and pain (Rao, 1986). Emotional symptoms are likely to include depression or euphoria (Minden & Schiffer, 1990; Rao, Huber, & Bornstein, 1992).

Because symptoms may be slowly progressive or fluctuating, many patients may be referred first to psychiatrists to rule out conversion disorder, which would impact on emotional symptoms and adjustment. Of note, the clinical course of multiple sclerosis is highly variable (Rao, 1986). If an individual is on a progressively deteriorating course, standard retraining techniques may be inappropriate. Rather, a focus on compensatory strategies and environmental modifications that are trained early on can be useful throughout many stages of the illness.

Treatment of Specific Emotional Deficits

This section focuses on particular emotional symptoms that may occur with a range of neurological disorders. Although treatment will vary depending on diagnosis, the basic approach to these symptoms is likely to be similar. Many of these approaches are borrowed from standard psychotherapy practice but are modified for use with individuals with neurological dysfunction. In all cases, the approach chosen will depend on the cognitive profile of the individual, as well as on the emotional symptom(s). Hibbard and colleagues (1990a), for example, argue that more cognitively impaired individuals respond better to behavioral approaches, whereas those with greater insight and cognitive functioning respond better to cognitive therapy approaches.

The psychopharmacological treatment of emotional disorders in persons with brain damage requires special consideration. For many individuals, treatment with medication may be contraindicated due to coexisting medical problems. In addition, the side effects of psychopharmacological agents may further interfere with cognitive and emotional functioning. For the clinical management of the patient, it is important to be aware of his or her medication status and to discuss with the prescribing physician the effects of these medications on functioning. For example, when treating depression, anticholinergic use (such as tertiary amine tricyclics) should be closely monitored for increased confusional state, slurred speech, blurred vision, and fatigue. Fluoxetine can cause sleep changes and headache, as well as increase seizure risk. All non-monoamine oxidase inhibitor antidepressants can cause sedation. Treatment of anger includes the use of serotonergic drugs, antiseizure medication, and benzodiazepines, which can cause fatigue and sedation. Another drawback to pharmacological management is that many people are already heavily medicated for coexisting conditions. Finally, not all individuals respond well to or are compliant with taking medication. For further discussion of pharmacological intervention, see Lisanby and Sackeim (Chapter 18, this volume).

Depression

Depression is a very frequent concomitant of acquired neurological dysfunction. For post-stroke depression, Hibbard and colleagues (e.g., Grober et al., 1993; Hibbard et al., 1990a,b) suggest that psychotherapy may be the treatment of choice. Psychotherapy allows persons with neurological dysfunction to learn new coping styles, improve social skills, and increase their sense of mastery and control, which can help prevent the recurrence of depression.

Cognitive therapy. Using the cognitive therapy model (Beck et al., 1979), Hibbard and colleagues (1990a) provide a series of principles specific to treatment of post-stroke depression that can be adapted for persons with other types of neurological dysfunction. These principles include the following: (*1*) level of cognitive functioning moderates treatment strategies used; (*2*) cognitive remediation enhances patients' ability to profit from therapy; (*3*) new learning and generalization are difficult for stroke patients; (*4*) patients' awareness of depressive symptomatology moderates the therapeutic strategy; (*5*) mourning is an important component of treatment; (*6*) premorbid personality, lifestyle, and interests provide a context for understanding current behavior; (*7*) understanding the discrepancy between actual and perceived losses is essential to treatment; (*8*) reinforcing even small therapeutic gains improves mood; (*9*) emphasis on the collaborative therapeutic relationship facilitates a working alliance; (*10*) to ensure continuity of treatment, session flexibility is essential; (*11*) fluctuations in medical status affect the course of treatment; (*12*) distortions of family members must be addressed in therapy; (*13*) family members' mourning must be addressed; and (*14*) family members are important therapeutic helpers. In conjunction with traditional cognitive therapy, these principles provide specific tools with which to address the depression following neurological impairment.

The cognitive therapeutic approach assumes that depression is caused by "dysfunctional thoughts" (Beck et al., 1979). Cognitive therapy focuses on identifying aspects of these thoughts that are irrational and challenging the distortions with more rational thinking. Importantly, cognitive therapy is an active, directive, and time-limited approach. In this approach, maladaptive assumptions developed from prior experience are identified (e.g., "If I don't do everything perfectly, then I'm a failure"). The therapy includes monitoring these negative thoughts; learning to recognize the connections among thoughts, feelings, and behavior; examining evidence for and against the distorted thoughts; substituting more realistic interpretations; and altering dysfunctional beliefs that can distort an individual's experiences.

Behavioral interventions. As in traditional cognitive therapy, behavioral strategies are also an important component of treating depression. It may be the primary approach for persons with severe cognitive deficits and/or limited awareness (Grober et al., 1993). Behavioral interventions may be incorporated into the therapeutic process. Role-playing coping responses can be used to enhance generalization, and assertiveness training can help patients regain a sense of competence.

Behavioral assignments, based on work explored in a session, are provided to test and challenge dysfunctional thinking. For example, if a person's belief is that "because I have a brain injury, I can't do anything well," then tasks that easily can be accomplished should be employed. Furthermore, assignments should target symptoms of depression (e.g., loneliness) and involve activities that were previously pleasurable (Stein & Raskin, 2000). As the person progresses, a feelings log or diary (Beck et al., 1979) is sometimes useful.

The grieving process. Recovering from depression after brain damage is analogous to the grieving process (Kubler-Ross, 1969) because it identifies losses that are not always obvious to the patient. Such losses include cognitive abilities, emotional control, work status, self-esteem, autonomy, sense of self, intimacy, pain-free health, control over how one spends time (e.g., going to appointments and contacting insurance companies), and plans for the future.

Anxiety and post-traumatic stress disorder

Anxiety occurs in a wide range of neurological conditions as a physiological result of injury and as a reaction to decreased cognitive resources.

Cognitive and behavioral strategies. Immediately following an injury or illness, daily functioning is often disrupted. Common tasks may be challenging or fatiguing, and the individual's confidence may become eroded. Often, the most common symptom reported by the patient is anxiety. Providing the patient with information about anxiety, along with reassurance of its reversible nature, may lead to increased insight. Behavioral strategies for anxiety management might include controlled/deep breathing; progressive muscle relaxation; frequent/brief walks or stretching when symptoms begin to manifest; and improved sleep patterns and overall amount of sleep.

Relaxation training. Relaxation training may be a useful method for reducing anxiety that occurs subsequent to neurological disorder. A connection is established between the abilities to enter a relaxed state under ideal circumstances and to generalize relaxation to other situations. Relaxation training may take the form of therapist-guided exercises in sessions or listening to similar exercises on commercially produced cassettes.

Systematic desensitization. Systematic desensitization is a behavioral approach that entails relaxation in conjunction with gradual exposure to trauma-related stimuli. In this way, individuals improve control over their reactions to these stimuli within treatment, which can then be generalized to daily life. One approach to systematic desensitization requires that descriptions of images, activities, or situations that elicit symptoms be recorded. These scenarios can be ranked or rated by degree of anxiety. While the patient is in a relaxed state, the therapist begins describing the triggers that produce anxiety. If the individual indicates symptoms of anxiety, the therapist ceases or decreases exposure to the trigger and facilitates relaxation. Persons with cognitive dysfunction may require a more structured approach toward anxiety reduction (e.g., written instructions and schedules) (Hovland & Raskin, 2000).

Anger

Increases in irritability and expressions of anger or frustration are frequently reported with many neurological conditions. Anger and frustration may be expressed as negative self-talk, verbal abusiveness, and/or physical aggressiveness. Stress and turmoil are created in the home, and significant problems at work may occur when individuals exhibit such behaviors. Disinhibition, common in brain damage, may result in impulsivity, distractibility, fatigue, and irritability. Premorbid personality and reactive emotional responses may also contribute to the expression of anger.

McKay, Rogers, and McKay (1989) suggest that anger can reduce stress by discharging or blocking awareness of painful levels of emotional or physical arousal. Anger may serve to dissipate painful affect, reduce or eliminate painful sensations, release tension, and be a response to perceived threats.

Cognitive therapy. Hovland and Mateer (2000) provide a comprehensive discussion of the treatment of anger after brain injury. The following treatment approaches are based largely on their work.

Early in treatment, if concerns arise regarding the potential for escalating aggression or violence, steps should be taken to make the environment safe via environmental management. This might include having potential weapons removed, removing alcohol or drugs, providing supervision, or contacting appropriate agencies. The family or significant others can be advised of environmental strategies, such as leaving the person when signs of anger develop or distracting the person by changing the focus of conversation or activity.

Behavioral therapies. Another approach to anger management has a more behavioral focus. The behavioral approach tends to be concrete, focuses on measurable behaviors, and is data based and hierarchical in nature. This systematic approach is of particular benefit for individuals whose irritability and anger may have a more organic than situational basis and who have difficulty with abstraction, memory, attention, or self-awareness.

Novaco (1979) described the stress inoculation approach to anger control as not attempting to suppress anger but rather to minimize maladaptive affects and maximize adaptive functioning. Novaco (1979) specified the following stages for this training: preparation for provocation, confrontation, coping with arousal, subsequent reflection, conflict unresolved, and conflict resolved. Wood (1984, 1987) described a large number of cases in which behavior therapy was used to manage behavioral disorders in brain-injured patients (including aggression). Only a few studies have documented the efficacy of behavioral intervention for anger control in brain-injured individuals (e.g., Lira, Carne, & Masri, 1983; McGlynn, 1990; Uomoto & Brockaway, 1992).

It is particularly helpful for the neuropsychologist, speech–language pathologist, and cognitive therapist to work in tandem to establish the connection between frustration and cognitive deficits. Under conditions of greater cognitive demand, frustration is likely to escalate. For example, the cognitive therapist may be addressing problems with distractibility, which could be tied to the patient's irritability. Problems with divided and alternating attention on tasks can adversely affect emotional homeostasis. Finally, it is important to provide information about the relationship between emotional and cognitive deficits to the client's significant other, family, friends, coworkers, and/or employer.

Much of the focus in treatment itself is on identifying what has been termed the *angry behavior cycle* (Goldstein et al., 1987). Sessions focus on recognizing anger cues, using relaxation techniques, and using self-evaluation and reward. Anger-provoking situations are role-played with the therapist, and information is gathered about behavior outside of sessions through completion of anger-management records.

Apathy and indifference

Apathy is described by Stuss and colleagues (Chapter 14, this volume) as an absence of responsiveness that is demonstrated by poor self-initiation of action. Apathy can be observed in overt behavior but also in more subtle ways. For example, during memory testing, the individual with neurological dysfunction may not provide a response in a recall paradigm but then may produce considerable information when prompted. There also may be a poverty of language when asked to provide biographical information or to describe pictorial stimuli in the absence of aphasia. In severe cases, apathy associated with depression can mimic dementia. In younger individuals, apathy is often mistaken for being lazy, malingering, or having a psychiatric disturbance (Lezak, 1995).

Stuss and colleagues (Chapter 14, this volume) suggest that apathy can be differentiated by symptomatology and underlying brain structure. For example, damage to any one of five frontal/subcortical circuits leads to a unique form of apathy.

Campbell and Duffy (1997) point out the importance of evaluating environmental and family contributions to apathy. Family therapy is recommended using a problem-centered model that includes education, clarification of roles, instruction in interpersonal communication, and techniques for problem-solving.

Rehabilitation approaches to apathy have included behavioral techniques. The individual can be given structured activities to perform at preset times so that it is not up to him or her to initiate activities. Opportunities for reward are provided. At the same time, the individual can be educated about the neurological cause of apathy. Increased awareness is then made a treatment goal. With this type of treatment, videotapes of the individual interacting in group settings or feedback from peer group members can be very helpful (Sohlberg et al., 1993).

Behavior modification of apathy was used successfully by Rosenthal and Meyer (1971) in a case study of a woman diagnosed with clinical abulia due to non-neurological causes. She was helped to set goals, use new problem-solving techniques, and increase environmental opportunities for reward.

Affective Deficits

Affect is expressed through the complex combination of verbal language, voice, prosody, face, gesture, and posture. When affective communication is impaired, there may be marked difficulty in the discrimination and/or production of a range of facial expressions. In addition, deficits in the perception and use of prosody, gesture, body posture, and body position may diminish an individual's participation in communication. Such patients may demonstrate difficulty in interpreting situational cues that signal emotional meaning.

Affective disorders occur in a variety of neurological conditions, including stroke, PD, traumatic brain injury, and SDAT. For example, patients with stroke and damage to the right cerebral hemisphere have demonstrated deficits within the facial (Borod, 1992), prosodic (Tompkins, 1995), and verbal (Borod, Bloom, & Haywood, 1998) channels of emotional communication. PD patients have reduced facial expression and articulatory deficits that limit their expression. Patients with traumatic brain injury, right-brain damage, and SDAT often demonstrate pragmatic communication disorders and deficits in discourse (Ferrand & Bloom, 1997).

Several traditional approaches from speech–language pathology may be employed to treat affective communication disorders. Augmentative and Alternative Communication (AAC) systems may be adapted to give patients access to the expression of a wide range of emotional responses (Silverman, 1995). Augmentative and Alternative Communication systems can take the form of lapboards, notebooks, or electronic devices that use synthesized speech. Prosodic deficits may be addressed with a variety of behavioral methods, for example, respiratory monitoring through visual feedback. Pragmatic language intervention may raise a patient's awareness of interpersonal communication cues (e.g., turn-taking or topic selection). Communication groups can provide an opportunity to practice communication strategies in new situations. Interpersonal communication approaches to remediation have been suggested by Davis and Wilcox (1985).

CONCLUSIONS

In summary, a number of approaches to rehabilitation have been applied to emotional processing deficits. These include cognitive remediation, behavior modification, speech–language therapy, and environmental management (e.g., caregiver participation and milieu approaches to treatment), as well as psychotherapy and psychopharmacology.

The treatment of emotional deficits needs to be applied concurrently with therapy for speech and language because auditory comprehension and expressive communication (i.e., verbal and nonverbal) seem to constrain emotional processing. For example, in stroke, a person with a left-hemisphere lesion and reduced receptive and expressive language would be a poor candidate for an affective treatment approach that relied on verbal mediation.

From a theoretical perspective, the approach taken here may have some application to the model of emotional processing proposed by Borod (Borod, 1993b; Borod et al., in press). Specifically, Borod (1993b) described a componential approach that addresses the issue of separate and related systems organized with respect to four different hierarchical levels of emotion: processing mode (i.e., appraisal, perception, arousal, experience, expression, and behavior); communication channel (i.e., facial, prosodic, lexical, gestural, and postural); emotional dimension (e.g., pleasant/unpleasant, aroused/nonaroused, and approach/avoidance); and discrete emotion (e.g., happiness, disgust, anger, and surprise). Within each level, there is the opportunity for interaction among individual elements or components.

We believe that processing modes are useful in cognitive rehabilitation (e.g., perception treated by cognitive remediation); communication channels are amenable to intervention by speech–language therapies (e.g., prosodic expression of emotion treated by visual feedback about respiration); emotional dimensions might be treated by pharmacological agents (e.g., a mood disorder treated by antidepressants); and discrete emotions may be best addressed by behavioral approaches (e.g., stress disorders treated by psychotherapy). The componential model is ripe for further testing and provides a promising approach for research in the treatment of emotional deficits from a neuropsychological perspective.

ACKNOWLEDGMENTS

This project was supported, in part, by a Trinity College Faculty Research Expense Grant to S.A.R., by a Hofstra University Research and Development Award to R.L.B., and by NIMH grant MH42172 to J.C.B.

REFERENCES

Adams, R. (1993). *Principles of Neurology*. New York: McGraw-Hill.

Anderson, J. (1996). ACT: A simple theory of complex cognition. *American Psychologist, 51*, 355–365.

Beck, A., Rush, J., Shaw, B., & Emery, G. (1979). *Cognitive Therapy for Depression*. New York: Guilford Press.

Ben-Yishay, Y., Rattok, J., Lakin, P., Piasetsky, E., Ross, B., Silver, S., Zide, E., & Ezrachi, O. (1985). Neuropsychological rehabilitation: Quest for a holistic approach. *Seminars in Neurology, 5*, 252–259.

Blonder, L., Burns, A. Bowers, D., Moore, R., & Heilman, K. (1993). *Brain and Cognition, 21*, 44–56.

Borod, J. (1992). Interhemispheric and intrahemispheric control of emotion: A focus on unilateral brain damage. *Journal of Consulting and Clinical Psychology, 60*, 339–348.

Borod, J. (1993a). Cerebral mechanisms underlying facial, prosodic, and lexical emotional expression: A review of neuropsychological studies and methodological issues. *Neuropsychology, 7*, 445–463.

Borod, J. (1993b). Emotion and the brain—Anatomy and theory: An introduction to the Special Section. *Neuropsychology, 7*, 427–432.

Borod, J. (1996). Emotional disorders/emotion. In J.G. Beaumont, P. Kenealy, & M. Rogers (Eds.), *The Blackwell Dictionary of Neuropsychology* (pp. 312–320). Oxford, England: Blackwell Publishers.

Borod, J., Bloom, R., & Haywood, C.S. (1998). Verbal aspects of emotional communication. In M. Beeman & C. Chiarello (Eds.), *Right Hemisphere Language Comprehension: Perspectives from Cognitive Neuroscience* (pp. 285–307). Mahwah, NJ: Lawrence Erlbaum Associates.

Borod, J., Pick, L., Hall, S., Sliwinski, M., Madigan, N., Obler, L., Welkowitz, J., Canino, E., Erhan, H., Goral, M., Morrison, C., & Tabert, M. (in press). Relationships among facial, prosodic, and lexical channels of emotional perceptual processing. *Cognition and Emotion*.

Borod, J., Welkowitz, J., Apert, M., Brozgold, A., Martin, C., Peselow, E., & Diller, L. (1990). Parameters of emotional processing in neuropsychiatric disorders: Conceptual issues and a battery of tests. *Journal of Communication Disorders, 23*, 247–271.

Brozgold, A., Borod, J., Martin, C., Pick, L., Alpert, M., & Welkowitz, J. (1998). Social functioning and facial emotional expression in neurological and psychiatric disorders. *Applied Neuropsychology, 5*, 15–23.

Buck, R., & Duffy, R. (1980). Nonverbal communication of affect in brain-damaged patients. *Cortex, 16*, 351–362.

Campbell, J., & Duffy, J. (1997). Treatment strategies in amotivated patients. *Psychiatric Annals, 27*, 44–49.

Chapey, R. (1986). *Language Intervention Strategies in Adult Aphasia*. Baltimore: William & Wilkins.

Cicerone, K., & Wood, J. (1987). Planning disorder after closed head injury: A case study. *Archives of Physical Medicine and Rehabilitation, 68*, 111–115.

Cummings, J. (1986). Subcortical dementia: Neuropsychology, neuropsychiatry, and pathophysiology. *British Journal of Psychiatry, 149*, 682–697.

Davis, G., & Wilcox, M. (1985). *Adult Aphasia Rehabilitation: Applied Pragmatics*. San Diego: College Hill Press.

Diller, L., & Gordon, W. (1981). Interventions for cognitive deficits in brain-injured adults. *Journal of Consulting and Clinical Psychology, 14,* 822–834.

Duffy, J. (1995). *Motor Speech Disorders: Substrates, Differential Diagnosis, and Management.* St. Louis: Mosby Year Book.

Ferrand, C., & Bloom, R. (1997). *Introduction to Organic and Neurogenic Disorders of Communication: Current Scope of Practice.* Boston, MA: Allyn and Bacon.

Goldstein, A., Glick, B., Reiner, S., Zimmerman, D., & Coultry, T. (1987). *Aggression Replacement Training: A Comprehensive Intervention for Agressive Youth.* Champaign, IL: Research Press.

Goodglass, H., & Kaplan, E. (1983). *Boston Diagnostic Aphasia Examination.* Philadelphia: Lea & Febiger.

Gordon, W. (1987). Methodological considerations in cognitive remediation. In M. Meier, A. Benton, & L. Diller (Eds.), *Neuropsychological Rehabilitation* (pp. 111–131). New York: Guilford Press.

Grober, S., Hibbard, M., Gordon, W., Stein, P., & Freeman, A. (1993). The psychotherapeutic treatment of post-stroke depression with cognitive–behavioral therapy. In W. Gordon (Ed.), *Advances in Stroke Rehabilitation* (pp. 215–241). Boston, MA: Andover Medical Publishers.

Haley, W., Brown, S., & Levine, E. (1987). Family caregiver appraisals of patient behavioral disturbance in senile dementia. *International Journal of Aging and Human Development, 25,* 25–34.

Helm-Estabrooks, N., Nicholas, M., & Morgan, A. (1989). *Melodic Intonation Therapy Program.* San Antonio, TX: Special Press.

Hibbard, M., Grober, S., Gordon, W., & Aletta, E. (1990a). Modification of cognitive psychotherapy for the treatment of post-stroke depression. *Behavior Therapist, 13,* 15–17.

Hibbard, M., Grober, S., Gordon, W., Aletta, E., & Freeman, A. (1990b). Cognitive therapy and the treatment of poststroke depression. *Topics in Geriatric Rehabilitation, 5,* 43–55.

Hornak, J., Rolls, E., & Wade, D. (1996). Face and voice expression identification in patients with emotional and behavioral changes following ventral frontal damage. *Neuropsychologia, 34,* 247–261.

Hovland, D., & Mateer, C. (2000). Treatment of irritability and anger. In S. Raskin & C. Mateer (Eds.), *Neuropsychological Management of Mild Traumatic Brain Injury.* New York: Oxford University Press.

Hovland, D., & Raskin, S. (2000). Anxiety and post-traumatic stress. In S. Raskin & C. Mateer (Eds.), *Neuropsychological Management of Mild Traumatic Brain Injury.* New York: Oxford University Press.

Kay, T. (1992). Neuropsychological diagnosis: Disentangling the multiple determinants of functional disability after mild traumatic brain injury. In L. Horn & N. Zasler (Eds.), *Rehabilitation of Post-Concussive Disorders,* Vol. 6 (pp. 109–127). Philadelphia: Henley and Belfus.

Kent, J., Borod, J., Koff, E., Welkowitz, J., & Alpert, M. (1988). Posed facial emotional expression in brain-damaged patients. *International Journal of Neuroscience, 43,* 81–87.

Kirsch, N., Levine, S., & Fallon-Krueger, M. (1987). The microcomputer as an "orthotic" device for patients with cognitive deficits. *Journal of Head Trauma Rehabilitation, 2,* 77–86.

Kubler-Ross, E. (1969). *On Death and Dying.* New York: Macmillan.

Lezak, M. (1995). *Neuropsychological Assessment.* New York: Oxford University Press.

Lira, F., Carne, W., & Masri, A. (1983). Treatment of anger and impulsivity in a brain damaged patient: A case study applying stress inoculation. *Clinical Neuropsychology*, *3*, 159–160.

Lubinski, R.(1981). Environmental language intervention. In R. Chapey (Ed.), *Language Intervention Strategies in Adult Aphasia* (pp. 162–185). Baltimore: Williams & Wilkins.

Luria, A. (1963). *Restoration of Function After Brain Injury*. New York: Pergamon Press.

Lyons, J. (1992). Communication use and participation in life for adults with aphasia in natural settings: The scope of the problem. *American Journal of Speech–Language Pathology*, *1*, 7–14.

Mayer, N., Keating, D., & Rapp, D. (1986). Skills, routines, and activity patterns of daily living: A functional nested approach. In B. Uzzell & Y. Gross (Eds.), *Clinical Neuropsychology of Intervention* (pp. 111–124). Boston: Martinus Nijhoff.

Mayeux, R., Stern, Y., Cote, L., & Williams, J. (1984). Altered serotonin metabolism in depressed patients with Parkinson's disease. *Neurology*, *34*, 642–646.

McGlynn, S. (1990). Behavioral approaches to neuropsychological rehabilitation. *Psychological Bulletin*, *108*, 420–441.

McKay, M., Rogers, P., & McKay, J. (1989). *When Anger Hurts*: *Quieting the Storm Within*. Oakland, CA: New Harbinger Publications.

Minden, S., & Schiffer, R. (1990). Affective disorders in multiple sclerosis: Review and recommendations for clinical research. *Archives of Neurology*, *47*, 98–104.

Montreys, C., & Borod, J. (1998). A preliminary evaluation of emotional experience and expression following unilateral brain damage. *International Journal of Neuroscience*, *96*, 269–283.

Myers, P. (1994). Communication disorders associated with right hemisphere damage. In R. Chapey (Ed.), *Language Intervention Strategies in Adult Aphasia*. Baltimore: Williams & Wilkins.

Myers, P. (1998). *Right Hemisphere Damage*: *Disorders of Communication and Cognition*. San Diego: Singular Publishing Group.

Novaco, R.W. (1979). The cognitive regulation of anger and stress. In P. Kendall & S. Hollon (Eds.), *Cognitive Behavioral Interventions*: *Theory, Research and Procedures* (pp. 241–285). Orlando: Academic Press.

Poser, C., Paty, L., Scheinberg, I., McDonald, F., Davis, G., Ebers, K., Johnson, W., Sibley, D., Silberberg, D., & Touretellote, W. (1993). New diagnostic criteria for multiple sclerosis: Guidelines for research protocols. *Annals of Neurology*, *13*, 227–231.

Raichle, M., Fiez, J., Videen, T., MacLeod, A., Pardo, J., Fox, P., & Petersen, S. (1994). Practice-related changes in human brain functional anatomy during nonmotor learning. *Cerebral Cortex*, *4*, 8–16.

Rao, S. (1986). Neuropsychology of multiple sclerosis: A critical review. *Journal of Clinical and Experimental Neuropsychology*, *8*, 503–542.

Rao, S., Huber, S., & Bornstein, R. (1992). Emotional changes with multiple sclerosis and Parkinson's disease. *Journal of Consulting and Clinical Psychology*, *60*, 369–712.

Raskin, S., & Gordon, W. (1992). The impact of different approaches to cognitive remediation on generalization. *NeuroRehabilitation*, *2*, 38–45.

Robinson, R., & Price, T. (1982). Post-stroke depressive disorders: A follow-up study of 103 patients. *Stroke*, *13*, 635–641.

Rosenthal, T., & Meyer, V. (1971). Case report: Behavioral treatment of clinical abulia. *Conditioned Reflex*, *6*, 22–29.

Ross, E. (1997). Right hemisphere syndromes and the neurology of emotion. In S. Schacter & O. Devinsky (Eds.), *Behavioral Neurology and the Legacy of Norman Geschwind* (pp. 183–191). Philadelphia: Lippincott-Raven.

Scott, S., Caird, F., & Williams, B. (1984). Evidence for an apparent sensory speech disorder in Parkinson's disease. *Journal of Neurology, Neurosurgery, and Psychiatry, 47*, 840–843.

Silverman, F. (1995). *Communication for the Speechless*. Boston: Allyn and Bacon.

Sohlberg, M., Johansen, A., Geyer, S., & Hoornbeek, A. (1993). *A Manual for Teaching Patients To Use Compensatory Memory Systems*. Puyallup, WA: Association for Neuropsychological Research and Development.

Sohlberg, M., & Mateer, C. (1989). *Introduction to Cognitive Rehabilitation*. New York: Guilford Press.

Sohlberg, M., & Raskin, S. (1996). Principles of generalization applied to attention and memory interventions. *Journal of Head Trauma Rehabilitation, 11*, 65–78.

Sohlberg, M., Sprunk, H., & Metzelaar, K. (1988). *Cognitive Rehabilitation, 6*, 36–41.

Starkstein, S., & Robinson, R. (1992). Neuropsychiatric aspects of cerebral vascular disorders. In S. Yudofsky & R. Hales (Eds.), *Textbook of Neuropsychiatry* (pp. 449–472). Washington, DC: American Psychiatric Press.

Stein, D., Brailowsky, S., & Will, B. (1995). *Brain Repair*. New York: Oxford University Press.

Stein, P., & Raskin, S. (2000). Treatment of depression. In S. Raskin & C. Mateer (Eds.), *Neuropsychological Management of Mild Traumatic Brain Injury*. New York: Oxford University Press.

Stokes, T., & Baer, D. (1977). An implicit technology of generalization. *Journal of Applied Behavioral Analysis, 10*, 349–367.

Tompkins, C. (1995). *Right Hemisphere Communication Disorders: Theory and Management*. San Diego, CA: Singular Publishing Group, Inc.

Uomoto, J., & Brockway, J. (1992). Anger management training for brain injured patients and their family members. *Archives of Physical Medicine and Rehabilitation, 73*, 674–679.

Whiteneck, G., Charlifue, S., Gerhart, K., Overholser, J., & Richardson, G. (1992). Quantifying handicap: A new measure of long-term rehabilitation outcomes. *Archives of Physical Medicine and Rehabilitation, 73*, 519–526.

Willer, B., & Corrigan, J. (1994). Whatever it takes: A model for community based services. *Brain Injury, 8*, 647–659.

Wilson, B., Baddeley, A., Evans, J., & Shiel, A. (1994). Errorless learning in rehabilitation of memory impaired people. *Neuropsychological Rehabilitation, 4*, 307–326.

Wood, R.L. (1984). Behavioral disorders following severe brain injury: Their presentation and psychological management. In N. Brooks (Ed.), *Closed Head Injury: Psychological, Social, and Family Consequences* (pp. 195–219). Oxford, England: Oxford University Press.

Wood, R.L. (1987). *Brain Injury Rehabilitation: A Neurobehavioral Approach*. Rockville, MD: Aspen Press.

17

Emotional Processing in Schizophrenia: A Focus on Affective States

CHRISTIAN G. KOHLER, RUBEN C. GUR, AND RAQUEL E. GUR

Schizophrenia has traditionally been viewed as a psychiatric illness with prominent clinical features of psychosis and cognitive dysfunction. Psychotic symptoms frequently consist of auditory hallucinations, paranoid or somatic delusions, and ideas of reference. Contrary to negative symptoms and cognitive dysfunction, psychotic—or "positive"—symptoms commonly fluctuate with the course of illness and respond to neuroleptic treatment.

Deficits in cognition, considered a stable hallmark of schizophrenia, have long been described, and in the early part of the twentieth century were used to differentiate schizophrenia from affective illnesses. Recent investigations have shown quite marked neuropsychological functioning deficits in schizophrenia, of a magnitude similar to performance of patients with brain injury (for review, see Heaton & Crowley, 1981). Neuropsychological impairment has been found in patients treated with medications (Braff et al., 1991), as well as in untreated patients with first-episode schizophrenia (Censits et al., 1997; Saykin et al., 1994). Neurocognitive deficits have been most consistently noted in abstraction and mental flexibility (Goldberg et al., 1989), attention–vigilance (Censits et al., 1997; Nuechterlein & Dawson, 1984; Saykin et al., 1994), and verbal memory and learning (Braff et al., 1991; Goldberg et al., 1989; Kareken et al., 1995; Saykin et al., 1991, 1994). While not as pervasive or severe, neuropsychological impairment has also been described in affective disorders, specifically depression.

Such disorders have generally been evaluated in middle-aged or elderly patients. Impairments have been reported in verbal memory and learning (Breslow, Kocsis, & Belkin, 1980; Brown et al., 1994; Stromgren, 1977; Weingartner, Gold, & Ballenger, 1981) and in attention (Brown et al., 1994; Caine, 1981; Cummings & Benson, 1984; Frith, Stevens, & Johnstone, 1983; King & Caine, 1990). Some investigators have found cognitive dysfunction to improve with treatment of depressed mood (Frith, Stevens, & Johnstone, 1983; Malone & Helmsley, 1977; McAllister & Price, 1982). This supports the initial terminology of "pseudodementia" (Kiloh, 1961), which distinguished reversible cognitive dysfunction in the setting of depression from progressive dementias. Others have, however, suggested cognitive dysfunction to be independent of mood changes (Gold, Weingartner, & Ballenger, 1979; Henry, Weingartner, & Murphy, 1973; Reuss, Silberman, & Post, 1979; Weingartner, Gold, & Ballenger, 1981).

Early descriptions of the phenomenology of schizophrenia included affective disturbance in emotional processing, such as abnormal expression and abnormal experience, as symptoms inherent to, but not always characteristic of, the illness. Kraepelin's binary model (1896) proposed an exclusivity of schizophrenia and affective phenomena and delineated a clear distinction between dementia praecox and manic depressive illness. By 1919, however, Kraepelin reported affective disturbances that were present at the onset of dementia praecox, "usually anxious, despondent, they weep and lament, would like to die," and became less prominent during later stages of the illness with more prominent somatic preoccupation and self-neglect.

Eugen Bleuler (1911), whose views have been influential in our understanding of schizophrenia, divided the phenomenology of schizophrenia into primary and secondary symptoms. Primary symptoms—disturbances in affect, association, ambivalence, and autism–were seen as partial, but necessary for the diagnosis. Secondary symptoms, which included not only delusions and hallucinations but also depressed mood, could be absent or could change without any alteration in the underlying process. He suggested that affective disturbances could be either part of the underlying disease process or alternatively psychological reactions to the illness. By midcentury, Kurt Schneider (1959) described first rank symptoms—hallucinations, delusions, thought broadcasting, and control—to be characteristic of the illness. In this model, which greatly influenced the conceptualization of schizophrenia in the United States and Europe, affective disturbances were viewed as secondary symptoms.

Within the past decade and with attempts to further characterize symptoms of schizophrenia, the concept of positive and negative symptoms was created (Andreasen & Olsen, 1982). Positive symptoms, which are often episodic in nature, consist of hallucinations, delusions, bizarre behavior, and thought disorder. Although positive symptoms are more easily identifiable and dramatic in nature, it is the negative symptoms that have been described as characteristic of schizophrenia since Bleuler's conceptualization of core symptoms. Negative symptoms are typically present with the first onset of illness (Fennig et al., 1996), tend to be chronic in nature, and may herald poorer outcome (Andreasen & Olsen, 1982). They are characterized by affective flattening, alogia, avolition, anhedonia, and inattention and are more pronounced in schizophrenia patients, particularly men, than in patients with other psychotic disorders (Husted, Beiser, & Iacono, 1995; Reddy, Mukherjee, & Schnur, 1992; Shtasel et al., 1992). Negative symptoms are thought to increase with duration of illness and may be worsened by neuroleptic medication with strong postsynaptic dopaminergic D_2 blockade, such as haloperidol, fluphenazine, and risperidone.

In this chapter, we examine current evidence for neural substrates of emotional dysfunction in schizophrenia in the domains of expression, experience, and recognition of emotion. Abnormal expression of emotional states usually consists of flattening of affect and inappropriate affect. Abnormal experience includes decreased intensity of emotional experience and mood states, ranging from depression to mania. Abnormal recognition is described as impaired ability to recognize facial expression of emotion. Clinically, it appears that all three are implicated in but by no means unique to schizophrenia, as other chapters in this volume describe emotional functioning in mood disorders (Davidson & Henriques, Chapter 11; Robinson & Manes, Chapter 10), brain-damaged patients (Borod et al., Chapter 4), and other neurological disorders (Heilman et al., Chapter 15).

CLINICAL MANIFESTATIONS OF DISORDERED EMOTIONS IN SCHIZOPHRENIA

Clinical Features

Expression

Diminished affect in the facial expression of emotion has been considered since Bleuler (1911) to be a core symptom in schizophrenia. Impairment commonly consists of flat or inappropriate affect and may precede the onset of psychosis by many years (Walker et al., 1993). It can be worsened by administration of neuroleptics with strong nigrostriatal dopaminergic blockade, which can produce extrapyramidal symptoms including pseudoparkinsonism and akinetic depression (Krakowski, Czobor, & Volavka, 1997; Rifkin, Quitkin, & Klein, 1975; Van Putten & May, 1978). Compared with healthy subjects, patients with depression, and patients with parkinsonism, schizophrenic patients have been described to express less emotions, with a propensity for negative rather than positive emotions (Brozgold et al., 1998; Martin et al., 1990). Several studies have suggested an independence between subjective ratings and facial display of emotions in schizophrenia (Berenbaum & Oltmann, 1992; Kring et al., 1993; Sison et al., 1996). People with schizophrenia have, however, been noted to be unreliable reporters of their emotional experiences (Jaeger et al., 1990), and affective flattening may indicate muted emotional experience.

A major difficulty in evaluating deficits of emotional expression in schizophrenia stems from the potential overlap of this, and other negative symptoms, with depression. McGlashan (1982) addressed the similarity and possible coexistence of negative and depressive symptoms. He distinguished between affective poverty ("aphanisis") and postpsychotic depression. The first occurred in patients who had recovered from an acute psychotic episode and shielded themselves from uncomfortable stimuli. Postpsychotic depression was characterized by sad, hopeless mood, psychomotor retardation with apathy, and neurasthenic complaints and was present in approximately 25% of patients at remission of the acute psychotic episode.

Investigators who attempted to explore the potential link between depressive symptoms and negative features of schizophrenia evaluated patients at different stages of the illness, ranging from acute schizophrenia (Kitamura & Suga, 1991; Ring et al., 1991) to acute exacerbation in chronic schizophrenia (Goldmann et al., 1992) and chronic stable schizophrenia (Craig et al., 1985; Kibel, Laffont, & Liddle, 1993; Kuck et al., 1992; Prosser et al., 1987), and included patient samples in which women were not represented or were grossly underrepresented (Craig et al., 1985; Kibel, Laffont, & Liddle, 1993; Kuck et al., 1992; Prosser et al., 1987). Although several studies found little or no association between depressive and negative features (Goldmann et al., 1992; Kibel, Laffont, & Liddle, 1993; Kuck et al., 1992), other studies (Craig et al., 1985; Kulhara et al., 1989; Prosser et al., 1987) found an association between negative and vegetative features of depression. Vegetative symptoms of depression consist of somatic and nonspecific behavioral disturbances, such as anergia, anhedonia, insomnia, and lack of appetite, and can be found in many psychiatric disorders. Kitamura and Suga (1991) reported an association between depressive ratings and negative ratings, specifically for avolition–apathy and anhedonia–asociality, and Ring et al. (1991) noted a correlation between negative and depressive symptoms, but only in male and not female patients. No study found a link between negative symptoms and depressive cognitions, which are more specific to depression and consist of sadness, anxiety, guilt, tension, and somatic concern. Because of the underrepresentation of women sex-specific effects cannot be ruled out.

In an attempt to evaluate whether these features are clinically separable, we examined the relationship between clinical ratings of characteristic symptoms of schizophrenia—negative and positive symptoms (Andreasen & Olsen, 1982)—and clinical ratings for depression in a large sample of schizophrenic patients. Patients were grouped into a high and low depression group according to ratings on the Hamilton Depression Rating Scale. Subjects with depression scored 18 or above on the 21-item Hamilton Depression Rating Scale, which indicates the presence of at least moderate severity of depressive symptoms (Baxter et al., 1985; Bench et al., 1993). The high and low depression groups, which are described in more detail below, did not differ in severity of negative symptoms. The lack of association argues that in schizophrenia negative symptoms are distinct from depression.

In our patient sample, as in other studies of emotional expression, there is a need for objective quantitative measures of affect expression. Even the more elaborate methods, however, that have detailed procedures for establishing reliability and validity (Ekman & Friesen 1976) ultimately rely on subjective ratings.

Experience

Emotional intensity. Historically, schizophrenia was thought to involve a decreased range of emotional experience. This was inferred from an inability to identify one's own emotional experience and an impairment in facial expression of emotions, or what is referred to as *flattening of affect.* A recent study (Schneider et al., 1995) has tested this hypothesis formally with a standardized mood induction procedure including happy and sad faces. The procedure was applied to 40 schizophrenic subjects and to healthy controls matched for sex. Patients exhibited impaired ability to respond to mood induction, particularly for happiness, irrespective of medication status (23 were taking neuroleptics and 17 were not) and sex. Performance on mood induction was positively correlated with hallucinations and negatively correlated with the negative symptom complex of anhedonia (Fig. 17.1).

Depression. After the introduction of antipsychotic medications in the treatment of schizophrenia, clinical reports appeared that described a dramatic increase in the incidence of depression and suicide (Beisser, 1961; Hussar, 1962). Apart from the explanation that many previously untreated patients were too disorganized to experience sad mood or to act on it, these reports coincided with the deinstitutionalization of patients, who were being exposed to the stresses of greater personal freedom and gradual reintegration into the community with variable success (Farberow, Shneidman, & Leonard, 1962). Experience with the antihypertensive agent reserpine, also used to treat schizophrenia and known to cause depression in some patients, led to the concern that depression might result from pharmacotherapy in schizophrenia. This led to the introduction of the term *pharmacogenic depression* (Galdi, 1983; Helmchen & Hippius, 1967). Several subsequent studies, however, have at least partially refuted an association. Indeed, there are reports of patients with schizophrenia who were treated with antipsychotic medications and showed improvement in both psychotic and depressive symptoms (Johnson, 1981;

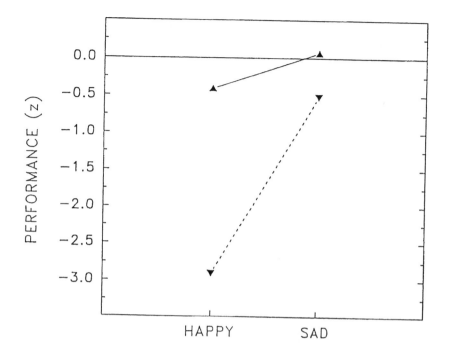

▼ EMOTION DISCRIMINATION
▲ MOOD INDUCTION

Figure 17.1. Specificity for discriminating and experiencing valence-specific emotions in schizophrenic patients. The z-scores are based on results with normal controls. (Reprinted with permission from Schneider et al., 1995.)

Knights & Hirsch, 1981; Koreen et al., 1993; McGlashan & Carpenter, 1976; Roth, 1970). A further suggestion was that treatment with antipsychotic medications may cause depressive symptoms due to extrapyramidal motor disturbances (Craig et al., 1985; Johnson, 1981; Rifkin, Quitkin, & Klein, 1975; Van Putten & May, 1978). This was termed *akinetic depression*.

The identification and treatment of depression in schizophrenia is clinically important because at least 10% of people with schizophrenia commit suicide (Miles, 1977), and the majority of these were depressed in the months preceding their deaths (Cohen et al., 1964; Planansky & Johnston, 1971; Roy, 1981). Depression occurs most commonly during the onset of psychosis (Bowers & Astrachan, 1967; House, Bostock, & Cooper, 1987; Johnson, 1981; Knights & Hirsch, 1981; Koreen et al., 1993; Mayer-Gross et al., 1955; McGlashan & Carpenter, 1976; Roth, 1970; Steinberg, Green, & Durrell, 1967; Stern, Pillsbury, & Sonnenberg, 1972). Reduction of acute symptoms and clinical stabilization are associated with decline of depressive symptoms (House, Bostock, & Cooper,

1987; Knights & Hirsch, 1981; Shanfield et al., 1970), which may reemerge during each relapse (Johnson, 1981; Koreen et al., 1993; Shanfield et al., 1970). McGlashan and Carpenter (1976) estimated that postpsychotic depression occurs in 25% of all psychotic episodes, although others have suggested a somewhat lower incidence. Depression is unusual with increasing chronicity of illness, perhaps because its symptoms are gradually replaced by negative symptoms (House, Bostock, & Cooper, 1987).

In an effort to separate the effects of depression from symptoms primarily attributable to schizophrenia, we compared a group of schizophrenia subjects with depression to a group without depression. Subjects with depression were scored 18 or above on the 21-item Hamilton Depression Rating Scale (Kohler et al., 1998a). There were 63 patients (35 men, 28 women) in the high ($\geq$18) depression group and 81 patients (52 men, 29 women) in the low (<18) depression group. The groups were compared on demographic and clinical variables and on eight neuropsychological domains (abstraction–flexibility, attention–vigilance, verbal memory, spatial memory, language, spatial functions, sensory functions, and fine manual motor skills). The two groups differed in age at onset of illness, severity of delusions (Tables 17.1 and 17.2), and performance in a single neuropsychological domain: attention (Figs. 17.2 and 17.3). The specific component of impaired attention was vigilance, with the poorest performance by women with higher depression scores. The presence of specific attentional impairment associated with depressive symptoms in schizophrenia is consistent with the hy-

Table 17.1. Demographic and Clinical Characteristics of Schizophrenic Groups with High and Low Depression Scores

	HIGH DEPRESSION GROUP (HAM-HI): MEAN ($\pm$SD)	RANGE	LOW DEPRESSION GROUP (HAM-LO): MEAN ($\pm$SD)	RANGE
Sex				
Male	35		52	
Female	28		29	
Race				
White	27		45	
Black	36		35	
Other	0		1	
Age at evaluation (yr)	30.0 (7.9)	17.1–44.8	29.8 (6.8)	16.7–44.0
Duration (yr)	6.5 (6.0)	0–24	7.8 (6.7)	0–29
Age at onset (yr)*	24.1 (7.2)	11–41	22.0 (5.4)	13–36
Hospitalizations (n)	1.9 (2.8)	0–57	3.4 (7.5)	0–12
Education (yr)	12.7 (2.4)	8–20	12.7 (1.9)	8–17

*p < 0.05.
HAM, Hamilton Depression Rating Scale.

Table 17.2. Clinical and Behavioral Features of Schizophrenia Groups with High and Low Depression Scores

	HIGH DEPRESSION GROUP (HAM-HI) MEAN (± SD)	LOW DEPRESSION GROUP (HAM-LO) MEAN (±SD)
Schizophrenia	47	70
Schizophreniform d/o	16	11
Never medicated	28	26
Previously medicated	35	55
21-item HAM		
Score*	22.6 (3.5)	11.6 (4.2)
Range	18–31	1–17
SANS		
Affect	2.5 (1.3)	2.3 (1.3)
Alogia	2.6 (1.4)	2.2 (1.5)
Avolition	2.6 (1.3)	2.5 (1.5)
Anhedonia	3.2 (1.0)	3.0 (1.4)
Attention	1.9 (1.4)	1.8 (1.5)
SAPS		
Hallucinations	2.8 (1.4)	2.4 (1.5)
Delusions**	3.6 (1.0)	2.9 (1.2)
Bizarre behavior	1.6 (1.3)	1.4 (1.3)
Thought disorder	2.0 (1.3)	2.0 (1.5)

*$P < 0.001$.

**$P = 0.007$.

HAM, Hamilton Depression Rating Scale; SANS, The Scale for the Assessment of Negative Symptoms; SAPS, The Scale for the Assessment of Positive Symptoms.

pothesis of frontal lobe dysfunction in depression because these regions have been implicated in attentional processes.

Mania. Unlike depression in schizophrenia, mania has been much less commonly described. In 1911, Bleuler postulated that any affective symptoms may occur in the setting of schizophrenia, provided that criteria for certain fundamental schizophrenic symptoms were met: splitting of cognition from emotion and behavior, formal thought disorder, flat or blunted affect, autism, and ambivalence.

Manic symptoms in the setting of schizophrenia may represent a schizomanic state or warrant the diagnosis of schizoaffective disorder. Patients with schizophrenia sometimes display manic symptoms (Tsuang & Loyd, 1988) and become agitated, irritable, impulsive, and insomniac as part of an acute psychotic exacerbation or in response to hallucinations and delusions. Usually these symptoms are temporary, and the behavioral picture lacks more typical manic symptoms (e.g., pressured speech, grandiosity, and elated mood). Kasanin (1933) coined the term "schizo-affective psychosis" to describe a group of patients with sudden onset in youth, prominent affective and schizophrenic symptoms, external

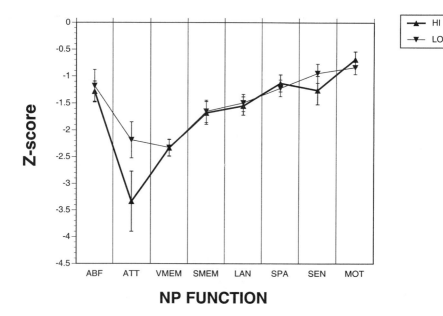

Figure 17.2. Neuropsychological profile of schizophrenia patients with high ($N = 63$) and low ($N = 81$) depression scores. The z-scores are based on results with normal controls. ABF, abstraction-flexibility; ATT, attention; VMEM, verbal memory; SMEM, spatial memory; LAN, language abilities; SPA, spatial abilities; SEN, sensory abilities; MOT, motor abilities.

stressor, and good premorbid adjustment. The initial description did not specify the relationship between schizoaffective disorder and affective disorders or schizophrenia.

The existence of schizoaffective disorder as a separate clinical entity has repeatedly been questioned. Over the years, different definitions for schizoaffective disorder have been proposed. Attempts to identify it as a variant of schizophrenia or an affective disorder based on clinical symptoms, genetics, and prognosis have yielded equivocal results (Lapensee, 1992). Schizoaffective disorder has been removed from the schizophrenia category since the introduction of the third edition of the *Diagnostic and Statistical Manual of Mental Disorders* (DSM-III). The diagnostic criteria were narrowed in the revised DSM-III by establishing the necessity of longitudinal, isolated psychotic symptoms. This is unchanged in DSM-IV. The primary difficulty in diagnosing schizoaffective disorder is differentiation from schizophrenia with atypical affective disorder and bipolar disorder or major depression with mood incongruent psychotic features. In schizoaffective disorder, affective symptoms are a prominent, if temporary, part of the illness. In contrast, in the affective illnesses, psychotic symptoms are limited to acute exacerbations.

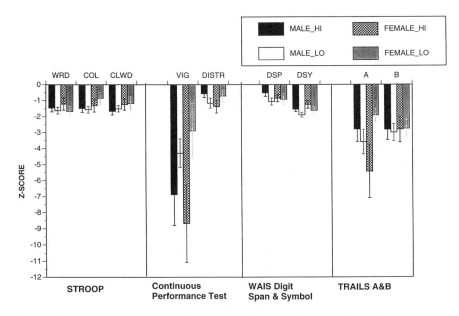

Figure 17.3. Attention subitems for male and female schizophrenia patients with high (MALE_HI, FEMALE_HI) and low (MALE_LO, FEMALE_LO) depression scores on subtests of attention. WRD, word condition; COL, color condition; CLWD, color word condition; VIG, vigilance; DISTR, distractibility; DSP, digit span; DSY, digit symbol. The z-scores are based on results with normal controls. Depressed and nondepressed schizophrenia patients differ in vigilance. (Reprinted with permission from Kohler et al., 1998a.)

Several hypothetical models have been formulated that attempt to place schizophrenic symptoms in the context of other psychiatric symptoms and make the binary distinction between affective and schizophrenic disorders obsolete. The "continuum model" (Crow, 1985) proposes purely affective and schizophrenic disorders to be at opposite ends of a spectrum rather than mutually exclusive. In the "hierarchical schema of symptoms" (Foulds & Bedford, 1975), disorders located in a pyramidal hierarchy exhibit not only illness-specific symptoms but also nonspecific symptoms of disorders located on lower, but not higher, pyramidal steps.

Recognition

Over the last 15 years a large body of literature has examined recognition of emotion in brain-related disorders and healthy people as measured by the ability to identify the emotional quality of facial expression. In healthy subjects, gender-related effects were reported for emotion recognition (Erwin et al., 1992; Natale, Gur, & Gur, 1983). Women showed better accuracy for brief exposures, and men were less sensitive to expressed sadness in female faces. Impairment of emotion recognition has been found in right-brain injuries (Adolphs et al., 1994; Borod et al., 1993), schizophrenia (Cutting 1981; Feinberg et al., 1986; Heimberg et al., 1992; Schneider et al., 1995; Walker, McGuire, & Bettes, 1984), depression (Feinberg et al., 1986; Gur et al., 1992), and Huntington's chorea (Jacobs, Shuren, & Heilman, 1995).

In schizophrenia, investigators using emotion recognition tasks found that schizophrenic patients performed more poorly than depressed patient groups and controls (Feinberg et al., 1986; Gessler et al., 1989; Schneider et al., 1992; Walker, McGuire, & Bettes, 1984; Zuroff & Colussy, 1986). In studies that included a control task such as facial recognition or age discrimination, however, investigators found impaired performance of schizophrenic patients on the control tasks as well (Borod et al., 1993; Feinberg et al., 1986). This supports the idea of a generalized deficit in facial processing in schizophrenia. In contrast, differential deficits for emotional discrimination were observed by Cutting (1981) and Novic (1984), who studied chronic schizophrenics and found a differential emotion discrimination deficit when compared with color, facial, and age recognition. Heimberg et al. (1992) likewise reported differential impairment in discrimination of happy and sad facial expression relative to age discrimination (Fig. 17.4). Improvement of performance has been reported in patients with major depression after treatment response (Mikhailova et al., 1996), however, the deficit may be stable in schizophrenia (Gaebel & Wolwer, 1992).

Treatment Interventions

Treatment for schizophrenia is in large part aimed at improvement and prevention of acute psychotic symptoms, which tend to respond to neuroleptics. Emotional dysfunction in schizophrenia has received limited attention, apparently because acute psychotic symptoms overshadow less dramatic symptomatology. In addition, emotional dysfunction, similar to neuropsychological impairment, can be viewed as a trait of the illness that may precede the onset of psychotic symptoms and may not change with treatment. This is underscored by increased evi-

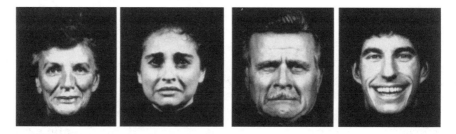

Figure 17.4. Sample items of faces with happy and sad expressions.

dence for neurodevelopmental aberrations in schizophrenia. For example, a retrospective study of childhood home videos obtained from adults currently suffering from schizophrenia showed difficulties in relatedness and slowed motor development (Walker et al., 1993).

Depression

Studies on treatment of depression in schizophrenia have suffered from the methodological limitations inherent in assessing and quantifying depression in schizophrenia. All studies evaluating the presence of depressed mood in patients with acute psychosis report improvement with remission regardless of the use of antidepressant medication. Most studies have centered on the treatment of depressive symptoms in chronic institutionalized patients, and only a few have examined the role of antidepressant treatment in patients suffering from an acute episode.

Two comprehensive reviews (Plasky, 1991; Siris, 1991) of the literature on depressive symptoms in schizophrenia evaluated over 30 publications and found only three articles that clearly support the benefit of antidepressant treatment. Many studies were difficult to interpret due to flawed designs. Plasky (1991) reviewed the literature on antidepressant use in schizophrenia by analyzing seven studies published between 1979 and 1990 and briefly reviewing several others. Some studies were limited by inadequate assessment of depression (Waehrens & Gerlach, 1980), small number of patients (Goff et al., 1990), retrospective chart review with no quantification of depressed mood (Siris, Rifkin, & Reardon, 1982), and comparative patient groups with markedly different psychosis scores (Prusoff et al., 1979). It appears that tricyclic antidepressants are beneficial for treating symptoms of depression in schizophrenia once the psychosis is stabilized (Prusoff et al., 1979; Siris et al., 1982, 1987), but can worsen psychotic symptoms (Dufresne, Kass, & Becker, 1988; Kramer, Vogel, & DiJohnson, 1989; Prusoff et al., 1979) and may have no effect on negative symptoms of schizophrenia (Becker, 1983; Waehrens & Gerlach, 1980).

Siris (1991) reviewed 29 studies published between 1972 and 1989 that describe the prevalence and treatment of secondary depression in schizophrenia, including nine double-blind studies of antidepressants. Six studies described standard criteria for the diagnosis of schizophrenia and scales to evaluate depression, consisting of the Diagnostic and Statistical Manual, Research Diagnostic Criteria, Feighner (1981), Hamilton Rating Scale for Depression, and Beck Depression Inventory. Only one study (Siris et al., 1987) showed unequivocal improvement of mood on antidepressant medication, as imipramine was superior to placebo with improvement of depressive symptoms in patients with schizophrenia or schizoaffective disorder who had stable psychotic symptoms. Other studies that show an apparent beneficial effect of antidepressant medication are flawed in the selection of patients who had previously responded to antidepressant treatment (see Siris et al., 1994) or had a high placebo response (Johnson, 1981). Studies indicating a beneficial effect of antidepressants included patients who were treated as outpatients or exhibited more stable psychotic symptoms. Siris (1991) concluded that antidepressants are without benefit for patients without clear depressive symptoms or with florid psychotic symptoms and of questionable or limited benefit for chronic inpatients and patients with unstable psychotic symptoms.

Over the last 10 years, atypical neuroleptics that affect serotonergic pathways have been used widely in the treatment of schizophrenia. Of this group of medications, clozapine and olanzapine have been investigated for specific antidepressant effects in schizophrenia and mood disorders (Ranjan & Meltzer, 1996; Weisler et al., 1997; Zarate, Tohen, & Baldessarini, 1995). In a large cohort of patients with acute exacerbation of chronic schizophrenia, at least an average dose of olanzapine was found to improve anxious and depressive symptoms compared with placebo and haloperidol. This effect was found to be independent of improvement in positive, negative, and extrapyramidal symptoms (Tollefson et al., 1998a,b). Likewise, clozapine has been described to have a beneficial effect on depressive symptoms (Abraham et al., 1997) and suicidality (Meltzer & Okayli, 1995).

Negative symptoms

Over the past 10 years, there has been an increasing understanding that negative symptoms represent characteristic symptoms of schizophrenia, which persist throughout the course of illness, are more common in men, and have marked consequences on the person's social and interpersonal functioning. While positive symptoms of schizophrenia—hallucinations, delusions, and disordered thinking—are responsive to treatment with standard neuroleptic medications, negative symptoms—flat affect, alogia, and anhedonia—are less readily treated, and in fact, may worsen as a side effect of dopaminergic blockade. About 10 years ago, Tandon, Greden, and Silk (1988) showed that trihexyphenidyl, a commonly used anticholinergic agent, improved negative symptoms in a small series of patients. Subsequent studies revealed standard haloperidol treatment to improve negative symptoms independent of positive symptoms (Palao et al., 1994) and even in previously neuroleptic naive schizophrenia patients (Labarca et al., 1993), although at a slower rate than positive symptoms. With the advent of atypical neuroleptics, clozaril (Miller et al., 1994) and, more recently, olanzapine (Tollefson & Sanger, 1997) were found to improve prominent negative symptoms compared with haloperidol and placebo; however, the effect on negative symptoms remains disputed (Buchanan et al., 1998). The effects of the newer, antipsychotic medications are thought to occur through complex pleotropic interactions targetting multiple neurotransmitters, including serotonin systems. Similarly, fluvoxamine, a specific serotonin reuptake inhibitor, has been reported to improve prominent negative symptoms compared with maprotiline, a noradrenergic antidepressant (Silver & Shmugliakov, 1998).

NEUROBIOLOGICAL STUDIES OF EMOTIONAL PROCESSING

The introduction of neurobiologic studies for advancing the understanding of emotion-related symptoms in schizophrenia has lagged behind neurocognitive research. Advanced methods in the study of emotional processing have been applied to schizophrenia, as summarized above. There are important gaps and a need for more research.

Brain metabolism and blood flow studies in patients with major depression have described decreased metabolism in the left inferior frontal lobe (positron emission tomography with fluorodeoxyglucose [FDG-PET]; Baxter et al., 1985; Dolan & Friston, 1989), left anterior cingulate (single photon emission computed tomography with hexamethyl-propylene amine oxime; Mayberg et al., 1994), and caudate nuclei (Baxter et al., 1985). Similar findings have been found for depressed patients with Parkinson's disease (Mayberg et al., 1990), Huntington's chorea (Mayberg et al., 1992), stroke (Robinson et al., 1984) and complex partial seizures (Bromfield et al., 1992). From these neuroimaging studies it appears that idiopathic depression and depression in other neurological disorders involve a disequilibrium of left compared with right anterior hemispheric structures, including limbic circuitry

We evaluated 79 patients who were grouped according to their ratings on the Hamilton Rating Scale for Depression: ≥18 was the cutoff between the schizophrenia depression and schizophrenia control groups. All patients underwent clinical and MRI evaluation, and a subsample of 37 underwent FDG-PET measurements of cerebral glucose metabolism (Kohler et al., 1998b). Patient groups with and without depression did not differ in the demographic variables of sex, race, age at evaluation, and education. Furthermore, there were no differences in the clinical variables of diagnosis (schizophrenia, schizophreniform), medication status (neuroleptic naive, previously medicated), age at onset of schizophrenia, duration of illness, or number of hospitalizations. Regarding symptoms, there was no main effect due to depression group, but there was a negative versus positive symptoms by subscale by depression group interaction ($F = 3.37$; df = 3,231; $P = 0.02$). This was because patients in the schizophrenia with depression group were rated higher on alogia and lower on delusions. No other subscale showed a difference between the groups, nor did the groups differ in ratings of quality of life.

The schizophrenia with depression group had larger bilateral temporal lobe volumes and decreased laterality (left minus right) of metabolism in the anterior cingulate. The neuroanatomic findings (Fig. 17.5) suggest that depression in

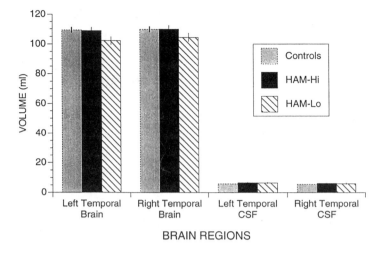

Figure 17.5. Temporal lobe brain and cerebrospinal fluid (CSF) volumes by depression group (high depression, $N = 40$; low depression, $N = 39$). Schizophrenia patients with depression have larger temporal lobe volumes. (Reprinted with permission from Kohler et al., 1998b.)

schizophrenia is associated with higher volume of the temporal lobe. Indeed, unlike their counterparts with low depression, whose temporal lobe volumes were significantly reduced compared with healthy controls, the high depression patients with schizophrenia had normal volumes. This finding further buttresses the position that depression in schizophrenia is distinct from primary negative symptoms. Our earlier studies have shown that deficit patients with schizophrenia have smaller temporal lobe volumes than nondeficit patients (Turetsky et al., 1995). Furthermore, in the current sample, the more depressed group had lower ratings on alogia and larger temporal lobe volumes. The association of depression with normal temporal lobe volumes in schizophrenia suggests that some integrity of the temporal lobe is necessary for the experience of depression, consistent with evidence for the role of the temporal lobe in emotional experience.

In the subsample of patients who had FDG-PET measures of cerebral glucose metabolism, the patient group with higher depression ratings had reduced left lateralization of metabolism in the anterior cingulate (Fig. 17.6). Whereas healthy subjects show relatively higher left hemispheric metabolism in this region, this gradient is somewhat diminished in the high depression group and increased in the low depression group. Thus, depression in schizophrenia seems associated with a relative decrease in left compared with right cingulate activity. This is consistent with evidence for greater right hemispheric involvement in dysphoric states in lesion studies (Gainotti, 1972; Robinson et al., 1984; Ross & Mesulam, 1979; Sackeim et al., 1982), as well as in studies of healthy people (Davidson et al., 1990; Davidson & Tomarken, 1989; Natale, Gur, & Gur, 1983; Sackeim,

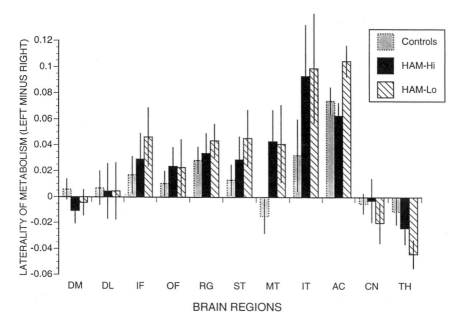

Figure 17.6. Laterality of 18-fluorodeoxuglucose (FDG) PET metabolism by depression group (high depression, $N = 19$; low depression, $N = 18$). Depressed schizophrenia patients have relative hypometabolism in the left anterior cingulate. DM, dorsal medial prefrontal; DL, dorsal lateral prefrontal; IF, inferior frontal; OF, orbital frontal; RG, rectal gyrus; ST, superior temporal; MT, midtemporal; IT, inferior temporal; AC, anterior cingulate; CN, caudate nucleus; TH, thalamus. (Reprinted with permission from Kohler et al., 1998b.)

Gur, & Saucy, 1978). The cingulum and mesial temporal regions form the limbic lobe (Broca, 1878), the instrumental part of the neural circuitry responsible for emotional processing (Papez, 1937). Our findings indicate that the neurobiology of depression in schizophrenia has features in common with major depression and depression associated with other brain disorders. Specifically, this involves altered function of frontal regions as measured by lateralized metabolism.

SUMMARY

In this chapter, we provide a historical overview of the concepts of emotional processing; clinical features of expression, experience, and recognition of emotions; and treatment interventions with a focus on affective states in the illness of schizophrenia. Although schizophrenia has been traditionally considered a disorder of cognition, disturbed affect has been implicated from the outset, and there is increased evidence for its major role. To the extent that disturbed affect is a core negative symptom, its presence in a patient is an ominous sign, foreboding poor course and treatment response. On the other hand, disturbed affect in the form of depression or, less frequently, manic symptoms may indicate a more palliable form of psychosis. To this extent we describe similarities in cognition and brain metabolism of depression in schizophrenia compared with idiopathic depression as well as depression in other brain-related disorders and link the presence of depression in schizophrenia with preserved temporal lobe volume, indicating preserved anatomy of limbic structures.

In the future, research in the area of emotional expression may include attempts at amelioration of affective flattening via rehabilitation and pharmacotherapy that target serotonergic neural substrates. Future investigations in emotional experience in schizophrenia may include further evaluation of whether depression during different phases of acute and chronic schizophrenia will more favorably respond to atypical rather than to typical antipsychotic or perhaps antidepressant medication. Conversely, it is not known whether mood stabilizers may ameliorate symptoms of mania in schizophrenia. With respect to emotion recognition, research may be directed at further investigations on the controversial concept of a specific emotion recognition deficit in schizophrenia by developing a visuospatial control task that differs in the component of emotion recognition only. Another question is whether deficits in emotional processing represent a stable deficit in schizophrenia or whether such deficits can be ameliorated via treatment of positive or negative symptoms of schizophrenia. Finally, neurobehavioral probes evaluating neuronal activation during emotional processing may further elucidate the question of whether emotion recognition represents a specific impairment in the illness of schizophrenia.

REFERENCES

Abraham, G., Nair, C., Tracy, J.I., Simpson, G.M., & Josiassen, R.C. (1997). The effects of clozapine on symptom clusters in treatment-refractory patients. *Journal of Clinical Psychopharmacology, 17*, 49–53.

Adolphs, R., Tranel, D., Damasio, H., & Damasio, A. (1994). Impaired recognition of emotion in facial expressions following bilateral damage to the human amygdala. *Nature, 372*, 669–672.

Andreasen, N.C., & Olsen, S. (1982). Negative versus positive schizophrenia. Definition and validation. *Archives of General Psychiatry, 39*(7), 789–794.

Baxter, L.R., Phelps, M.E., Mazziotta, J.C., Schwartz, J.M., Gerner, R.H., Selin, C.E., & Sumida, R.M. (1985). Cerebral metabolic rates for glucose in mood disorders. *Archives of General Psychiatry, 42*, 441–447.

Becker, R.E. (1983). Implications of the efficacy of thiothixine and a chlorpromazine-imipramine combination for depression in schizophrenia. *American Journal of Psychiatry, 140*, 208–211.

Beisser, A.R. (1961). Study of suicide in mental hospitals. *Diseases of the Nervous System, 22,* 365–369.

Bench, C.J., Friston, K.J., Brown, R.G., Frackowiak, R.S.J., & Dolan, R.J. (1993). Regional cerebral blood flow in depression measured by positron emission tomography: The relationship with clinical dimensions. *Psychological Medicine, 23,* 579–590.

Berenbaum, H., & Oltmann, T.F. (1992). Emotional experience and expression in schizophrenia and depression. *Journal of Abnormal Psychiatry, 101,* 37–44.

Bleuler, E. (1911). *Dementia Praecox oder die Gruppe der Schizophrenien.* Leipzig: Aschaffenburgs Handbuch, Deutike.

Borod, J.C., Martin, C.C., Alpert, M., Brozgold, A., & Welkowitz, J. (1993). Perception of facial emotion in schizophrenic and right brain-damaged patients. *The Journal of Nervous and Mental Disease, 181,* 494–502.

Bowers, M.B., & Astrachan, B.M. (1967). Depression in acute schizophrenic psychosis. *American Journal of Psychiatry, 123,* 976–979.

Braff, D.L., Heaton, R., Kuck, J., Cullum, M., Moranville, J., Grant, I., & Zisook, S. (1991). The generalized pattern of neuropsychological deficits in outpatients with chronic schizophrenia with heterogeneous wisconsin card sorting test results. *Archives of General Psychiatry, 48,* 891–898.

Breslow, R., Kocsis, J., & Belkin, B. (1980). Memory deficits in depression: Evidence utilizing the Wechsler Memory Scale. *Perceptual and Motor Skills, 51,* 541–542.

Broca P (1878). Anatomie comparée des circonvolutions cérébrales. Le grand lobe limbique et la scissure limbique dans la serie des mammiféres. *Revue Anthropologique, 2,* 384–498.

Bromfield, E.B., Altshuler, L., Leiderman, D.B., Balish, M., Ketter, T.A., Devinsky, O., Post, R.M., & Theodore, W.H. (1992). Cerebral metabolism and depression in patients with complex partial seizures. *Archives of Neurology, 49,* 617–623.

Brown, R.G., Scott, L.C., Bench, C.J., & Dolan, R.J. (1994). Cognitive function in depression: Its relationship to the presence and severity of intellectual decline. *Psychological Medicine, 24,* 829–847.

Brozgold, A.Z., Borod, J.C., Martin, C.C., Pick, L.H., Alpert, M., & Welkowitz, J. (1998). Social functioning and facial emotional expression in neurological and psychiatric disorders. *Applied Neuropsychology, 5,* 15–23.

Buchanan, R.W., Breier, A., Kirkpatrick, B., Ball, P., & Carpenter, W.T. (1998). Positive and negative symptom response to clozapine in schizophrenia patients with and without the deficit syndrome. *American Journal of Psychiatry, 155,* 751–760.

Caine, E.D. (1981). Pseudodementia: Current concepts and future directions. *Archives of General Psychiatry, 38,* 1359–1364.

Censits, D.M., Ragland, J.D., Gur, R.C., & Gur, R.E. (1997). Neuropsychological evidence supporting a neurodevelopmental model of schizophrenia: A longitudinal study. *Schizophrenia Research, 24,* 289–298.

Cohen, S., Leonard, C.V., Farberow, N.L., & Shneidman, E. (1964). Tranquilizers and suicide in the schizophrenic patient. *Archives of General Psychiatry, 11,* 312–321.

Craig, T.J., Richardson, M.A., Pass, R., & Bregman, Z. (1985). Measurement of mood and affect in schizophrenic inpatients. *American Journal of Psychiatry, 142,* 1272–1277.

Crow, T.J. (1981). Positive and negative schizophrenia symptoms and the role of dopamine. *British Journal of Psychiatry, 139,* 251–254.

Crow, T.J. (1985). The two syndrome concept: Origins and current status. *Schizophrenia Bulletin, 11,* 471–486.

Cummings, J.L., & Benson, F. (1984). Subcortical dementia: Review of an emerging concept. *Archives of Neurology, 41,* 874–879.

Cutting, J. (1981). Judgment of emotional expression in schizophrenics. *British Journal of Psychiatry, 139,* 1–6.

Davidson, R.J., Ekman, P., Saron, C.D., Senulis, J.A., & Forest, W.V. (1990). Approach–withdrawal and cerebral asymmetry: Emotional expression and brain physiology. *Journal of Personality and Social Psychology, 58,* 330–341.

Davidson, R.J., & Tomarken, A.J. (1989). Laterality and emotion: An electrophysiological approach. In F. Boller & J. Grafman (Eds.), *Handbook of Neuropsychology,* Vol. 3 (pp. 419–441). Amsterdam: Elsevier.

Dolan, R.J., & Friston, K.J. (1989). Positron emission tomography in psychiatric and neuropsychiatric disorders. *Seminars in Neurology, 9(4),* 330–337.

Dufresne, R.L., Kass, D.J., & Becker, R.E. (1988). Bupropion and thiothixene versus placebo and thiothixene in the treatment of depression in schizophrenia. *Drug Development Research, 12,* 259–266.

Ekman, P., & Friesen, W. (1976). *Pictures of Facial Affect.* Palo Alto, CA: Consulting Psychologists Press.

Erwin, R.J., Gur, R.C., Gur, R.E., Skolnick, B.E., Mawhinney-Hee, M., & Smailis, J. (1992). Facial emotion discrimination: I. Task construction and behavioral findings in normals. *Psychiatry Research, 42,* 231–240.

Farberow, N.L., Shneidman, E.S., & Leonard, C.V. (1962). Suicide: Evaluation and treatment of suicide risk among schizophrenic patients in psychiatric hospitals. *VA Medical Bulletin, MB-8.*

Feighner, J.P. (1981). Nosology of primary affective disorders and application to clinical research. *Acta Psychiatrica Scandinavica, Supplementum, 290,* 29–41.

Feinberg, T.E., Rifkin, A., Schaffer, C., & Walker, E. (1986). Facial discrimination and emotional recognition in schizophrenia and affective disorders. *Archives of General Psychiatry, 43,* 276–279.

Fennig, S., Bromet, E.J., Galambos, N., & Putnam, K. (1996). Diagnosis and six-month stability of negative symptoms in psychotic disorders. *European Archives of Psychiatry and Clinical Neuroscience, 246,* 63–70.

Foulds, G.A., & Bedford, A. (1975). Hierarchy of classes of personal illness. *Psychological Medicine, 5,* 181–192.

Frith, C.D., Stevens, M., & Johnstone, E.C. (1983). Effects of ECT and depression on various aspects of memory. *British Journal of Psychiatry, 142,* 610–617.

Gaebel, W., & Wolwer, W. (1992). Facial expression and emotional face recognition in schizophrenia and depression. *European Archives of Psychiatry and Clinical Neuroscience, 242(1),* 46–52.

Gainotti, G. (1972). Emotional behavior and hemispheric side of the lesion. *Cortex, 8,* 41–55.

Galdi, J. (1983). The causality of depression in schizophrenia. *British Journal of Psychiatry, 142,* 621–625.

Gessler, S., Cutting, J., Frith, C.D., & Weinman, J. (1989). Schizophrenic inability to judge facial emotion: A controlled study. *British Journal of Clinical Psychology, 28,* 19–29.

Goff, D.C., Brotman, A.W., Wates, M., & McCormick, S. (1990). Trial of fluoxetine added to neuroleptics for treatment-resistant schizophrenic patients. *American Journal of Psychiatry, 147,* 492–494.

Gold, F.W., Weingartner, H., & Ballenger, J.C. (1979). Effects of 1-desamino-8-Darginine vasopressin on behaviour and cognition in primary affective disorder. *Lancet,* *2,* 992–994.

Goldberg, T.E., Weinberger, D.R., Pliskin, N.H., Berman, K.F., & Podd, M.H. (1989). Recall memory deficits in schizophrenia: A possible manifestation of prefrontal dysfunction. *Schizophrenia Research, 2,* 251–257.

Goldman, R.S., Tandon, R, Liberzon, I., & Greden, J.F. (1992). Measurement of depression and negative symptoms in schizophrenia. *Psychopathology, 25,* 49–56.

Gur, R.C., Erwin, R.J., Gur, R.E., Zwil, A.S., Heimberg, C., & Kraemer, H.C. (1992). Facial emotion discrimination: II. Behavioral findings in depression. *Psychiatry Research, 42,* 241–251.

Heaton, R.K., & Crowley, T.J. (1981). Effects of psychiatric disorders and their somatic treatments on neuropsychological test results. In S.B. Filskov & T.J. Boll (Eds.), *Handbook of Clinical Neuropsychology* (pp. 481–525). New York: Wiley-Interscience.

Heimberg, C., Gur, R.E., Erwin, R.J., Shtasel, D.L., & Gur, R.C. (1992). Facial emotion discrimination: III. Behavioral findings in schizophrenia. *Psychiatry Research, 42,* 253–265.

Helmchen, H., & Hippius, H. (1967). Depressive Syndrome im Verlauf neuroleptischer Therapie. *Nervenarzt, 38,* 445.

Henry, G.M., Weingartner, H., & Murphy, D.L. (1973). Influence of affective states and psychoactive drugs on verbal learning and memory. *American Journal of Psychiatry, 130,* 966–971.

House, A., Bostock, J., & Cooper, J. (1987). Depressive syndromes in the year following onset of a first schizophrenic illness. *British Journal of Psychiatry, 151,* 773–779.

Hussar, A.E. (1962). Effect of tranquilizers on medical mortality and morbidity in mental hospitals. *Journal of the American Medical Association, 179,* 682–686.

Husted, J.A., Beiser, M., & Iacono, W.G. (1995). Negative symptoms in the course of first-episode affective psychosis. *Psychiatry Research, 56,* 145–154.

Jacobs, D.H., Shuren, J., & Heilman, K.H. (1995). Impaired perception of facial identity and facial affect in Huntington's disease. *Neurology, 45,* 1217–1218.

Jaeger, J., Bitter, I., Czobor, P., & Volavka, J. (1990). The measurement of subjective experience in schizophrenia: The subjective deficit syndrome scale. *Comprehensive Psychiatry, 31,* 216–226.

Johnson, D.A.W. (1981). Studies of depressive symptoms in schizophrenia: I, The prevalence of depression and possible causes; II, A two-year longitudinal study of symptoms; III, A double-blind trial of placebo against orphenadrine; IV, A double-blind trial of nortriptyline for depression in chronic schizophrenia. *British Journal of Psychiatry, 139,* 89–101.

Kareken, D.A., Gur, R.C., Mozley, P.D., Mozley, L.H., Saykin, A.J., Shtasel, D.L., & Gur, R.E. (1995). Cognitive functioning and neuroanatomic volume measures in schizophrenia. *Neuropsychology, 9,* 211–219.

Kasanin, J. (1933). The acute schizoaffective psychosis. *American Journal of Psychiatry, 90,* 97–126.

Kibel, D.A., Laffont, I., & Liddle, P.F. (1993). The composition of the negative features of chronic schizophrenia. *British Journal of Psychiatry, 162,* 744–750.

Kiloh, L.G. (1961). Pseudo-dementia. *Acta Psychiatrica Scandinavica, 37,* 336–351.

King, D.A., & Caine. E.D. (1990). In J.L. Cummings (Ed.), *Depression in Subcortical Dementia* (pp. 218–230). New York: Oxford University Press.

Kitamura, T., & Suga, R. (1991). Depressive and negative symptoms in major psychiatric disorders. *Comprehensive Psychiatry, 32,* 88–94.

Knights, A., & Hirsch, S.R. (1981). "Revealed" depression and drug treatment for schizophrenia. *Archives of General Psychiatry, 38*, 806–811.

Kohler, C.G., Gur, R.C., Swanson, C.S., Petty, R., & Gur, R.E. (1998a). Depression in Schizophrenia: I. Association with neuropsychological deficits. *Biological Psychiatry, 43*, 165–172.

Kohler, C.G., Swanson, C.S., Gur, R.C., Harper Mozley, L., & Gur, R.E. (1998b). Depression in schizophrenia: II. MRI and PET findings. *Biological Psychiatry, 43*, 173–180.

Koreen, A.R., Siris, S.G., Chakos, M., Alvir, J., Mayerhoff, D., & Lieberman, J. (1993). Depression in first-episode schizophrenia. *American Journal of Psychiatry, 150*, 1643–1648.

Kraepelin, E. (1919). *Dementia Praecox and Paraphrenia* [R.M. Barcley & G.M. Robertson, translators]. Edinburgh: E.&S. Livingstone, 1971.

Krakowski, M., Czobor, P., & Volavka, J. (1997). Effect of neuroleptic treatment on depressive symptoms in acute schizophrenia episodes. *Psychiatry Research, 71*, 19–26.

Kramer, M.S., Vogel, W.H., & DiJohnson, C. (1989). Antidepressants in "depressed" schizophrenic inpatients. *Archives of General Psychiatry, 46*, 922–928.

Kring, A., Kerr, S.L., Smith, D.A., & Neale, J.M. (1993). Flat affect in schizophrenia does not reflect diminished subjective experience of emotion. *Journal of Abnormal Psychology, 2*, 77–106.

Kuck, J., Zisook, S., Moranville, J.T., Heaton, R.K., & Braff, D.L. (1992). Negative symptomatology in schizophrenic outpatients. *Journal of Nervous and Mental Disease, 180*, 510–515.

Kitamura, T., & Suga, R. (1991). Depressive and negative symptoms in major psychiatric disorders. *Comprehensive Psychiatry, 32*, 88–94.

Kulhara, P., Avasthi, A., Chadda, R., Chandiramani, K., Mattoo, S.K., Kota, S.K., & Joseph, S. (1989). Negative and depressive symptoms in schizophrenia. *British Journal of Psychiatry, 154*, 207–211.

Labarca, R., Silva, H., Jerez, S., Ruiz, A., Forray, M.I., Gysling, K., Andres, M.E., Bustos, G., Castillo, Y., & Hono, J. (1993). Differential effects of haloperidol on negative symptoms in drug-naive schizophrenic patients: Effects on plasma homovanillic acid. *Schizophrenia Research, 9(1)*, 29–34.

Lapensee, M.A. (1992). A review of schizoaffective disorder: I. Current concepts. *Canadian Journal of Psychiatry* [*Revue Canadienne de Psychiatrie*], *37(5)*, 335–346.

Malone, J.R.L., & Helmsley, D.R. (1977). Lowered responsiveness and auditory signal detectability during depression. *Psychological Medicine, 7*, 717–722.

Martin, C.C., Borod, J.C., Alpert, M., Brozgold, A., & Welkowitz, J. (1990). Spontaneous expression of facial emotion in schizophrenic and right-brain-damaged patients. *Journal of Communication Disorders, 23*, 287–301.

Mayberg, H.S., Lewis, P.J., Regenold, W., & Wagner, H.N. Jr. (1994). Paralimbic hypoperfusion in unipolar depression. *Journal of Nuclear Medicine, 35*, 929–934.

Mayberg, H.S., Starkstein, S.E., Peyser, C.E., Brandt, J., & Dannals, R.F. (1992). Paralimbic frontal lobe hypometabolism in depression associated with Huntington's disease. *Neurology, 42*, 1791–1797.

Mayberg, H.S., Starkstein, S.E., Sadzot, B., Preziosi, T., Andrezejewski, P.L., Dannals, R.F., Wagner H.N. Jr., & Robinson, R.G. (1990). Selective hypometabolism in the inferior frontal lobe in depressed patients with Parkinson's disease. *Annals of Neurology, 28*, 57–64.

Mayer-Gross, W., Slater, E., & Roth, M. (1955). *Clinical Psychiatry*. Baltimore: Williams & Wilkins.

McAllister, T.W., & Price, T.R.P. (1982). Severe depressive pseudodementia with and without dementia. *American Journal of Psychiatry, 139*, 626–629.

McGlashan, T.H. (1982). Aphanisis: The syndrome of pseudodepression in chronic schizophrenia. *Schizophrenia Bulletin, 2*, 118–134.

McGlashan, T., & Carpenter, W.T. (1976). An investigation of the postpsychotic depressive syndrome. *American Journal of Psychiatry, 133*, 4–19.

Meltzer, H.Y., & Okayli, G. (1995). Reduction of suicidality during clozapine treatment of neuroleptic-resistant schizophrenia: Impact on risk–benefit assessment. *American Journal of Psychiatry, 152*, 183–90.

Mikhailova, E.S., Vladimirova, T.V., Iznack, A.F., Tsusulkovskaya, E.J., & Sushko, N.V. (1996). Abnormal recognition of facial expression of emotions in depressed patients with major depression disorder and schizotypal personality disorder. *Biological Psychiatry, 40*, 697–705.

Miles, C. (1977). Conditions predisposing to suicide: A review. *Journal of Nervous and Mental Disease, 164*, 231–246.

Miller, D.D., Perry, P.J., Cadoret, R.J., & Andreasen, N.C. (1994). Clozapine's effect on negative symptoms in treatment refractory schizophrenics. *Comprehensive Psychiatry, 35(1)*,8–15.

Natale, M., Gur, R.E., & Gur, R.C. (1983). Hemispheric asymmetries in processing emotional expressions. *Neuropsychologia, 21*, 555–565.

Novic, J., Luchins, D.J., & Perline, R. (1984). Facial affect recognition in schizophrenia. Is there a differential deficit? *British Journal of Psychiatry, 144*, 533–537.

Nuechterlein, K.H., & Dawson, M.E. (1984). Information processing and attentional functioning in the developmental course of schziophrenic disorders. *Schizophrenia Bulletin, 10*, 160–203.

Palao, D.J., Arauxo, A., Brunet, M., Marquez, M., Bernardo, M., Ferrer, J., & Gonzalez-Monclus, E. (1994). Positive versus negative symptoms in schizophrenia: Response to haloperidol. *Progress in Neuropsychopharmacology and Biological Psychiatry, 18*, 155–164.

Papez, J.W. (1937). A proposed mechanism of emotion. *Archives of Neurology and Psychiatry, 38*, 725–743.

Planansky, K., & Johnston, R. (1971). The occurrence and characteristics of suicidal preoccupation and acts in schizophrenia. *Acta Psychiatrica Scandinavica, 47(4)*, 473–483.

Plasky, P. (1991). Antidepressant usage in schizophrenia. *Schizophrenia Bulletin, 17*, 649–657.

Prosser, E.S., Csernansky, J.G., Kaplan, J., Thiemann, S., Becker, T.J., & Hollister, L.E. (1987). Depression, parkinsonian symptoms, and negative symptoms in schizophrenics treated with neuroleptics. *Journal of Nervous and Mental Disease, 175*, 100–105.

Prussoff, V.A., Williams, D.A., Weissman, M.M., & Astrachan, B.M. (1979). Treatment of secondary depression in schizophrenia. *Archives of General Psychiatry, 36*, 569–575.

Ranjan, R., & Meltzer, H.Y. (1996). Acute and long-term effectiveness of clozapine in treatment-resistent psychotic depression. *Biological Psychiatry, 40*, 253–258.

Reddy, R., Mukherjee, S., & Schnur, D.B. (1992). Comparison of negative symptoms in schizophrenia and poor-outcome bipolar patients. *Psychological Medicine, 22*, 361–365.

Reuss, V.I., Silberman, E., & Post, R.M. (1979). *d*-Amphetamine: Effects on memory in a depressed population. *Biological Psychiatry, 4*, 345–356.

Rifkin, A., Quitkin, F., & Klein, D.F. (1975). Akinesia. *Archives of General Psychiatry, 332*, 672–674.

Ring, N., Tantam, D., Montague, L., Newby, D., Black, D., & Morris, J. (1991). Gender differences in the incidence of definite schizophrenia and atypical psychosis—Focus on negative symptoms of schizophrenia. *Acta Psychiatrica Scandinavica, 84*, 489–496.

Robinson, R.G., Kubos, K.L., Starr, L.B., Rao, K., & Price, T.G. (1984). Mood disorders in stroke patients. *Brain, 107*, 81–93.

Ross, E.D., & Mesulam, M.-M. (1979). Dominant language functions of the right hemisphere? Prosody and emotional gesturing. *Archives of Neurology, 36*, 144–148.

Roth, S. (1970). The seemingly ubiquitous depression following acute schizophrenic episodes, a neglected area of clinical discussion. *American Journal of Psychiatry, 127*, 51–58.

Roy, A. (1981). Depression in the course of chronic undifferentiated schizophrenia. *Archives of General Psychiatry, 38*, 296–297.

Sackeim, H.A., Greenberg, M., Weiman, A., Gur, R.C., Hungerbuhler, J., & Geschwind, N. (1982). Hemispheric asymmetry in the expression of positive and negative emotions. Neurologic evidence. *Archives of Neurology, 39*, 210–218.

Sackeim, H.A., Gur, R.C., & Saucy, M.C. (1978). Emotions are expressed more intensely on the left side of the face. *Science, 202*, 434–436.

Saykin, A.J., Gur, R.C., Gur, R.E., Mozley, D., Mozley, L.H., Resnick, S.M., Kester, D.B., & Stafiniak, P. (1991). Neuropsychological function in schizophrenia: Selective impairment in memory and learning. *Archives of General Psychiatry, 48*, 618–624.

Saykin, A.J., Shtasel, D.L., Gur, R.E., Kester, D.B., Mozley, L.H., Stafiniak, P., & Gur, R.C. (1994). Neuropsychological deficits in neuroleptic naive patients with first-episode schizophrenia. *Archives of General Psychiatry, 51*, 124–131.

Schneider, K. (1959). *Klinische Psychopathologie* [M.W. Hamilton, translator]. New York: Grune & Stratton.

Schneider, F., Gur, R.C., Gur, R.E., & Shtasel, D.L. (1995). Emotional processing in schizophrenia: Neurobehavioral probes in relation to psychopathology. *Schizophrenia Research, 17*, 67–75.

Schneider, F., Koch, J.D., Mattes, R., & Heimann, H. (1992). The recognition of emotions from the facial expression in divided visual half field presentations in schizophrenic and depressive patients. *Nervenarzt, 63*, 545–550.

Shanfield, S., Tucker, G.J., Marrow, M., & Detre, T. (1970). The schizophrenic patient and depressive symptomatology. *Journal of Nervous and Mental Disease, 151*, 203–210.

Shtasel, D.L., Gur, R.E., Gallacher, F., Heimberg C., & Gur, R.C. (1992): Gender differences in the clinical expression of schizophrenia. *Schizophrenia Research, 7*, 225–231.

Silver, H., & Shmugliakov, N. (1998). Augmentation of fluvoxamine but not maprotiline improves negative symptoms in treated schizophrenia: Evidence for a specific serotonergic effect from a double-blind study. *Journal of Clinical Psychopharmacology, 18*, 208–211.

Siris, S.G. (1991). Diagnosis of secondary depression in schizophrenia. *Schizophrenia Bulletin, 17(1)*, 75–97.

Siris, S.G., Bermanzohn, P.C., Mason, S.E., & Shuwall, M.A. (1994). Maintenance imipramine therapy for secondary depression in schizophrenia. *Archives of General Psychiatry, 51*, 109–115.

Siris, S.G., Morgan, V., Fagerstrom, R., Rifkin, A., & Cooper, T.B. (1987). Adjunctive imipramine in the treatment of post-psychotic depression: A controlled trial. *Archives of General Psychiatry, 44*, 533–539.

Siris, S.G., Rifkin, A.E., & Reardon, G.T. (1982). Response of postpsychotic depression to adjunctive imipramine or amitryptiline. *Journal of Clinical Pychiatry, 43*, 485–486.

Siris, S.G., Rifkin, A.E., Reardon, G.T., Doddi, S.R., Strahan, A., & Hall, K.S. (1986).

Stability of the post-psychotic depressive syndrome. *Journal of Clinical Psychiatry, 47,* 86–88.

Sison, C.E., Alpert, M., Fudge, R., & Stern, R.M. (1996). Constricted expressiveness and psychophysiological reactivity in schizophrenia. *Journal of Nervous and Mental Disease, 184,* 589–597.

Steinberg, H.R., Green, R., & Durell, J. (1967). Depression occurring during the course of recovery from acute schizophrenic symptoms. *American Journal of Psychiatry, 124,* 699–702.

Stern, M.J., Pillsbury, J.A., & Sonnenberg, S.M. (1967). Postpsychotic depression in schizophrenics. *Comprehensive Psychiatry, 123,* 976–979.

Stromgren, L.S. (1977). The influence of depression on memory. *Acta Psychiatrica Scandinavica, 56,* 109–128.

Tandon, R., Greden, J.F., & Silk, K.R. (1988). Treatment of negative schizophrenic symptoms with trihexyphenidyl. *Journal of Clinical Psychopharmcology, 8,* 212–215.

Tollefson, G.D., & Sanger, T.M. (1997). Negative symptoms: A path analytic approach to a double blind, placebo, and haloperidol-controlled clinical trial with olanzapine. *American Journal of Psychiatry, 154,* 466–474.

Tollefson, G.D., Sanger, T.M., Beasley, C.M., & Tran, P.V. (1998a). A double-blind, controlled comparison of the novel antipsychotic olanzapine versus haloperidol or placebo on anxious and depressive symptoms accompanying schizophrenia. *Biological Psychiatry, 43,* 803–810.

Tollefson, G.D., Sanger, T.M., Lu, Y., & Thieme, M.E. (1998b). Depressive signs and symptoms in schizophrenia: A prospective blinded trial of olanzapine and haloperidol. *Archives of General Psychiatry, 55,* 250–258.

Tsuang, M.T., & Loyd, D.W. (1988). Other psychotic disorders. In R. Michels (Ed.), *Psychiatry.* Philadelphia: J.B. Lippincott.

Turetsky, B.T., Cowell, P.E., Gur, R.C., Grossman, R.I., Shtasel, D.L., & Gur, R.E. (1995). Frontal and temporal lobe brain volumes in schizophrenia: Relationship to symptomatology and clinical subtype. *Archives of General Psychiatry, 52,* 1061–1070.

Van Putten, T., & May, P.R. (1978). Akinetic depression in schizophrenia. *Archives of General Psychiatry, 35,* 1101–1107.

Waehrens, V.A., & Gerlach, J. (1980). Antidepressant drugs in anergic schizophrenia. *Acta Psychiatrica Scandinavica, 61,* 438–444.

Walker, E.F., Grimes K.E, Davis, D.D., & Smith A.J. (1993). Childhood precursors of adult-onset schiozophrenia: Facial expressions of emotion. *American Journal of Psychiatry, 150,* 1654–1660.

Walker, E.F., McGuire, M., & Bettes, B. (1984). Recognition and identification of facial stimuli by schizophrenics and patients with affective disorders. *British Journal of Clinical Psychology, 23,* 37–44.

Weingartner, H., Gold, B., & Ballenger, J.D. (1981). Effects of vasopressin on human memory functions. *Science, 211,* 601–613.

Weisler, R.H., Ahearn, E.P., Davidson, J.R., & Wallace, C.D. (1997). Adjunctive use of olanzapine in mood disorders: Five case reports. *Annals of Clinical Psychiatry, 9,* 259–262.

Zarate, C.A., Tohen, M., & Baldessarini, R.J. (1995). Clozapine in severe mood disorders. *Journal of Clinical Psychiatry, 56,* 411–417.

Zuroff, D.C., & Colussy, S.A. (1986). Emotion recognition in schizophrenic and depressed patients. *Journal of Clinical Psychology, 42,* 411–417.

18

Therapeutic Brain Interventions in Mood Disorders and the Nature of Emotion

SARAH H. LISANBY AND HAROLD A. SACKEIM

The introduction of convulsive therapy (ECT) in the 1930s and psychotropic medications in the 1950s changed the face of therapeutics in psychiatry. Before the development of these somatic treatments, the predominant view was that the major forms of psychopathology reflected irreversible structural degeneration of the brain and that little could be done to ameliorate symptoms. The discovery of effective somatic therapies did more than undo this therapeutic nihilism. It provided fertile ground for nosological refinement and for the generation of hypotheses regarding the mechanisms of action of the treatments and the underlying pathophysiology of specific disorders (Fink, 1979; Klein et al., 1980).

We attempt to summarize the implications of the knowledge gained in the treatment of mood disorders for theories about the neurobiological regulation of emotion. The four brain interventions examined include: (*1*) psychopharmacological treatments, (*2*) ECT, (*3*) functional neurosurgery, and (*4*) repetitive transcranial magnetic stimulation (rTMS). These interventions have mood-altering effects but differ in their mechanisms of action and degree of anatomical specificity. Other brain interventions, including light therapy and sleep deprivation, have contributed to our understanding of mood systems but are beyond the scope of this chapter.

PSYCHOPHARMACOLOGICAL TREATMENTS

Pharmacological Dissection

The differential efficacy of pharmacological treatments has been fundamental in subtyping mood disorders and generating a refined nosology. The first distinction was between unipolar and bipolar disorders. Traditional antidepressant medications, such as tricyclic antidepressants (TCAs), monoamine oxidase inhibitors (MAOIs), and selective serotonin reuptake inhibitors (SSRIs), effectively treat the depressed phase of bipolar disorder but may provoke hypomania or mania. These agents rarely provoke these reactions in patients with an established unipolar course. Mood-stabilizing agents, principally lithium carbonate, and/or a variety of anticonvulsant medications (e.g., carbamazepine and sodium valproate) are effective antimanic agents (Goodwin & Jamison, 1990). Other research confirmed that unipolar and bipolar disorders differ in familial transmission, onset, and clinical course (Angst, Felder, & Frey, 1979; Gershon et al., 1982). These findings provided *prima facie* evidence that the pathophysiologies of depressed and manic states were distinct. Additionally, bipolar and unipolar patients differ in key symptomatic manifestations during the depressed phase. For example, psychomotor retardation is more common in bipolar than in unipolar depression (Sobin & Sackeim, 1997).

Differential pharmacological response has been used to subtype unipolar depression. Patients with delusional or psychotic depression respond poorly to monotherapy with antidepressant medications (TCAs, MAOIs, or SSRIs) (Chan et al., 1987; Glassman, Kantor, & Shostak, 1975). Such patients also have a poor response to monotherapy with antipsychotic medication (Spiker et al., 1985) but show robust rates of response to combination treatment with an antidepressant and antipsychotic medication (Perry et al., 1982; Spiker et al., 1985) or ECT (Sobin et al., 1996). This distinction between delusional and nondelusional depression is supported by differences in other aspects of phenomenology, family history, and suicide rate (Glassman & Roose, 1981; Roose et al., 1983). The pharmacological evidence implies that abnormalities in dopaminergic systems are more central to delusional than to nondelusional depression.

Among nondelusional depressed patients, further distinctions may be drawn. Atypical depression presents with increased sleep (hypersomnia), increased appetite (hyperphagia), marked fatigue ("leaden paralysis"), and/or rejection sensitivity. These patients respond well to MAOIs and perhaps to SSRIs, but have low response rates to TCAs (Liebowitz et al., 1984, 1988; Quitkin, 1992; Quitkin et al., 1988). This suggests that noradrenergic dysregulation is less relevant to atypical than to typical major depression, and the former may have more prominent abnormalities in serotonin and/or dopamine transmission.

Finally, there is evidence to distinguish melancholic or severe depression from nonmelancholic or less severe presentations (for review, see Rush & Weissenburger, 1994). Melancholic, endogenous, or vegetative features among inpatients have predictive value regarding response to TCAs (Abou-Saleh & Coppen, 1983; Gibbons, Clark, & Davis, 1982; Kiloh, Ball, & Garside, 1962; Reisby et al., 1977). Presently there is controversy as to whether SSRIs are inferior to TCAs in the treatment of severe, melancholic depression (Roose et al., 1994). In part because of this controversy and its neurobiological implications, newer antidepressant agents, such as venlafaxine and mirtazapine, were designed to target multiple neurotransmitter systems (e.g., norepinephrine and serotonin) in an attempt to be more effective for a broader range of depressed patients than the SSRIs.

These examples of pharmacological dissection illustrate that the pathophysiology of mood disorders is likely to be heterogeneous. It is hazardous to claim that the mechanisms involved in a treatment intervention are necessarily related to the etiology or pathophysiology of the disorder being treated. For example, no one contends that depressed patients respond to ECT because the lack of a seizure is intrinsic to their pathophysiology. Individuals sharing certain phenomenological features, however, often respond to different pharmacological regimens. In some cases, there are also established differences in familial transmission, clinical course, and associated biological abnormalities.

Given the heterogeneous pathophysiology of affective disorders, the generalizability of neurobiological studies of normal variation in mood to clinical samples becomes tenuous. A central aim of mood provocation studies in normal samples is to relate biological effects to global descriptors of mood, such as depression, anxiety, and elation. Given the likely heterogeneity of depressed patient groups, the relevance of such data and the models they generate for understanding mood disorders are highly inferential.

Phases of Mood Disturbance

A key principle in the biological treatment of mood disorder is that effective somatic treatments suppress symptom manifestations but have little impact on the underlying disorder. This perspective originally emanated from study of the pharmacological prevention of relapse and recurrence. A classic set of studies demonstrated that approximately 50% of patients will relapse within a 6-month period if antidepressant medication or ECT is discontinued at the point of clinical response (Imlah, Ryan, & Harrington, 1965; Kay, Fahy, & Garside, 1970; Mindham, Howland, & Shepherd, 1973; Seager & Bird, 1962). Among medication-resistant patients who respond to ECT, our ongoing placebo-controlled research suggests that this relapse rate actually may be closer to 85% in the absence of continued somatic therapy. In contrast, there is overwhelming evidence that continuing the antidepressant regimen that produced remission reduces the 6-month relapse rate to about 20%.

These and related findings call for a distinction among three treatment phases: acute, continuation, and maintenance (Frank et al., 1990). Acute phase treatment aims to relieve symptoms. Continuation phase treatment, typically defined as from 6 to 12 months following symptomatic response, aims to suppress symptoms until the underlying episode spontaneously remits (Prien & Kupfer, 1986). The presumption is that the average duration of episodes is approximately 6 to 9 months, but this is subject to considerable individual variation. Maintenance treatment aims to prevent the recurrence of a new episode after the original episode has resolved (Frank et al., 1991).

Robust evidence from pharmacological trials supports these distinctions. Approximately 50% or more of patients with unipolar major depression will experience a recurrence within their lifetime. Long-term maintenance treatment with antidepressant regimens that produced the acute phase clinical response are effective in preventing recurrence (Frank et al., 1990; Prien et al., 1984). The efficacy of lithium carbonate in preventing episodes of both depression and mania is, in many respects, more impressive than its efficacy as acute treatment, particularly for depression (Calabrese, Bowden, & Woyshville, 1995).

The differential activity of psychopharmacological agents in the different phases of treatment suggests that attention be paid to the neurobiological disturbances (state, episode, and trait markers) specific to these phases. Distinctions may be made among the neural alterations associated with acute affective symptoms (state), the vulnerability to manifest symptoms through a sustained, but self-limited, period (episode), and the vulnerability to experience affective episodes (trait). During acute phase treatment, medications act on neural substrates responsible for symptom expression (state). A more fundamental biological disturbance, however, goes unabated despite treatment, only to resolve spontaneously (episode). Finally, another class of biological disturbance triggers single or recurrent episodes (trait).

Neurobiological investigations are only beginning to make these distinctions and to outline candidate markers for the distinct phases of mood disturbance. For example, measures of the activity of the hypothalamic–pituitary–adrenal axis or hypothalamic–pituitary–thyroid axis commonly show dysfunction during the state of major depression (Carroll, 1982; Prange, Garbutt, & Loosen, 1987). There is evidence that while most patients show normalization in some of these measures following response to acute phase treatment, continued abnormality is predictive of relapse (Holsboer, 1995). Consequently, such measures have some sensitivity as episode markers. Potential episode or trait markers include global and topographic disturbances in regional cerebral blood flow (rCBF), which in some cases have been found to persist independent of remission status (Nobler et al., 1994; Sackeim et al., 1990). There is evidence that specific neuropsychological profiles also characterize mood disorder patients independent of symptomatic status and are seen in children of bipolar probands before the onset of affective episodes (Decina et al., 1983; Sackeim et al., 1992a). These likely reflect trait markers.

It is common in basic emotion research to distinguish between state and trait neurobiological factors. For example, among normal individuals, Davidson (1995) has associated persistent lateralized electroencephalographic (EEG) patterns to individual differences in emotional reactivity to provocations, thus linking a lateralized trait phenomenon to a propensity for specific affect states.

Effects of Pharmacological Agents on the Regulation of Emotion

Antidepressant agents are not euphoriants. Normal subjects administered TCAs, MAOIs, SSRIs, or other effective antidepressants do not experience elation. This is supported by the fact that such medications are rarely the objects of abuse. Furthermore, euphoriants or stimulants, like amphetamine, have only a minor role in the treatment of major depression (Hare, Dominian, & Sharpe, 1962; Thase & Rush, 1995). Only in the case of bipolar disorder is there a propensity for antidepressant agents to trigger hypomania or mania. Similarly, antimanic agents, such as lithium and anticonvulsants, do not elicit depressed mood in normal subjects.

One implication of these observations is that the systems subserving the states of depression and mania in clinical samples are not, in ordinary circumstances, mutually inhibitory. In unipolar depression, suppressing symptoms with antidepressant medication does not provoke euphoria, regardless of the intensity of treatment. This would contradict one version of the original valence hypothesis, at least with respect to mood disorders. This hypothesis suggested that mutually inhibitory neural systems regulate the expression of positive and negative mood states (Sackeim et al., 1982). The evidence from pharmacology is that, for the most part, one class of symptoms can be suppressed without provoking the other.

The effect of antidepressant and antimanic agents on normal variations in mood has received surprisingly little attention. Anecdotal evidence suggests that antidepressant medications do not seem to interfere with the normal dysphoric response to negative life events. Likewise, there is no evidence that mood-stabilizing agents, such as lithium or the anticonvulsants, reduce the normal range of happiness or sadness. These observations imply that psychotropic medications effective in the treatment of mood disorder act at a neurobiological level responsible for symptom manifestation, leaving the neural systems responsible for normal mood reactivity intact. In turn, this suggests that there are fundamental differences in the neural systems that regulate normal variation in mood and that are dysregulated during the state of major depression and mania. This implies that studies of physiological alterations during normal states of sadness and happiness are of limited relevance to understanding the pathophysiology of major depression and mania (and vice versa). It is noteworthy that the initial tomographic brain imaging studies of mood provocation in normal people and of the resting state in major depression and mania have yielded dramatically different profiles of rCBF effects (for a review of clinical studies, see George et al., 1995a; Pardo, Pardo, & Raichle, 1993; Sackeim & Prohovnik, 1993; Schneider et al., 1994).

A number of pharmacological interventions can induce euphoria in normal subjects. These are the most common drugs of abuse and include stimulants, cocaine, and opioids. Barbiturates and alcohol are classified as central nervous system depressants but are commonly abused, like benzodiazepines, due to their anxiolytic properties. As reviewed elsewhere (Sackeim, 1986), there have been concerted attempts for several decades to identify pharmacological agents that reliably induce clinical depression or simply depressed mood state in normal subjects. These efforts have mostly failed. This would suggest a fundamental, as yet unidentified, difference in the substrates regulating depressed and elated mood states in normal individuals.

Mechanisms of Action and the Pathophysiology of Mood Disturbance

Antidepressants differ widely in their intrinsic pharmacological properties. TCAs, MAOIs, SSRIs, and a variety of newer compounds, however, possess roughly equivalent efficacy for nonpsychotic, nonatypical, major depression (Burke & Preskorn, 1995). Although there are numerous examples of patients who respond to one but not another type of antidepressant within or outside of the same class, this is the exception rather than the rule. Does this suggest that there is a common mode of action across these agents despite differing pharmacological profiles, or are there multiple avenues to relieve symptoms?

The possibility of a common mode of antidepressant action, despite differences in pharmacological effects, should not be discounted. Almost all effective antidepressants share a similar time course of action and result in a common set of neurobiological changes, such as downregulation of the postsynaptic β_2-adrenergic receptor and/or upregulation of the postsynaptic serotonin $5HT_2$ receptor and the gamma-aminobutyric acid (GABA) $GABA_b$ receptor (Gerner & Bunney, 1986; Heninger & Charney, 1987; Lloyd, Morselli, & Bartholini, 1987). The major neurotransmitter systems implicated in the treatment of mood disorders, noradrenergic, dopaminergic, serotonergic, and GABAergic, strongly interact. Cerebrospinal fluid studies of transmitter metabolite levels have shown considerable overlap in the effects of different classes of pharmacological agents (Potter & Manji, 1993).

Nonetheless, there is also compelling evidence to support specificity in the mode of action of pharmacological treatments in achieving antidepressant response. Dietary tryptophan depletion rapidly decreases brain levels of tryptophan (precursor to serotonin), serotonin, and 5-hydroxyindoleacetic acid (5-HIAA, a metabolite of serotonin). In formerly depressed patients who were successfully treated with an SSRI, tryptophan depletion results in rapid, transient relapse (Bremner et al., 1997; Delgado et al., 1990). Tryptophan depletion also disrupts the response to light therapy in seasonal affective disorder (Neumeister et al., 1997). It does not, however, appear to worsen symptoms in untreated depressed patients (Delgado et al., 1994), nor does it provoke relapse in patients who have responded to a TCA (Heninger, Delgado, & Charney, 1996) or ECT (Cassidy et al., 1997). There is initial evidence for a double dissociation between serotonergic and noradrenergic manipulations; transient relapse in patients who responded to a TCA, but not to an SSRI, may be provoked by depleting noradrenergic stores (Delgado et al., 1993).

This experimental reversal of therapeutic effects contingent on the form of treatment that produced the response provides impressive evidence for specificity in mechanisms of action. It suggests that SSRIs differ from TCAs and ECT in how antidepressant effects are accomplished. In turn, this suggests that multiple neurobiological substrates (or nodes within a network) can be altered to suppress depressive symptoms. Given this diversity in the modes of therapeutic action, one must entertain the possibility that multiple physiological alterations may result in a unitary presentation of depressed mood in normal individuals and/or clinical depression.

ELECTROCONVULSIVE THERAPY

Convulsive therapy involves the deliberate induction of a generalized, grand mal seizure for therapeutic purposes and is the biological treatment with the longest history of continuous use in psychiatry. Indications include major depression, acute mania, and schizophrenia (Weiner et al., 1990). It is generally acknowledged that convulsive therapy is the most potent antidepressant treatment and that a substantial number of patients with medication-resistant depression show considerable benefit from its use (Prudic et al., 1996). Similarly, the short-term efficacy of convulsive therapy in mania is well established and may equal or exceed its potency as an antidepressant (Mukherjee, Sackeim, & Schnur, 1994). Given the substantial evidence implicating dysregulation of distinct neurobiological systems in major depression and mania, the efficacy of ECT in both conditions requires consideration (Post et al., 1986).

When convulsive therapy was introduced in the mid-1930s, seizure induction was accomplished through systemic injection of proconvulsant agents. Electroconvulsive therapy involves the application to the scalp of a time-varying electrical stimulus of sufficient intensity to produce a generalized seizure. Electroconvulsive therapy replaced chemical induction because of its greater medical safety and control over the timing and likelihood of seizure. In the 1950s, it was appreciated that application of the electrical stimulus to the left or right hemisphere (i.e., left unilateral [LUL] or right unilateral [RUL] ECT), resulted in distinct short-term cognitive sequelae (Sackeim, 1992). For example, each form of ECT results in a material-specific amnestic syndrome, with greater verbal loss following LUL ECT and greater nonverbal memory loss following RUL ECT (Sackeim, 1992). The magnitude and consistency of the differences in transient neuropsychological effects between LUL and RUL ECT are sufficiently robust that the nature and direction of language lateralization can be reliably determined on a patient-by-patient basis (Geffen, Traub, & Stierman, 1978; Pratt & Warrington, 1972). Bilateral (BL) ECT, with symmetrical placement of stimulating electrodes over frontotemporal areas, results in the cognitive deficits associated with both forms of unilateral ECT, perhaps to a more severe and persistent degree (Sackeim, 1992; Sackeim et al., 1993b). The capacity to manipulate the site of brain stimulation by the positioning of extracranial electrodes in ECT offers one method to investigate the neural systems dysregulated in mood disorders.

Efficacy of Electroconvulsive Therapy: Generalized or Localized Effects?

For decades, the field of ECT held the view that a generalized seizure was necessary and sufficient to treat major depression. How the seizure was produced was considered irrelevant (Small, 1974). Furthermore, it was thought that the quantity of electricity used to produce the seizure did not impact on efficacy but did contribute to cognitive side effects (Sackeim, Devanand, & Nobler, 1995). A large body of literature had shown that markedly suprathreshold electrical stimulation intensifies side effects without additional benefit (Ottosson, 1960; Scott et al., 1992; Weiner et al., 1986b).

Competing hypotheses have been put forth to explain the view that generalized seizure activity is central to the therapeutic effects of ECT. One hypothesis was that for therapeutic effects to be achieved, widespread, generalized changes in brain neurochemistry were necessary. The alternative hypothesis was that localized brain systems were involved, but their neurobiology could only be altered with ECT by engagement of a generalized seizure. Drawing a link between hypothalamic dysfunction and the vegetative symptoms of melancholic depression (sleep and appetite disturbance, diurnal variation, reduced libido), many theorists argued that the ultimate source of ECT's therapeutic effects resulted from neurochemical changes in the diencephalon (Abrams, 1997; Abrams & Taylor, 1976; Fink, 1990).

There is substantial evidence that a generalized seizure is critical in obtaining therapeutic effects with ECT. A series of studies contrasted "sham ECT" (the repeated administration of general anesthesia) with real ECT. This work established that in the treatment of major depression (for review, see Sackeim, 1989) or acute mania (Sikdar et al., 1994), real ECT is considerably more effective than sham.

This type of study controls for psychological factors surrounding ECT, including the high expectations for remission, and indicates that the passage of electricity and/or the production of a seizure are central to efficacy. Other work went a step further and compared ECT with subconvulsive electrical stimulation, which was found to be substantially less effective (Fink, Kahn, & Green, 1958; Ulett, Smith, & Glesser, 1956). Ottosson (1960) provided one of the most influential pieces of evidence that the generalized seizure is critical. He found that pretreatment with lidocaine, which reduced seizure expression, resulted in inferior clinical outcome. Finally, electrical and chemical seizure induction appeared to have equal efficacy, suggesting that methods of seizure elicitation are irrelevant to beneficial effects (Small, 1974).

Despite this wealth of evidence, recent research has challenged the view that a generalized seizure is both necessary and sufficient for antidepressant effects (Sackeim et al., 1993b). This research implies that the current paths traversed by the electrical stimulus, and the current density within those paths, fundamentally impact on the efficacy of the treatment (Sackeim, 1994a). Consequently, there is now convincing evidence for neuroanatomical specificity in the neural systems that must be altered for ECT to exert antidepressant effects.

Technical Factors and the Efficacy of Electroconvulsive Therapy

Until recently, standard ECT practice involved administering the same electrical dosage to all patients. Methods to quantify the threshold for a generalized seizure were only developed in the last decade (Sackeim et al., 1987c). The field also lacked information on the extent of individual differences in seizure threshold and the factors that determine this variability (Sackeim et al., 1994; Sackeim, Devanand, & Prudic, 1991; Weiner et al., 1990).

It is now evident that there are marked individual differences in seizure threshold (Lisanby et al., 1996; Sackeim et al., 1994; Sackeim, Devanand, & Prudic, 1991). Fixed dosage regimens often result in grossly suprathreshold stimulation and increased cognitive side effects. Another consequence of this practice was a failure to appreciate that, combined with electrode positioning, electrical dosage could have a profound effect on efficacy.

The first study to address this issue used a double-blind, randomized design in which patients with major depression were treated with either BL or RUL ECT, with electrical intensity maintained just above seizure threshold (Sackeim et al., 1987a). The surprising outcome of this work was that RUL ECT given just above threshold was notably deficient as an antidepressant. Seventy percent of patients randomized to BL ECT were classified as responders, whereas only 28% of RUL ECT patients were so classified. These findings led to the hypothesis that the efficacy of RUL ECT was highly sensitive to dosage. Robin and de Tissera (1982) raised the possibility that electrical dosage impacts on speed of clinical response. A subsequent study tested both propositions. Patients with major depression were randomized to receive either BL or RUL ECT with stimulus intensity just above seizure threshold (low dose) or stimulus intensity 2.5 times the seizure threshold (high dosage) (Sackeim et al., 1993b). Only 17% of patients receiving RUL ECT at low intensity responded, but increasing the stimulus intensity of RUL ECT markedly improved the response rate. This work also demonstrated that speed of response is enhanced with higher stimulus intensity for both BL and RUL ECT. In ongoing research at Columbia University, the dose–response function for RUL ECT is being more carefully defined.

Why Is Low Dosage Right Unilateral Electroconvulsive Therapy Ineffective?

Research has established that dramatic differences in antidepressant effects are obtained by varying electrode positioning and stimulus dosage. This implies that the current paths traversed by the ECT stimulus determine rates of response, implicating specificity in the anatomy of the neural systems involved in the therapeutic effects of ECT. It is possible to induce generalized seizures that reliably lack efficacy. Thus, while a generalized seizure may be necessary, it is not sufficient. Exploring why alterations of stimulus intensity impact on the efficacy of RUL ECT provides a new approach to elucidate the mechanisms of action of ECT. Three hypotheses, discussed below, have been offered to account for the effects of stimulus intensity on the efficacy of RUL ECT (Sackeim, 1994a).

Bilateral seizure generalization

In unilateral ECT, current density is relatively evenly distributed across the anterior two-thirds of the stimulated hemisphere and approximately three times greater in the stimulated than nonstimulated hemisphere (Weaver, Williams, & Rush, 1976). Although LUL and RUL ECT both produce bilaterally generalized seizures, EEG seizure expression is often greater on the side of stimulation (d'Elia & Perris, 1970). Other physiological indices are compatible with a profound asymmetry in functional brain activity. Following unilateral ECT, there is a marked decrease in rCBF in anterior regions on the side of stimulation, with little or no change in the opposite hemisphere (Nobler et al., 1994; Silfverskiöld & Risberg, 1989). Similarly, there is an increase in delta activity in the resting EEG, most marked over the stimulated hemisphere (Sackeim et al., 1996). Deficits in learning and memory largely reflect disruption of processing in the stimulated hemisphere (Sackeim, 1992; Sackeim et al., 1993b).

Some have taken the position that the efficacy of RUL ECT is enhanced at higher stimulus intensity because the increased electrical dosage results in greater bilateral seizure generalization, making RUL more like BL ECT (Weiner & Coffey, 1986). A critical implication of this view is that bilateral neurobiological alterations are necessary to achieve antidepressant effects, contradicting ideas that lateralization in the regulation of emotion has relevance for therapeutics, at least in the context of ECT. This position predicts that physiological and neuropsychological asymmetries are reduced when the stimulus intensity of RUL ECT is increased. The available evidence does not support these predictions. In fact, EEG asymmetries during and following seizure induction appear to be somewhat enhanced at high relative to low intensity RUL ECT (Krystal et al., 1993; Krystal, Weiner, & Coffey, 1995; Sackeim et al., 1996). Left-sided neglect in the acute postictal period, an indicator of right hemisphere disruption, is more consistent and profound with high intensity than low intensity RUL ECT (Sackeim et al., 1992b). High intensity RUL ECT does not result in greater acute or short-term retrograde amnesia for verbal material but increases the amnesia for nonverbal information (Sackeim et al., 1993b).

Stimulation of deep subcortical structures

At equivalent electrical intensity, BL ECT results in substantially greater current density in diencephalic regions than RUL ECT (Weaver et al., 1976). Increasing the stimulus intensity of RUL ECT results in greater current density and perhaps seizure expression in deep subcortical regions. In agreement with classic views emphasizing hypothalamic effects, it has been argued that this effect accounts for the increased efficacy of higher dosage RUL ECT (Abrams, 1986, 1997).

Assessment of this possibility is difficult due to the absence of direct markers of electrical stimulation or seizure propagation to the diencephalon. Nonetheless, some indirect measures of hypothalamic activity have been examined. ECT results in an acute surge of plasma hormones, such as prolactin, oxytocin, and vasopressin, whose release is mediated by the hypothalamus. Manipulations of electrode placement and stimulus intensity impact on the magnitude of the release of specific hormones (Devanand et al., 1998; Lisanby et al., 1998a; Zis et al., 1996). Variations in the magnitude of these hormone surges may not, however, correlate with efficacy (Devanand et al., 1998; Lisanby et al., 1998a). Likewise, ECT produces consistent short-term changes in measures of the hypothalamic–pituitary–adrenal axis, and these changes are also unrelated to efficacy (Devanand et al., 1987, 1991). One could hypothesize that the development of transcortical slow wave (delta) activity in the interictal EEG reflects an effect on thalamic pacemakers. This has also, however, been found to be unrelated to efficacy (Sackeim et al., 1996).

Anticonvulsant action and functional activity in prefrontal cortex

It is well established that ECT is a powerful anticonvulsant (Post et al., 1986; Sackeim et al., 1983a). Repeated treatment with ECT results in a progressive rise in seizure threshold and a reduction in both seizure duration and intensity of seizure expression (Sackeim et al., 1987b). Electroconvulsive therapy results in acute and short-term topographically distributed changes in functional brain activity. There is a decrease in cortical rCBF and regional cerebral metabolic rate for glucose and a marked increase in slow wave activity in the EEG (Ackermann, Engel, & Baxter, 1986; Nobler et al., 1994; Weiner et al., 1986a).

Electroconvulsive shock in animal models of epilepsy has shown marked anticonvulsant properties equaling or exceeding numerous anticonvulsant medications (Babington & Wedeking, 1975; Post et al., 1986) and has been used occasionally in the clinical treatment of seizure disorders (Caplan, 1946; Sackeim et al., 1983a; Schnur et al., 1989). Electroconvulsive shock increases concentrations of specific inhibitory neurotransmitters and peptides on a regional basis. The most likely candidates underlying the anticonvulsant action of ECT include GABA, endogenous opioid, adenosine, and neuropeptide Y (Sackeim, Devanand, & Nobler, 1995; Woldbye et al., 1996).

One theory posits that the anticonvulsant effects of ECT underlie both its antidepressant and antimanic properties (Post et al., 1986; Sackeim et al., 1983a). Unlike conventional antidepressant medications, some anticonvulsants have established antimanic properties and some degree of antidepressant effects. Electroconvulsive therapy has marked efficacy in both conditions.

A version of the anticonvulsant hypothesis focuses on the topographic distribution of the increase in inhibitory neurotransmission and the reduction in functional brain activity that accompany ECT. This theory argues that the spatial distribution of these effects is determined more by the sites of seizure initiation than by seizure propagation. It is claimed that at low dosage, RUL ECT results in seizures that initiate in the motor cortex. At higher dosages, prefrontal cortical regions are more likely to be sites of seizure initiation with RUL ECT (Sackeim & Mukherjee, 1986). Reduction in functional activity in prefrontal regions is considered essential to the therapeutic effects of ECT in mood disorders (Sackeim, 1994a).

The known variability in seizure threshold across cortical regions may explain the finding that manipulation of the stimulus intensity of RUL ECT alters the sites of seizure initiation. Within the cortex, the primary motor area has the lowest threshold for seizure induction (Sackeim & Mukherjee, 1986). Because current density with RUL ECT is relatively evenly distributed over the anterior two-thirds of the stimulated hemisphere, primary motor cortex is the likely site of seizure initiation when minimal dosage is used. With a large enough increase in dose, current density should be sufficient to trigger self-sustaining seizure activity from prefrontal regions. In contrast, current density with BL ECT is greatest near the prefrontal pole and drops sharply along the anteroposterior dimension (Hayes, 1950). The fact that seizures are initiated with BL ECT in prefrontal regions regardless of the stimulus intensity may explain why electrical intensity has little impact on the efficacy of BL ECT.

Recent brain imaging studies support the theory that reduction of functional activity in prefrontal cortical regions is linked to the efficacy of ECT. The rCBF reductions seen acutely and 1 week following ECT typically show an antero-posterior gradient, with greatest reductions at the prefrontal pole. Most importantly, this topographic alteration appears to be strongly correlated with therapeutic response in both major depression and mania (Nobler et al., 1994). Likewise, the development of slow wave EEG activity in prefrontal sites shows topographic specificity in relation to antidepressant effects (Sackeim et al., 1996). Furthermore, relative to high dosage RUL ECT, low dosage RUL ECT is considerably less likely to enhance prefrontal slow wave activity. Based on such evidence supporting the importance of frontal changes, one group has attempted to concentrate current density in prefrontal regions, using a bifrontal electrode placement. Preliminary findings suggest that bifrontal ECT may be more effective than the traditional frontotemporal BL placement and may also result in reduced amnestic side effects (Lawson et al., 1990; Letemendia et al., 1993).

In summary, the available evidence supports the idea that ECT exerts antide-pressant, and possibly antimanic, effects through its anticonvulsant properties, particularly the reduction of functional activity in prefrontal cortical regions. The emphasis on the role of prefrontal regions is a top-down perspective, suggesting that functional suppression in prefrontal areas modulates activity in limbic, striatal, thalamic, and hypothalamic regions (Sackeim, 1994a). It should be noted, however, that anticonvulsant theories, and the specific formulation emphasizing effects in prefrontal regions, are far from proven. The relevant evidence is largely correlational, showing associations between the topographic changes in post-ECT brain imaging measures of functional activity and manipulations of treatment technique and clinical outcome.

To more directly test these views, key experiments are needed. It may be possible to block the anticonvulsant properties of ECT with pharmacological manipulations (Tortella & Long, 1985, 1988). If therapeutic efficacy is unaltered under such conditions, the anticonvulsant theory would be compromised. It should also be possible to develop powerful devices that elicit localized seizure activity with rTMS (Sackeim, 1994b) and at the same time use rTMS to limit seizure propagation, protecting specific brain systems. Comparing efficacy in patients randomized to different sites of seizure provocation/inhibition could be a powerful tool to further define the anatomy of the neural systems subserving the profound therapeutic effects of ECT.

The Efficacy of Electroconvulsive Therapy and Lateralization in the Regulation of Emotion

A large body of evidence has documented a special role for right hemisphere mechanisms in the expression and reception of emotion (e.g., Borod et al., 1986;

Heilman, Scholes, & Watson, 1975; Sackeim, Gur, & Saucy, 1978). Various versions of the valence hypothesis (Sackeim et al., 1982) suggest that euphoric and dysphoric mood states reflect alteration of distinct lateralized systems (Davidson, 1995; Liotti & Tucker, 1995; Robinson et al., 1988; Sackeim, 1991). Unilateral ECT results in marked asymmetries in measures of brain activity, neurological signs (Kriss et al., 1978), and neuropsychological changes indicative of disruption of lateralized neural systems (Sackeim, 1992). Consequently, the comparison of LUL and RUL ECT in antidepressant and antimanic effects is of considerable interest.

LUL ECT results in considerably more prolonged postictal disorientation than RUL ECT (Daniel & Crovitz, 1982). This fact, and the view that patients prefer the nonverbal memory deficits following RUL ECT relative to the verbal deficits of LUL ECT, led to the virtually exclusive use of RUL ECT for unilateral treatment (Weiner et al., 1990). It was not differential efficacy that led to this practice.

A small group of studies compared LUL and RUL ECT in therapeutic properties (Abrams, Swartz, & Vedak, 1989; Cohen, Penick, & Tarter, 1974; Costello et al., 1970; Cronin et al., 1970; Decina et al., 1985; Deglin, 1973; Fleminger et al., 1970; Halliday et al., 1968; Small et al., 1993; Sutherland, Oliver, & Knight, 1969). Most of these studies used nonoptimal ECT technique and were characterized by other methodological problems. The overriding impression from this work is that both LUL and RUL ECT exert marked antidepressant effects. Although the evidence is inconsistent (Abrams, Swartz, & Vedak, 1989), there are some indications that RUL ECT may be somewhat superior to LUL ECT in the treatment of major depression (Cohen, Penick, & Tarter, 1974; Cronin et al., 1970; Fleminger et al., 1970; Halliday et al., 1968; Small et al., 1993). This would be compatible with the idea that suppression of functional activity within anterior regions of the right hemisphere has antidepressant effects (Sackeim et al., 1982).

Whether there is a difference between LUL and RUL ECT in acute mania is less certain. Initial studies suggested that RUL ECT leads to a worsening of manic symptoms (Small et al., 1985, 1993). In a large retrospective study, however, Black, Winokur, and Nasrallah (1987) found no difference between RUL and BL ECT. In a small random-assignment trial, Mukherjee, Sackeim, and Lee (1988) found that LUL, RUL, and BL ECT were equally effective in medication-resistant manic patients.

As summarized above, recent research indicates that the spatial distribution of current density in the brain strongly determines the efficacy of ECT (Sackeim et al., 1993b). Brain imaging studies examining the topography of changes in rCBF and EEG slow wave activity have linked reductions in functional activity in bilateral prefrontal regions to the efficacy of ECT for both major depression and acute mania (Nobler et al., 1994; Sackeim et al., 1996). Studies contrasting LUL and RUL ECT generally indicate that both exert marked antidepressant effects yet produce qualitative differences in the nature of cognitive side effects. This pattern of findings leads to two alternative hypotheses about the role of lateralized mood systems in the pathophysiology of mood disorders and the mechanisms of therapeutic action of ECT.

The first hypothesis is perhaps the most straightforward. Despite a wealth of evidence concerning lateralization in the regulation of normal mood and in the precipitation of mood disturbance following brain damage (for review, see Sackeim, 1991), the pathophysiology of major mood disorders may not have significant lateralized components. Indeed, it is conceivable that depression may initiate with some degree of asymmetry in patterns of functional brain activity but that, once these states have become autonomous, chronic, and/or severe, the fundamental disturbances are bilateral. It is noteworthy that in large-scale studies of patients receiving ECT, rCBF abnormalities reflected dysregulation of bilateral networks involving prefrontal, superior temporal, and anterior parietal cortical regions (Sackeim et al., 1990, 1993a). More generally, tomographic resting studies of mood disorders have repeatedly demonstrated abnormalities in prefrontal regions, but findings of frontal asymmetry have been more the exception than the rule (Sackeim & Prohovnik, 1993). Effective forms of ECT, unilateral or bilateral, may initiate seizures in prefrontal cortex, and it may be that, despite an asymmetrical initiation with unilateral ECT, tight coupling between left and right prefrontal regions invariably leads to intense bilateral prefrontal expression of seizures and subsequent bilateral reduction in functional activity. This hypothesis accounts for the findings of asymmetry in physiological and neuropsychological measures by noting that such asymmetries largely reflect asymmetrical impact on more posterior areas. For example, it is generally thought that the material-specific amnesia observed following LUL and RUL ECT reflects ipsilateral disruption of medial temporal lobe structures. This hypothesis suggests that lateralization in the regulation of emotion has little to do with the pathophysiology of major mood disorders or their treatment with ECT.

As discussed below, the initial research on nonconvulsive rTMS suggests that this intervention has antidepressant properties that may depend on the brain region stimulated. Indeed, there are suggestions that dysregulated lateralized systems play a key role in the therapeutic effects of rTMS (Pascual-Leone et al., 1996b). If subsequent research confirms these observation, the tenability of the hypothesis just offered will be questionable. This is not to say that there is overlap in the mechanisms of action of rTMS and ECT. Instead, it is quite likely that these interventions differ in how they modulate functional brain activity (Sackeim, 1994b). The lesson from rTMS, however, may be that it is a more focal intervention capable of selectively altering functional activity in prefrontal regions, with less impact on homologous, contralateral cortex. A second hypothesis would stipulate that functional suppression in right prefrontal regions may be necessary and sufficient to produce antidepressant effects with ECT (and perhaps in left prefrontal regions for antimanic effects). Present forms of unilateral ECT, because of patterns of current shunting and intrinsic coupling of prefrontal regions, produce bilateral effects in the critical regions and misleadingly suggest that lateralization of function is unimportant with respect to therapeutics. Testing these two rival hypotheses is of considerable theoretical and practical importance and may become possible with the development of methods to deliver more focal forms of ECT.

FUNCTIONAL NEUROSURGERY

Overview

Functional neurosurgery is directed at altering the physiology of specific neural systems for the treatment of psychopathology (Diering & Bell, 1991). This goal should be distinguished from the surgical resection of abnormal tissue, such as a tumor, which may produce secondary psychiatric symptoms (Lisanby et al., 1998b). Previously referred to as *psychosurgery,* functional neurosurgery is finding new applications for mood, anxiety, and other psychiatric disorders (Yudofsky & Ovsiew, 1990). Although originally used extensively for schizophrenia, functional neurosurgery has generally been found to be more effective for major depression and obsessive compulsive disorder (Ballantine & Giriunas, 1979).

History of Functional Neurosurgery for Psychiatric Disorders

Early studies by Papez (1937) identified limbic circuits (regions of the frontal lobes, cingulate cortex, and subcortical structures) as central to emotion regulation, and it is these limbic structures that are the targets of most neurosurgical approaches to psychiatric disorders.

First performed by Moniz (1936), frontal leukotomy was introduced in the United States by Freeman and Watts (1942) (reviewed by Diering & Bell, 1991; Swayze, 1995). The original procedure involved blind ablation of white matter tracts underlying prefrontal cortex, whereas the Lyerly (1939) bilateral leukotomy involved ablation of white matter under direct visualization. Other techniques involved selective ablation of Brodmann's areas 9, 10, and 46 ("topectomy"; Pool et al., 1949, 1956) and the severing of fibers connecting these areas with the cingulate gyrus (Scoville, 1949). Efficacy was difficult to determine due to methodological limitations, such as the lack of stereotactic guidance (May, 1974).

Technical refinements led to more focal lesions (Fulton, 1951) and stereotactic procedures (Spiegel, Wycis, & Freed, 1950). More targeted procedures included the thalamotomy (Spiegel, Wycis, & Freed, 1950), cingulotomy (Cassidy, Ballantine, & Flanagan, 1965; Livingston, 1953; Whitty et al., 1952), subcaudate tractotomy (Knight, 1965), and limbic leukotomy (combination of cingulotomy and subcaudate tractotomy; Kelly, Richardson, & Mitchell-Heggs, 1973). Several of these early procedures represent precursors of techniques used today (Ballantine & Giriunas, 1979; Ballantine et al., 1987).

Postsurgical Affective Symptoms

Affective symptoms have been described following surgical ablation of limbic structures for the treatment of nonpsychiatric, as well as psychiatric, conditions. Apathy and lack of initiative are well-described aspects of frontal lobe syndromes following frontal leukotomy (Hakola et al., 1993). Depressive symptoms following temporal lobectomy for epilepsy may relate to degeneration of subcortical structures secondary to deafferentation (Parashos, 1993). Davidson et al. (1996) reported distinct alterations in emotional arousal following right and left temporal lobectomy. Transient depression has been reported following thalamotomy (especially left-sided) in the treatment of movement disorders, supporting the role of thalamolimbic connections in mood symptoms (Angelini et al., 1982; Broggi, Angelini, & Giorgi, 1980).

Modern Stereotactic Neurosurgical Procedures for Psychiatric Disorders

Modern stereotactic approaches have reduced morbidity and produce only transient effects on attention, without reported long-term effects on neurological status, higher brain functions, or personality (Corkin, Twitchell, & Sullivan, 1979; Maxwell, 1993). Three of the more common procedures (cingulotomy, subcaudate tractotomy, and anterior capsulotomy) are described below (for review, see Mindus & Jenike, 1992). Other procedures include amygdalotomy, hypothalamotomy, thalamotomy, and various combinations of limbic structures (Ballantine & Giriunas, 1979).

Anterior cingulotomy

Anterior cingulotomy refers to the bilateral severing of the anterior supracallosal fibers of the anterior cingulate, thereby altering connections within the limbic system. This procedure has been reported to have therapeutic effects in mood disorders (Ballantine et al., 1967, 1987), anxiety disorders (Jenike et al., 1991), and pain (Foltz & White, 1962). Efficacy is generally higher in major depression (about 60%) than in obsessive compulsive disorder, and appears after considerable postsurgery delay. Ballantine et al. (1977) reported that 75% of 154 patients with mood disorder were improved after bilateral cingulotomy. A retrospective review by Jenike et al. (1991) found that 25%–30% of obsessive compulsive disorder patients benefitted substantially from cingulotomy. This benefit in obsessive compulsive disorder is thought to be due to interruption of abnormal fronto-striatal-thalamic activity, as suggested by positron emission tomography (PET) studies (Martuza et al., 1990). The claim that destruction of the anterior cingulate is associated with antidepressant effects is compatible with findings from sleep deprivation (Wu et al., 1992), ECT (Scott et al., 1994), and pharmacological treatment (Bench et al., 1995) indicating reduced functional activity in this region concomitant with antidepressant response.

Stereotactic subcaudate tractotomy

Stereotactic subcaudate tractotomy (SST) transects the subcaudate region of the orbital gyrus, thereby interrupting thalamo-anterior cingulate fibers (Bartlett, Bridges, & Kelly, 1981; Bridges, 1994; Broseta et al., 1979; Burrows 1994; Sramka et al., 1992). Knight's procedure (1965, 1969, 1973) involved the implantation of radioactive yttrium (^{90}y) beads. About 70%–80% of depressed patients were improved, with success rates of around 50% in anxiety disorders (Broseta et al., 1979; Corkin, Twitchell, & Sullivan, 1979; Martuza et al., 1990). Bridges et al. (1994) reviewed the results in over 1300 SST procedures and suggested that unipolar depression and a history of good response to ECT were associated with good SST outcome.

Anterior capsulotomy

Anterior capsulotomy transects the anterior limb of the internal capsule, severing thalamo-orbitofrontal fibers (Hay, 1993). This may be accomplished via radiofrequency heat lesions (Bingley et al., 1973) or stereotactic gamma irradiation (Leksell & Backlund, 1979; Rylander, 1979). Improvement in obsessive compulsive disorder has been reported (Bingley et al., 1973) with about a 70% success rate (Martuza et al., 1990). There is some evidence of personality change, lack of initiative, and mood elevation following capsulotomy (Hay, 1993; Martuza et al., 1990; Sachdev 1995), and concern about long-term distal effects in cortex, following large lesions produced with gamma irradiation.

Conclusions

The literature on the use of surgical ablation to treat mood disorders is small, and, because all procedures other than gamma irradiation involve breaching the skull, there has been little opportunity for sham controlled comparisons. The retrospective nature of the clinical reports limits certainty about the claims of therapeutic properties. At the same time, it should be recognized that reports of significant improvement in a substantial percentage of treatment-refractory patients deserves attention.

In general, the literature on functional neurosurgery in mood disorders supports the role of limbic structures in the regulation of emotion. Although the specific anatomical targets for the various neurosurgical approaches have varied, all the procedures affect limbic networks, directly or indirectly. This may result in alterations in the relative activity (e.g., neurophysiological or neurochemical) of various nodes in this network. In addition, transection of frontolimbic and thalamocingulate connections may alter serotonergic and dopaminergic transmission at sites remote from the lesion (Corkin, Twitchell, & Sullivan, 1979). The association between the time course of mood changes and the appearance of thalamic atrophy following frontal leukotomy supports the importance of distal effects.

Neuroimaging studies may help establish links between the modulation of disordered networks and the clinical efficacy of stereotactic functional neurosurgery for mood disorders as has been demonstrated in the case of pallidotomy for Parkinson's disease (Eidelberg et al., 1996, 1997). Such work may provide another means to isolate the relevant circuits dysregulated in major depression and may help to select patients likely to respond to particular surgical interventions. Recently, chronically indwelling electrical stimulators have been used in lieu of neurosurgery to achieve functional alteration of networks for therapeutic benefit in central pain syndromes and movement disorders. This approach has been applied to psychiatric disorders in the past (Escobedo, Fernandez-Guardiolo, & Solís, 1973) and may have future applications.

REPETITIVE TRANSCRANIAL MAGNETIC STIMULATION

Overview

Many of the current tools used to study the neurobiology of emotion are limited in their ability to establish causal links among changes in regional brain function and mood. Repetitive transcranial magnetic stimulation (rTMS) holds promise as a new paradigm to examine the nature of the neural systems regulating emotional processes and to identify their functional interrelations. The ability of rTMS to stimulate brain areas noninvasively is a significant advance beyond techniques that require the invasive method of direct cortical or transcranial electrical stimulation. Evidence suggests that rTMS may have focal excitatory or inhibitory cortical effects, offering the capacity to probe both the anatomical localization and the neurophysiological alterations that result in mood change. Research with this new tool has contributed to our understanding of the neural organization of emotion and has potential in the clinical treatment of mood disorders.

Description of the Technique

Magnetic stimulators capitalize on the ability of time-varying magnetic fields to induce eddy currents in biological tissue via the principle of electromagnetic induction. The magnetic stimulator stores electrical current and then discharges it in brief pulses through a stimulating coil. Each pulse produces a magnetic field around the coil. When the resultant magnetic field is adjacent to a conducting medium, such as nervous tissue, an electrical current is induced that results in neuronal depolarization. This technique has been used to stimulate peripheral nerves (Bickford & Fremming, 1965; Polson, Barker, & Freeston, 1982) and more recently the central nervous system (Barker, 1985, 1987). Early magnetic stimulators delivered single magnetic pulses at limited repetition rates (≤ 0.3 Hz), referred to as *single pulse TMS*. Stimulation frequencies above 1 Hz available with the new generation of stimulators are referred to as *repetitive TMS*.

Magnetic fields pass through scalp and skull without the impedance encountered by direct electrical stimulation, permitting enhanced control over the site and intensity of stimulation. The focality of stimulation with rTMS depends on coil design and orientation relative to neuronal fibers (Amassian et al., 1992; Cohen et al., 1990; Maccabee et al., 1993). The most focal coils have a resolution of about 0.5 cm, as demonstrated in selective stimulation of the cortical representation of neighboring muscle groups in the motor strip (Brasil-Neto et al., 1992). The strength of the magnetic field falls off rapidly with increasing distance from the coil. Depth of stimulation, even at high intensity, is estimated to be 2 cm below the scalp, reflecting stimulation of the underlying cortex near the gray–white junction (Rudiak & Marg, 1994). This does not mean that rTMS does not have remote or transsynaptic effects. For example, George et al. (1996) found an increase in thyrotropin stimulating hormone following dorsolateral prefrontal cortex (DPLFC) rTMS, suggesting subcortical effects. Acquiring ^{15}O-PET during rTMS, Paus et al. (1997) reported that rTMS to the frontal eye field resulted in dose-dependent distal effects in superior parietal and medial parieto-occipital regions, consistent with visual system connectivity.

Mood Effects in Normal Volunteers

There is preliminary evidence for regionally specific mood effects of rTMS in normal subjects. Three studies found that rTMS of the left DLPFC transiently induced dysphoria, whereas right DLPFC rTMS elevated mood in normal volunteers (Dearing et al., 1996; George et al., 1996; Pascual-Leone, Catalá, & Pascual, 1996a). Dearing et al. (1996) found significant effects as early as 20 minutes post-stimulation, whereas George et al. (1996) found the peak mood change at 5–8 hours. The mood changes in normal volunteers have been small in magnitude and not well replicated. For example, in a recent study of 50 normal volunteers receiving rTMS to the left DLPFC, Nedjat et al., (1998) reported three cases of transient hypomania, highlighting the complexity of the topic but also supporting potential mood-modulatory effects of rTMS.

Clinical Effects of Repetitive Transcranial Magnetic Stimulation in Mood Disorders

Recent trials suggest that rTMS has therapeutic properties for major depression. Four studies found that single pulse TMS reduces depressive symptoms (Grisaru et al., 1994; Höflich et al., 1993; Kohbinger et al., 1995; Padberg et al., 1998). Although left DLPFC rTMS is reported to induce transient sadness in normal volunteers, recent studies show notable antidepressant effects when rTMS is delivered to the left DLPFC in depressed patients. Initial open-trial studies (Catalá, Rubio, & Pascual-Leone, 1996; George et al., 1995b) have been replicated in two blinded, sham-controlled studies. Pascual-Leone et al. (1996b) reported that 5 days of left DLPFC rTMS had marked antidepressant effects in 11 of 17 medication-resistant patients with psychotic depression. In another blinded, sham-controlled, crossover trial, George et al. (1997) found that daily left DLPFC rTMS had significant but modest antidepressant effects in outpatients with major depression. The optimal laterality and frequency of stimulation are not presently known. Evidence suggests that slow frequencies of rTMS (1 Hz) applied to the right DLPFC may also be therapeutic (Klein et al., 1999).

The time course and laterality of rTMS-induced mood effects in patients and normal volunteers differ. The mood effects of rTMS in normal volunteers have been observed acutely following a single rTMS session, whereas therapeutic benefit in patients with major depression has been reported following 1–2 weeks of daily stimulation. The acute effects of a single rTMS session in 11 patients with major depression has recently been examined. Left prefrontal rTMS appeared to elevate mood acutely, whereas right-sided stimulation acutely worsened mood in one case (B.D. Greenberg, personal communication, August 1997).

There is preliminary evidence that right but not left prefrontal rTMS may be of benefit in mania (Grisaru et al., 1998), suggesting that the antimanic effects show a laterality opposite to the antidepressant effect. Right DLPFC rTMS has also been reported to improve mood in obsessive compulsive disorder (Greenberg et al., 1997).

The Effects of Repetitive Transcranial Magnetic Stimulation on Mood

The preliminary suggestions that slow TMS and rTMS have antidepressant properties have generated considerable interest in the clinical and research commu-

nities. The finding that rTMS may produce rapid antidepressant effects in severely ill patients may result in the development of new treatment options. The
side-effect profile of nonconvulsive rTMS is more benign than that of ECT. To
date, the only major identified risk of rTMS is the possibility of seizure induction (Wassermann, 1998). Considerable work needs to be done, however, before
rTMS can be claimed to have clinical utility. For example, the evidence from the
initial studies suggests that the antidepressant effects are short-lived (Pascual-
Leone et al., 1996b). It is unknown whether more sustained effects can be
achieved by use of this intervention as a continuation treatment or in combination with antidepressant medications.

Regardless of ultimate clinical utility, the initial findings are striking in suggesting that repetitive stimulation of a specific lateralized cortical area results in
antidepressant effects, whereas stimulation with similar parameters over the same
area in normal subjects transiently induces dysphoria. If confirmed, the interpretation of this seeming paradox will be contingent on understanding of the local and distal physiological effects of rTMS in illness and in health.

rTMS physiological effects demonstrate some degree of frequency depen-
dency, which has yielded new information about dynamic changes in the excitability of motor pathways. For example, manipulations of frequency and intensity produce distinct patterns of facilitation and inhibition of motor responses
with distinct time courses (Jennum, Winkel, & Fuglsang-Fredericksen, 1995;
Pascual-Leone et al., 1994; Wassermann et al., 1996). Ten minutes of 1 Hz rTMS
has been shown to inhibit corticospinal excitability, whereas higher frequencies
(≥ 5 Hz) enhanced excitability for up to 30 minutes (Pascual-Leone & Tormos,
1997). These neurophysiological effects may relate to clinical applications of different rTMS frequencies. Frequency-dependent phenomena are seen in other areas (e.g., long-term potentiation and long-term depression in hippocampal slice
preparations) and result in differing physiological consequences. The possibility
of selectively producing post-stimulation excitation (disinhibition) or inhibition
in focal areas has remarkable potential for the mapping of brain–behavior relations and for developing targeted treatments.

The very preliminary evidence suggesting that both high frequency rTMS to the
left DLPFC and slow TMS to the right DLPFC have antidepressant properties raises
a new hypothesis regarding the role of lateralized neural systems in therapeutics,
at least in the context of rTMS. The hypothesis that high frequencies enhance activity and low frequencies inhibit functional brain activity is far from proven.
Nonetheless, one may speculate that enhanced functional activity in left or suppressed activity in right prefrontal areas may reduce depressive symptoms. Altering the lateralized balance of functional activity in a specific direction may be more
at issue than whether the particular intervention is inhibitory or excitatory.

Finally, the initial rTMS studies call for caution when generalizing from studies of therapeutics to discussions of the neural bases of normal variations in mood.

Stimulation with the same parameters over the same cortical site appears to have differing effects on mood in normal and clinical samples. Key here will be the determination of whether the physiological consequences of rTMS differ in depressed and normal subjects or whether the mood effects are opposite in direction despite similar alterations of neurophysiology. The first possibility would suggest that the neurophysiological disturbances accompanying the depressed state provide a fundamentally different substrate for rTMS effects. The latter may suggest intrinsic differences between depressed patients and healthy individuals in neural systems that regulate mood.

CONCLUSIONS

By their nature, the various somatic treatments for mood disorders differ in their likelihood of addressing anatomical or biochemical aspects of mood regulation. Physical interventions, like ECT, neurosurgery, and rTMS, allow for experimental manipulations that further understanding of the neuroanatomical bases of therapeutic effects. The fact that the most recent antidepressant medications were designed to target one or more chemical systems indicates a degree of neurochemical specificity in this approach to therapeutics.

Across these interventions, it is now clear that there is anatomical and biochemical specificity in how neural systems can be altered to suppress the symptoms of major depression and acute mania. It is also evident from much of this work that therapeutic effects may be achieved by either intervention at different nodes of a complex mood regulatory system or modulation of distinct networks. Furthermore, while links may be sought between the mechanisms of action of these therapeutic interventions and the pathophysiology of the disorders, the necessity of such linkage is not obvious. Effective treatments do not necessarily act on or reverse the underlying pathological abnormalities (e.g., Nobler et al., 1994; Sackeim et al., 1996). While the study of therapeutics is rich in offering hypotheses regarding the basic regulation of emotional processes, it is also evident that caution is needed in generalizing from one arena to the other. The possibility that different neurophysiological alterations are associated with clinical disorders and normal variation in mood and/or that patients with mood disorders have distinct patterns of neural representation of affective processes requires serious consideration.

REFERENCES

Abou-Saleh, M.T., & Coppen, A. (1983). Classification of depression and response to antidepressive therapies. *British Journal of Psychiatry, 143,* 601–603.

Abrams, R. (1986). A hypothesis to explain divergent findings among studies comparing the efficacy of unilateral and bilateral ECT in depression. *Convulsive Therapy, 2,* 253–257.

Abrams, R. (1997). *Electroconvulsive Therapy.* New York: Oxford University Press.

Abrams, R., Swartz, C.M., & Vedak, C. (1989). Antidepressant effects of right versus left unilateral ECT and the lateralization theory of ECT action. *American Journal of Psychiatry, 146,* 1190–1192.

Abrams, R., & Taylor, M.A. (1976). Diencephalic stimulation and the effects of ECT in endogenous depression. *British Journal of Psychiatry, 129,* 482–485.

Ackermann, R.F., Engel, J., Jr., & Baxter, L. (1986). Positron emission tomography and autoradiographic studies of glucose utilization following electroconvulsive seizures in humans and rats. *Annals of the New York Academy of Sciences, 462,* 263–269.

Amassian, V.E., Eberle, L., Maccabee, P.J., & Cracco, R.Q. (1992). Modeling magnetic coil excitation of human cerebral cortex with a peripheral nerve immersed in a brain-shaped volume conductor: The significance of fiber bending in excitation. *Electroencephalography and Clinical Neurophysiology, 85,* 291–301.

Angelini, L., Nardocci, N., Bono, R., & Broggi, G. (1982). Depression after stereotactic thalamotomy in patients with abnormal movements. *Italian Journal of Neurological Sciences, 3,* 301–310.

Babington, R.G., & Wedeking, P.W. (1975). Blockade of tardive seizures in rats by electroconvulsive shock. *Brain Research, 88,* 141–144.

Ballantine, H.T., Bouckoms, A.J., Thomas, E.K., et al. (1987). Treatment of psychiatric illness by stereotactic cingulotomy. *Biological Psychiatry, 22,* 807.

Ballantine, H.T., Cassidy, W.L., Flanagan, N.B., & Marino, R. (1967). Stereotaxic anterior cingulotomy for neuropsychiatric illness and intractable pain. *Journal of Neurosurgery, 26,* 488–495.

Ballantine, H.T., & Giriunas, I.E. (1979). Advances in psychiatric surgery. In T. Rasmussen & R. Marino R. (Eds.), *Functional Neurosurgery.* New York: Raven Press.

Ballantine, H.T., Levy, B.S., Dagi, T., & Giriunas, I.B. (1977). Cingulotomy for psychiatric illness: report of 13 years' experience. In W.H. Sweet, S. Obrador, & J.G. Martin-Rodríguez, (Eds.), *Neurosurgical Treatment in Psychiatry, Pain, and Epilepsy* (pp. 333–354). Baltimore: University Park Press.

Barker, A.T. (1985). Non-invasive magnetic stimulation of the human motor cortex. *Lancet, I* (8437) 1106–1107.

Barker, A.T. (1987). Magnetic stimulation of the human brain and peripheral nervous system: An introduction and the results of an initial clinical evaluation. *Neurosurgery, 20(1),* 100–109.

Bartlett, J., Bridges, P., & Kelly, D. (1981). Contemporary indications for psychosurgery. *British Journal of Psychiatry, 8,* 269.

Bench, C.J., Frackowiak, R.S., & Dolan, R.J. (1995). Changes in regional cerebral blood flow on recovery from depression. *Psychological Medicine, 25,* 247–261.

Bickford, R.G., & Fremming, B.D. (1965). Neuronal stimulation by pulsed magnetic fields in animals and man. *Digest of the 6th International Conference on Medical Electronics and Biological Engineering* (p. 112).

Bingley, T., Leksell, L., Meyerson, B.A., & Rylander, G. (1973). Stereotactic anterior capsulotomy in anxiety and obsessive-compulsive states. In L.V. Laitinen & K.E. Livingston (Eds.), *Surgical Approaches in Psychiatry* (pp. 159–164). Baltimore: University Park Press.

Black, D.W., Winokur, G., & Nasrallah, A. (1987). Treatment of mania: A naturalistic study of electroconvulsive therapy versus lithium in 438 patients. *Journal of Clinical Psychiatry*, *48*, 132–139.

Borod, J. C., Koff, E., Perlman Lorch M., & Nicholas, M. (1986). The expression and perception of facial emotion in brain-damaged patients. *Neuropsychologia*, *24*, 169–180.

Brasil-Neto, J.P., McShane, L.M., Fuhr, P., Hallett, M., & Cohen, L.G. (1992). Topographic mapping of the human motor cortex with magnetic stimulation: Factors affecting accuracy and reproducibility. *Electroencephalography and Clinical Neurophysiology*, *85*, 9–16.

Bremner, J.D., Innis, R.B., Ng, C.K., Staib, L.H., Salomon, R.M., Bronen, R.A., Duncan, J., Southwick, S.M., Krystal, J.H., Rich, D., Zubal, G., Dey, H., Soufer, R., & Charney, D.S. (1997). Positron emission tomography measurement of cerebral metabolic correlates of yohimbine administration in combat-related posttraumatic stress disorder. *Archives of General Psychiatry*, *54*, 246–254.

Bridges, P.K., Bartlett, J.R., Hale, A.S., Poynton, A.M., Malizia, A.L., & Hodgkiss, A.D. (1994). Psychosurgery: Stereotactic subcaudate tractomy. An indispensable treatment. *British Journal of Psychology*, *165*, 599–611.

Broggi, G., Angelini, L., & Giorgi, C. (1980). Neurological and psychological side effects after stereotactic thalamotomy in patients with cerebral palsy. *Neurosurgery*, *7*, 127–134.

Broseta, J., Barcia-Salorio, J.L., Roldan, P., & Barbera, J. (1979). Stereotactic subcaudate tractotomy: Long-term results and measuring of effects on psychiatric symptoms. In E.R. Hitchcock & H.T. Ballantine (Eds.), *Modern Concepts in Psychiatric Surgery* (pp. 241–252). New York: Elsevier/North-Holland Biomedical Press.

Burke, M.J., & Preskorn, S.H. (1995). Short-term treatment of mood disorders with standard antidepressants. In F.E. Bloom & D.J. Kupfer (Eds.), *Psychopharmacology: The Fourth Generation of Progress* (pp. 1053–1066). New York: Raven Press.

Burrows, G.D., Norman, T.R., & Judd, F.K. (1994). Definition and differential diagnosis of treatment-resistant depression. *International Clinical Psychopharmacology*, *9(S2)*, 5–10.

Calabrese, J.R., Bowden, C., & Woyshville, M.J. (1995). Lithium and anticonvulsants in the treatment of bipolar disorder. In F.E. Bloom & D.J. Kupfer (Eds.), *Psychopharmacology: The Fourth Generation of Progress* (pp. 1099–1111). New York: Raven Press.

Caplan, G. (1946). Electrical convulsion therapy in treatment of epilepsy. *Journal of Mental Science*, *92*, 784–793.

Carroll, B.J. (1982) The dexamethasone suppression test for melancholia. *British Journal of Psychiatry*, *140*, 292–304.

Cassidy, F., Murry, E., Weiner, R.D., & Carroll, B.J. (1997). Lack of relapse with tryptophan depletion following successful treatment with ECT. *American Journal of Psychiatry*, *154*, 1151–1152.

Cassidy, W.L., Ballantine, H.T., & Flanagan, N.B. (1965). Frontal cingulotomy for affective disorders. *Biological Psychiatry*, *8*, 269.

Catalá, M.D., Rubio, B., & Pascual-Leone, A. (1996). Lateralized effect of rapid-rate transcranial magnetic stimulation of dorsolateral prefrontal cortex on depression. *Neurology*, *46*, A327.

Chan, C.H., Janicak, P.G., Davis, J.M., Altman, E., Andriukaitis, S., & Hedeker, D. (1987). Response of psychotic and nonpsychotic depressed patients to tricyclic antidepressants. *Journal of Clinical Psychiatry*, *48*, 197–200.

Cohen, B.D., Penick, S.B., & Tarter, R.E. (1974). Antidepressant effects of unilateral electric convulsive shock therapy. *Archives of General Psychiatry, 31,* 673–675.

Cohen, L.G., Roth, B.J., Nilsson, J., Dang, N., Panizza, M., Bandinelli, S., Friauf, W., & Hallett, M. (1990). Effects of coil design on delivery of focal magnetic stimulation. Technical considerations. *Electroencephalography and Clinical Neurophysiology, 75,* 350–357.

Corkin, S., Twitchell, T.E., & Sullivan, E.V. (1979). Safety and efficacy of cingulotomy for pain and psychiatric disorder. In E.R. Hitchcock & H.T. Ballantine, H.T. (Eds.), *Modern Concepts in Psychiatric Surgery* (pp. 253–274). New York: Elsevier/North-Holland Biomedical Press.

Costello, C.G., Belton, G.P., Abra, J.C., & Dunn, B.E. (1970). The amnesic and therapeutic effects of bilateral and unilateral ECT. *British Journal of Psychiatry, 116,* 69–78.

Cronin, D., Bodley, P., Potts. L., Mather, M.D., Gardner, R.K., & Tobin, J.C. (1970). Unilateral and bilateral ECT: A study of memory disturbance and relief from depression. *Journal of Neurology, Neurosurgery, and Psychiatry, 33,* 705–713.

Daniel, W.F., & Crovitz, H.F. (1982). Recovery of orientation after electroconvulsive therapy. *Acta Psychiatrica Scandinavia, 66,* 421–428.

Davidson, R.A., Smith, B.D., Tamny, T.R., & Fedio, P.(1996). Emotional arousal in temporal lobectomy: Autonomic and performance effects of success and failure feedback. *Journal of Clinical and Experimental Neuropsychology, 18,* 249–258.

Davidson, R.J. (1995). Cerebral asymmetry, emotion, and affective style. In R.J. Davidson & K. Hugdahl (Eds.), *Brain Asymmetry* (pp. 361–387). Cambridge, MA: MIT Press.

Dearing, J.E., George, M.S., Greenberg, B.D., Wassermann, E.M., Schlaepfer, T.E., & Post, R.M. (1996). Effects of Prefrontal Repetitive Transcranial Magnetic Stimulation (rTMS) on Mood and Anxiety in Healthy Volunteers: A Replication Study. *APA New Research Program,* Abstract NR182. Washington, DC: American Psychiatric Association.

Decina, P., Kestenbaum, C.J., Farber, S., Kron, L., Gargan, M., Sackeim, H.A., & Fieve, R.R. (1983). Clinical and psychological assessment of children of bipolar probands. *American Journal of Psychiatry, 140,* 548–553.

Decina, P., Sackeim, H.A., Prohovnik, I., Portnoy, S., & Malitz, S. (1985). Case report of lateralized affective states immediately after ECT. *American Journal of Psychiatry, 142,* 129–131.

Deglin, V.L. (1973). A clinico-experimental study of unilateral electroconvulsive seizures. *Zhurnal Nevropatologii I Psikhiatrii, 73,* 1609–1621.

Delgado, P.L., Charney, D.S., Price, L.H., Aghajanian, G.K., Landis, H., & Heninger, G.R. (1990). Serotonin function and the mechanism of antidepressant action. Reversal of antidepressant-induced remission by rapid depletion of plasma tryptophan. *Archives of General Psychiatry, 47,* 411–418.

Delgado, P.L., Miller, H.L., Salomon, R.M., Licinio, J., Heninger, G.R., Gelenberg, A.J., & Charney, D.S. (1993). Monoamines and the mechanism of antidepressant action: Effects of catecholamine depletion on mood of patients treated with antidepressants. *Psychopharmacological Bulletin, 29,* 389–396.

Delgado, P.L., Price, L.H., Miller, H.L., Salomon, R.M., Aghajanian, G.K., Heninger, G.R., & Charney, D.S. (1994). Serotonin and the neurobiology of depression. Effects of tryptophan depletion in drug-free depressed patients. *Archives of General Psychiatry, 51,* 865–874.

d'Elia, G., & Perris, C. (1970). Comparison of electroconvulsive therapy with unilateral and bilateral simulation. *Acta Psychiatrica Scandinavia, 215,* 9–29.

Devanand, D.P., Decina, P., Sackeim, H.A., Hopkins, N., Novacenko, H., & Malitz, S. (1987). Serial dexamethasone suppression tests in initial suppressors and nonsuppressors treated with electroconvulsive therapy. *Biological Psychiatry, 22,* 463–472.

Devanand, D.P., Lisanby S., Lo, E.-S., Fitzsimons, L., Cooper, T.B., Halbreich, U., & Sackeim, H.A. (1998). Effects of electroconvulsive therapy on plasma vasopressin and oxytocin. *Biological Psychiatry, 44,* 610–616.

Devanand, D.P., Sackeim, H.A., Lo, E.S., Cooper, T., Huttinot, G., Prudic, J., & Ross, F. (1991). Serial dexamethasone suppression tests and plasma dexamethasone levels. Effects of clinical response to electroconvulsive therapy in major depression. *Archives of General Psychiatry, 48,* 525–533.

Diering, S.L., & Bell, W.O. (1991). Functional neurosurgery for psychiatric disorders: A historical perspective. *Stereotactic and Functional Neurosurgery, 57,* 175–194.

Eidelberg, D., Moeller, J.R., Ishikawa, T., Dhawan, V., Spetsieris, P., Silbersweig, D., Stern, E., Woods, R.P., Fazzini, E., Dogali, M., & Beric, A. (1996). Regional metabolic correlates of surgical outcome following unilateral pallidotomy for Parkinson's disease. *Annals of Neurology, 39,* 450–459.

Eidelberg, D., Moeller, J.R., Kazumata, K., Antonini, A., Sterio, D., Dhawan, V., Spetsieris, P.H., Alterman, R., Kelly, P.J., Dogali, M., Fazzini, E., & Beric, A. (1997). Metabolic correlates of pallidal neuronal activity in Parkinson's disease. *Brain, 120,* 1315–1324.

Escobedo, R., Fernández-Guardiola, R., & Solís, G. (1973). Chronic stimulation of the cingulum in humans with behaviour disorders. In L.V. Laitinen & K.E. Livingston (Eds.), *Surgical Approaches in Psychiatry* (pp. 65–68). Baltimore: University Park Press.

Fink, M. (1979). *Convulsive Therapy: Theory and Practice.* New York: Raven Press.

Fink, M. (1990). How does ECT work? *Neuropsychopharmacology, 3,* 77–82.

Fink, M., Kahn, R.L., & Green, M.A. (1958). Experimental studies of convulsive and drug therapies in psychiatry: Theoretical implications. *Archives of Neurology and Psychiatry, 80,* 733–734.

Fleminger, J.J., Horne, D.J. de, Nair, N.P., & Nott, P.N. (1970). Differential effect of unilateral and bilateral ECT. *American Journal of Psychiatry, 127,* 430–436.

Foltz, E.L., & White, L.E. (1962). Pain "relief" by frontal cingulotomy. *Journal of Neurosurgery, 19,* 89–100.

Frank, E., Kupfer, D.J., Perel, J.M., Cornes, C., Jarrett, D.B., Mallinger, A.G., Thase, M.E., McEachran, A.B., & Grochocinski, V.J. (1990). Three-year outcomes for maintenance therapies in recurrent depression. *Archives of General Psychiatry, 47,* 1093–1099.

Frank, E., Prien, R.F., Jarrett, R.B., Keller, M.B., Kupfer, D.J., Lavori, P.W., Rush, A.J., & Weissman, M.M. (1991). Conceptualization and rationale for consensus definitions of terms in major depressive disorder. Remission, recovery, relapse, and recurrence. *Archives of General Psychiatry, 48,* 851–855.

Freeman, W., & Watts, J.W. (1942). *Psychosurgery: In the Treatment of Mental Disorders and Intractable Pain.* Springfield, IL: Charles C. Thomas.

Fulton, J.F. (1951). *Frontal Lobotomy and Affective Behavior: A Neurophysiological Analysis.* New York: W.W. Norton & Company.

Geffen, G., Traub, E., & Stierman, I. (1978). Language laterality assessed by unilateral ECT and dichotic monitoring. *Journal of Neurology, Neurosurgery, and Psychiatry, 41,* 354–359.

George, M.S., Ketter, T.A., Parekh, P.I., Horwitz, B., Herscovitch, P., & Post, R.M.

(1995a). Brain activity during transient sadness and happiness in healthy women. *American Journal of Psychiatry, 152,* 341–351.

George, M.S., Wasserman, E.M., Kimbrell, T.A., Little, J.T., Williams, W.E., Danielson, A.L., Greenberg, B.D., Hallett, M., & Post, R. (1997). Daily left prefrontal rTMS improves mood in depression a placebo-controlled crossover trial. *American Journal of Psychiatry, 154,* 1752–1756.

George, M.S., Wassermann, E.M., Williams, W.A., Callahan, A., Ketter, T.A., Basser, P., Hallett, M., & Post, R.M. (1995b). Daily repetitive transcranial magnetic stimulation (rTMS) improves mood in depression. *NeuroReport, 6*(14), 1853–1856.

George, M.S., Wassermann, E.M., Williams, W.A., Steppel, J., Pascual-Leone, A., Basser, P., Hallett, M., & Post, R.M. (1996). Changes in mood and hormone levels after rapid-rate transcranial magnetic stimulation (rTMS) of the prefrontal cortex. *Journal of Neuropsychiatry and Clinical Neurosciences, 8,* 172–180.

Gerner, R.H., & Bunney, W.E., Jr. (1986). Biological hypothesis of affective disorders. In P.A. Berger & H.K.H. Brodie (Eds.), *American Handbook of Psychiatry, Vol. 8* (pp. 265–301). New York: Basic Books.

Gershon, E.S., Hamovit, J., Guroff, J.J., Dibble, E., Leckman, J.F., Sceery, W., Targum, S.D., Nurnberger, J.I. Jr., Goldin, L.R., & Bunney, W.E., Jr. (1982). A family study of schizoaffective, bipolar I, bipolar II, unipolar, and normal control probands. *Archives of General Psychiatry, 39,* 1157–1167.

Gibbons, R.D., Clark, D.C., & Davis, J.M. (1982). A statistical model for the classification of imipramine response in depressed inpatients. *Psychopharmacology, 78,* 185–189.

Glassman, A.H., Kantor, S.J., & Shostak, M. (1975). Depression, delusions, and drug response. *American Journal of Psychiatry, 132,* 716–719.

Glassman, A.H., & Roose, S.P. (1981). Delusional depression: A distinct clinical entity? *Archives of General Psychiatry, 38,* 424–427.

Goodwin, F.K., & Jamison, K.R. (1990). *Manic-Depressive Illness.* New York: Oxford University Press.

Greenberg, B.D., George, M.S., Martin, J.D., Benjamin, J., Schlaepfer, T.E., Altemus, M., Wassermann, E.M., Post, R.M., & Murphy, D.L. (1997). Effect of prefrontal repetitive transcranial magnetic stimulation in obsessive-compulsive disorder: A preliminary study. *American Journal of Psychiatry, 154,* 867–869.

Grisaru, N., Yarovslavsky, U., Abarbanel, J., Lamberg, T., & Belmaker, R.H. (1994). Transcranial magnetic stimulation in depression and schizophrenia. *European Neuropsychopharmacology 4,* 287–288.

Halliday, A.M., Davison, K., Browne, M.W., & Kreeger, L.C. (1968). A comparison of the effects on depression and memory of bilateral E.C.T. and unilateral E.C.T. to the dominant and non-dominant hemispheres. *British Journal of Psychiatry, 114,* 997–1012.

Hare, E.H., Dominian, J., & Sharpe, L.(1962) Phenelzine and dexamphetamine in depressive illness: A comparative trial. *British Medical Journal, 1,* 9–12.

Hay, P., Sachdev, P., Cumming, S., Smith, J.S., Lee, T., Kitchener, P., & Matheson, J. (1993). *Acta Psychiatrica Scandinavica, 87,* 197–207.

Hayes, K.J. (1950). The current path in ECS. *Archives of Neurology and Psychiatry, 63,* 102–109.

Heilman, K.M., Scholes, P., & Watson, R. (1975). Auditory affective agnosia. *Journal of Neurology, Neurosurgery, and Psychiatry, 38,* 69–72.

Heninger, G.R., & Charney, D.S. (1987). Mechanisms of action of antidepressant treatments: Implications for the etiology and treatment of depressive disorders. In H.Y. Meltzer (Eds.), *Psychopharmacology: The Third Generation of Progress* (pp. 535–544). New York: Raven Press.

Heninger, G.R., Delgado, P.L., & Charney, D.S. (1996). The revised monoamine theory of depression: A modulatory role for monoamines, based on new findings from monoamine depletion experiments in humans. *Pharmacopsychiatry, 29,* 2–11.

Höflich, G., Kasper, S., Hufnagel, A., Ruhrmann, S., & Möller, H.J. (1993). Application of transcranial magnetic stimulation in treatment of drug-resistant major depression— A report of two cases. *Human Psychopharmacology, 8,* 361–365.

Hokola, H.P.A., Puranen, M., Repo, L., & Tiihonen, J. (1993). Long-term effects of bilateral frontal lobe lesions from neuropsychiatric and neuroradiological aspects. *Dementia, 4,* 109–112.

Holsboer, F. (1995). Neuroendocrinology of mood disorders. In F.E. Bloom & D.J. Kupfer (Eds.), *Psychopharmacology: The Fourth Generation of Progress* (pp. 957–970). New York: Raven.

Imlah, N.W., Ryan, E., & Harrington, J.A. (1965). The influence of antidepressant drugs on the response to electroconvulsive therapy and on subsequent relapse rates. *Neuropsychopharmacology, 4,* 438–442.

Jenike, M.A., Baer, L., Ballantine, H.T., Martuza, R.L., Synes, S., Giriunas, I., Buttolph, L., & Cassem, N.H. (1991). Cingulotomy for refractory obsessive-compulsive disorder. *Archives of General Psychiatry, 48,* 548–555.

Jennum, P., Winkel, H., & Fuglsang-Fredericksen, A. (1995). Repetitive magnetic stimulation and motor evoked potentials. *Electroencephalography and Clinical Neurophysiology, 97,* 96–101.

Kay, D.W., Fahy, T., & Garside, R.F. (1970). A 7-month double-blind trial of amitriptyline and diazepam in ECT-treated depressed patients. *British Journal of Psychiatry, 117,* 667–671.

Kelly, D., Richardson, A., & Mitchell-Heggs, N. (1973). Stereotactic limbic leucotomy: Neurophysiological aspects and operative technique. *British Journal of Psychiatry, 123,* 133–140.

Kiloh, L.G., Ball, J.R.B., & Garside, R.F. (1962). Prognostic factors in treatment of depressive states with imipramine. *British Medical Journal, 1,* 1225–1229.

Klein, D., Gittelman, R., Quitkin, F., & Rifkin, A. (1980). *Diagnosis and Drug Treatment of Psychiatric Disorders: Adults and Children.* Baltimore: Williams & Wilkins.

Klein, E., Kreinin, I., Mecz, L., Marmur, S., Chistyakov, A., & Feinsod, M. (1999). Therapeutic efficacy of prefrontal repetitive transcranial magnetic stimulation in major depression: A double-blind controlled study. *Archives of General Psychiatry, 56,* 315–320.

Knight, G. (1965). Stereotactic tractotomy in the surgical treatment of mental illness. *Journal of Neurology, Neurosurgery, and Psychiatry, 28,* 304.

Kohbinger, H., Höflich, G., Hufnagel, A., Möller, H., & Kasper, S. (1995). Transcranial magnetic stimulation (TMS) in the treatment of major depression—A pilot study. *Human Psychopharmacology, 10,* 305–310.

Kriss, A., Blumhardt, L.D., Halliday, A.M., & Pratt, R.T. (1978). Neurological asymmetries immediately after unilateral ECT. *Journal of Neurology, Neurosurgery, and Psychiatry, 41,* 1135–1144.

Krystal, A.D., Weiner, R.D., & Coffey, C.E. (1995). The ictal EEG as a marker of adequate stimulus intensity with unilateral ECT. *Journal of Neuropsychiatry and Clinical Neurosciences, 7,* 295–303.

Krystal, A.D., Weiner, R.D., McCall, W.V., Shelp, F.E., Arias, R., & Smith, P. (1993). The effects of ECT stimulus dose and electrode placement on the ictal electroencephalogram: An intraindividual crossover study. *Biological Psychiatry, 34,* 759–767.

Lawson, J.S., Inglis, J., Delva, N.J., Rodenburg, M., Waldron, J. J., & Letemendia, F.J. (1990). Electrode placement in ECT: Cognitive effects. *Psychological Medicine, 20,* 335–344.

Leksell, L., & Backlund, E.-O. (1979). Stereotactic gammacapsulotomy. In E.R. Hitchcock & H.T. Ballantine (Eds.), *Modern Concepts in Psychiatric Surgery.* New York: Elsevier/North-Holland Biomedical Press.

Letemendia, F.J., Delva, N.J., Rodenburg, M., Lawson, J.S., Inglis, J., Waldron, J.J., & Lywood, D.W. (1993). Therapeutic advantage of bifrontal electrode placement in ECT. *Psychological Medicine, 23,* 349–360.

Liebowitz, M.R., Quitkin, F.M., Stewart, J.W., McGrath, P.J., Harrison, W.M., Markowitz, J.S., Rabkin, J.G., Tricamo, E., Goetz, D.M., & Klein, D.F. (1988). Antidepressant specificity in atypical depression. *Archives of General Psychiatry, 45,* 129-137.

Liebowitz, M.R., Quitkin, F.M., Stewart, J.W., McGrath, P.J., Harrison, W.M., Rabkin, J.G., Tricamo, E., Markowitz, J.S., & Klein, D.F. (1984). Phenelzine vs. imipramine in atypical depression: A preliminary report. *Archives of General Psychiatry, 41,* 669–677.

Liotti, M., & Tucker, D.M. (1995). Emotion in asymmetric corticolimbic networks. In R.J. Davidson & K. Hugdahl (Eds.), *Brain Asymmetry* (pp. 389–423). Cambridge, MA: MIT Press.

Lisanby, S.H., Devanand, D.P., Nobler, M.S., Prudic, J., Mullen, L., & Sackeim, H.A. (1996). Exceptionally high seizure threshold: ECT device limitations. *Convulsive Therapy, 12,* 156–164.

Lisanby, S.H., Devanand, D.P., Prudic, J., Pierson, D., Nobler, M.S., Fitzsimons, L., & Sackeim, H.A. (1998a). Prolactin response to ECT: Effects of electrode placement and stimulus dosage. *Biological Psychiatry, 43,* 146–155.

Lisanby, S.H., Kohler, C., Swanson, C.L., & Gur, R.E. (1998b). Psychosis secondary to brain tumor. *Seminars in Clinical Neuropsychiatry, 3,* 12–22.

Livingston, K.E. (1953). Cingulate cortex isolation for the treatment of psychoses and psychoneuroses. *Research Public Association of Nervous and Mental Disorders, 31,* 374–378.

Lloyd, K.G., Morselli, P.L., & Bartholini, G. (1987). GABA and affective disorders. *Medicine and Biology, 65,* 159–165.

Lyerly, J.G. (1939). Transection of the deep association fibers of the prefrontal lobes in certain mental disorders. *South Surgeon, 8,* 426–434.

Maccabee, P.J., Amassian, V.E., Eberle, L.P., & Cracco, R.Q. (1993). Magnetic coil stimulation of straight and bent amphibian and mammalian peripheral nerve in vitro: Locus of excitation. *Journal of Physiology, 460,* 201–219.

Martuza, R.L., Chiocca, E.A., Jenike, M.A., Giriunas, I.E., & Ballantine, H.T. (1990). Stereotactic radiofrequency thermal cingulotomy for obsessive compulsive disorder. *Journal of Neuropsychiatry, 2,* 331–336.

Maxwell, R.E. (1993). Behavioral modification. In M.L.J. Apuzzo (Ed.), *Brain Surgery: Complication Avoidance and Management* (pp. 1557–1565). New York: Churchill Livingstone.

May, P.R.A. (1974). Treatment of schizophrenia, III: a survey of the literature on prefrontal leukotomy. *Comprehensive Psychiatry, 15,* 375–388.

Mindham, R.H.S., Howland, C., & Shepherd, M. (1973). An evaluation of continuation therapy with tricyclic antidepressants in depressive illness. *Psychological Medicine, 3*, 5–17.

Mindus, P., & Jenike, M.A. (1992). Neurosurgical treatment of malignant obsessive compulsive disorder. *Psychiatric Clinics of North America, 15*, 921–938.

Moniz, E. (1936). Les premières tentatives opératoires dans le traitement de certaines psychoses. *Encéphale, 31*, 1–29.

Mukherjee, S., Sackeim, H.A., & Lee, C. (1988). Unilateral ECT in the treatment of manic episodes. *Convulsive Therapy, 4*, 74–80.

Mukherjee, S., Sackeim, H.A., & Schnur, D.B. (1994). Electroconvulsive therapy of acute manic episodes: A review of 50 years' experience. *American Journal of Psychiatry, 151*, 169–176.

Nedjat, S., Folkerts, H.W., Michael, N.D., & Arolt, V. (1998). Evaluation of side effects after rapid-rate transcranial magnetic stimulation over the left prefrontal cortex in normal volunteers. *Electroencephalography and Clinical Neurophysiology, 107*, 96P.

Neumeister, A., Praschak-Rieder, N., Besselmann, B., Rao, M.L., Gluck, J., & Kasper, S. (1997). Effects of tryptophan depletion on drug-free patients with seasonal affective disorder during a stable response to bright light therapy. *Archives of General Psychiatry, 54*, 133–138.

Nobler, M.S., Sackeim, H.A., Prohovnik, I., Moeller, J.R., Mukherjee, S., Schnur, D.B., Prudic, J., & Devanand, D.P. (1994). Regional cerebral blood flow in mood disorders, III. Treatment and clinical response. *Archives of General Psychiatry, 51*, 884–897.

Ottosson, J.O. (1960). Experimental studies of the mode of action of electroconvulsive therapy. *Acta Psychiatrica Scandinavica Supplement, 145*, 1–141.

Padberg, F., Zwanzger, P., Thoma, H., Haag, C., Kathmann, N., Hampel, H., & Möller, H.J. (1998). TMS in major depression: Impact of frequency and intensity on the therapeutic effect in pharmacotherapy-refractory patients. *Electroencephalography and Clinical Neurophysiology, 107*, 96P.

Papez, J.W. (1937). A proposed mechanism of emotion. *Archives of Neurology and Psychiatry, 38*, 725–743.

Parashos, I.A., Oxley, S.L., Boyko, O.B., & Krishnan, K.R.R. (1993). In vivo quantitation of basal ganglia and thalamic degenerative changes in two temporal lobectomy patients with affective disorder. *Journal of Neuropsychiatry and Clinical Neurosciences, 5*, 337–341.

Pardo, J.V., Pardo, P.J., & Raichle, M.E. (1993). Neural correlates of self-induced dysphoria. *American Journal of Psychiatry, 150*, 713–719.

Pascual-Leone, A., Catalá, M.D., & Pascual, A.P. (1996a). Lateralized effect of rapid-rate transcranial magnetic stimulation of the prefrontal cortex on mood. *Neurology, 46*, 499–502.

Pascual-Leone, A., Rubio, B., Pallardó, F., & Catalá, M.D. (1996b). Beneficial effect of rapid-rate transcranial magnetic stimulation of the left dorsolateral prefrontal cortex in drug-resistant depression. *Lancet, 348*, 233–237.

Pascual-Leone, A., & Tormos, J.M. (1997). TMS effects measured electrophysiologically in humans. *Biological Psychiatry, 41*, 75S.

Pascual-Leone, A., Valls-Solé, J., Wassermann, E.M., & Hallett, M. (1994). Responses to rapid-rate transcranial stimulation of the human motor cortex. *Brain, 117*, 847–858.

Paus, T., Jech, R., Thompson, C.J., Comeau, R., Peters, T., & Evans, A.C. (1997). Transcranial magnetic stimulation during positron emission tomography: A new method for studying connectivity of the human cerebral cortex. *Journal of Neuroscience, 17*, 3178–3184.

Perry, P.J., Morgan, D.E., Smith, R.E., & Tsuang, M.T. (1982). Treatment of unipolar depression accompanied by delusions. *Journal of Affective Disorders*, *4*, 195-200.

Polson, M.J.R., Barker, A.T., & Freeston, I.L. (1982). Stimulation of nerve trunks with time-varying magnetic fields. *Medical and Biological Engineering and Computing*, *20*, 243–244.

Pool, J.L., Collins, L.M., Kessler, E., Vernon, L.J., & Feiring, E. (1949). Surgical procedure. In F.A. Mettler (Ed.), *Selective Partial Ablation of the Frontal Cortex: A Correlative Study of Its Effects on Human Psychotic Subjects by the Columbia-Greystone Associates* (pp. 34–47). New York: Paul B. Hoeber.

Pool, J.L., Ransohoff, J., Greenberg, I.M., Correll, J., Gaard, R., & Spear, W. (1956). Surgical procedure. In Lewis, N.D.C., Landis, C., & King, H.E. *Studies in Topectomy* (pp. 9–14). New York: Grune & Stratton.

Post, R.M., Putnam, F., Uhde, T.W., & Weiss, S. R. (1986). Electroconvulsive therapy as an anticonvulsant. Implications for its mechanism of action in affective illness. *Annals of the New York Academy of Sciences*, *462*, 376–388.

Potter, W.Z., & Manji, H.K. (1993). Are monoamine metabolites in cerebrospinal fluid worth measuring? *Archives of General Psychiatry*, *50*, 653–656.

Prange, A.J., Jr., Garbutt, J.C., & Loosen, P.T. (1987). The hypothalamic–pituitary–thyroid axis in affective disorders. In H.Y. Meltzer (Ed.), *Psychopharmacology: The Third Generation of Progress* (pp. 629–636). New York: Raven Press

Pratt, R.T., & Warrington, E.K. (1972). The assessment of cerebral dominance with unilateral ECT. *British Journal of Psychiatry*, *121*, 327–328.

Prien, R.F., & Kupfer, D. (1986). Continuation drug therapy for major depressive episodes: How long should it be maintained? *American Journal of Psychiatry*, *143*, 18–23.

Prien, R., Kupfer, D., Mansky, P., Small, J., Tuason, V., Voss, C., & Johnson, W. (1984). Drug therapy in the prevention of recurrences in unipolar and bipolar affective disorders. *Archives of General Psychiatry*, *41*, 1096–1104.

Prudic, J., Haskett, R.F., Mulsant, B., Malone, K.M., Pettinati, H. M., Stephens, S., Greenberg, R., Rifas, S.L., & Sackeim, H.A. (1996). Resistance to antidepressant medications and short-term clinical response to ECT. *American Journal of Psychiatry*, *153*, 985–992.

Quitkin, F.M. (1992). Relationship of serotonin in atypical depression. Presented at the 3rd I.T.E.M.-Labo Symposium on Strategies in Psychopharmacology. *Laboratory Symposium* (Abstract). Paris, Feb. 26–28.

Quitkin, F.M., Stewart, J.W., McGrath, P.J., Liebowitz, M.R., Harrison, W.M., Tricamo, E., Klein, D.F., Rabkin, J.G., Markowitz, J.S., & Wager, S.G. (1988). Phenelzine versus imipramine in the treatment of probable atypical depression: Defining syndrome boundaries of selective MAOI responders. *American Journal of Psychiatry*, *145*, 306–311.

Reisby, N., Gram, L.F., Bech, P., Nagy, A., Petersen, G.O., Ortmann, J., Ibsen, I., Dencker, S.J., Jacobsen, O., Krautwald, O., Sondergaard, I., & Christiansen, J. (1977). Imipramine: Clinical effects and pharmacokinetic variability. *Psychopharmacology*, *54*, 263-272.

Robin, A., & de Tissera, S. (1982). A double-blind controlled comparison of the therapeutic effects of low and high energy electroconvulsive therapies. *British Journal of Psychiatry*, *141*, 357–366.

Robinson, R.G., Boston, J.D., Starkstein, S.E., & Price, T.R. (1988). Comparison of mania and depression after brain injury: Causal factors. *American Journal of Psychiatry*, *145*, 172–178.

Roose, S.P., Glassman, A.H., Attia, E., & Woodring, S. (1994). Comparative efficacy of selective serotonin reuptake inhibitors and tricyclics in the treatment of melancholia. *American Journal of Psychiatry, 151,* 1735–1739.

Roose, S.P., Glassman, A.H., Walsh, B.T., Woodring, S., & Vital-Herne, J. (1983). Depression, delusions, and suicide. *American Journal of Psychiatry, 140,* 11591162.

Rudiak, D., & Marg, E. (1994). Finding the depth of magnetic brain stimulation: A reevaluation. *Electroencephalography and Clinical Neurophysiology, 93,* 358–371.

Rush, A.J., & Weissenburger, J.E. (1994). Melancholic symptom features and DSM-IV. *American Journal of Psychiatry, 151,* 489–498.

Rylander, G. (1979). Stereotactic radiosurgery in anxiety and obsessive-compulsive states: Psychiatric aspects. In E.R. Hitchcock & H.T. Ballantine (Eds.), *Modern Concepts in Psychiatric Surgery* (pp. 235–240). New York: Elsevier/North-Holland Biomedical Press.

Sachdev, P., & Hay, P. (1995). Does neurosurgery for obsessive-compulsive disorder produce personality change? *Journal of Nervous and Mental Disease, 183,* 408–413.

Sackeim, H.A. (1986). A neuropsychodynamic perspective on the self: Brain, thought, emotion. In L.M. Hartman & K.R. Blankstein (Eds.), *Perception of Self in Emotional Disorder and Psychotherapy* (pp. 51–83). New York: Plenum.

Sackeim, H. A. (1989). The efficacy of electroconvulsive therapy in treatment of major depressive disorder. In S. Fisher & R.P. Greenberg (Eds.), *The Limits of Biological Treatments for Psychological Distress: Comparisons with Psychotherapy and Placebo* (pp. 275–307). Hillsdale, NJ: Erlbaum.

Sackeim, H.A. (1991). Emotion, disorders of mood, and hemispheric specialization. In B.J. Carroll & J.E. Barrett (Eds.), *Psychopathology and the Brain* (pp. 209–242). New York: Raven Press.

Sackeim, H.A. (1992). The cognitive effects of electroconvulsive therapy. In W.H. Moos, E.R. Gamzu, & L.J. Thal (Eds.), *Cognitive Disorders: Pathophysiology and Treatment* (pp. 183–228). New York: Marcel Dekker.

Sackeim, H.A. (1994a). Central issues regarding the mechanisms of action of electroconvulsive therapy: Directions for future research. *Psychopharmacological Bulletin, 30,* 281–308.

Sackeim, H.A. (1994b). Magnetic stimulation therapy and ECT. *Convulsive Therapy, 10,* 255–258.

Sackeim, H.A., Decina, P., Epstein, D., Bruder, G.E., & Malitz, S. (1983a). Possible reversed affective lateralization in a case of bipolar disorder. *American Journal of Psychiatry, 140,* 1191–1193.

Sackeim, H.A., Decina, P., Kanzler, M., Kerr, B., & Malitz, S. (1987a). Effects of electrode placement on the efficacy of titrated, low-dose ECT. *American Journal of Psychiatry, 144,* 1449–1455.

Sackeim, H.A., Decina, P., Portnoy, S., Neeley, P., & Malitz, S. (1987b). Studies of dosage, seizure threshold, and seizure duration in ECT. *Biological Psychiatry, 22,* 249–268.

Sackeim, H.A., Decina, P., Prohovnik, I., & Malitz, S. (1987c). Seizure threshold in electroconvulsive therapy. Effects of sex, age, electrode placement, and number of treatments. *Archives of General Psychiatry, 44,* 355–360.

Sackeim, H.A., Decina, P., Prohovnik, I., Malitz, S., & Resor, S.R. (1983b). Anticonvulsant and antidepressant properties of electroconvulsive therapy: A proposed mechanism of action. *Biological Psychiatry, 18,* 1301–1310.

Sackeim, H.A., Devanand, D.P., & Nobler, M.S. (1995). Electroconvulsive therapy. In F. Bloom & D. Kupfer (Eds.), *Psychopharmacology: The Fourth Generation of Progress* (pp. 1123–1142). New York: Raven.

Sackeim, H.A., Devanand, D.P., & Prudic, J. (1991). Stimulus intensity, seizure threshold, and seizure duration: Impact on the efficacy and safety of electroconvulsive therapy. *Psychiatric Clinics of North America, 14*, 803–843.

Sackeim, H.A., Freeman, J., McElhiney, M., Coleman, E., Prudic, J., & Devanand, D.P. (1992a). Effects of major depression on estimates of intelligence. *Journal of Clinical and Experimental Neuropsychology, 14*, 268–288.

Sackeim, H.A., Greenberg, M.S., Weiman, A.L., Gur, R.C., Hungerbuhler, J.P., & Geschwind, N. (1982). Hemispheric asymmetry in the expression of positive and negative emotions: Neurologic evidence. *Archives of Neurology, 39*, 210–218.

Sackeim, H.A., Gur, R.C., & Saucy, M.C. (1978). Emotions are expressed more intensely on the left side of the face. *Science, 202*, 434–436.

Sackeim, H.A., Long, J., Luber, B., Moeller, J.R., Prohovnik, I., Devanand, D.P., & Nobler, M.S. (1994). Physical properties and quantification of the ECT stimulus: I. Basic principles. *Convulsive Therapy, 10*, 93–123.

Sackeim, H.A., Luber, B., Katzman, G.P., Moeller, J.R., Prudic, J., Devanand, D.P., & Nobler, M.S. (1996). The effects of electroconvulsive therapy on quantitative electroencephalograms. Relationship to clinical outcome. *Archives of General Psychiatry, 53*, 814–824.

Sackeim, H.A., & Mukherjee, S. (1986). Neurophysiological variability in the effects of the ECT stimulus. *Convulsive Therapy, 2*, 267–276.

Sackeim, H.A., Nobler, M.S., Prudic, J., Devanand, D.P., McElhinney, M., Coleman, E., Settembrino, J., & Maddatu, V. (1992b). Acute effects of electroconvulsive therapy on hemispatial neglect. *Neuropsychiatry, Neuropsychology, and Behavioral Neurology, 5*, 151–160.

Sackeim, H.A., & Prohovnik, I. (1993). Studies of brain imaging in mood disorders. In J.J. Mann & D. Kupfer (Eds.), *The Biology of Depressive Disorders: Part A: A Systems Perspective* (pp. 205–258). New York: Plenum.

Sackeim, H.A., Prohovnik, I., Moeller, J.R., Brown, R.P., Apter, S., Prudic, J., Devanand, D.P., & Mukherjee, S. (1990). Regional cerebral blood flow in mood disorders: I. Comparison of major depressives and normal controls. *Archives of General Psychiatry, 47*, 60–70.

Sackeim, H.A., Prohovnik, I., Moeller, J.R., Mayeux, R., Stern, Y., & Devanand, D.P. (1993a). Regional cerebral blood flow in mood disorders: II. Comparison of major depression and Alzheimer's disease. *Journal of Nuclear Medicine, 34*, 1090–1101.

Sackeim, H.A., Prudic, J., Devanand, D.P., Kiersky, J.E., Fitzsimons, L., Moody, B.J., McElhiney, M.C., Coleman, E.A., & Settembrino, J.M. (1993b). Effects of stimulus intensity and electrode placement on the efficacy and cognitive effects of electroconvulsive therapy. *New England Journal of Medicine, 328*, 839–846.

Schneider, F., Gur, R.C., Jaggi, J.L., & Gur, R.E. (1994) Differential effects of mood on cortical cerebral blood flow: A [133]xenon clearance study. *Psychiatry Research, 52*, 215–236.

Schnur, D.B., Mukherjee, S., Silver, J., Degreef, G., & Lee, C. (1989). Electroconvulsive therapy in the treatment of episodic aggressive dyscontrol in psychotic patients. *Convulsive Therapy, 5*, 353–361.

Scott, A.I., Dougall, N., Ross, M., O'Carroll, R.E., Riddle, W., Ebmeier, K.P., & Goodwin, G.M. (1994). Short-term effects of electroconvulsive treatment on the uptake of 99mTc-exametazime into brain in major depression shown with single photon emission tomography. *Journal of Affective Disorders, 30*, 27–34.

Scott, A.I., Rodger, C.R., Stocks, R.H., & Shering, A.P. (1992). Is old-fashioned electroconvulsive therapy more efficacious? A randomised comparative study of bilateral brief-pulse and bilateral sine-wave treatments. *British Journal of Psychiatry, 160,* 360–364.

Scoville, W.B. (1949). Selective cortical undercutting as a means of modifying and studying frontal lobe function in man: Preliminary report of forty-three operative cases. *Journal of Neurosurgery, 61,* 65–73.

Seager, C.P., & Bird, R.L. (1962). Imipramine with electrical treatment in depression: A controlled trial. *Journal of Mental Science, 108,* 704–707.

Sikdar, S., Kulhara, P., Avasthi, A., & Singh, H. (1994). Combined chlorpromazine and electroconvulsive therapy in mania. *British Journal of Psychiatry, 164,* 806–810.

Silfverskiöld, P., & Risberg, J. (1989). Regional cerebral blood flow in depression and mania. *Archives of General Psychiatry, 46,* 253–259.

Small, I.F. (1974). Inhalant convulsive therapy. In M. Fink, S. Kety, J. McGaugh, & T.A. Williams (Eds.), *Psychobiology of Convulsive Therapy* (pp. 65–77). Washington, DC: Winston & Sons.

Small, J.G., Milstein, V., Kellams, J.J., Miller, M.J., Woodham, G. C., & Small, I.F. (1993). Hemispheric components of ECT response in mood disorders and schizophrenia. In C.E. Coffey (Ed.), *The Clinical Science of Electroconvulsive Therapy* (pp. 111–123). Washington, DC: American Psychiatric Press.

Small, J.G., Small, I.F., Milstein, V., Kellams, J.J., & Klapper, M.H. (1985). Manic symptoms: An indication for bilateral ECT. *Biological Psychiatry, 20,* 125–134.

Sobin, C., Prudic, J., Devanand, D.P., Nobler, M.S., & Sackeim, H.A. (1996). Who responds to electroconvulsive therapy? A comparison of effective and ineffective forms of treatment. *British Journal of Psychiatry, 169,* 322–328.

Sobin, C., & Sackeim, H. A. (1997). The psychomotor symptoms of depression. *American Journal of Psychiatry, 154,* 4–17.

Spiegel, E.A., Wycis, H.T., & Freed, H. (1950). Thalamotomy in mental disorders. *Archives of Neurology and Psychiatry, 64,* 595–598.

Spiker, D.G., Weiss, J.C., Dealy, R.S., Griffin, S.J., Hanin, I., Neil, J.F., Perel, J.M., Rossi, A.J., & Soloff, P.H. (1985). The pharmacological treatment of delusional depression. *American Journal of Psychiatry, 142,* 430–436.

Sramka, M., Pogady, P., Csokova, Z., & Pogady, J. Long-term results in patients with stereotaxic surgery for psychopathologic disorders. *Bratislavske Lekarske Listy, 93,* 364–366.

Sutherland, E.M., Oliver, J.E., & Knight, D.R. (1969). E.E.G., memory, and confusion in dominant, non-dominant, and bi-temporal E.C.T. *British Journal of Psychiatry, 115,* 1059–1064.

Swayze, V.W. (1995). Frontal leukotomy and related psychosurgical procedures in the era before antipsychotics (1935–1954): A historical overview. *American Journal of Psychiatry, 152,* 505–515.

Thase, M.E., & Rush, A.J. (1995). Treatment-resistant depression. In F.E. Bloom & D.J. Kupfer (Eds.), *Psychopharmacology: The Fourth Generation of Progress* (pp. 1081–1098). New York: Raven Press.

Tortella, F.C., & Long, J.B. (1985). Endogenous anticonvulsant substance in rat cerebrospinal fluid after a generalized seizure. *Science, 228,* 1106–1108.

Tortella, F.C., & Long, J.B. (1988). Characterization of opioid peptide-like anticonvulsant activity in rat cerebrospinal fluid. *Brain Research, 456,* 139–146.

Ulett, G., Smith, K., & Gleser, G. (1956). Evaluation of convulsive and subconvulsive shock therapies utilizing a control group. *American Journal of Psychiatry*, *112*, 795–802.

Wassermann, E.M. (1998). Report on risk and safety of repetitive transcranial magnetic stimulation (rTMS): Suggested guidelines from the International Workshop on Risk and Safety of rTMS June 1996. *Electroencephalography and Clinical Neurophysiology*, *108*, 1–16.

Wassermann, E.M., Grafman, J., Berry, C., Hollnagel, C., Wild, K., Clark, K., & Hallett, M. (1996). Use and safety of a new repetitive transcranial magnetic stimulator. *Electroencephalography and Clinical Neurophysiology*, *101*, 412–417.

Weaver, L., Williams, R., & Rush, S. (1976). Current density in bilateral and unilateral ECT. *Biological Psychiatry*, *11*, 303–312.

Weiner, R.D., & Coffey, C.E. (1986). Minimizing therapeutic differences between bilateral and unilateral nondominant ECT. *Convulsive Therapy*, *2*, 261–265.

Weiner, R.D., Fink, M., Hammersley, D., Moench, L., Sackeim, H. A., & Small, I. (1990). *The Practice of ECT: Recommendations for Treatment, Training and Privileging*. Washington, DC: American Psychiatric Press.

Weiner, R.D., Rogers, H.J., Davidson, J.R., & Kahn, E.M. (1986a). Effects of electroconvulsive therapy upon brain electrical activity. *Annals of the New York Academy of Sciences*, *462*, 270–281.

Weiner, R.D., Rogers, H.J., Davidson, J.R., & Squire, L.R. (1986b). Effects of stimulus parameters on cognitive side effects. *Annals of the New York Academy of Sciences*, *462*, 315–325.

Whitty, C.W.M., Duffield, J.E., Tow, P.M., & Carins, H. (1952). Anterior cingulectomy in the treatment of mental disease. *Lancet*, *1*, 475–481.

Woldbye, D.P., Greisen, M.H., Bolwig, T.G., Larsen, P.J., & Mikkelsen, J.D. (1996). Prolonged induction of c-fos in neuropeptide Y– and somatostatin-immunoreactive neurons of the rat dentate gyrus after electroconvulsive stimulation. *Brain Research*, *720*, 111–119.

Wu, J.C., Gillin, J.C., Buchsbaum, M.S., Hershey, T., Johnson, J.C., & Bunney, W.E., Jr. (1992). Effect of sleep deprivation on brain metabolism of depressed patients. *American Journal of Psychiatry*, *149*, 538–543.

Yudofsky, S., & Ovsiew, F. (1990). Neurosurgical and related interventions for the treatment of patients with psychiatric disorders. *Journal of Neuropsychiatry*, *2*, 253–255.

Zis, A.P., Yatham, L.N., Lam, R.W., Clark, C.M., Srisurapanont, M., & McGarvey, K. (1996). Effect of stimulus intensity on prolactin and cortisol release induced by unilateral electroconvulsive therapy. *Neuropsychopharmacology*, *15*, 263–270.

Index

AB (Aprosodia Battery), 84*t,* 88–89
Abulia
  apathy and, 341
  behavioral therapy for, 355
Acoustical analysis, computerized, 89, 95
Activation, 397
Activities of daily living (ADL), in post-
    stroke depression, 248, 249*f*
Affect
  definition of, 47
  disorders of. *See* Affective disorders
  expression of, 426
  flattening of, 436
  positive, 269–270
  positive *vs.* negative, 145
  states/traits, 139, 140*t*–141*t*
Affective Auditory Verbal Learning Test, 97
Affective deficits
  rehabilitation for, 426–427
Affective disorders. *See also specific affective*
    disorders
  basal ganglia dysfunction and, 385
  in neurological conditions, 426
Age, changes with, 19, 91
Aggression
  amygdala and, 219
  controlled-instrumental, 13, 320
  cortisol and, 327
  epilepsy and, 377

heart rate and, 329, 331
impulsive-emotional, 320, 325
  biological *vs.* psychological/
    environmental factors, 334
  hormones, 332*t*
  neurobiological effects, 333
  neurochemistry, 332*t*
  neuropsychology, 331–333, 332*t*
  norepinephrine and, 326
  psychophysiology, 332*t*
  stressful life events and, 333–334
neurobiological influences, 321
neuropsychology, 321, 325
  brain imaging studies, 323–324
  brain lesion studies, 323
  tests, 322–323
psychophysiology
  electroencephalogram, 330, 331
  heart rate and, 329, 331
reactive, definition of, 322
risk factors, 321–322
testosterone and, 326–327
types
  affective/defensive *vs.* predatory,
    320–321
  neurobiological variables, 321
  reactive *vs.* proactive, 320–321
  validity of, 321
Agitations, 40, 41

Agnosia, 47, 197
Akinetic mutism, 344, 347, 352
Alcoholic violence, cortisol and, 327
Alexia, left hemisphere cortical dysfunction
    and, 369
Alzheimer's disease
  apathy in
    decreased right temporal perfusion in, 345
    methylphenidate for, 353–354
  emotional deficits, 420
  end-stage, amantadine for, 353
Amantadine, for apathy, 352–353, 354
Amnesia, 68
Amphetamines, for apathy, 352
Amygdala
  ablation, 376, 393
  activation, 184
  anatomy, 197
  atrophy, in Huntington's disease, 382
  consolidation effect and, 173
  cortices, 197
  emotion-cognition connection and,
    219–220
  lesions, 170, 197–198
    apathy and, 344
    emotional communication and, 374–375
    facial expression recognition and,
      204–205
  neural connections, 44, 63, 197
  norepinephrine in, 170
  role, 197–198
    in aggression, 219, 377
    in conditioning, 203–204
    in depression, 393
    in development, 204
    in emotional experience, 198
    in encoding, 170, 183
    in facial expression processing, 375
    in facial expression recognition,
      198–200, 199f–201f, 202–203
    in fear conditioning, 376
    in learning, 170, 204
    in social judgment, 197–198
  in secondary mania, 242
  stimulation
    electrical, 218–219
    rage and, 376
  visceral feedback hypothesis and, 388–390
Amytal injection. See Wada test
Anagenesis, 48
Anencephaly, 56
Anger
  behavioral therapy for, 424–425
  cognitive therapy for, 424

expression of, 424
frustration and, 180
stress reduction and, 424
Anger behavior cycle, 425
Angular gyrus, deficits, in violent behavior,
    324
Anterior asymmetry, 12
Anterior capsulotomy, 473
Anterior cingulotomy, 472–473
Antidepressants. See also specific
    antidepressants
  for bipolar disorder, 457
  for depression, 457
    after traumatic brain injury, 261–262
    in schizophrenia, 443–444
  mechanisms of action, 461–462
  for mood disorders, 460–461
  repetitive transcranial magnetic stimulation
    as, 124–125
  tricyclic. See Tricyclic antidepressants
Antimanic agents, for mood disorders,
    460–461
Antisocial behavior, temporal lobe deficits
    and, 324
Anxiety
  anxious apprehension, 12
  anxious arousal, 12
  classification, 298
  cognitive biases, 310–312
  cognitive impairments, 312–313
  cognitive studies, 310–313
  lesion studies, 308–310
  neuropsychological studies, 302–308,
    305t–307t
    behavioral paradigms for, 306–308
    electrophysiological paradigms for,
      303–306, 305f, 306f
    hemodynamic paradigms for, 303–306
  in Parkinson's disease, 380
  prevalence, 298
  state vs. trait, 300–301
  stress and, 301–302
  treatment
    behavioral, 423
    cognitive, 423
    relaxation, 423
    systematic desensitization, 423–424
  types of, 299–301, 300t, 313
  vs. panic, 62
Apathy
  abulia and, 341
  in Alzheimer's disease, 345, 353–354
  causes of, 342, 343t
    dementia, 345

localized brain dysfunction, 342–345
  psychiatric disorders, 345–346
characteristics of, 340, 425
definitions of, 13, 340–342, 356
diagnosis of, 425–426
executive
  forms of, 348
  pharmacotherapy for, 352
extreme. *See* Akinetic mutism
social, 350
states, conceptualizations of, 346–351
  comparison of, 350–351
  in disturbed arousal, 347
  in frontal system dysfunction, 347–350
treatment, 351, 356
  behavioral, 355–356
  pharmacotherapy, 351–355
  rehabilitative, 355–356, 425–426
Aphasia
  depression in, 249–250
  left hemisphere cortical dysfunction and,
    368–369, 369
Appraisals
  components of, 165–166
  conscious/controlled, 168
  current
    bias content of emotional memories and,
      179
    missing information and, 179–181
  in depression, 169
  dispositional attributions in, 169
  fast/automatic, 166, 171
    encoding and, 167–168
    separate processing pathway for, 170
  frontal lobe and, 170–171
  functions, 164
  of self-relevance, 165–166
  slow, 166
  of stimulus, viewing time and, 167
Appraisal theory, 153–154
Apprehension, anxious, 299–301, 300*t*
Approach–avoidance, modular theory of
  emotional expression and, 7–8, 396–398
Aprosodia Battery (AB), 84*t*, 88–89
Aquinas, Thomas, 33
Aristotle, 33, 52, 142
Arousal
  anxious, characteristics of, 300–301, 300*t*
  assessment tools for, 89
  control, hemispheric asymmetrical, 8, 396
  disturbed, apathy in, 347
  modular theory of emotional expression
    and, 394–396
  peripheral autonomic, assessment of, 396

Assessment, emotional, 96–97. *See also*
  Arousal; Emotional experience;
  Expression; Perception
  literature review, 81–82, 83*t*–85*t*, 86–93
  neuroimaging
    baseline for, 126–127
    statistical analysis for, 127
    study design for, 127
  test batteries and related studies, 83*t*–85*t*
Association, reminiscence effect and,
    173
Attention
  automatic capture, by emotion, 166–167
  biases, in anxiety, 311
  mediation of, 394
  in schizophrenia, 441*f*
Atypical neuroleptics, for apathy, 352
Augmentative and Alternative
  Communication systems, 426
Automatic evaluation effect, 166–167
Autonomic arousal, 3, 4, 8, 89
Avoidance behaviors, frontal lobe and,
    398
Awareness, 46, 50

Background and general techniques, 4–7
BAS (Behavioral Approach System), 269
Basal ganglia
  in depression, 393
  diseases, 377, 399. *See also* Huntington's
    disease; Parkinson's disease
    emotional communication in, 384
    emotional experience in, 385
    emotional perception in, 92
    progressive supranuclear palsy, 383
    striatonigral degeneration, 384
    Wilson's disease, 383–384
  emotional expression and, 223
  lesions
    affective disorders and, 385
    apathy from, 343–344, 350
Basic emotion models, 147–148
Basotemporal cortex
  lesions, mania and, 242
  in secondary mania, 242
Battery of Emotional Expression and
    Comprehension (BEEC), 89–90
Beck Depression Inventory, 81, 380
BEEC (Battery of Emotional Expression and
    Comprehension), 89–90
Behavior, emotional, 398
Behavioral Approach System (BAS), 269
Behavioral Inhibition System (BIS), 269
Behavioral studies, of anxiety, 306–308

Behavioral therapy
   for anger, 424–425
   for anxiety, 423
   for apathy, 355–356
   for depression, 422–423
   for post-traumatic stress disorder, 423
   stategies, 422–423
Between-group analysis, 107
Biases, cognitive, in anxiety, 310–312
Biology *vs.* culture debate, 143
Bipolar disorder
   after stroke
      diagnosis of, 245–246
      lesion location in, 245, 246*t*
   cerebral glucose metabolism in, 283–286,
      285*f*, 286*f*
   mania, 10
   pharmacotherapy, 383
BIS (Behavioral Inhibition System), 269
Blood flow, regional cerebral. *See* Regional
      cerebral blood flow
Blood oxygen level-dependent functional
      magnetic resonance imaging (BOLD),
      119–120
Bodily processes, 47
BOLD (blood oxygen level-dependent
      functional magnetic resonance
      imaging), 119–120
Brain. *See also specific brain structures*
   in anxiety *vs.* depression, 305–306
   basal lateral circuits, 376
   blood flow. *See* Regional cerebral blood
      flow
   dysfunction, *vs.* structural abnormality,
      109–110
   hemispheres. *See also* Left hemisphere;
      Right hemisphere
      anterior/posterior dimensions in, 272
      asymmetry of. *See* Hemispheric
         asymmetry
      laterality of. *See* Laterality
   imaging studies. *See also specific imaging
      methods*
      in aggression, 323–324
      of ECT efficacy, 469–470
   injury
      evaluation of emotional experience in,
         91
      traumatic. *See* Traumatic brain injury
   lesions, aggression and, 323
   localized dysfunction, apathy and, 342–345
   metabolism, positron emission tomography
      of, 118
   processing levels, 42–43, 56

regional function studies, inconsistencies
      in, 298–299
   structure
      abnormal, *vs.* dysfunction, 109–110
      computed tomography, 112
      subcortical. *See* Subcortical structures
Brain lesion method, 3, 5
Brain stem
   circuitry, 57–58
   integrative mechanisms, in emotional
      processing, 61–62
   pontine, 56
   pontine level, 56
   subsystems, in emotional processing,
      60–61
Brief Psychiatric Rating Scale, 96
Broca's aphasia, 226
Bromocriptine
   for akinetic mutism, 352
   for apathy, 353
Buck slides, 94

Capgras syndrome, 350
Capsulotomy, anterior, 473
Caregiver participation, in rehabilitation,
      416
Cartesian impasse, 33, 40, 41, 52
Catastrophic reaction, 239–240
Category error, 40
Caudality
   anterior *vs.* posterior brain structures, 4
Center-Periphery debate, 143–144
Central details, 167, 168
Cerebellar diaschisis, 112
Cerebral blood flow. *See* Regional cerebral
      blood flow
Cerebral cortex dysfunction, 399
Cerebral glucose metabolism. *See* Glucose
      metabolism, cerebral
Cerebral inactivation, 271–273
Cerebral metabolism, methodological issues,
      278–279
Cerebrospinal fluid (CSF)
   norepinephrine, in antisocial behavior,
      325–326
   serotonin, in antisocial behavior, 325–326
   volumes, in depression with schizophrenia,
      445–446, 446*f*
Cerebrovascular disease, 11
Channels of emotional communication
   facial, 4, 81, 95, 426
   general, 4, 90, 95, 426, 427
   gestural, 4, 81, 95
   lexical/verbal, 4, 81, 95, 426

postural, 4, 81
prosodic/intonational, 4, 81, 95, 426
quantification of features, 95
scenic, 6, 81
Chimeric Faces Task (CFT), 307–308
Chorea, Huntington's, 382–383
Cingulate gyrus, 215–216, 349
Cingulotomy, anterior, 472–473
Circuit models, 146–147
Citalopram, for post-stroke depression,
    253–254
Clinical implications, 3–4, 14–17
Clonidine, for secondary mania, 244
Clozaril, for schizophrenia negative
    symptoms, 444
Cognition
    affective, 47–48, 49f, 50
    in anxiety, 310–313
    brain processing
        levels of, 42–43
        speed of, 43–44
    corticolimbic mechanisms of, 66–68
    definition of, 46
    domains. See Emotion
    impairments, in anxiety, 312–313
    motivation and, 45
    philosophical conceptualizations, 33–42
    rational, 47–48, 49f, 50
    syncretic vs. analytic, 47–48
    vs. emotion, 42, 97–98
Cognition-emotion debate, 142
Cognition system, vs. emotional system,
    220–221, 222t
Cognitive functions, emotional stimuli and,
    97–98
Cognitive knowledge, 42
Cognitive psychology, memory and,
    165
Cognitive rehabilitation, 414–416
    functional skills training, 414
    process approach, 414–416
Cognitive systems, emotional systems and,
    218–220
Cognitive therapy
    for anger, 424
    for anxiety, 423
    for depression, 422
    for post-traumatic stress disorder, 423
    principles, 422
Cognizance, 50
Communication, emotional
    in basal ganglia diseases, 384
    channels of. See Channels of emotional
        communication

deficits
    in left hemisphere cortical dysfunction,
        368–369
    in right hemisphere cortical dysfunction,
        370–372
    disorders, mechanisms of, 385–387
    in Huntington's disease, 382
    limbic system dysfunction and, 374–375
    in Parkinson's disease, 378–380
Compensation training, 415
Componential approach to emotional
    processing, 4, 6, 10, 16, 81, 82, 90,
        427
Componential models
    profile of, 151t
    synthesis with other models, 150–152
    types of, 149–150
Comprehension
    disorders, in right hemisphere cortical
        dysfunction, 370–371
    left hemisphere cortical dysfunction and,
        368–369
Computed tomography (CT), 112
Computerized Speech Laboratory, 95
Conditioning, amygdala role in, 203–204
Consciousness, 51–52
Convulsive therapy. See Electroconvulsive
    therapy
Corpus callosum deficits, in violent behavior,
    324
Cortical/subcortical, 4
Cortical systems
    anatomy/physiology of, 65–69
    dysfunction, and emotional deficits
        left hemisphere, 368–370
        right hemisphere, 370–374
    in post-stroke mood disorders, 252
Corticobulbar dysfunction, 374
Corticolimbic evolution, archicortical/
    paleocortical routes of, 65–66
Cortisol, violence and, 327
Crying, pathological, 240
CSF. See Cerebrospinal fluid
CT (computed tomography), 112
Cues
    affective, bias from, 174–175
    for retrieval process, 174
Cultural issues, 21

Dacrystic epilepsy, emotional changes in, 377
Darwin, Charles, 143, 147
Darwinists, 34
Dementia. See also Alzheimer's disease
    apathy in, 345

Depression
  akinetic, 437
  apathy in, 345–346
  appraisals in, 169
  after brain injury. *See* Traumatic brain
      injury, depression after
  with comprehension deficits, diagnosis of,
      248–249
  delusional *vs.* nondelusional, 457
  in elderly, 276
  emotional expression and perception, 93
  after functional neurosurgery, 472
  internal expression assessment in, 96
  left frontal activity and, 270
  melancholic *vs.* severe, 457–458
  negative ruminative self-evaluation and,
      172
  neurobiology
      electroencephalogram studies, 273–277
      evoked potential studies, 277–278
      glucose metabolism in, 283–286, 285*f,*
          286*f*
      physiologic brain changes, 393
      regional abnormalities, 286–288
      regional cerebral blood flow, 281–283
  in Parkinson's disease. *See* Parkinson's
      disease, depression in
  pharmacogenic, 436–437
  postpsychotic, 435
  sadness and, 180
  scales for evaluating, 96
  in schizophrenia. *See* Schizophrenia,
      depression in
  self-concept and, 175–176
  after stroke. *See* Stroke, depression after
  after traumatic brain injury. *See* Traumatic
      brain injury, depression after
  treatment, 422
      behavioral interventions for, 422–423
      cognitive therapy for, 422
      electroconvulsive, 462
      repetitive transcranial magnetic
          stimulation for, 476–478
      vegetative symptoms, 435
Descartes, Rene, 33, 142–143
Development, amygdala role in, 204
Developmental-evolutionary perspective, 5
Dewey, John, 36, 37
Dextroamphetamine, for post-TBI depression,
      262
*Diagnostic and Statistical Manual of Mental
      Disorders* (DSM-III-R), 245
*Diagnostic and Statistical Manual of Mental
      Disorders* (DSM-IV), 298

Diaschisis, 242
Dichotic listening, 5
Diencephalic theories, of emotional
      expression, 390–391
Diencephalon, 57. *See also* Hypothalamus;
      Thalamus
Differential Emotions Scale, 96
Dimensional emotion models
  modular theory and, 391
  multidimensional, 145–146
  profile of, 151*t*
  synthesis with other models, 150–152
  unidimensional, 145
  vs. discrete model, 4, 7
Discourse production, 17, 371
Discrete emotion models
  description of, 146–148
  profile of, 151*t*
  synthesis with other models, 150–152
  vs. dimensional model, 4
Dopamine reduction, in Parkinson-associated
      depression, 381
Dopaminergic drugs, for apathy, 352,
      353–354
Dorsal circuit, 67
Dorsolateral prefrontal circuit, in apathy,
      348–349
Dorsomedial thalamic nucleus, damage,
      apathy and, 344
Drives
  definition of, 48
  limbic mechanisms, 71–73
Drugs. *See also specific drugs or classes of
      drugs*
  memory-impairing, 170
Dualism, 33–34
Dysphoria, in Parkinson's disease, 381

Ecological realism, 46
Ecological validity, 97
Ecphoric process, 174–175
ECT. *See* Electroconvulsive therapy
EEG. *See* Electroencephalography
Elation, 11, 240–242
Elderly depression, EEG patterns in, 276
Electroconvulsive therapy (ECT)
  anticonvulsant effects, 466–468
  bilateral seizure generation in, 465–466
  efficacy
      in deep subcortical structures, 466
      generalized *vs.* localized effects,
          463–464
      lateralization in emotional regulation
          and, 468–471

of low dosage right unilateral method,
464–468
in prefrontal cortex, 468
technical factors and, 464–465
historical aspects, 456, 462–463
indications, 462
left unilateral, 463, 469
for mood disorder, 458
for post-TBI depression, 262
right unilateral
low dosage, inefficacy of, 465–468
nonverbal memory deficits after, 469
vs. left unilateral, 463
Electroencephalography (EEG)
aggression/violence, 330, 331
in anxiety, 304–305, 305*f*, 306*f*
of depression, 274–277
of induced sadness, 274
methodological issues, 273–274
quantitative, 112, 113*t*, 114
Elicitation of emotional expression
procedures for, 94
research on, 153–154
Eliminative materialists, 111
Emotion
automatic capture of attention by, 166–167
brain processing system. *See* Emotional
processing systems
cerebral hemispheric specialization
theories, evidence for, 3–4
communication. *See* Communication,
emotional
continuum, terminology for, 145
control, descending projections for,
68–69
current, evaluations of past episodes and,
175–182
definition of, 3, 18, 80, 138–139
delimitation of, 139, 140*t*–141*t*, 142
descriptions of, 367
differentiation
endogenous viewpoint, 153–154
exogenous viewpoint, 153
dimensions and emotion type, 7
dimensions *vs.* discrete emotions, 10
domains, 139, 398. *See also* Emotional
experience
episodic nature of, 137–138
expression of. *See* Expression
function of, 20
global neural processing mode changes
and, 195
guidance of encoding, 165–172
historical aspects of, 31

influence
on memory, 164, 165, 184–185
on subjective experience of
remembering, 181–182
information
postevent elaboration/consolidation of,
172–174
retrieval, neural mechanisms in,
182–184
knowledge of, 42, 196–197. *See also*
Appraisals
environmental factors and, 208–209
neural structures in, 208
somatosensory cortices and, 205–206,
207*f*, 208
memory and, hierarchic anatomy of, 70–71
motivation and, 45
negative, right hemisphere and, 217
neuroimaging. *See* Neuroimaging of emotion
neuropsychological theories. *See*
Neuropsychological theories
perception, tests of, 97
philosophical conceptualizations, 33–42
positive, 7, 20, 21
psychological functions and, 155–156
psychological models. *See also*
Dimensional emotion models;
Discrete emotion models
current, description of, 144–150
historical aspects of, 142–144
recognition, in schizophrenia, 441–442, 442*f*
recollective experience and, 182
regulation, by pharmacologic agents,
460–461
rehabilitation, 4–14
retrieval process and, 174–184
social, 20, 21
somatic changes from, 195
subcortical bases, 60–64, 69–70, 215–216
subjective experience of. *See* Affect
subject matter of, 195
survival value of, 195
systems-level theory, 195
theoretical models, 21
treatment of, 418–427
valence, 7
vs. cognition, 10, 42, 97–98, 142
vs. feelings, 139, 143
withdrawal-related, frontal asymmetry and,
8, 270–271
Emotional disorders, 11–14. *See also specific
emotional disorders*
with brain damage, historical aspects of,
239–240

Emotional disorders (*continued*)
　with common neurological disorders,
　　419–421
　treatment of, 418–421
Emotional experience. *See also* Affect
　appraisals. *See* Appraisals
　assessment tools for
　　New York Emotion Battery, 90–91
　　related studies, 89, 91
　brain disorders and, 367–368
　constructive processes in, 164
　defects, 399
　duration of, 180, 367
　evaluation of subjective experience, 91,
　　95–96
　extended, memory for, 180
　left hemisphere cortical dysfunction and,
　　370
　limbic system dysfunction and, 375–377
　mechanisms, 387
　　central theories, 390–398
　　feedback theories, 387–390
　mediation, limbic circuits and, 368
　negative
　　recall of, 176
　　rehearsal of, 172
　positive, recall of, 176
　in psychological disorders. *See under*
　　specific psychological disorders
　recreating, importance of, 163–164
　in right hemisphere cortical dysfunction, 372
　self-defining, control over, 178
　significance, reevaluation of, 178–179
　theories, 399–400
Emotional incontinence, 240
Emotional labililty, 240
Emotional memory system
　deficits, neuropsychological mechanisms
　　of, 373
　implicit, 44
　in right hemisphere cortical dysfunction,
　　372–373
Emotional processing systems
　cognitive systems and, 218–220
　common language, need for, 21
　componential nature of, 221–224, 222*t*.
　　See also Componential approach to
　　emotional processing
　hierarchical organization of, 224–227, 427
　lateralization of, 206
　levels of, 42–43
　modalities, 4
　modes. *See also* Arousal; Emotional
　　experience; Expression; Perception

multiple, via multiple channels, 84*t*–85*t*,
　89–93
multiple, via single channel, 84*t*, 88–89
single, via multiple channels, 82,
　83*t*–84*t*, 86–88
somatosensory cortices and, 205–206,
　207*f*, 208
speed of, 43–44
neural mechanisms/substrates, 3, 18
neurological assessment. *See* Assessment,
　emotional
neuropsychological studies
　background, 4–7
　brain organization and, 4
　general techniques, 4–7
parameters of, 4
processing modes, 4, 427
vs. cognition system, 220–221, 222*t*
Emotional situations/scenes, assessment of,
　84*t*, 89
Emotional states, 138
Emotional Stroop Task, 97
Emotive knowledge, 32
Empiricism, 33–34
Encephalitis, limbic, 376
Encephalization, 57, 59
Encoding
　amygdala and, 183
　amygdala function in, 170
　duration of emotional events, 180
　frontal lobe and, 170–171
　guidance, by emotion, 165–172
　of memories, 164–165
　neural mechanisms of, 169–171
　schema-guided, 168–169
　vividness of memory and, 181–182
English neorealism, 37–38
Environmental factors, knowledge of emotion
　and, 208–209
Epilepsy
　aggression and, 377
　aggression in, 219
　mood disturbances in, 271
　violence and, 323
Epinephrine, 389
Epistemics, 32
Epistemology, 32
Event-related potentials (ERPs)
　in aggression/violence, 330, 331
　in anxiety, 304
Evoked potentials
　depression studies, 277–278
　methodological issues, 277
Experimental affect battery, 93

Experimental studies, 3
Expression
    assessment tools for, 88–93
        Aprosodia Battery, 88–89
        Battery of Emotional Expression and
            Comprehension, 89–90
        experimental affect battery, 93
        New York Emotion Battery, 90–91
        related studies, 88, 91–93
    deficits, in right cortical dysfunction,
        371–372
    elicitation. See Elicitation of emotional
        expression
    evaluation procedures, 94–96
    external, observations of, 94–95
    facial. See Facial expression
    left hemisphere cortical dysfunction and,
        369
    literature on, 83t–84t, 88
    rating procedures for, 90–91
    in schizophrenia, 434–436
    subcortical structures and, 91–92, 215–216
The Expression of Emotion in Man and
    Animals (Darwin), 143, 147

FAB (Florida Affect Battery), 87
Facial Action Coding System (FACS), 92, 95
Facial asymmetry, 5
Facial expression
    deficits
        frontal lobe damage and, 224
        in Parkinson's disease, 378–379
        in right hemisphere cortical dysfunction,
            371
        in schizophrenia, 434–436
        in stroke, 223
    discrimination defects, right hemisphere
        damage and, 386
    of fear, amygdala and, 375
    knowledge of emotion and, 196
    processing
        in Huntington's disease, 382
        somatosensory cortices and, 205–206,
            207f, 208
    recognition
        amygdala and, 198–200, 199f–201f,
            202–203
        amygdala damage and, 204–205
        in schizophrenia, 441–442, 442f
    unilateral facial manipulation, 94
Facial feedback hypothesis, 387–388
"Faculty" doctrines, 142
Fear
    conditioning, amygdala and, 63, 203–204

facial expression, impaired recognition of,
    198, 201f
Feedback theories, of emotional expression,
    387–390
Feelings. See also Affect;
    Emotional experience
    knowledge-by-acquaintance, 46
    subjective, 95–96, 155
    vs. emotions, 40, 139, 143
Flattening of affect, 436
Florida Affect Battery (FAB), 87
Fluency tests, 98
Fluvoxamine, for schizophrenia negative
    symptoms, 444–445
fMRI. See Functional magnetic resonance
    imaging
Formalization, of language, 44–45
Friedes Neuropsychological Personality
    Survey, 96
Frontal leukotomy, 471
Frontal lobe
    affective appraisals and, 170–171
    asymmetry, withdrawal-related emotions
        and, 270
    attentional-arousal systems and, 395
    avoidance behaviors and, 398
    bilateral cortical dysfunction, 373–374
    dementia, apathy in, 345
    dorsolateral, 397
    glucose metabolism, violent behavior and,
        324
    intentional control of emotion and, 223–224
    left, inactivation, depression and, 272
    lesions
        aggression and, 323–324
        apathy and, 342–343, 347–350, 355
        episodic memory retrieval and, 183
        facial emotional expressions and, 224
        manual grasp response and, 398
        memory deficits in, 73–74
Frontal lobe syndrome, 323, 325
Frontotemporal lobar dysfunction, apathy in,
    345
Frustration, anger and, 180
Functional communication, 97
Functional imaging
    of blood flow and energy metabolism, 110
    brain structural abnormality, vs.
        dysfunction, 109–110
    information from multiple conceptual
        levels, 109
    interpretation of, 110–111
    paradigms, 106–109
    problems, common, 125–127

Functional imaging (*continued*)
  techniques, 22, 112, 127. *See specific
    functional imaging techniques*
  with transcranial magnetic stimulation,
    125, 126*f*
Functionalists, 111
Functional magnetic resonance imaging
    (fMRI)
  blood oxygen level-dependent, 119–120
  inversion recovery, 119
    serial perfusion technique, 120–121,
      121*f*
  serial perfusion, 120–121, 121*f*
  spin labeling, 119, 120
  vs. other imaging methods, 112, 113*t*
Functional neurosurgery
  definition of, 471
  historical aspects, 471–472
  in mood disorders, 473–474
  postsurgical affective symptoms, 472
  stereotactic procedures for, 472–473
Functional skills training, 414

GAD (generalized anxiety disorder), 301, 303
Gelastic seizures, 20
Gender differences, 19–20, 117–118, 117*f*
Generalization of treatment, 418
Generalized anxiety disorder (GAD), 301,
    303
Geriatric Depression Screening Scale, 96
Gestures, in right hemisphere cortical
    dysfunction, 371
"Ghost in the machine," 48, 49*f*, 50
Gibson, James J., 46
Glucogen, violence and, 328
Glucose metabolism, cerebral
  in depression
    bipolar *vs.* unipolar, 283–286, 285*f*, 286*f*
    with schizophrenia, 445, 446–447, 447*f*
  electroconvulsive therapy and, 467
  in Huntington's disease, 383
Grieving process, for depression after brain
    injury, 423
Guilt, shame and, 180

Haloperidol, for schizophrenia negative
    symptoms, 444
Halstead-Reitan Neuropsychological Test
    Battery, 322
Hamilton Depression Rating Scale scores
  in post-stroke depression, 253–254, 254*f*
  in schizophrenia, 436
Heart rate, violence and, 329, 331
Hemiparkinson's disease, 92–93, 380–381

Hemispheres
  interhemispheric, 4
  intrahemispheric, 4
Hemispheric asymmetry
  in anxiety, 304–305, 305*f*, 306*f*
  arousal control and, 5, 396
  in depression, EEG studies of, 275–277
  in emotional expression, 226–227
    cortical structures and, 227–229
    subcortical structures and, 227–229
  in emotional representation, 7, 216–218,
    219
  prosodic, 370
  in regional cerebral blood flow, in induced
    mood states, 279–281
  right-hemispheric specialization for
    emotion, theoretical basis for, 7
  valence, pharmacotherapy and, 393–394
Hemispheric valence hypothesis, 7, 393
Herpes simplex infection, emotional changes
    in, 376
5-HIAA. *See* Serotonin
Hierarchic integration, Jacksonian, 57, 58
Hippocampus
  anticipatory functions, 63, 64
  in emotional expression, 215–216
  memory and, 182, 183
HMPAO, 114
Hormones, violence and, 326–328
Huntington's disease
  emotional communication in, 382
  emotional experience in, 382–383
Hypoglycemia, violence and, 327–328
Hypothalamus
  in autonomic components of emotion,
    223
  in emotion, 220
  in emotional expression, 215–216
  emotional expression and, 390–391
  functions, 62, 197
  ventromedial, 62

IAPS (International Affective Picture
    System), 94
Inclinations, 40
Indifference, treatment of, 425–426
Indifference reaction, 240. *See also* Apathy
Individual differences, 19–20
Inflammatory disease, emotional changes in,
    376
Instincts, 48
Insulin, violence and, 327–328
Interceptors, 46–47
Interhemispheric factor, 4. *See* Laterality

Interictal phenomenon, emotional changes in, 376–377
International Affective Picture System (IAPS), 94
Interrater reliability, 95
Intrahemispheric factor, 4

Jacksonian hierarchic integration, 57, 58
James, William, 34, 35–36, 37, 143–144
James-Lange theory, 139

Klüver-Bucy syndrome, 344
Knowledge
    of emotion, 196–197
    hierarchy, 50
    levels of, 50–52
Knowledge-by-acquaintance, 46, 48, 50
Knowledge-by-description, 46, 48, 50

Labeling, of emotional states, 148
Language
    formalization of, 44–45, 52
    left hemisphere cortical dysfunction and, 368–369
    ordinary, analysis of, 39–42
    role of, 50–51
"Language games," 39–40
Laterality. See also Hemispheric asymmetry
    definition of, 4
    electroconvulsive therapy efficacy and, 468–471
    experimental behavioral techniques, 5
    in parkinsonian motor symptoms, 92–93, 380–381
Lateralization, in emotional regulation, 4, 468–471
Laughing, pathological, 240
Learning, amygdala role in, 170, 204
LeDoux resolution, of Zajonc-Lazarus debate, 43–44
Left hemisphere
    cortical dysfunction, 368–370
    deficits
        in aggression, 323
        in violent behavior, 324
    emotion production and, 217, 269
    lesions
        anxiety and, 308–310
        catastrophic-depressive reaction, 392
        emotional communication and, 386
        emotional disorders in, 240
        emotional expression and, 183
        emotional reactivity in, 226–227
        with stroke-related depression, 248
        unilateral neglect syndrome and, 228–229

Levodopa, for depression in Parkinson's disease, 381
Lexical models, 148
Lexical/verbal emotion, 4. See also Channels of emotional communication
Limbic system
    back projections, 72–73
    drive mechanisms, 71–73
    dysfunction, 399
        emotional communication and, 374–375
        emotional experience and, 375–377
    emotional functions of, 216
    forward projections, 72–73
    mechanisms of, 70
    structures. See also Amygdala; Hippocampus
        anticipatory, 63–64
        integrative influences on emotion and cognition, 61–62
        surgical ablation of, affective symptoms after, 471
"Logical atoms," 38
Luria-Nebraska Neuropsychological Battery, 322

Magnetic resonance imaging (MRI)
    of amygdala damage, 198, 199f
    BOLD technique, 108
    conventional, 112
    functional. See Functional magnetic resonance imaging
    within-individual analysis, 108
Magnetic resonance spectroscopy (MRS), 121–122
Mania
    bipolar disorder, and, 11
    electroconvulsive therapy for, 462
    in schizophrenia, 439–441
    after stroke. See Stroke, mania after
    after traumatic brain injury. See Traumatic brain injury, mania after
Maximally Discriminative Facial Movement Coding System, 95
Meaning, pragmatic theory of, 35
Meaning oriented models
    description of, 148–149, 151t
    synthesis with other models, 150–152
Melodic Intonation Therapy, 415
Memory
    of action vs. appearance, 168
    of central details, 168
    circuits, 67
    construction process, emotion and, 175–176

Memory (*continued*)
    corticolimbic mechanisms of, 66–68
    declarative or explicit, 44
    deficits, in frontal lobe lesions, 73–74
    distortions/biases, 165
    emotional, current appraisals and, 179
    emotional influences on, 164, 165,
        184–185
    field perspective, 181
    improved, viewing time and, 167
    norepinephrine and, 170
    observer perspective, 181
    of peripheral details, 168
    reference/procedural or associative, 64
    rehearsal and, 172–173
    reminiscence effect and, 173
    retrograde deficits, in right hemisphere
        cortical dysfunction, 372–373
    of schema-relevant information, 168
    usefulness of, 163–164
    vividness, 181–182
    working/declarative or configural, 64
Mesencephalic reticular formation (MRF),
    395–396
Mesencephalon, 57
Methylphenidate
    for apathy, 353–354
    for post-TBI depression, 262
Mind-body debate, 142–143
Minnesota Multiphasic Inventory (MMPI),
    81, 392
MMPI-2, 95
Modal emotions, 149–150
Modular theory of emotional expression,
    391–398
    approach–avoidance and, 396–398
    approach and withdrawal, 7–8
    arousal and, 8, 394–396
    motor activation and, 396–398
    motor direction, 7–8
    valence and, 7, 391–394
Monism, 33–34
Monoamine oxidase inhibitors
    for bipolar disorder, 457
    for depression, 457
    for Parkinson-associated depression, 381
Mood
    as emotional component, 40
    laterality in parkinsonian motor symptoms
        and, 380–381
    left hemisphere cortical dysfunction and,
        370
    regulation, retrieval and, 177–179

    repetitive transcranial magnetic stimulation
        effects on normal volunteers, 475–476
    in right hemisphere cortical dysfunction, 372
    vs. emotion, 47
Mood and Anxiety Symptom Questionnaire,
    305, 307*f*
Mood disorders
    bipolar. *See* Bipolar disorder
    with brain injury, 262–263
    mania. *See* Mania
    neurobiology of, 459–460
    pathophysiology of, 458, 461–462
    phases of, 458–460
    post-stroke, cortical *vs.* subcortical lesions
        in, 252
    psychiatric populations, 17
    psychopharmacology
        mechanisms of action, 461–462
        neurobiological studies of, 459
    repetitive transcranial magnetic stimulation
        for, 476–478
    treatment interventions, 478
    unipolar. *See* Depression
Mood induction procedures, 94, 98
Motivation
    definition of, 45–46
    emotion, cognition and, 45
    intrinsic, 74–75
    ventral medial frontal and orbital frontal
        cortices, 171
Motivational-emotional system, 45–46
Motive persistence, 73–74
Motor activation, modular theory of
        emotional expression and, 15,
        396–398
Motor direction, 7
MRF (mesencephalic reticular formation),
    395–396
MRI. *See* Magnetic resonance imaging
MRS (magnetic resonance spectroscopy),
    121–122
Multidisciplinary approach to rehabilitation,
    15, 416
Multiple sclerosis, emotional deficits,
    420–421
Murderers, brain imaging studies, 324
Mutism
    akinetic, 344, 347, 352
    model of, 351

Naturalistic observation approach, 88
Negative affect, 269–270
Neglect of the left half of space, 240

Neocortical, 4
Neural mechanisms
    in emotional information retrieval, 182–184
    in emotional processing, 3, 81
Neurobehavioral Rating Scale, 96
Neuroanatomy, evolutionary, 57–59
Neurobiological studies. *See under specific disorders*
Neurobiological systems-level theory of emotion, 9–10
Neurochemistry, of violence, 325–326
Neuroimaging of emotion, 106
    baseline for, 126–127
    functional. *See* Functional imaging
    statistical analysis for, 127
    study design for, 127
    techniques, common problems of, 125–127
Neuroleptics
    for apathy, 354
    atypical, for depression treatment, in schizophrenia, 444
Neurological epistemology, 32
Neuromotor programs, 147
Neuropharmacology, of Parkinson's disease, 381–382
Neuropsychological tests
    for aggression, 322–323
    compendium of, 80, 81–93
    for emotional processing, 81–93
Neuropsychological theories of emotion, 7–11
    current, 218–229, 222t. *See also* Cognitive systems; Emotional processing systems
    componential nature of emotional processing system, 221–224, 222t. *See also* Componential approach to emotional processing
    distinction between emotional and cognition systems, 220–221, 222t
    hierarchical organization of emotional system, 224–227
    left/right and cortical/subcortical dichotomies in emotion and, 4, 227–229
    relationship of emotional and cognition systems, 97–98, 218–220
    historical development, 214–218
Neuropsychologist, role on rehabilitation team, 417t
Neuroscientists
    compendium of, 80, 81–93
    eliminative materialists, 111
    for emotional processing, 81–93
    functionalists, 111
    reductive materialists, 111

Neurosurgery, functional. *See* Functional neurosurgery
Neurotransmitters, in apathy, 352
New York Emotion Battery (NYEB), 90–91
Noetic approach, for cognitive rehabilitation, 415–416
Norepinephrine
    cerebrospinal fluid levels, in antisocial behavior, 325–326
    memory and, 170
    in Parkinson's disease, 381
Normative data, 81–93
Nortriptyline, for post-stroke depression, 253, 254f
Nucleus basalis, 70
NYEB (New York Emotion Battery), 90–91

Observation
    of external expression, 94–95
    of internal states and dispositions, 95–96
Obsessive-compulsive disorder (OCD)
    anxious apprehension in, 301
    with depression, rCBF in, 303
Occupational therapist, role on rehabilitation team, 417t
Olanzapine, for schizophrenia negative symptoms, 444
Orbitofrontal cortex
    lesions
        mania and, 242
        motivational deficits and, 171
    in secondary mania, 242–243
Orbitofrontal lobotomy, 349

PAG (periaqueductal gray), 61
Pain
    cues, retrieval bias from, 175
    past, memories of, 177–178
PANAS model, 145
Panic
    regional cerebral blood flow in, 303–304
    survival value of, 298
    vs. anxiety, 62
Parameters of emotional processing, 4
Parkinson's disease (PD)
    depression in, 254–255, 262, 380
        diagnosis of, 380
        mechanism of, 257–258
        prevalence of, 255, 255f
        relationship to cognitive impairment, 256–257, 256f
        treatment of, 258
    emotional communication in, 378–380

Parkinson's disease (PD) (*continued*)
  emotional deficits, 420
  emotional experience in, 380–382
  emotional expression and perception in,
      92–93, 223
  neuropharmacology, 381–382
  unilateral hemispheric pathology in, 92–93
Pathological emotionalism, 240
Pathological laughing or crying, 240
PD. *See* Parkinson's disease
Peirce, C.S., 35
Pemoline, for post-TBI depression, 262
Perception
  assessment tools for, 87–88
    Aprosodia Battery, 88–89
    Battery of Emotional Expression and
        Comprehension, 89–90
    experimental affect battery, 93
    New York Emotion Battery, 90–91
    Perception of Emotions Test, 86
    Profile of Nonverbal Sensitivity, 82, 86
    related studies, 87, 88, 91–93
    Victoria Emotion Perception Test, 86
  disorders, in right hemisphere cortical
      dysfunction, 370–371
  emotional, 4, 81
  motivated, physiology of, 72–73
  right hemisphere and, 269
  subcortical lesion effects on, 91–92
Perception of Emotions Test (POET), 86
Periaqueductal gray (PAG), 61
Peripheral autonomic arousal, assessment, 396
Peripheral details, 167, 168
Perisylvian lesions, catastrophic-depressive
      reaction in, 392
Personality Assessment Inventory, 95
PET. *See* Positron emission tomography
Pharmacotherapy. *See also specific*
        pharmacotherapeutic agents
  for mood disorders. *See under specific*
        mood disorders
  for regulation of emotion, 460–461
Physiatrist, role on rehabilitation team, 417*t*
Physical abuse, impulsive-emotional
      aggression and, 333–334
Physical therapist, role on rehabilitation team,
      417*t*
Plato, 33, 142
POET (Perception of Emotions Test), 86
PONS (Profile of Nonverbal Sensitivity), 82,
      86
Portland Adaptability Inventory, 96
Positive emotions, 20, 21
Positivism, 37–39, 41–42

Positron emission tomography (PET)
  blood flow studies, 116–118, 117*f*
  brain metabolism studies, 118
  coincidence detection, 116
  vs. other imaging methods, 112, 113*t*
  vs. SPECT, 116
Post-Stroke Depression Rating Scale, 96
Post-traumatic stress disorder
  behavioral therapy for, 423
  cognitive therapy for, 423
  relaxation training for, 423
  systematic desensitization for, 423–424
Pragmatics, 17, 96, 417, 426
Pragmatism, 34–37
Pragnosia, 96
Prefrontal cortex
  in depression, 393
  functional activity, electroconvulsive
      therapy and, 468
Primary affects, 47, 48
Primes, 46, 48
Process approach, for cognitive rehabilitation,
      414–416
Processing modes, 4, 81–82
Profile of Nonverbal Sensitivity (PONS), 82,
      86
Progressive supranuclear palsy (PSP), 383
Prosody
  assessment tools for
    Aprosodia Battery, 88–89
    Battery of Emotional Expression and
        Comprehension, 89–90
    experimental affect battery, 93
    Florida Affect Battery, 87
    New York Emotion Battery, 90–91
    Perception of Emotions Test, 86
    Profile of Nonverbal Sensitivity, 82. 83
    related studies, 87, 91–93
    Victoria Emotion Perception Test, 86
  emotional
    left hemisphere damage and, 386
    right hemisphere damage and, 386–387
    in Parkinson's disease, 92–93, 379–380
    positron emission tomography of, 118
Pseudobulbar affect, 240
PSP (progressive supranuclear palsy), 383
Psychiatric disorders, apathy in, 345–346
Psychiatrist, role on rehabilitation team, 417*t*
Psychic akinesia, 343–344
Psychological functions, emotional effects on,
      155–156
Psychological models of emotion, 144, 156
  componental, 149–150
  dimensional, 145–146

discrete, 146–148
meaning oriented, 148–149
research foci, current, 153–156
synthesis of, 150–152
Psychometrics, 21–22, 82, 97
Psychomotor seizures, emotional changes in, 376–377
Psychopharmacological treatment, of emotional disorders, 421
Psychopharmacological treatments, in mood disorders, 457–462
Psychosis, schizo-affective, 438
Psychostimulants, for post-TBI depression, 262
Psychosurgery. *See* Functional neurosurgery
Psychotherapist, role on rehabilitation team, 417t

Quantification of features in evaluation of emotion
computerized voice analysis, 95
discourse analysis, 95
facial muscle action units, 95

Rabies, emotional changes in, 376
Radical empiricism, metaphysics of, 35
Rating procedures for emotional expression, 94–95
Rationalism, 33–34
rCBF. *See* Regional cerebral blood flow
Reaction modalities, patterning of, 154–155
"Reaction triad" of emotion, 8, 138
Recall
bias, from ecphoric processes, 174–175
depression and, 169
remember/know procedure, 182
reminiscence effect and, 173
Recreational therapist, role on rehabilitation team, 417t
Reductive materialists, 111
Reflexes, 48
Regional cerebral blood flow (rCBF)
in depression, 281–283
with obsessive compulsive disorder, 303
electroconvulsive therapy and, 467
energy metabolism and, 110
in induced sadness states, 279–281
methodological issues, 278–279
in panic disorder, 303–304
positron emission tomography for, 116–118, 117f
Region of interest analysis, 107
Rehabilitation
for affective deficits, 426–427

for apathy, 355–356
assessment techniques, 416–417
caregiver participation in, 416
cognitive, approaches for, 414–416
cognitive remediation, 414
communication abilities, 417
for emotional deficits, 427
generalization strategies for, 418
multidisciplinary treatment, 15, 416, 417t
process approach to, 414
team, professional roles in, 416, 417t
Rehearsal, of emotional information, 172–173
Relative judgment theory, 351
Relaxation training, 423
Relevance detectors, 138
Remediation. *See* Rehabilitation
Remembering, subjectivity of, 181–182
Remember/know procedure, 182
Reminiscence effect, 173
Repetitive transcranial magnetic stimulation (rTMS), 470, 474. *See also* TMS
clinical effects in mood disorders, 476–478
description of, 475
mood effects, on normal volunteers, 475–476, 476–478
Research
future directions for, 18–21
research considerations, 18–21
Reserpine
for dysphoria in Parkinson's disease, 381
for schizophrenia, 436
Retraining, 415
Retrieval
bias in, 184
of emotional knowledge, 196–197, 200, 202f
of knowledge, 195
of memories, 164–165
as mood regulation, 177–179
neural mechanisms in, 182–184
as self-regulation, 176–177
Right hemisphere
activity
in anxiety, 308
in panic disorder, 304
cortical dysfunction
bilateral frontal lobe, 373–374
communication deficits in, 370–372
corticobulbar, 374
dominance for emotion, 7, 216–217
emotion and, 217
in emotional behavior, 226
emotional processing and, 7, 205

Right hemisphere (*continued*)
lesions, 205
anxiety and, 308–310
emotional communication and, 386
emotional disorders in, 240
emotional expression and, 183
secondary mania and, 243
in motor activation, 397–398
perception and, 269
stroke lesions, 250–251
Rorschach test, 95
rTMS. *See* Repetitive transcranial magnetic
stimulation
Russell, Bertrand, 37–38, 42
Ryle, Gilbert, 40–41

SAD (seasonal affective disorder), 284, 462
Sadness. *See also* Depression
depression and, 180
electroencephalogram studies
in induced states, 274
methodological issues, 273–274
induced, regional cerebral blood flow in,
279–281
left frontal activity and, 270
Scene, 6, 81
Schemas, emotional, memory of, 168
Schizophrenia
apathy in
behavioral therapy for, 355
diagnosis of, 345–346
attention in, 441*f*
clinical characteristics, with depression,
438–439, 438*t*, 439*t*
clinical features, 434–442
"continuum model," 441
demographics, with depression, 438–439,
438*t*
depression in, 436–439, 438*t*, 439*t*, 443–444
akinetic, 437
cerebral blood flow in, 445
cerebrospinal fluid volumes in, 445–446,
446*f*
glucose metabolism in, 445, 446–447,
447*f*
negative symptoms and, 435, 444–445
pharmacogenic, 436–437
treatment of, 437–438, 443–444
emotional deficits in, 16, 93
emotional disorders in, 434–436
emotional experience in
intensity of, 436, 437*f*
neuropsychology of, 436–441, 437*f*,
438*t*, 439*t*, 440*f*, 441*f*

emotional expression in, 93, 434–436, 448
emotional processing, neurobiological
studies of, 445–447, 445–448, 446*f*,
447*f*
mania in, 439–441
neuropsychological features in, 440*f*
neuropsychological functioning deficits in,
432–433
phenomenology of, 433
recognition of emotion in, 93, 441–442,
442*f*
suicide in, 436, 437
symptoms
clinical ratings of, 435–436
cognitive deficits, 432
hierarchical schema of, 441
negative, 434, 444–445
positive, 433–434, 444
primary, 433
psychotic or positive, 432
secondary, 433
treatment, 442–443
for depression, 443–444
of negative symptoms, 444–445
of positive symptoms, 444
Seasonal affective disorder (SAD), 284, 462
Seizures
emotional changes in, 376–377
generalized, in electroconvulsive therapy,
463–464
violence and, 323
Selective serotonin reuptake inhibitors
(SSRIs)
for bipolar disorder, 457
for depression, 457
for Parkinson-associated depression, 381
Self-attribution theory of emotion, 42–43
Self awareness, in pharmacotherapy for
apathy, 354
Self-concept
in emotional appraisals, 169
memory retrieval and, 176–177
positive, building/maintaining, 177
Self-evaluation, negative ruminative cycle of,
172
Senile dementia of Alzheimer's disease,
treatment of, 420
Septal lesions, emotional experience and, 376
Serotonin (5-HIAA)
cerebrospinal fluid levels
in antisocial behavior, 325–326
in Parkinson's disease-associated
depression, 257
in Parkinson's disease, 381

Serotonin-reuptake inhibitors (SSRIs)
  for Huntington's disease, 383
  for post-stroke depression, 253–254
Sex differences. *See* Gender differences
SFE (Social Functioning Examination),
      259–260, 259*f*
Shame, guilt and, 180
Single-case study, 107
Single photon emission computed
      tomography (SPECT)
  ligand, 114–115
  in manic patients, 114–115
  perfusion, 115, 115*f*
  radiotracers, 114
  vs. other imaging methods, 112, 113*t*
  vs. PET, 116
Single pulse transcranial magnetic
      stimulation, 475
Skin conductance, violence and, 328–329,
      331
SMA damage (supplementary motor area),
      apathy in, 348
Social affordances, 46
Social apathy, 350
Social awareness, in pharmacotherapy for
      apathy, 11, 354
Social cognitive neuroscience approach, 165
Social constructivist models, 149
Social emotions, 10, 20, 21
Social functioning, 20–21
Social Functioning Examination (SFE),
      259–260, 259*f*
Social functioning inventories, 81
Social psychology, memory and, 165
Social skills training, 14, 20, 97
Social worker, role on rehabilitation team,
      417*t*
Sociocultural issues, 10
Sociopaths, aggression in, 219
Somatic anxiety (anxious arousal),
      characteristics of, 300–301, 300*t*
Somatosensory cortices, 9, 205–208
  facial expression processing and, 205–206,
      207*f*, 208
Soul
  conceptualization of, 33, 52
  tripartite, 142
SPECT. *See* Single photon emission
      computed tomography
Speech language pathologist, role on
      rehabilitation team, 417*t*
Speech-language therapy, approaches for,
   .   414–416
SSRIs. *See* Serotonin-reuptake inhibitors

SST (stereotactic subcaudate tractotomy), 473
STAI (State-Trait Anxiety Inventory), 304,
      307
Startle response, 68–69
State-Trait Anxiety Inventory (STAI), 304,
      307
Statistical analysis, for neuroimaging of
      emotion, 127
Stereotactically normalizing, 107
Stereotactic subcaudate tractotomy (SST), 473
Stimulus
  automatic classification, 167–168
  evaluation, 166
Stress
  anxiety and, 301–302
  definition of, 301
  reduction, anger and, 424
  right-hemispheric processing in, 308
  sources, 301–302
Stress inoculation approach, 425
Striatonigral degeneration, 384
Stroke
  bipolar disorder after, 245–246, 246*f*
  depression after, 246–247, 262
    lesion location and, 241–242, 241*f*,
      250–252, 250*f*, 251*f*, 272
    longitudinal course of, 247
    mechanisms of, 252–253
    prevalence of, 247
    relationship to impairment, 248–250,
      249*f*
    severity, 272
    treatment of, 253–254, 254*f*
  emotional changes in, 392–393
  emotional deficits, treatment of, 419–420,
      426–427
  lesion location
    bipolar disorder and, 245, 246*f*
    depression and, 241–242, 241*f*
  mania after, 240–241, 262
    lesion location and, 241–242, 241*f*
    mechanism of, 242–243
    risk factors for, 242, 243
    treatment of, 243–244
  mood disorders after, cortical *vs.*
      subcortical lesions in, 252
  unilateral right-hemisphere basal ganglia,
      92
  vocal/facial expression defects in, 223
Stroop paradigm, 166–167
Structured Assessment of Depression in
      Brain-Damaged Individuals, 96
Study design, for neuroimaging of emotion,
      127

Subcortical structures
deep, electroconvulsive stimulation of, 466
in emotional expression, 215–216
lesions, emotional expression/perception
and, 91–92
in post-stroke mood disorders, 252
Subcortical (diencephalic) theories, of
emotional expression, 390–391
Subjective experience. *See* Emotional
experience
Subjective feelings
definition of, 155
measurement of, 95–96, 155
Subtyping in clinical disorders, 19, 21
Suicide, in schizophrenia, 436, 437
Superior parietal gyrus, deficits, in violent
behavior, 324
Supplementary motor area damage (SMA),
apathy in, 348
Survival, evolutionary, 166
Symptom Check List-90, 81
Systematic desensitization, 423–424
Systems-level theory of emotion, 9, 195

Tachistoscopic viewing, 5
Talairach atlas, 107
TBI. *See* Traumatic brain injury
Techniques, general, 4–7
Telencephalon. *See also* Basal ganglia
evolutionary neuroanatomy, 57, 58
network architecture of, 59
Temporal lobe
in depression with schizophrenia, 445–446,
446*f*
dysfunction, violence and, 323
lesions
in aggression, 323–324
antisocial behavior and, 324
Temporal lobectomy, 173, 393
Temporal lobe epilepsy
emotional changes in, 91, 376–377
limbic drive mechanisms, 71–73
questionnaire, 96
"Tender-minded" philosophies, 34
Test batteries, 81–93
Test reliability, 97
Test validity, 97
Testosterone, violent behavior and, 326–327
Thalamus
in depression, 393
emotional expression and, 390–391
intralaminar nuclei of, 397
modality-specific sensory systems, 394
Thematic Apperception Test, 95

Theoretical perspectives, 7–11
"Tick-rate" hypothesis, 173
Transcranial magnetic stimulation (TMS),
108–109. *See also* rTMS
electromagnetic coil, 122–123
with functional imaging, 125, 126*f*
induced changes in normal mood, 123–124
repetitive, as antidepressant, 124–125
Traumatic brain injury (TBI)
apathy in, pharmacotherapy for, 352
depression after, 263
grieving process for, 423
impairment variables and, 260–261
lesion location and, 260, 261*f*
longitudinal course of, 258–259
risk factors for, 259–260, 259*f*
treatment of, 261–262
depression in, 258
impairment variables and, 260–261
lesion location and, 260, 261*f*
longitudinal course of, 258–259
risk factors for, 259–260, 259*f*
treatment of, 261–262
emotional deficits, 419
mania after
impairment variables and, 244
lesion location and, 245
mechanism of, 245
prevalence of, 244
Trazodone, for post-stroke depression, 253
Tricyclic antidepressants
for bipolar disorder, 457
for depression, 457
for Parkinson-associated depression, 258,
381
for schizophrenia-associated depression,
443
Trihexyphenidyl, for schizophrenia negative
symptoms, 444
Truth, pragmatic theory of, 35–36
Tryptophan depletion, dietary, 461–462

Unilateral neglect syndrome, 228

Valence model
description, 7–8, 216–217
modular theory of emotional expression
and, 391–394
reversed valence effect, 17
transcranial magnetic stimulation studies,
123–124
Ventral circuit, 67
Ventral medial frontal cortex lesions,
motivational deficits and, 171

Ventral pallidum, 223
Ventral striatum, 223
Ventromedial frontal cortices, 197
Verbal labels, of emotional states, 150
VERT (Victoria Emotion Perception Test), 86
Vertical integration, 57, 69, 74
Verticality
    cortical *vs.* subcortical/limbic brain
        structures, 4
Victoria Emotion Perception Test (VERT),
    86
Vienna Circle, 38–39
Violence
    aggressive. *See* Aggression
    controlled-instrumental, 320
    hormones and, 326–328, 332*t*
        cortisol, 327
        glucogen, 328
        insulin, 327–328
        testosterone, 326–327
    hypoglycemia and, 327–328
    impulsive-emotional, 320
    neurochemistry, 325–326, 332*t*
    neuropsychology, 325, 331–333, 332*t*
    pervasiveness of, 320
    psychophysiology, 332*t*
        description of, 328–331
        electroencephalogram, 330, 331

event-related potentials, 330, 331
heart rate, 329, 331
prospective research, 330–331
skin conductance, 328–329, 331
Viral disease, emotional changes in, 376
Visceral feedback hypothesis, 388–390
Vocational counselor, role on rehabilitation
    team, 417*t*
Voluntary call initiation, 69

Wada test
    hemispheric differences in, 392
    left hemisphere, 271
    in secondary mania, 243
"Weapon focus," 167, 168
Whitehead, Alfred North, 37–38
Wilson's disease, 383–384
Wisconsin Card Sorting Task, in Parkinson
    Disease-associated depression,
    256–257, 256*f*
Within-group analysis, 107–108
Within-individual analysis, 108
Wittgenstein, Ludwig, 38, 39–40

Zajonc-Lazarus debate
    arguments in, 43
    LeDoux resolution of, 43–44
Zung Depression Inventory, 380